Connecting for Patients

Interdisciplinary Care Transitions and Collaboration

BARBARA KATZ, RN, MSN

Vice President, Clinical Program Development
VNA Community Healthcare, Inc.
Guilford, CT
President, BK Healthcare Consulting, LLC

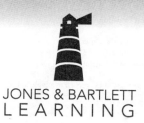

JONES & BARTLETT
LEARNING

World Headquarters
Jones & Bartlett Learning
5 Wall Street
Burlington, MA 01803
978-443-5000
info@jblearning.com
www.jblearning.com

Jones & Bartlett Learning books and products are available through most bookstores and online booksellers. To contact Jones & Bartlett Learning directly, call 800-832-0034, fax 978-443-8000, or visit our website, www.jblearning.com.

Substantial discounts on bulk quantities of Jones & Bartlett Learning publications are available to corporations, professional associations, and other qualified organizations. For details and specific discount information, contact the special sales department at Jones & Bartlett Learning via the above contact information or send an email to specialsales@jblearning.com.

Production Credits
VP, Product Management: Amanda Martin
Director of Product Management: Matt Kane
Product Manager: Teresa Reilly
Product Specialist: Christina Freitas
Production Manager: Carolyn Rogers Pershouse
Vendor Manager: Molly Hogue
Marketing Communications Manager: Katie Hennessy
Product Fulfillment Manager: Wendy Kilborn
Composition: S4Carlisle Publishing Services
Project Management: S4Carlisle Publishing Services
Cover Design: Kristin E. Parker
Rights & Media Specialist: John Rusk
Media Development Editor: Troy Liston
Cover Image (Title Page, Chapter Opener):
© Manop Phimsit/EyeEm/Getty Images
Printing and Binding: McNaughton & Gunn
Cover Printing: McNaughton & Gunn

Library of Congress Cataloging-in-Publication Data
Names: Katz, Barbara, RN, author.
Title: Connecting care for patients : interdisciplinary care transitions and
  collaboration / Barbara Katz.
Description: Burlington, Massachusetts : Jones & Bartlett Learning, [2020] |
  Includes bibliographical references and index.
Identifiers: LCCN 2018028554 | ISBN 9781284129427 (pbk. : alk. paper)
Subjects: | MESH: Transitional Care--organization & administration | Patient
  Readmission | Professional-Patient Relations | Interprofessional Relations
  | United States
Classification: LCC R727.3 | NLM W 84.7 | DDC 610.69/6--dc23 LC record available at https://lccn.loc.gov/2018028554

6048

Printed in the United States of America
22 21 20 19 18   10 9 8 7 6 5 4 3 2 1

To my husband Jerry, my sons Brendan, Connor, and Scott, and their families who provided unconditional support during the writing of this book. Also to my wonderful colleagues at VNA Community Healthcare, especially CEO Janine Fay, and all the other friends and colleagues in my own "health neighborhood" who provided advice and encouragement and who generously shared their personal stories, opinions, and ideas.

–Barbara Katz

Brief Contents

Contents

Chapter 4 Leading for Connected Care—The Senior Management Role 111

Chapter 5 Middle Managers and Connected Care 149

Chapter 6 Care Coordination and Communication on the Front Lines—The Clinician Role 195

Chapter 7 Experiencing Connected Care—The Patient Role 235

Chapter 8 Pulling Together for the Patient—Teamwork in Health Care 283

Chapter 9 Digital Connections, Communication, and Collaboration 325

Preface

These days, conversations about health care—whether between professionals or with patients, former patients, or family caregivers—frequently turn to the issue of fragmentation, lack of care coordination, and situations where some vital patient care task has "fallen through the cracks." In those instances where the care experiences being described are patient centered and fully coordinated, people often seem surprised and describe these positive situations as unusual, or even remarkable. This perceived lack of continuity, coordination, and wholeness in health care is the reason this book was written.

The writing of the book occurred during what may be one of the most tumultuous periods in recent American history, and certainly in the history of the U.S. healthcare system. While pundits expounded, politicians argued, and health professionals toiled away in the trenches of patient care, the problems of healthcare fragmentation continued but were not left unnoticed. The Affordable Care Act was debated, dissected, reviled, defended, and attacked during this period, but at the time of this writing at least some of it is still in force. Value-based payment model testing continues with no clear winning strategies declared. Research on the issues of more coordinated chronic care management picked up momentum.

Retail health and consumer directed care, which are both fragmenting and connecting strategies, became more widespread during the period this book was written. The surprise announcement that corporate giants Amazon, Berkshire Hathaway, and JP Morgan Chase were taking health care redesign for their employees into their own hands shook the healthcare establishment to its core. Fragmentation of care was one stated reason for this game-changing decision, verifying that this issue continues to be a vital one.

During this period, there was an explosion of technology in the form of telemedicine, artificial intelligence, more sophisticated electronic medical records, the use of avatars to perform some care tasks, wearables, and sophisticated patient-tracking devices. While touted as a panacea for disconnection, it has gradually become clear that without a strong guiding human hand with a patient-centered systems view, the technology drives us and often produces unintended consequences. Newer research into the root causes of clinician burnout, which has become endemic, identified poorly designed and managed technology, especially electronic medical records as a culprit in some cases.

This book is the culmination of my own experiences as a nurse, a manager in many healthcare settings, a patient, a healthcare consultant, a mother, a caregiver for elderly parents, and an advocate within a family caregiver support network. In almost every instance when I have mentioned the topic of the book I was writing, the response by both laypeople and professionals has been, "Yes, that's a really big problem." Many of the people I talked with had ideas for improvement, which have also been incorporated into the book.

The ideas in the book first originated from a seminar called "Connecting the Dots," which was delivered at a regional home healthcare conference. The session, with its emphasis on practical tools and techniques for fighting care disconnects and creating a more seamless experience for both home healthcare clinicians and patients struck a chord with the audience.

Home health care, in particular, is a healthcare industry segment where care disconnects are particularly glaring, because the home is an uncontrolled environment, the patient and family can be themselves without the control or management of health professionals, and gaps and cracks in care all too readily come to light.

During the writing of the book, I spoke with a wide variety of health professionals, patients, executives, family caregivers, and people who have friends and neighbors who are grappling with illness and disability. Almost all of these people encouraged me to delve deeper and work harder to look for solutions to the fragmentation problem. When asked why this was so important, three reasons emerged:

- Fragmented care harms patients and can actually cause death and serious disability—this is a problem that those of us in the business of saving lives cannot afford to ignore.
- Fragmented care is a source of anger, angst, and stress for health professionals who may feel so frustrated that they leave their chosen profession.
- Fragmented care wastes money. It is well documented that health care is a major drain on the U.S. economy and money wasted

by inefficient health care could be used to improve the quality of life for all Americans.

A key premise of this book is that we can't wait for some idealized, integrated health system or new payment model to connect care for patients. It may be many years, and possibly never, before integrated delivery systems become the norm. In the meantime, there are plenty of strategies, tools, and tactics that can be applied by any CEO, manager, clinician, or patient advocate to make care more connected and satisfying for patients and clinicians.

These tools, such as patient self-management support, motivational interviewing, care transition interventions, and techniques for humanizing technology, are now used only in pockets of the healthcare industry. One goal of this book is to help familiarize a wider range of nurses and other professionals with practical, patient-centered approaches that can be incorporated into daily clinical practice. Another goal is to help nursing and other health professional students equip themselves to provide optimal levels of care in a complex and demanding healthcare environment.

My hope is that in some small way this work makes life on the front lines of health care a little easier for both dedicated and hardworking clinicians and the patients they serve.

Barbara Katz, RN, MSN

Reviewers

David Au, PhD
Assistant Professor of Healthcare
  Management
Department of Management and Healthcare
  Administration
Valdosta State University
Valdosta, GA

Paul J. Azar III, MD, MS
Adjunct Professor
University of Louisiana at Lafayette
Lafayette, LA

Lauren Bates, DNP, RN
Instructor of Nursing
Morehead State University
Morehead, KY

Susan Beck, MSN, CNS, RN, PhD-C
Assistant Professor
Bloomsburg University
Bloomsburg, PA

Janet Bischof, PhD, RN, NE-BC, CNE
Associate Professor/Director
Wheeling Jesuit University
Wheeling, WV

Carolyn Blake, MAEd, MPH, MT(ASCP)
Instructor
Kent Intermediate School District
Grand Rapids, MI

Faith Breen, PhD
Professor of Management
Prince George's Community College
Largo, MD

Karen J. Buhr, PhD
Assistant Professor of Health Policy &
  Administration
Penn State Mont Alto
Mont Alto, PA

Gail L. Bullard, DHEd, MSHA, RN, LBBH
Program Coordinator, Assistant Professor
Ferris State University
Big Rapids, MI

Kelly Callahan, BSN, RN
Coordinator, Health Learning Resource
  Center/PN Instructor
University of Arkansas Fort Smith
Fort Smith, AR

Rachel W. Cozort, PhD, RN, CNE
Associate Professor
Pfeiffer University
Misenheimer, NC

C. Christine Delnat, MSN, RN
Assistant Professor
St. Mary-of-the-Woods College
West Terre Haute, IN

**Karen McMillen Dielmann, DEd, PHR,
  SHRM-CP**
Assistant Professor and Program Director
Pennsylvania College of Health Sciences
Lancaster, PA

Retta Evans, PhD, MCHES
Associate Professor and Graduate Program
  Director
University of Alabama at Birmingham
Birmingham, AL

S. Kim Genovese, PhD, RN-BC, CNE
Associate Professor of Nursing
College of Nursing and Health Professions
Valparaiso University
Valparaiso, IN

Maureen T. Greene, PhD, RN
Nurse Research Coordinator
Ascension Healthcare Wisconsin
Port Washington, WI

**Sheila Grossman, PhD, APRN,
FNP-BC, FAAN**
Professor & Director of Faculty Scholarship
and Mentoring
Marion Peckham School of Nursing & Health
Studies
Fairfield, CT

Robin Ann Harvan, EdD
Professor and Director of Health Sciences
Programs
MCPHS University
Boston, MA

James D. Hess, EdD
Chair and Director
Oklahoma State University
Tulsa, OK

Lanis L. Hicks, PhD
Professor Emerita
Health Management & Informatics,
School of Medicine
University of Missouri
Columbia, MO

**Marianne Jankowski, DHSc, MBA,
MSPH, RRT**
Chair
Health Services Professions Department
The Chicago School
Chicago, IL

Dr. Melissa Kagarise, DHSc
Associate Professor
Saint Francis University
Loretto, PA

George C. Karahalis, MHA, LFACHE
Adjunct Assistant Professor
School of Business
The Citadel, The Military College
of South Carolina
Charleston, SC

Pamela R. Kelly, DHA, MBA/HCM
Professor
Liberty University
Lynchburg, VA

Nancy Kupper, RN, MSN
Associate Professor
Tarrant County College
Fort Worth, TX

Cindy K. Manjounes, MS, EdD, PhD
Campus Dean and Professor
Lindenwood University
Belleville, IL

Warren G. McDonald, PhD
Professor and Chair, Department of Health
Administration
Methodist University
Fayetteville, NC

Brinda McKinney, PhD, MSN, RN
BSN Program Director
Arkansas State University
Jonesboro, AR

**Deb McQuilkin, DNP, MEd, RN, NEA-BC,
FACMPE**
Associate Professor
University of South Carolina
Columbia, SC

Kimberly McVicar, MSA
Assistant Professor
Health Administration Program
Ferris State University
Big Rapids, MI

Lynn D. Mohr, PhD, APRN, PCNS-BC, CPN
Assistant Professor
Rush University College of Nursing
Chicago, IL

CHAPTER 1

Connected Care—Closing the Gaps and Filling the Cracks in Health Care

▶ Introduction

This text is about connecting the elements of care in our complex healthcare world to create the best outcomes for our patients and to achieve organizational and professional success for ourselves. While most works on this topic have taken the 25,000-foot view and concentrated on national policy issues and health system issues, or have focused on specialty areas of care coordination and case management, this text comes from, and is aimed at, the front lines of health care where care is closest to the patient. The goal here is to raise awareness of the serious consequences of fragmented health care and to distill evidence-based best practices in care coordination, care transitions, and collaboration to achieve better outcomes, better patient experience, and lower costs.

The text poses a systemic solution to healthcare fragmentation. This solution is called **connected care**. It incorporates care coordination attitudes and actions into the job of every nurse and every other health professional and embeds it into the structure and processes of health care and community organizations. Connected care is a comprehensive, systems approach to connecting care activities and achieving better outcomes for patients. It is a philosophy, a set of principles, structures, best practices, strategies, and tools that overcome care fragmentation. The foundation of connected care is patient centeredness. The pillars of connected care are care transitions, care coordination, communication, teamwork, and collaboration.

The connected care approach links disparate elements of care coordination, care transitions, case management, and various collaborative strategies to achieve patient goals and to provide a seamless, safe, and transparent experience for patients. It connects all elements of care through clinician consistency and information sharing at each step in care.

Connected care also includes electronic information exchange, tracking, and information gathering at each step during care. The core daily work of connected care is patient and family caregiver education and completion of all patient-related follow-up tasks so that patients receive the services, medical information, supplies, community resources, and equipment they need.

Also in this chapter, we further analyze the elements of connected care and look at the principles, structures, processes, measures, and tools that you, the reader, can use to create your own culture of connected care. Nurses, with their strong history of championing patient-centered care principles and practices, will be leaders in the implementation of connected care.

▶ Connected Care—And Not: Some Stories

A Disconnected Care Experience Helps Fuel Medicare Transformation

In March 2016, the *New York Times* ran a profile of Dr. Patrick Conway, then chief medical officer and deputy administrator for innovation and quality for Centers for Medicare and Medicaid Services (CMS). The article focused on how his experience as a practicing pediatrician has informed his work with CMS. The article describes how Conway's experience is highly relevant to the theme of this text: "His zeal to improve care is rooted in personal experience. He said he was frustrated by the fragmented care that his father received when he was dying of cancer in 2007. He promised his father that he would devote his life to trying to change the healthcare system. His father told him, 'You can't. It's too hard. But you are persistent. If anyone can, it would be you'" (Pear, 2016, p. A9).

Conway went on to lead the Center for Medicare and Medicaid Innovation (CMMI) and was a key force in attempting to remodel the healthcare system during the Obama administration. He was responsible for launching many of the new value-based payment programs that emphasize payment for results and for providing creative care models that have rapidly pushed healthcare organizations toward more integration and collaboration.

A Health System Executive Experiences "Dis-integrated Care"

Shortly after the article about Conway appeared in the *New York Times*, an executive from a large medical group practice spoke at a regional healthcare conference about his newly minted accountable care organization.

He proudly described the high-level organizational structure, the multiple clinical initiatives, and the technology that the system was using to create a cutting-edge integrated care model.

The focus was on member facilities and physicians, contracts, technology, and metrics. There was little discussion about where the patient, family caregivers, or other healthcare providers fit into this hugely complex system. When asked about patient focus, his reply indicated that the area would need more work.

He went on to say that his experience with his parents was actually motivating him to develop more patient-centered systems within his organization. He explained that his mother had been treated for congestive heart failure at a highly regarded metropolitan hospital. The hospital was not in his integrated delivery system, but it did have many of the same programs in place. When his mother was discharged from the hospital, she came home with reams of written instructions, newly prescribed oxygen, multiple prescriptions that needed to be filled, and a long list of specialty follow-up appointments to be made. The needed medical equipment hadn't arrived and there didn't seem to be anyone immediately available to help connect the dots for the family. The executive, who had been trained as a health professional, talked about how he and his father felt overwhelmed and despairing. His voice caught as he talked.

This is the stark contrast between the ideal of integrated care and the reality. The executive's speech ended on a positive note. The hospital had actually made a referral to home health care and the agency started care 24 hours later, but the executive and his family had not been fully informed about this process and didn't know who to call in the interim. His parents finally did get some help coordinating care when the home health agency provided nursing case management services and developed a comprehensive care plan with the help of the primary care physician and cardiologist.

The nurse case manager was able to coordinate the fragmented elements of care his parents were receiving for a safer and more satisfying patient experience. What was not accomplished at the system level was accomplished by an individual nurse.

🔍 CASE STUDY

Cracks and Gaps in a Complex Case

A home healthcare agency received a referral from a local skilled nursing facility (SNF) for a 50-year-old woman who had suffered a series of progressively more serious and debilitating heart attacks that had necessitated multiple hospitalizations, SNF stays, and home healthcare episodes. The referral came via a faxed referral form from the SNF. The referral form was handwritten—both within the lines and sideways on the page. About a third of it was unreadable. There was some information about a wound, but wound care orders were not clearly indicated. The SNF did not call the home care agency to suggest this was a high-risk case that required special attention. When the home care nurse opened the case, she found that this patient could barely get out of her chair and was a serious fall risk. She also had an unhealed pressure ulcer and was incontinent, making wound care very difficult.

The home care agency then struggled to coordinate care for an overwhelmed spouse/caregiver, to manage the patient's deteriorating condition, and to make sense of disjointed orders from multiple physicians. Within a few days, the patient was readmitted to the hospital.

Needless to say, the home healthcare staff speculated, and not in a kind way, about the care that had been provided in the SNF and the lack of communication on discharge. Instead of leaving things there, the agency had a member of the executive team call the SNF administrator to debrief the case and to see if there were ways to avoid similar situations in the future.

A meeting of the home care management team, the home care nurse, and the SNF administrator and clinical team was arranged. The nursing director came prepared with some immediate improvements, including a "heads-up" document that could be sent to home care intake to alert staff to important care considerations.

The SNF team described the care that had been given in the facility and the home health team was better able to understand the course of the patient's stay and some of the factors that had influenced the discharge process. They found that the patient had come home from the hospital

(continues)

🔍 CASE STUDY   *(continued)*

with the pressure ulcer and that the patient's husband had aggressively pushed to have the patient discharged before the facility staff felt she was ready. Ultimately, the SNF and the home healthcare agency forged a better working relationship in the service of patients, but only after being jolted into awareness of their disconnection through a poor patient outcome.

What Can We Learn from These Stories?

These situations illustrate the reality of disconnection and connection in the daily delivery of health care to patients. The perspective is different in each story (e.g., Dr. Conway, at the national level, the executive at the health system level, and two local healthcare organizations managing a patient transition at the local level). Yet, despite these differing perspectives, the patient and family experience was remarkably similar—that is, fragmented and less than satisfactory. Each of the players in these scenarios had different solutions to the problem.

Dr. Conway helped create new payment models that are still, to some extent, driving the healthcare system toward greater patient focus and integration. The medical practice executive used his own negative experience to allocate care coordination resources and guide his system toward a more connected patient experience. The home healthcare agency and the skilled nursing facility developed a better collaborative working relationship and tools for communication about high-risk patient situations.

▶ The Quality Chasm and Connected Care

Disconnected care and the distress and harm that it causes patients had been a national problem for a long time, but it wasn't until the start of the 21st century that an authoritative national body tackled the problem. The Institute

of Medicine (IOM), in its landmark work, *Crossing the Quality Chasm* (2001), detailed how the American healthcare system had failed to produce quality outcomes and had failed to satisfy patient needs and to manage costs. Much of the document focuses on fragmentation and disconnection in the health system, its negative consequences, and possible remedies.

In the introduction the authors stated: "Indeed, between the health care that we *now have* and the health care that we *could have* lies not just a gap, but a chasm" (IOM, 2001, p. 1). The authors go on to say, "Yet physician groups, hospitals, and other health care organizations operate as silos, often providing care without the benefit of complete information about the patient's condition, medical history, services provided in other settings, or medications prescribed by other clinicians" (p. 4).

The IOM proposed a series of rules and structural changes to bridge the quality chasm. Among many recommendations advanced by the IOM, some are particularly relevant to the connected care approach:

- The patient is the center of control
- Cooperation among clinicians
- Shared knowledge and free flow of information (IOM, p. 8)
- Redesign of care processes based on best practices (IOM, p. 12)

The goal of this text is to help practicing nurses and other clinicians apply these principles and find practical solutions to this problem of healthcare fragmentation and its negative consequences. Nurses, who are perceived as the most trusted health professionals (Gallup.com, 2016), are essential to solving this problem. As one patient, interviewed in a study about hospital care coordination, said, "Nurses, it's up to them to make sure things are going ok" (Beaudin, Lammers, & Pedroja, 1999, p. 21).

For the purposes of this text, we relabel fragmentation as "disconnection" and consolidate the wide variety of systems, structures, and best practices that embody the IOM principles into the concept of connected care, which will be the theme throughout the text. We will begin to explore how organizations can create structures and nurses, doctors, family caregivers, and community professionals can develop the mindset and skills necessary to practice the type of communication, collaboration, teamwork, and care coordination that produces true connected care for patients. The chapter includes some exercises and activities to help you, the reader, begin to assess your organization's level of connected care competence and to identify areas for improvement.

▶ Where Are We Now? The Current Status of Care Connection and Disconnection

Crossing the Quality Chasm— National Progress

In the years since the IOM Quality Chasm study was published, the healthcare community has taken the care fragmentation problem seriously. Solutions have been developed and tested at both the policy and practice levels. Nursing in particular has been at the forefront of creating policies, methods, and tools that better coordinate care for patients. Nurses have also advocated for systemic solutions to disconnection.

The passage of the Affordable Care Act (ACA) tremendously accelerated the drive toward more connected care. As part of its mandate to lower costs and improve health outcomes, the CMS, in 2015, implemented an aggressive timeline for remodeling the healthcare system through payment reform. Specifically, CMS instituted a "volume to value" shift in which providers are paid, not for delivering more care, but for achieving better results (CMS, 2015). Connected care principles, practices, and measures are an integral part of this shift.

Value in this new approach to care is embodied in a concept known as "The Triple Aim" (**FIGURE 1-1**). First coined by Dr. Don Berwick, former administrator of CMS, in an article in *Health Affairs* (Berwick, Nolan, & Whittington, 2008), the aim describes three goals for American health care:

- Improve the health of patient populations (groups of patients with like characteristics).
- Improve the patient experience.
- Lower per capita costs.

As volume shifts toward value, payments are being linked to achievement of Triple Aim goals; and new delivery system and payment models are emerging. More recently, the Triple

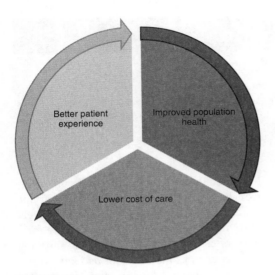

FIGURE 1-1 The Triple Aim

Data from Berwick, D., Nolan, T., & Whittington, J. (2008). The triple aim: Care, health, and cost. *Health Affairs, 27*(3), 759–769. doi:10.1377/hlthaff.27.3

Aim concept has been expanded to incorporate the goal of improving the clinician experience. The new construct is called the Quadruple Aim (Bodenheimer & Sinsky, 2014). While the quadruple aim concept has not been universally adopted, it is gaining ground as a core principle of value-based care.

The new payment models are collectively known as **value-based payment**. Generating and testing these models has been the work of CMMI.

At the time of this writing, with the election of President Donald Trump and the uncertain future of at least parts of the ACA, the future of these integration initiatives is unclear. However, since integration is supported by many insurers and employer groups, the predicted demise of value-based payment and integrated care strategies may be premature.

While value-based payment models may not survive in their current form, the pressures of high costs, patient dissatisfaction, and persistent patient safety problems will almost certainly drive a continued move toward care integration strategies.

The current model of government-sponsored, value-based payment initiatives employs a variety of methods to achieve more connected care for patients:

- **Creating care coordination and care transition codes and payments** for managing patients with chronic conditions allowing physicians and Advanced Practice Registered Nurses (APRNs) to bill Medicare for care coordination activities (CMS, 2016a)
- **Support for new organizational structures**, such as patient-centered medical homes (PCMHs) (National Committee on Quality Assurance [NCQA], 2018), which are advanced primary care medical practices that provide extended services and care coordination for patients
- **A policy level focus on connected care initiatives** through the National Quality Strategy: "Promoting effective communication and coordination of care" is one of the six National Quality Strategy priorities (Agency for Healthcare Research and Quality [AHRQ], 2017)
- **Medicare-sponsored, and in some cases, mandated, alternative payment models (APMs)** that encourage connected care (joint replacement bundles, chronic care bundling, Medicare shared savings programs) (CMS, 2018a)
- **Measures shared across industry segments**, such as the Improving Medicare Post-Acute Care Transformation Act (IMPACT Act), which mandates a set of common patient outcome measures across postacute settings including skilled nursing facilities, long-term acute care hospitals, and home health care (CMS, 2014)

CMS is clearly not leaving care coordination to chance. Through its various payment innovation models it is creating some forced connections between previously separated industry segments. Some people would call these collaborations "shotgun marriages" but they are likely to be an enduring element of our newly remodeled healthcare system.

How Far Have We Come? A Current Snapshot

A September 2016 headline in the online reporting source, Bloomberg News, reads "US Health Care System Ranks as One of the Least Efficient." The article described the United States as ranking 50th out of 55 nations in healthcare efficiency. In a quote from Paul Ginsburg, professor at the University of Southern California and director of the Center for Health Policy at the Brookings Institution in Washington, DC, the article describes the key reason for this inefficiency: "The U.S. system tends to be more fragmented, less organized and coordinated, and that's likely to lead to inefficiency" (Du & Lieu, 2016).

Data from a 2011 Commonwealth Fund survey of American views of the healthcare system found that most felt that the healthcare system needed fundamental change. Many cited breakdowns in care coordination, including lost medical tests or lack of information about test results, meager communication between physicians, poor physician continuity, and inadequate patient education (Stremikis, Schoen, & Fryer, 2011).

A 2016 article in *Fierce Healthcare* cited a study by CRICO Strategies that detailed how miscommunication—the most basic form of disconnection—caused 2,000 deaths and $1.7 billion in malpractice claims in a single year (Budryk, 2016).

The news isn't all bad, however. In a 2015 report to Congress, the Agency for Healthcare Research and Quality noted that providers had improved discharge processes, providing more patients with discharge instructions. The report also noted that more providers have adopted health information technologies (AHRQ, 2015).

The Chartbook on Care Coordination notes that from 2005 to 2013 the percentage of heart failure patients who received written discharge instructions increased from 57.4% to 94.6%, while hospital readmissions (a key measure of care connection and integration) have declined (AHRQ, 2016a).

At the time of this writing, 17 years after the publication of *Crossing the Quality Chasm*, it is fair to say that we have generated and tested many solutions and made some progress toward reducing care fragmentation. However, our progress has not been nearly fast enough or complete enough. Nurses and other health professionals continue to struggle with highly complex care systems that are seldom fully patient centered and coordinated.

Far too often, these dysfunctional work systems require health professionals to take laborious, and sometimes heroic, action to connect the dots for patients. Stories in both professional journals and the popular press continue to detail the realities of a fragmented healthcare system.

A certified diabetes educator, Stacey DeFillipo, CDE, RD, describes progress toward better coordinated care this way:

> Rating our system on coordinating care on a scale of 1-10: five years ago a 2, now a 5. The 5 is an average as some systems are doing well (an 8) and others are still a 2. Care Coordination/Care Management Teams—these are growing by leaps and bounds in health systems and are working well to reduce readmissions. Outpatient care managers working in the primary care practice are responsible to follow up and help patients released from the hospital. They are really helping patients understand their health and health care. (DeFillipo, personal communication, 2017)

▶ Dissecting Fragmentation and Disconnected Care

The Root Causes of Disconnection

A 2009 article in the *Annals of Family Medicine* describes healthcare fragmentation in eloquent terms: "Underlying the current healthcare failings is a critical underappreciated problem: fragmentation-focusing and acting on the parts without adequately appreciating their relation to the evolving whole. This unbalance, this brokenness, is at the root of the more obvious healthcare crises of unsustainable cost increases, poor quality, and inequality. Fragmentation is at the heart of the ineffectiveness of our increasingly frantic efforts to nurture improvement" (Stange, 2009, p. 100).

Disconnection is now deeply rooted in the current culture of American health care, but this was not always the case. Until the 20th century, the healthcare system was relatively simple and coordinated. Families cared for sick people at home and called in the local family physician when things got more serious or complicated. Sometimes the local public health nurse was also called into service for preventive health teaching, to provide care during public health emergencies such as flu epidemics, or to assist the family doctor in delivering babies at home. Sometimes, the patient might consult a specialist, but typically care was simple, coordinated, and transparent.

In *The Fragmentation of U.S. Healthcare, Causes and Solutions,* Einar Elhauge (2010) states, "Just as too many cooks can spoil the broth, too many decision makers can spoil health care" (p. 1).

In essence, this is what happened to the U.S. healthcare system as specialization, new knowledge, new drugs, diagnostic equipment, information systems, and more healthcare organizations multiplied, and complexity became an essential part of the healthcare fabric.

Absent any coordinating mechanism, these different elements simply became healthcare "silos" (organizations or departments that are isolated from each other and interested only in their own work). Each silo is focused on its own payment model, clinical tasks, and patient population and is disconnected from the rest of the patient's healthcare delivery system. A good example occurs among elderly patients with chronic illness (Bushardt, Massey, Simpson, Ariail, & Simpson, 2008). In many cases,

patients are seen by multiple physicians, each of whom prescribes drugs for the chronic illness that he or she is treating without regard for, or without even knowing about, what others have prescribed. This lack of coordination often leads to duplicate drug use, higher costs to the insurer and the patient, and a higher incidence of drug-related complications such as falls.

Nurses, like other health professionals, have been caught in their own narrow healthcare silos, focused on performing specialized tasks. Senior managers in healthcare organizations have not always provided the structure, training, or processes that allow front line nurses to practice connected care (Dubree, 2013).

There is a vast amount of literature that analyzes the causes of disconnection in our healthcare system. Most of these factors are well known:

- **Fee-for-service payment structures**. The traditional American healthcare payment system has traditionally rewarded volume of care delivered but has not paid for many care connection activities or for actual health results (Adler & Hoagland, 2012). Many physicians and APRNs in fee-for-service environments limit their care activities to quick, billable visits or procedures.

  The time pressures of a busy practice and limited payment for connected care activities create little incentive to make the many phone calls and send the emails and letters needed to create a seamless care experience for patients, who are then left to coordinate things themselves. Indeed, many primary care professionals describe their work as "running on the hamster wheel" (Schumann, 2013). These fee-for-service structures have been self-perpetuating in part because they have been quite rewarding to certain segments of the healthcare industry such as pharmaceutical companies, medical device manufacturers, and specialty physicians who perform a high volume of expensive invasive procedures.

- **Health professional mindset**. Volume-driven, fee-for-service payments have sometimes created a mechanical, assembly line view of care. In the fee-for-service environment, the organization designs workflows and processes to maximize the efficiency of the health professionals who practice in it and the payment system that funds it. Many professionals in fee-for-service environments are focused on their own specialized tasks and the one patient in front of them at any given point in time.

Health professionals in these settings often have neither the time nor the energy to think about the next step in care, whether it be with another health professional or the family caregiver. This approach, in which each health professional prescribes different medications, orders different tests, and makes different recommendations without regard to what the rest of the patient's healthcare "team" is doing, leads to confusion, medical errors, and lack of a reasonable and rational care plan for patients.

The result is upset, angry, and over-whelmed patients and family caregivers and health professionals who sometimes are unaware of, or surprised at, patient dissatisfaction as well as wasted healthcare dollars and poor outcomes.

- **Professional "turf wars."** As each profession fights to carve out power and increase status, influence, and reimbursement for its members alone, it inhibits collaboration and can actually alienate other members of the healthcare team. Coordinated care is not possible when health professionals misunderstand or resent each other and choose not to work as a team. For example, a home care agency developed an APRN home visiting program targeted to frail elderly patients who could not get out of the house for medical appointments. While many physicians supported the service, some doctors, although they did not do home visits, refused to refer or collaborate with the APRN for fear of losing revenue and total control of the patient's care. The

recent controversy over expanding the scope of practice for APRNs in the Veterans Health Administration is a good example of this issue (Permut, 2016).

- **Resources dedicated to specialization and not to primary care.** As specialty care has expanded, primary care has declined, leaving many patients without a physician whose primary interest is in treating the whole person (Cassel & Reuben, 2011). Increasingly, specialists and primary care doctors don't communicate with each other, resulting in duplicate medications being prescribed, duplicate tests ordered, and physicians giving conflicting information to patients.

  With the rise of the hospitalist specialty, in which physicians with special training in hospital medicine manage all hospitalized patients, many primary care physicians stopped seeing their own patients in the hospital. This system, while providing patients with more expert hospital medical care, has broken the link between the hospital and the next step in care—that is, postacute care or discharge to the patient's home and continuity and follow-up with the patient's primary care doctor.

  In recent years, yet another specialty, the "extensivist" (a physician who coordinates care and follows patients from the inpatient to the outpatient setting) has developed to bridge the gap from hospital to outpatient setting (Powers, Milstein, & Jain, 2016). While some see this as a welcome development that fills a needed care gap, others see it as yet another level of complexity in the healthcare system and another chunk of responsibility taken away from the primary care physician.

- **Regulations that drive fragmentation.** The current Medicare and Medicaid payment structures pay for narrowly defined services and do not easily coordinate payments between them. For example, the many parts of Medicare (Parts A, B, C, D) all pay for different types of services, are highly complex, and are imperfectly coordinated (Elhauge, 2010). Strict rules about professionals operating only within their own discipline and payment system, while protecting patients against fraud and abuse, sometimes limit professional collaboration.

- **Competition and consolidation**. In many healthcare markets, large health systems are rapidly consolidating their reach by expanding and buying up medical practices and ambulatory care facilities to ensure that they gain a larger market share and maintain or increase revenue. Theoretically, getting care from one health system should produce a more seamless, integrated experience.

    Sometimes, however, this consolidation is more about market share, physician alliances, contracts between facilities, and health information systems than about a more connected patient care experience. This competition/consolidation drive can leave patients caught in the middle as some of their doctors align with one system and some with another. Systems for communications across and between delivery systems are typically nonexistent, further creating disconnected care for patients. Patients may also choose to escape higher costs, such as health system facility fees, by going outside the boundaries of an integrated delivery system, contributing to a more fragmented care experience.

- **Certain types of health consumerism**. The emerging retail consumer model of health care can be a force that creates more care disconnection. Patients with a desire for convenience and control may opt to receive episodic, point-of-service care in urgent care centers, retail clinics, and via telemedicine. Although in some cases these services are integrated into a primary care or integrated delivery system, they frequently have minimal connection with the patient's primary care physician or primary medical record (Pollack, Gidengil, & Mehrotra, 2010). In

these cases, patients who unwittingly choose a more disconnected form of health care in the name of convenience may end up taking on a heavier burden of care coordination themselves.

Patients who use multiple pharmacies to fill their prescriptions provide another example of patient-generated disconnected care. Good patient personal health records or health information systems (interoperability) that consolidate information from multiple sources are probably the ultimate solution to this type of disconnection.

- **Health disparities and social determinants of health**. Disconnected care affects patients and families at all socioeconomic levels and across all racial and ethnic groups, but it is clearly worse for those who are handicapped by mental illness, poverty, low health literacy, language barriers, no or poor insurance coverage, and the difficult lifestyle and sense of helplessness that may accompany these problems (Bradley & Taylor, 2016). In a broken and confusing healthcare system, patients and families without the ability to effectively organize and "work the system" may be unable to connect the elements of care themselves. Healthcare organizations and professionals, who insist that their only business is medical care and who do not take any responsibility for finding ways to help patients with issues such as transportation, obtaining prescriptions, or getting food into the house, foster the biggest disconnect of all—treating the illness and not the patient.

FIGURE 1-2 illustrates the root causes of disconnected care and the symptoms that they produce.

A Patient-Level View of Disconnected Care

There has been progress toward more connected care through policy and payment changes, and professional care coordination is more widespread

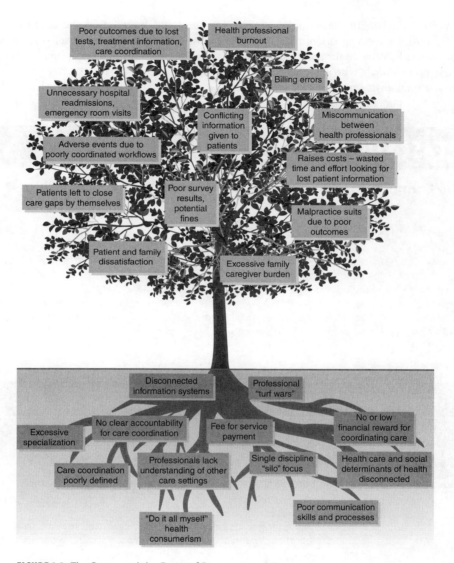

FIGURE 1-2 The Roots and the Fruits of Disconnected Care

ASK YOURSELF

- Which symptoms (fruits) of disconnection do you see in your organization?
- Which of the root causes of disconnected care described in this chapter are at work in your organization?

than ever, but the benefits have not always filtered down to the average patient with serious healthcare needs. What looks coordinated and aligned to professionals, who see things through the lens of their own profession or program, often looks fragmented and confusing to patients. This issue has been well documented in both the professional and popular press, with many stories featuring the negative results of disconnected care experiences (Rabin, 2013).

⌕ CASE STUDY

Who Connects the Dots for an Elderly Patient with Chronic Illness?

Let's look at the experience of a hypothetical patient with several chronic diseases who moves in and out of the formal healthcare system as her symptoms are controlled or worsen. Mrs. Habib is a 77-year-old woman with four chronic conditions: diabetes, congestive heart failure (CHF), chronic obstructive pulmonary disease (COPD), and osteoporosis. She has a primary care physician and sees five other specialists. She takes 15 prescription and nonprescription medications. She has had one emergency room visit, two hospitalizations, and one observation stay in the last six months. She has also had a hip replacement hospitalization and a postop skilled nursing facility stay and two home care episodes of care during this time period. Her family caregivers are her 79-year-old husband, who also has several chronic illnesses, and her 50-year-old daughter, who works full time and has two teenage children. **TABLE 1-1** illustrates the complexity of the patient's personal healthcare system.

TABLE 1-1 A Patient's Six-Month Journey Through the Care Continuum

Care Providers and Coordinators	July to December	Patient Information, Medical Records
1. Hospital	▪ Two hospital inpatient stays for heart failure, one inpatient stay for hip replacement surgery, two emergency room visits for heart failure, and one observation stay. ▪ Emergency room (ER) care coordinator notifies primary care physician (PCP) of visit. ▪ Hospital nurse care coordinator coordinates skilled nursing facility (SNF) admission, post hip replacement. ▪ For home discharges, care coordinator gives patient instructions and sends referral to home care agency. ▪ Hospital arranges postdischarge PCP visit.	▪ Hospital sends electronic referrals to SNF and home care agency. ▪ SNF and home care agency access hospital records via hospital electronic medical record (EMR) portal. ▪ Hospital notifies PCP of admissions and ER visits by phone call. ▪ Hospital sends PCP the discharge summary for one inpatient stay.

Care Providers and Coordinators	July to December	Patient Information, Medical Records
2. Orthopedic surgeon	■ Surgeon sees patient for one preoperative visit. ■ Surgeon performs surgery. ■ Surgeon sees patient for two postop visits.	■ Orthopedic practice EMR, not connected to hospital EMR, no patient portal. ■ Orthopedic office sends a paper report to PCP office.
3. SNF	■ Patient has 15-day inpatient stay following hip replacement. ■ SNF physician manages medical care while patient is in the facility. ■ Social worker coordinates discharge plan.	■ SNF records on paper. ■ Discharge summary faxed to PCP office. ■ Referral form (W10) faxed to home health agency.
4. PCP office	■ Sees patient monthly. ■ Saw patient for one post hospital discharge visit. ■ Patient missed one scheduled post hospital visit. ■ Had one post SNF follow-up visit. ■ One hip replacement preop visit and postop visit for cardiopulmonary symptom exacerbation.	■ PCP EMR is not connected to hospital EMR. ■ No patient portal (patient access to EMR). ■ PCP office faxes preop info on paper to orthopedic office. ■ All instructions and information are given to the patient on paper.
5. PCP office registered nurse (RN) care coordinator	■ RN calls patient regularly to check on symptom control. ■ RN calls patient daily after hospital discharge. ■ RN stays in contact with SNF during inpatient stay there. ■ RN coordinates care with home health agency.	■ RN documents in PCP office EMR, but RN notes are not shared with any other providers.
6. Cardiologist	■ Sees patient for three office visits and two hospital visits.	■ Cardiology EMR connected to hospital EMR. ■ Cardiologist faxes one paper report to PCP. ■ No patient portal into practice EMR.
7. Pulmonologist	■ Sees patient for one office visit and one hospital visit.	■ Pulmonology EMR connected to hospital EMR. ■ Patient portal 1 into practice EMR. ■ Pulmonologist does not communicate with PCP.

(continues)

TABLE 1-1 A Patient's Six-Month Journey Through the Care Continuum   *(continued)*

Care Providers and Coordinators	July to December	Patient Information, Medical Records
8. Endocrinologist (+certified diabetes educator [CDE])	■ Sees patient for three office visits.	■ Endocrinology EMR connected to hospital EMR. ■ Patient portal 2. ■ One note faxed to PCP.
9. Gynecologist	■ One preventive visit.	■ Gynecology EMR, uses patient portal 1. ■ No communication with PCP.
10. Medicare advantage plan high-risk case manager	■ Three phone calls to engage patient, who refuses.	■ Advantage plan electronic record with claims data. ■ Care coordinator does not have access to PCP office or hospital medical records.
11. State home care support program	■ Coordinates placement of nonmedical personal care assistant and emergency call button.	■ State agency patient record. ■ Care coordinators cannot access medical records.
12. Pharmacy 1	■ Fills 12 of 15 medications.	■ Pharmacy computer system. ■ Portal to insurer. ■ No access to medical records or to other pharmacy records.
13. Pharmacy 2	■ Fills 3 of 15 medications (prices lower).	■ Pharmacy computer system. ■ Portal to insurer. ■ No access to medical records or to other pharmacy records.
14. Laboratory	■ Draws and processes lab tests for all providers. ■ Reports results to providers.	■ Laboratory computer system. ■ Patient portal 3. ■ Electronic reports sent to specialists, paper reports faxed to PCP.
15. Home healthcare agency	■ Patient has two 30-day episodes of care with pre-discharge nurse liaison visit. ■ RN case management, physical therapy, home health aide, social work, telemonitoring.	■ Electronic referral from hospital. ■ Home care EMR. ■ Portal to hospital EMR for inpatient stay. ■ Portal to records of cardiologist.

Care Providers and Coordinators	July to December	Patient Information, Medical Records
	■ Social worker helps with application for state-funded nonmedical home care and stress management for overwhelmed caregivers.	■ Exchange paper reports with state home care support program. ■ Fax care plan and supplemental orders to PCP and specialists. ■ Give patient and family paper instructions and medication list.
16. Family caregivers (husband and adult daughter)	■ Go to all medical appointments. ■ Call clinicians when symptoms get worse. ■ Make follow-up appointments. Get patient to lab and medical appointments. ■ Ensure all clinicians get medical information from others. ■ Stay with patient in hospital. Ensure care coordinator makes a good discharge plan. ■ Coordinate scheduling and oversight of personal care assistant (PCA) with nonmedical agency. ■ Calls in prescription refills. ■ Barter with state home care program care coordinator for more personal care support services. ■ Visit elder law attorney for financial planning.	■ Home medication list. ■ Home medical notebook. ■ File with instructions from all providers. ■ List of providers and phone numbers. ■ List of websites and passwords for three patient portals. ■ Printouts of information from patient portals. ■ Files with administrative paperwork from SNF, home care, state home care support agency, nonmedical care agency.
17. Nonmedical home care agency	■ Do home assessment. ■ Schedule and oversee personal care. ■ Install and manage emergency alert system.	■ Nonmedical agency patient record. ■ No connection with other records.

Questions to Answer:
- There is plenty of care coordination here, but who is accountable for connecting all the dots for the patient?
- Who is talking to whom in this system?
- How many different medical records exist for this patient?
- How do the various medical records tell the patient story – or not?
- What would happen to this patient if there was no family caregiver and no nurse care coordinator in the PCP office?

As the table indicates, keeping track of all these visits, inpatient stays, laboratory tests, medications, and home treatments requires considerable family caregiver time and a high level of organizational skill. The family gets some help from the care coordinator in the primary care physician's office and the home healthcare nurse (when the patient is receiving home care), but in essence the responsibility falls on them. This level of effort puts a considerable burden on another chronically ill older adult (Mr. Habib) and on the couple's adult daughter who is trying to juggle a job, her own family, and her parents' needs.

This is a view seldom seen or appreciated by most of the health professionals involved in Mrs. Habib's care, with the possible exception of the home healthcare case manager (who is actually in the home with the family) and the primary care physician and nurse care coordinator (who see Mrs. Habib regularly over time). Such a broad view of a patient's healthcare services and caregiving support is necessary to real connected care.

FIGURE 1-3 shows how parts of one patient's healthcare neighborhood connect and disconnect. This diagram details in graphic form organizational connections for Mrs. Habib, whose six-month healthcare journey was detailed in Table 1-1.

Disconnected Care and Access to Care Management Services

Why, if we have so many care coordination professionals and care management programs, is the experience so disjointed for patients? One reason is that patients have access to care management or care coordination only when they are eligible for those services as part of their insurance coverage or through a facility or program where they receive care.

For example, a patient with a serious chronic illness might get care management services through a nurse care coordinator embedded in a primary care medical practice if that practice is a primary care medical home (i.e., a medical practice that offers extended services including care coordination). Another way a patient might get care management services is through an insurance program such as a Medicare Advantage plan or a Medicaid high-risk patient care coordination program. These care management services are highly dependent on eligibility.

If the patient changes insurance, or changes primary care physicians, her access to care management may disappear. If you happen to be a patient with chronic illness who is covered by traditional Medicare, unless your primary care physician offers practice level care coordination, you are very likely to be left to your own devices when it comes to care coordination since traditional Medicare has no mechanism to coordinate care for its insured population.

A recent study published in the online *American Journal of Managed Care* described a poll of 1,000 seniors, 85% of whom have one or more chronic conditions. Of those polled, 34% reported that a family member coordinates their care, and 35% said no one does, indicating a serious gap in care coordination for a high need population (Caffrey, 2016).

Even episodic care coordination through discharge planning or episode-specific care coordination (say, ambulatory surgery) has become less available to patients as care has moved out of formal healthcare settings into ambulatory care and lengths of stays in inpatient facilities have become shorter.

In summary, unless a patient or family pays out of pocket for a health advocate or care manager, the patient only gets this assistance when an institution or insurer thinks it is necessary, not when the patient feels confused and overwhelmed by the complexities of his or her healthcare needs.

Health Professionals' Experiences with Disconnected Care

"Everybody has a story," said an RN, college professor, and mother of a son with a serious chronic illness, when discussing the issues of disconnected care. In researching this book,

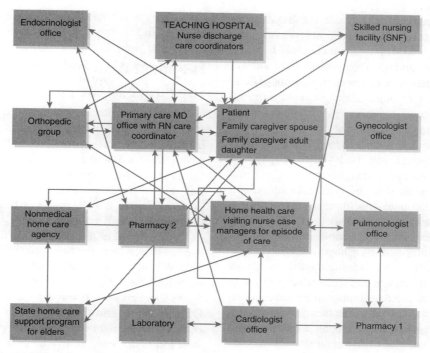

FIGURE 1-3 Mrs. Habib's Healthcare Community

I found that most of the patients and health professionals who I interviewed agreed. Few people volunteered stories of satisfying and well-organized care. Most described wide variation in their experience with different parts of the care process. Some could describe at least one excellent experience, say with a nurse navigator in a cancer center, and other examples of horrendous experiences with multiple physicians prescribing conflicting treatments and medications with little to no communication, with the nominal "care connector," the primary care physician.

While some professionals operate comfortably in task-oriented healthcare silos, many others experience frustration, anger, stress, and ultimately burnout. A recent online survey received (by the author) from the American Nurses Association illustrates this point. The survey, which solicited ideas for continuing education programs, contained multiple stress management–related topics such as "Nurse PTSD," "Combatting Stress,"

and "Effective Strategies for Nurses to Achieve Work Life Balance" (ANA, 2016). In the original IOM Quality Chasm Report, the authors note, "Poor designs set the workforce up to fail, no matter how hard they try" (p. 4).

Healthcare Organizations and Disconnected Care

Healthcare organizations are both victims and agents of disconnected care. Caught in a tornado of change as the healthcare system shifts from a volume to a value model, healthcare executives often describe their position as having one foot on the dock (fee-for-service payment) and one foot in the canoe (value-based payment).

The political turmoil of the 2016 presidential election has created possibly more forces for disconnection as the system resets itself for a new reality. Added to these major forces is the continuing drive by both federal and state agencies to cut costs and reduce fraud. While on one hand, the CMMI pushes for creative ideas, collaboration, and the development and testing of new models of care, the other divisions of CMS create new regulations that demand more resources, more bureaucratic structures, and in many cases more rigidity.

As government payers, employers, and insurers struggle to control healthcare costs, payment rates are dropping, margins are shrinking, and business as usual has become more difficult. At an organizational level, the symptoms of disconnection are common but not always recognized. Complaints about "miscommunication"—patients getting conflicting instructions, dollars being wasted on missed appointments, patients not understanding when to report changing symptoms, having wrong phone numbers, lacking patient follow-up, and patients receiving medical bills with errors—are examples of disconnection in daily clinical life. Most organizations see these as "just the way things are," not as symptoms of a deeper and more serious problem. Without a connected care measurement system, symptoms of disconnected care only come to light during complaint reviews, quality audits, state surveys, case conferences, and formal and informal conversations among staff and managers.

Many organizations, overwhelmed by conflicting demands and regulatory changes, take their eye off the ball of connected care while they hunker down and try to survive the change tornado. Others continue to move forward with collaboration and coordination efforts, and despite a less than ideal climate, generate solutions and innovations.

Fragmentation and Connection: The Push and the Pull

Our American healthcare system and our healthcare organizations are a volatile mix of fragmented and connected care delivery structures, payment models, and activities. Some of these forces push toward connection, while others pull toward fragmentation. There is progress on many fronts, but the forces of fragmentation are very much alive and well.

One helpful tool in visualizing these dynamic forces is force field analysis (**FIGURE 1-4**). This tool, developed by organizational psychologist Kurt Lewin (1951), visualizes dynamic forces that drive toward, and oppose, change. Organizations and teams use it to achieve change management goals by identifying negative forces that must be overcome or positive forces that must be strengthened for change to occur. The force field model is useful in visualizing the forces that impact connected care in your professional world.

ACTIVITY

1. Think about the bigger healthcare system in your own community and your own state.
2. Create your own force field analysis using the diagram as a guide.

ASK YOURSELF

1. How many disconnected care stories do you hear at work? Is this a widespread problem?
2. How well is your organization weathering the forces of change and providing new ways to offer connected care to patients?

▶ Measuring Connected Care

Care Coordination: A Key Element of Connected Care Measurement

Care coordination has become a generic term for the various care connection activities developed

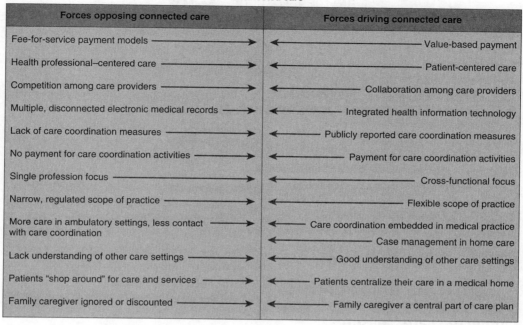

Connected care

Forces opposing connected care	Forces driving connected care
Fee-for-service payment models	Value-based payment
Health professional–centered care	Patient-centered care
Competition among care providers	Collaboration among care providers
Multiple, disconnected electronic medical records	Integrated health information technology
Lack of care coordination measures	Publicly reported care coordination measures
No payment for care coordination activities	Payment for care coordination activities
Single profession focus	Cross-functional focus
Narrow, regulated scope of practice	Flexible scope of practice
More care in ambulatory settings, less contact with care coordination	Care coordination embedded in medical practice
	Case management in home care
Lack understanding of other care settings	Good understanding of other care settings
Patients "shop around" for care and services	Patients centralize their care in a medical home
Family caregiver ignored or discounted	Family caregiver a central part of care plan

FIGURE 1-4 Force Field Analysis Graphic

to solve healthcare fragmentation and a key focus for measurement. Care coordination, however, is a difficult concept to pin down. A 2007 analysis of healthcare quality improvement strategies (McDonald et al., 2007) identified over 40 definitions of care coordination. Two of the most commonly used definitions come from the National Quality Forum (NQF) and the AHRQ:

- The NQF describes care coordination as "a function that helps ensure that the patient's needs and preferences for health services and information sharing across people, functions, and sites are met over time" (NQF, 2006, p. 1).
- The AHRQ definition of care coordination is "the deliberate organization of patient care activities between two or more participants (including the patient) involved in a patient's care to facilitate the appropriate delivery of health care services" (McDonald et al., 2007, p. 1).

The authors of the AHRQ (2014) Care Coordination Atlas, a work designed to describe and summarize useful care coordination measures, describe the rapid evolution of the field of care coordination over the three-year period from the first edition (AHRQ, 2010) to the 2014 version. While the field has moved forward in the years between the two editions, the authors indicate that continued ambiguity in care coordination definitions and lack of consensus around a single conceptual model still persists (AHRQ, 2014). Fuzzy definitions have not, however, been a barrier to the development of multiple care coordination strategies, roles, software, products, and services. Almost daily, healthcare news journals, commercially sponsored white papers, free webinars, blogs, and product announcements flood professional email inboxes, claiming to have found the ultimate solution to the problem of disconnected care (**FIGURE 1-5**).

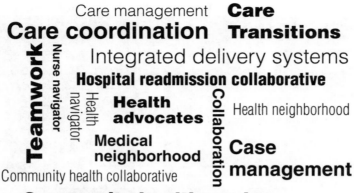

FIGURE 1-5 Word Cloud of Care Coordination Terms and Programs

▶ What Would It Look Like if We Did It Right?

Connected Care Measures

Formal measurement efforts have focused on two elements of connected care: care coordination and care transitions. In recent years, the development of care coordination measures has been the focus of intense effort by policy makers, academicians, and care coordination specialty groups. As these measures have migrated into accreditation, public reporting, and value-based payment models, they have also become of vital interest to administrators and clinicians.

The NQF (2006) has developed a list of endorsed care coordination measures including:

- Hospital readmission rates
- Percentage of patients who received a transition record at the time of discharge
- Number of unintentional medication discrepancies per patient (NQF, 2014)
- Patient age experience of care coordination using the Consumer Assessment of Health Care Providers and Systems (CAPHS) survey (CMS, 2016b)

Nursing, because of its widespread involvement in care coordination, and especially in specialty care coordination roles, has also developed

measurement models that build on those of NQF, ARHQ, and other theorists (American Nurses Association [ANA], 2013).

Care coordination measures are used in a variety of important ways:

- **Public reporting**—Medicare reports many care coordination measures (such as hospital readmission rates) on its website (Medicare, 2018). This public reporting system provides patients, families, and professionals with comparative data about healthcare organization performance. Examples are the Medicare Hospital Compare and Medicare Home Care Compare websites (Medicare, 2018). Both feature readmission rates and patient satisfaction data comparing organizations against state and national benchmarks.

- **Value-based payment**—CMS has included care coordination measures in the standards for new, alternative payment models such as accountable care organizations (i.e., groups of providers that work and are paid together to provide care for a group of patients) (CMS, 2018b) and bundled payment (i.e., payment for all elements of care provided for a single diagnosis or surgery) programs. These measures include hospital readmission rates, health information systems standards, and CAPHS measures. In these settings, measures are used to determine payments.

- **Cross sector measurement mandated by legislation**—The IMPACT Act of 2014 (CMS, 2014), which creates a unified measurement system across postacute settings, includes several care coordination measures such as 30-day readmission rates, postdischarge medication reconciliation, and transfer of health information and care preferences when an individual transitions to a different setting. Some of these measures are currently mandated, while others are still in development.

What Does It Take to Perform Well on These Measures?

The NQF (2010) has identified five domains for care coordination measurement and created a list of associated care coordination best practices for achieving higher scores on key measures. These domains and associated best practices provide a roadmap for organizations that plan to improve their level of connected care:

- Healthcare home—a single location where the patient receives primary care and where his or her primary medical record is kept
- A proactive plan of care and follow-up
- Communication among providers and across settings
- Information systems that link and share vital patient information
- Care transitions (modified from NQF, 2010, pp. 7–38)

Using the NQF best practices that are part of these domains, healthcare organizations can create a self-assessment of their own connected care effectiveness.

Organizational Connected Care Measures

For most organizations, connected care measures will be part of their accreditation requirements, and if they are Medicare participants,

part of their publicly reported measures. Organizations may develop their own operational goals for connected care. Following is an example of home health agency connected care measures and goals:

- **Outcome measure.** A home healthcare agency has a 30-day readmission rate of 16%. The agency goal is to improve its score to the level of the state benchmark, 15%.
- **Patient experience measure.** The same home healthcare agency scores 82% on the Home Health Consumer Assessment of Healthcare Providers and Systems (HHCAHPS) national survey question: "How well did the team communicate with patients?" The agency goal is to achieve or surpass the state benchmark score (85%).
- **Internal process measure.** The agency has found that patients are being readmitted because of poor instructions given at the end of the home care episode of care. The agency's goal is to reduce by 50% readmissions due to poor instructions. The agency will measure performance by calling patients two days after discharge, checking their understanding of discharge instructions using a standardized form and asking patients to rate the quality of the discharge instructions that they received.
- **Nursing consistency measure.** The agency has a standard of having no more than three nurses visit a patient during an episode of care. The electronic medical record is used to generate monthly reports that flag patients with too many nurses on the case.

ASK YOURSELF

- What are the official care coordination quality measures for your industry segment?
- How well is your organization performing on care coordination measures?
- What are your organization's target improvement goals for these measures?

▶ Beyond Care Coordination: Connected Care

While care coordination can be extraordinarily helpful to patients, it is often narrowly focused on strategies employed by health professionals within the structure of the healthcare system. It is often layered on top of a fragmented, disconnected system, as opposed to being embedded into the work of all professionals.

Few healthcare organizations extend their care coordination activities outside the boundaries of their own walls into the real patient world of care coordination activities that exist in families, friendship networks, community groups, faith communities, mobile applications, and social media.

Because it is unlikely that our healthcare culture or payment system will fully transform itself to an integrated model providing coordinated services to all patients anytime soon, a more comprehensive approach that can be adopted by healthcare organizations, large and small, would be very helpful in improving the care experience for patients. Connected care is such an approach.

Why Connected Care Is Vital

Numerous studies have documented the negative impact of care fragmentation. One study, which reviewed over 500,000 healthcare claims from commercially insured patients, found that more fragmented care demonstrated less use of clinical best practices, cost more, and generated more avoidable hospital admissions (Frandsen & Joynt, 2015).

Patient harm, including disability and death, for patients who have been the victims of high-risk fragmented care is well documented as are the malpractice risks associated with disconnected care (Budryk, 2016). For organizations, disconnected care can generate citations or sanctions on state surveys, producing thousands of dollars in fines, a public relations nightmare, and expensive corrective action. Even with so much evidence about the negative impact of fragmented care, executives and clinicians, consumed by a tidal wave of regulatory changes, market demands, and competing internal priorities, do not always focus on connected care approaches.

These constant distractions leave little time or energy to think about connecting with other providers or to consider the next steps in care in a way that creates a safe and seamless experience for patients. Yet, despite these obstacles, there are excellent reasons to make connected care an organizational strategic goal and to embed it into the daily fabric of clinical work:

- It is a key national health priority and a key part of the National Quality Strategy (AHRQ, 2015).
- It can lower costs and help organizations succeed with new payment models.
- It reduces patient harm by eliminating miscommunication, medical errors, and fragmented follow-up.
- It can improve patient satisfaction by creating a seamless experience.
- It may lower survey, accreditation, and malpractice risk for healthcare organizations.
- It is a key factor in reducing health professional dissatisfaction and burnout that results from the inability to provide good quality care in a fractured and dysfunctional healthcare system.

The impact of connected care—or its opposite, disconnected care—influences every aspect of a healthcare organization's performance. Many people characterize organizations that practice effective connected care as "having their act together" or "running a tight ship." Having this type of reputation can have a positive impact on organizational growth. The potential positive impacts of connected care on achieving Quadruple Aim goals and on employee satisfaction justify the level of effort and allocation of resources necessary to create a culture of connected care.

Crossing Your Own Quality Chasm: Organizational Connected Care Solutions

We described connected care as a systems approach to creating a safe and seamless patient experience. Connected care requires a healthcare culture change in which healthcare organization operations and individual health professional behaviors are aligned around creating a seamless care experience for patients. In this way it is somewhat like the patient safety culture movement, which seeks to embed patient safety attitudes and actions into every aspect of a healthcare organization's operations (Oh, 2012). Culture change starts with a set of guiding principles.

Connected Care Principles

- It's all about them (patients and caregivers), not just about us (health professionals).
- We're all in this together.
- We share relevant information to meet patient needs.
- We do the right things right.

(Modified from IOM, 2001)

It's all about them, not just about us. Connected care is about collaboration with the patient, not just adherence by the patient. In the connected care model, professionals filter all their actions through a patient lens.

Professionals co-create care plans with patients and work to incorporate patient goals. In the best case scenario, patients and professionals are mutually respectful of each other's expertise and effort, and work together as a team to achieve patient goals. Using the skills of active listening and motivational interviewing, professionals help patients articulate what is important to them and then take action to help them achieve their needs and wants. Professionals constantly ask themselves how their actions impact the patient experience and they ask patients for their perceptions and opinions in a very straightforward way: "How do you think we are doing on planning your discharge?"

This principle also applies to helping patients deal with what they don't know; namely, the pitfalls they might encounter at the next step in care and how to cope with them. For example, a nurse care coordinator, helping a patient prepare for discharge after a skilled nursing facility stay, would ask how the patient will get food, what types of transportation she has access to, and how much real help she will have when she gets home.

The family caregiver or other care partner is the second patient in connected care. He or she is often the patient's most ardent advocate and frequently carries the heaviest burden in the care coordination effort. Professionals must do detective work to find out who is in the patient's formal and informal care support system and then develop mechanisms for communicating with these vital helpers. Because this work is patient directed, patients may sometimes choose not to participate in connected care. After using reasonable means to create a collaborative partnership, health professionals must respect this choice.

We're all in this together. Connected care is all about collaboration and teamwork, not just between people in the same organization or profession and those who have the right degrees or certifications.

Nurses talking only to nurses and doctors talking only to doctors doesn't always produce coordinated results. The first step is to look outside your narrow professional silo and see the relevant parts of the patient web of care. To collaborate effectively, professionals must put aside status concerns, professional turf issues, jargon, and insider information. Collaboration of this type starts with dialogue about what each profession can do for the patient and by creating a common language for discussing patient care.

We share relevant information to meet patient needs. Connected care at risky handoff points, such as transitions between care settings, starts with thinking about the patient's next stop along the continuum of care, what the people in that care setting need to know, and what they can do to help. All too often, professionals assume that the information they find most convenient to give is the information that the next step in care needs. This is often not true. If agencies and organizations communicate about what they need to properly care for the patient and then the referring agency provides that information, care transitions will be smoother and more seamless for patients.

A good way to do this is to have periodic conversations about "what do you need from us?" with referral sources or collaborating agencies. A good example is the use of a standard referral form for communicating patient information and orders for home health care. When a skilled nursing facility, a medical office, or a hospital refers a patient to home care, the care coordinator or physician office typically uses a standard referral form to convey patient information and initial orders for care. If the form is faxed, the agency typically needs a phone call or an email "heads up" to ensure that the faxed form is not lost.

The form should provide patient demographics, key diagnoses, medications, brief information about patient treatment and condition, a list of services requested, and specific medical orders for wound care, home treatment, monitoring, or other services. Without these elements, the referral is incomplete and the home care agency must track down the referring clinician to clarify pieces of information.

We do the right things right. Organizations that value connected care devote attention and resources to creating patient-centered, lean and effective work processes that reduce handoffs, eliminate unnecessary complexity, and ensure teamwork between professionals and across departments. Using data from patient satisfaction surveys, outcome measures, chart reviews, readmissions debriefings, patient conversations, and workflow observations, the part of the healthcare organization responsible for quality identifies key work processes that impact care connections and may need improvement. Typically these are:

- Admission processes
- Referring the patient to outside care organizations
- Appointment and phone call processes
- Internal care transitions
- Coordinating the work of multiple health professionals and support staff
- Communicating and managing orders with primary care and other physicians
- Discharge processes

Using process improvement teams, tools, and techniques, the organization reduces waste, streamlines process steps, improves communication, meets patient requirements, reduces labor and staff frustration, and reduces the number of things that "fall through the cracks."

▶ Key Elements of Connected Care

Connected care consists of a foundation (patient centeredness) plus the five pillars mentioned earlier (care transitions, care coordination, communication, teamwork, and collaboration). There are also some additional elements that integrate and unify the patient experience (**FIGURE 1-6**). Let's examine each of these key elements in more depth:

1. **The organization is aligned around connected care principles and practices.** Ideally, connected care should be a key organizational goal. It should be supported by senior management through inclusion in the organizational strategic plan, regular management attention, resource allocations, giving time for connected care activities, and having measures that track achievement of connected care goals.

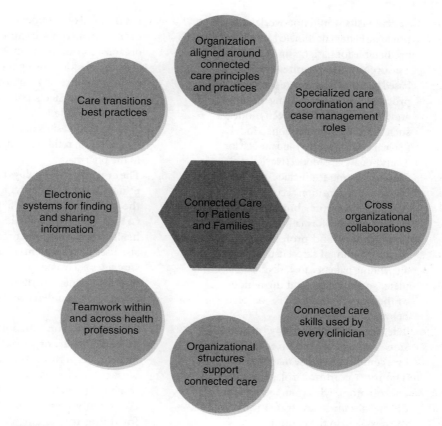

FIGURE 1-6 Connected Care Key Elements

2. **Organizational structures support connected care.** Some organizations are actually built to provide connected care for patients and families:

   - **Patient-centered medical homes** are one such structure. A PCMH is defined by the National Committee on Quality Assurance (NCQA) as "a model of care that emphasizes care coordination and communication to transform primary care into what patients want it to be" (NCQA, 2018).

   - **Medical neighborhoods** are groups of primary care providers and specialists who see the same patients and have collaborative care arrangements (Greenberg et al., 2014; Patient Centered Primary Care Collaborative, 2017).

   - **Accountable care organizations** are groups of providers who band together to provide care to a population of patients, usually with a value-based payment model that pays for results and not for more services (CMS, 2018b).

   In traditional healthcare organizations, structures can be altered to provide more connected care to patients. For example, a home health agency combined its nursing and therapy scheduling teams so that patient visits would not overlap and would be better coordinated and more predictable for patients and families.

3. **The organization applies evidence-based best practices to care transitions processes.** This means using the tools and techniques from proven models such as the Care Transitions Model™ (Coleman & Min, 2006) and the Naylor Transitional Care Model (Naylor et al., 2004). These models include processes for ensuring transition accountability, educating patients about self-care, sharing patient information with other organizations and professionals in the continuum of care, ensuring that all pending patient care tasks are complete, and ensuring that the handoff to the next step in care is complete before ending services.

4. **The organization employs professionals who have specialized skills in care coordination/case management.** The most common roles are care coordinators, who manage patient discharges and care transitions to the next step in the continuum; case managers, who implement complex patient care plans over extended periods of time; and liaison nurses, who come into the hospital from postacute settings (SNFs and home health care) to facilitate patient transitions to the next step in care (Evans, 2015).

   These professionals act as role models, consultants, and resources for other health professionals, who are not specialists but who incorporate care connection strategies into their daily work.

5. **Connected care skills are used by every clinician and every employee.** To create a true connected care culture, every employee must be accountable for monitoring and connecting the elements of care for patients and families. "That's not my job" is emphatically

not the kind of statement that should ever be heard in a connected care organization. Each employee must be accountable for "closing the loop" to ensure that care tasks are completed in a way that meets patient needs. A good example is calling a patient back with lab results or ensuring that a medication refill is promptly called to the pharmacy.

6. **The organization employs interdisciplinary teamwork strategies such as the AHRQ Team STEPPS® program (AHRQ, 2016b) to build effective healthcare teams.** The organization also uses internal team collaboration strategies such as single professional interdisciplinary conferencing and complex case conferences for clinical teams.

7. **The organization collaborates with other healthcare organizations.** The healthcare organization develops working relationships with other related organizations in its healthcare community. One common method for doing this is participation in hospital readmission collaborative groups (i.e., meetings between hospitals and postacute facilities to analyze complex cases and improve care transition processes to reduce readmissions) (Bradley et al., 2013). Other cross-functional groups may have different goals such as the development of patient education materials.

   In highly integrated delivery systems, group "huddles" or team meetings that include partners from each part of the care continuum from hospital to SNF, medical practice, and home care, are held to discuss care strategies for high-risk patients. No matter what the stated purpose of the group, relationships develop between health professionals who attend. These relationships can later be helpful when one organization needs the help of another to connect elements of care for a patient.

While none of these efforts approaches fully aligned connected care, it does illustrate how a community of willing health and community service providers can work together through formal and informal efforts to connect the elements of care for high-risk patients. This is the raw stuff of connected care.

8. **Electronic systems are used to share information and to track patients across the care continuum.** Information systems are as connected as possible. While few settings in the United States have fully interoperable information systems, there are ways to connect some electronic elements of the patient's story. Most organizations have the ability to use secure email to communicate with other health professionals in other settings. Many hospitals provide electronic referral portals where postacute providers can access patient information from the hospital record. Some integrated delivery systems use shared electronic databases or electronic patient tracking systems (that show which facility or provider is currently caring for the patient) with their preferred provider partners. Many hospitals, physicians, and outpatient facilities provide patient portals (i.e., password-protected websites that allow patients to see a portion of their own medical records) into their electronic medical record, so that patients can access their own medical information and share it with all members of their health team, if they choose.

Integrating these strategies into a coherent whole is the key challenge in implementing a true connected care culture. This text explores each of these elements in greater detail.

Collaboration in a Real Healthcare Community

Without a broader view of the various providers of health care and supportive services in a community, it is difficult to provide connected care for patients. In a healthcare community without strong integrated delivery systems, connections between organizations must be intentional and both informal (through personal relationships) and formal (through structured networking groups or improvement collaborative meetings). **FIGURE 1-7** and the following case study paint a picture of the various resources that interact with or are available to patients in a real healthcare community.

🔍 CASE STUDY

Connected Care Activities in a Real Healthcare Community

The following list provides examples of collaboration that occurs in the community depicted in Figure 1-7:

- The large teaching hospital in the community uses an electronic medical record that allows skilled nursing facilities and home care agencies to receive referrals electronically and to read selected parts of the patient hospital record.
- Patients who choose to use the hospital electronic medical record patient portal can see portions of their own medical record and retrieve medical test results online.

(continues)

- The hospital sponsors a monthly collaborative meeting of hospital case managers and staff from skilled nursing facilities and home care agencies where participants work together to reduce readmissions by sharing case study information, learn about hospital care coordination initiatives, and develop relationships that often lead to better collaboration on patient cases in the field.
- There are numerous healthcare and eldercare networking groups in the community, in which participants educate each other about their particular specialized care service and educate the public about how to better use the healthcare system.
- Several accountable care organizations (ACOs) in the community use a single online system that tracks patients through the care continuum and allows ACO providers to report back to and collaborate with the ACO care managers.

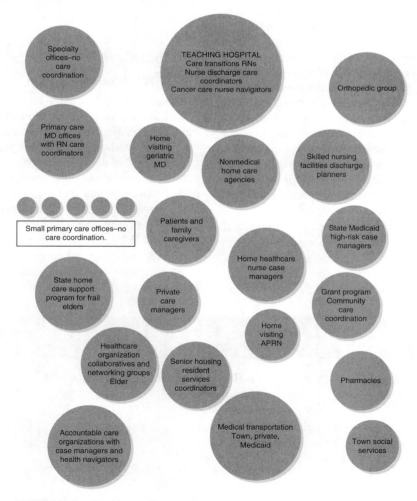

FIGURE 1-7 One Healthcare Community

- A statewide grant program funded a local skilled nursing facility to provide care coordination to patients who have complex serious illnesses and no access to care coordination. Through outreach to providers, the care coordinator has been able to connect the elements of care for many patients without other resources.

Who Provides Connected Care?

Connected care requires the active engagement and collaboration of healthcare and human services professionals and from every level of the healthcare organization from executive to front line staff. It also requires teamwork with health and human services professionals in community agencies. **FIGURE 1-8** illustrates the circle of support required to provide effective connected care to patients and their family caregivers. These roles range from that of a senior executive, who must align his organization around connected care goals, to the resident services coordinator in elderly housing who must find support for a high-risk patient who is discharged home without adequate support.

▶ Nursing and Connected Care

How Nurses Impact Connected Care

Nursing, as the largest healthcare profession (Bureau of Labor Statistics, 2015) with a presence in every segment of the healthcare industry, is essential to achieving connected care. Nurses are typically present at every step of the patient journey. Patients often see nurses as logical care connectors. Nurses foster connected care in four fundamental ways:

- Providing connected care for patients as part of front line nursing practice
- Practicing in specialized care coordination, care transitions, and case management roles
- Achieving system change for better care connections through management, executive, and policy roles

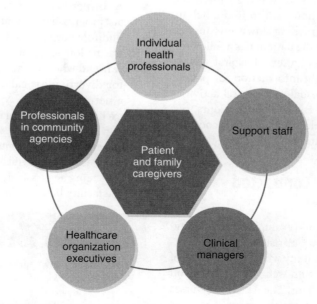

FIGURE 1-8 Working Together for Connected Care

- Acting as informal connected care advisors for personal networks of family, friends, neighbors, and professional colleagues

The American Nurses Association Congress on Nursing Practice and Economics (2012) describes the essential role of the registered nurse in the daily practice of care coordination, which is one core element of connected care:

> Patient-centered care coordination is a core professional standard and competency for all registered nursing practice. Based on a partnership guided by the healthcare consumer's and family's needs and preferences, the registered nurse is integral to patient care quality, satisfaction, and the effective and efficient use of health care resources. Registered nurses are qualified and educated for the role of care coordination, especially with high risk and vulnerable populations. (p. 1)

Nurses in their historic role as the "glue" in the healthcare system often instinctively weave connected care principles into their daily routine. Getting food for the waiting patient and family, making a phone call to find a helpful benefit program, tracking down missing lab tests, ensuring that the patient has a follow-up medical appointment after a hospital stay, or assembling the right information for patient self-care are all normal and natural activities that help connect the dots for patients, but aren't typically labeled as formal care coordination or care transitions.

Some Nursing Connected Care Activities

Parish nursing is a good example of community-based connected care. Parish nurses are members of a faith community who help members of their congregation with wellness activities and health-related problems. The American Nurses Association recognizes parish nursing as a type of specialty practice and describes it this way: "Today the parish nurse plays many roles: integrator of faith and health, health educator and counselor, referral advisor, health advocate, support-group developer, and volunteer coordinator. Besides congregations, settings for parish nurses include long-term care, hospice, day care, soup kitchens, schools, seminaries, and other faith-based community settings" (Patterson, 2010).

Nurses make up the largest proportion of professionals with job titles such as care coordinator and case manager. Indeed, nurses have made a concerted effort to define these roles as nursing-specific competencies.

Most nurses, even if they are not in a formal care coordination role, act as informal advisors for family and friends who have no access to care coordination services. This informal role often involves providing basic information about how the health system works, who to call for what, advising about which health facilities and doctors have the best reputation, and providing "insider" information about how to manage healthcare and insurance company bureaucracy. Consider the informal requests for care coordination help that one nurse (the author) managed in the last several months:

- A former neighbor, whose husband has fast progressing dementia, emailed for help finding a hospital bed for her husband who was no longer mobile.
- A friend who was facing a colon resection for diverticulitis called for help to find a network surgeon covered by her state exchange insurance plan.
- A friend called to ask whether he and his father, who lived in a nursing home, had the right to refuse a referral to hospice care which was being aggressively recommended, by the facility medical director.

ASK YOURSELF

What nursing activities do you do on a daily basis as part of your regular nursing practice or in your private life to help connect pieces of care for your patients, family, and friends?

Who Needs Connected Care?

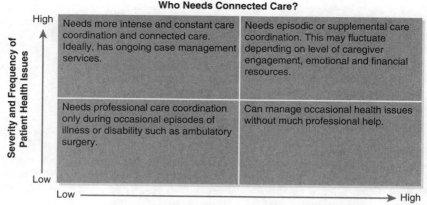

FIGURE 1-9 Who Needs Connected Care?

These types of nursing connected care activities, while not formal or official, help people without other resources connect the dots for themselves.

Who Needs Connected Care?

Not everyone who uses the healthcare system needs help with connected care (**FIGURE 1-9**). Many people now manage their own care using notebooks, calendars, mobile devices, online medical records, patient portals, tracking apps, retail health clinics, telemedicine, and online medical information.

Many patients fall into a middle range where they need connected care after surgery or during treatment for a serious illness such as chemotherapy for cancer treatment. Once the intense phase of the illness is over, these patients can go back to coordinating their own care. For frail, elderly patients with multiple serious chronic illnesses, and especially those with weaker caregiver support and/or socioeconomic barriers to health, more continuous connected care is essential to better outcomes, especially in reducing medication errors and hospital readmissions.

It is important to note that the target population for connected care is both the patient and his or her network of family caregivers and informal support helpers who surround

the patient throughout the care journey. Supporting the caregiver so he or she can continue helping coordinate patient care is an essential, and often missed, element of successful connected care.

Visualizing Connected Care in Daily Work

To create a connected care culture, clinicians must be able to visualize how connected care looks in clinical practice and internalize this vision into their own practice. **FIGURE 1-10** lists the key elements of a connected care organization. We can also visualize connected care by looking at a few examples:

One or more health professionals, usually in a primary care setting, works with the patient to create a care plan that incorporates patient goals, self-care and care coordination ability, social determinants of health, and level of caregiving support. Many times this is far from reality on the front lines of health care. Most care plans are developed by a single professional, looking at the patient through the lens of his or her role (e.g., "nursing care plan," "social work care plan"). Methods of charting can help to better integrate information from all disciplines and alleviate this problem. Incorporating patient goals into care planning is a relatively new idea for most professionals and requires

Check off all the elements of connected care that you recognize in your organization.

1. ❑ Your organization creates a patient-driven care plan that incorporates an assessment of patient's self-care ability and patient goals and includes strategies to address these abilities and goals.
2. ❑ The patient-driven care plan is used by all professionals who care for the patient as the core of their own specialized care plans.
3. ❑ Key professionals involved in the patient's care, or discharge, keep the patient's primary care provider(s) informed and ensure follow-up with primary care clinicians.
4. ❑ Information about the patient (the patient story) flows smoothly from one part of the care continuum to the next and ultimately back to the patient and caregivers at home.
5. ❑ Every health professional, not just care coordination specialists, take accountability for ensuring that there is consistent follow-up of patient care tasks and handoffs. Patients get test results, medical equipment, appointments, insurance information, and referrals that they need in a timely and coordinated way.
6. ❑ All members of the care team give patients consistent information and they respond effectively to patient questions.
7. ❑ All employees who care for or provide service to the patient coordinate their activities and work as a team.
8. ❑ The organization has structures and processes to deal with high-risk handoff points such as transitions of care to and from inpatient settings.
9. ❑ The patient's family caregivers and other key helpers are treated as important members of the team.
10. ❑ The patient's entire "web of care" including community organizations and formal and informal caregivers is included in your organization's connected care communication.

FIGURE 1-10 Connected Care Clinical Self-Assessment

some training in techniques such as active listening and motivational interviewing.

The patient-driven care plan is used by all professionals who care for patients as the core of their own specialized care plans. This means that each specialty or inpatient professional would be obligated to communicate with the patient, family, or primary care physician about how his or her specialized care plan might impact the core, patient goal–directed care plan.

Everyone involved in the patient's care coordinates with the patient's primary care medical practice. In most settings, this means ensuring that the patient has a primary care physician and communicating with that physician about the patient's status. A phone call to notify the physician that the patient has gone into the hospital is an example.

Home care, hospitals, and skilled nursing facilities often adopt a standard that their staff must help the patient make an appointment with his or her primary care physician within seven days of discharge. This appointment is vital, because it allows the primary care clinician to modify the care plan based on a recent inpatient stay and it provides an opportunity to reconcile medications that the patient was previously taking with those that were prescribed at discharge.

Every health professional, not just care coordination specialists, take accountability for connecting the elements of care for patients and ensuring that no information or activities "fall through the cracks." This is the sometimes tedious job of the care coordination element of connected care—ensuring that test results come back and that they are reviewed, that a course of action is developed and that the patient is informed, verifying correct family and doctor phone numbers, asking about how the patient will get medical supplies at home, and so forth.

Medication reconciliation (reconciling differences between medications prescribed in different settings or by different doctors to achieve one, current, and accurate medication list) is another vital (maybe the most vital) activity in this area. It also involves assessing and probing for potential gaps and cracks in care before a care transition. For example, a patient may insist that he is fully able to prepare his own medications at home, but when asked to demonstrate how he sets up his weekly pill box is unable to sort the medications correctly.

The organization has structures and processes to deal with high-risk handoff points such as transitions of care to and from outpatient settings. Care transitions are the highest risk parts of the care continuum, where the most errors and patient harm typically occur. The organization should recognize these high-risk handoff points and have structures in place to manage them.

For example, SNFs and home care agencies should have procedures for ensuring that when a patient is sent to the emergency room or is admitted to the hospital there is a process for communicating the medication list and other relevant patient information. Intake and admission is another high-risk point. One way to handle this is to have a clinical liaison from the receiving facility or agency visit the patient in the inpatient facility to assess care needs and to educate the patient and family about the next step in care.

Information about the patient (the patient story) flows smoothly from one part of the care continuum to the next and ultimately back to the patient at home. While this problem is often framed as a problem of health information systems interoperability, it is much more about the end goal of communication than the means of achieving it. This means that each health professional informs the next step in the care continuum about what he or she needs to know about the patient to provide effective care.

It also involves "telling the patient story" so that the patient becomes a real person with real problems and not just a collection of physical findings, diagnoses, and lab tests to those who read the medical record. It would also mean that each time the patient leaves the health setting and goes home to self-manage, he or she gets the education, information, and resources to care for himself or herself correctly and to know when to call for further help.

All employees who care for or provide service to the patient coordinate their activities and work as a team. Nothing makes patients and families more upset and confused than having different staff members and health professionals providing disjointed services and getting a different set of explanations and instructions from each member of the care team. For example, in an outpatient surgery center, all members of the clerical, medical, and nursing staff should be clear on the preoperative, surgical, recovery room, and discharge steps in care.

Each person in the process chain should prepare the patient for the next step: "First I will do some preliminary testing, then you will see the doctor and then you will sit with the booking secretary. It should take about an hour in total."

All members of the care team should provide consistent and reliable information and should respond effectively to patient questions. All team members should be using the same language and giving instructions that mesh. Written instructions should be clear and unambiguous. Ideally, there should be a set of frequently asked questions available. A good way to test for this problem of disjointed instructions or coordination is to ask a friend or family member to review the steps in your process and read your patient instructions. Care disconnects will become immediately visible to someone who is not part of the process.

The patient's family caregivers and other key helpers are treated as important members of the team. As in the case study of Mrs. Habib's medical care system and journey through the care continuum, family caregivers and other patient helpers are key members of the care team and they usually carry the heaviest care coordination burden for very ill patients. The healthcare organization must identify who these care support people are, what their roles are, how much they are available to help, and what information and resources they need to support the patient. For example, in large families, each adult child may have a specific role to play in his or her parent's care. When the patient gives permission, the family caregiver should be an integral part of any patient decision making and patient education activities. In some cases, the family caregiver may be so stressed and overwhelmed that he or she must actually be treated as "the second patient."

The patient's entire "web of care," including support people in community organizations, are included in the patient chain of communication. Health professionals all too often focus only on the patient and not on other care helpers who may be helping the patient with self-management support. This is especially vital for patients who have little or no family caregiving support. For example, a frail elderly person who has no family and lives in subsidized housing may have no support other than the building resident services coordinator, who is seldom, if ever, in the chain of healthcare communication. One way to uncover this information is to ask questions like "Who, besides your family, might help you when you go home?" If there are other people involved, the health professional could ask the patient for permission to include these helpers in care planning. Other resources for patient support that are often overlooked are neighbors and private paid helpers such as companions, homemakers, and personal care assistants.

ASK YOURSELF

Based on the assessment results, what goals could you set for improving connected care in your organization, department, and personal practice?

▶ Chapter Summary

Health care in the United States has suffered from care fragmentation and disconnection due to a fee-for-service payment system, excessive

specialization, health professional "silo" mindset, health professional "turf wars," and regulations that promote fragmentation and some aspects of consumer health choices. This fragmentation has produced adverse events for patients including patient injuries, deaths, readmissions, and excessive, wasteful healthcare expenditures. Connected care is an approach to reducing fragmentation and disconnection that incorporates care coordination techniques, but also embeds connected care activities into the work of every health professional. Nurses because of their broad, patient-centered view and their presence in every part of the healthcare system are uniquely positioned to practice connected care.

The healthcare industry has made a concerted effort, which has been accelerated by the Affordable Care Act, to create more connected care, to improve payments for care coordination, to better measure care connection activities, and to educate health professionals in connected care techniques. While some of these efforts have proved effective, the United States still ranks poorly on health outcome measures and efficiency. More work remains to be done. Health professionals must apply a set of connected care principles and practices to their daily work life to better connect the dots for patients and to achieve better health outcomes, lower costs, and improved patient satisfaction.

References

Adler, L., & Hoagland, W. (2012). What is driving US health care spending? Bipartisan Policy Center. Retrieved from http://bipartisanpolicy.org/library/what-driving-us-health-care-spending-americas-unsustainable-health-care-cost-growth/

Agency for Healthcare Research and Quality. (2010). Care coordination atlas. Retrieved from https://archive.ahrq.gov/professionals/systems/long-term-care/resources/coordination/atlas/care-coordination-measures-atlas.pdf

Agency for Healthcare Research and Quality. (2014). Care coordination atlas. Retrieved from http://www.ahrq.gov/professionals/prevention-chronic-care/improve/coordination/atlas2014/index.html

Agency for Healthcare Research and Quality. (2015). Annual progress report to Congress: National Strategy for Quality Improvement in Health Care. Retrieved from http://www.ahrq.gov/workingforquality/reports/annual-reports/nqs2015annlrpt.htm

Agency for Healthcare Research and Quality. (2016a). *National Healthcare Quality and Disparities Report chartbook on care coordination.* Pub. No. 16-0015-2-EF. Rockville, MD: AHRQ.

Agency for Healthcare Research and Quality. (2016b). Team STEPPS®: Strategies and tools to enhance performance and patient safety. Retrieved from http://www.ahrq.gov/professionals/education/curriculum-tools/teamstepps/index.html

Agency for Healthcare Research and Quality. (2017). About the national quality strategy. Retrieved from http://www.ahrq.gov/workingforquality/about.htm

American Nurses Association Congress on Practice and Economics, Position Statement: Care Coordination and Nurses Central Role, June 11, 2012 https://www.nursingworld.org/~4afbf2/globalassets/practiceandpolicy/health-policy/cnpe-care-coord-position-statement-final--draft-6-12-2012.pdf

American Nurses Association. (2016, December). Online survey received via email.

Beaudin, C. L., Lammers, J. C., & Pedroja, A. (1999). Patient perceptions of coordinated care: The importance of organized communication in hospitals. *Journal for Healthcare Quality, 21*(5), 18–23. doi:10.1111/j.1945-1474.1999.tb00985

Berwick, D., Nolan, T., & Whittington, J. (2008). The triple aim: Care, health, and cost. *Health Affairs, 27*(3), 759–769. doi:10.1377/hlthaff.27.3

Bodenheimer, T., & Sinsky, C. (2014). From triple to quadruple aim: Care of the patient requires care of the provider. *The Annals of Family Medicine, 12*(6), 573–576. doi:10.1370/afm.1713

Bradley, E., & Taylor, L. (2016). How social spending affects health outcomes. Robert Wood Johnson Foundation, Culture of Health. Retrieved from http://www.rwjf.org/en/culture-of-health/2016/08/how_social_spending.html

Bradley, E., Sipsma, H., Curry, L., Mehrotra, D., Horwitz, L. I., Krumholz, H. (2013). Quality collaboratives and campaigns to reduce readmissions: What strategies are hospitals using? *Journal of Hospital Medicine, 8*(11), 601–608. doi:10.1002/jhm.2076

Budryk, Z. (2016). Health care miscommunication cost 1.7B—and nearly 2000 lives. *Fierce Healthcare.*

Bureau of Labor Statistics. (2015). TED: The Economics Daily. Registered nurses have highest employment in healthcare occupations; anesthesiologists earn the most. Retrieved from https://www.bls.gov/opub/ted/2015/registered-nurses-have-highest-employment-in-healthcare-occupations-anesthesiologists-earn-the-most.htm

Bushardt, R., Massey, E., Simpson, T., Ariail, J., & Simpson, K. (2008). Polypharmacy: Misleading, but manageable. *Clinical Interventions in Aging, 3*(2), 383–389. https://www.ncbi.nlm.nih.gov/pmc/articles/PMC2546482/

Caffrey, M. (2016). Poll finds major care coordination gaps among seniors. *American Journal of Managed Care.* Retrieved from http://www.ajmc.com/focus-of-the-week/1216/poll-finds-major-care-coordination-gaps-among-seniors

Cassel, C., & Reuben, D. (2011). Specialization, subspecialization, and subsubspecialization in internal medicine. *New England Journal of Medicine, 364,* 1169–1173. doi:10.1056/NEJMsb1012647

Centers for Medicare and Medicaid Services. (2014). Impact Act of 2014 and cross setting measures. Retrieved from www.cms.gov/Medicare/Quality-Initiatives-Patient-Assessment-Instruments/Post-Acute-Care-Quality-Initiatives/IMPACT-Act-of-2014-and-Cross-Setting-Measures.html

Centers for Medicare and Medicaid Services, CMS.gov. (2015). Better care. smarter spending. healthier people: paying providers for value, not volume. *Media Release Database Fact- Sheet.* Retrieved from: www.cms.gov/Newsroom/MediaReleaseDatabase/Fact-sheets/2015-Fact-sheets-items/2015-01-26-3.html

Centers for Medicare and Medicaid Services. (2016a). Medicare Learning Network, Chronic Care Management Services. Retrieved from https://www.cms.gov/Outreach-and-Education/Medicare-Learning-Network-MLN/MLNProducts/Downloads/ChronicCareManagement.pdf

Centers for Medicare and Medicaid Services. (2016b). Consumer assessment of healthcare providers & systems (CAHPS). Retrieved from www.cms.gov/Research-Statistics-Data-and-Systems/Research/CAHPS

Centers for Medicare and Medicaid Services. (2018a). Alternative payment models in the quality payment program as of February 2018. Retrieved from www.cms.gov/Medicare/Quality-Payment-Program/Resource-Library/Comprehensive-List-of-APMs.pdf

Centers for Medicare and Medicaid Services. (2018b). Accountable Care Organizations, Retrieved from https://www.cms.gov/Medicare/Medicare-Fee-for-Service-Payment/ACO/

Coleman, E., & Min, S. J. (2006), The care transitions intervention. Results of a randomized controlled trial. *Archives of Internal Medicine, 166*(17), 1822–1828. doi:10.1001/archinte.166.17.1822

Du, L., & Lieu, W. (2016). US health care system ranks as one of the least efficient. Retrieved from https://www.bloomberg.com/news/articles/2016-09-29/u-s-health-care-system-ranks-as-one-of-the-least-efficient

Dubree, M. (2013). Why "breaking down" traditional care silos is difficult, but necessary. Advisory Board Nursing Executive Center. National Meeting Video Series. Retrieved from https://www.advisory.com/research/nursing-executive-center/multimedia/video/2013/2012-2013-national-meeting-videos/vanderbilt-1

Elhauge, E. (Ed.). (2010). *The fragmentation of US health care, causes and solutions.* Cambridge: Oxford University Press.

Evans, M. (2015). Demand grows for care coordinators. *Modern Healthcare.* Retrieved from http://www.modernhealthcare.com/article/20150328/MAGAZINE/303289980

Frandsen, B., Joynt, K., Rebitzer, J. B., & Jha, A. K. (2015). Fragmentation, quality, and costs among chronically ill patients. *American Journal of Managed Care, 21*(5), 355–362. http://www.ajmc.com/journals/issue/2015/2015-vol21-n5/care-fragmentation-quality-costs-among-chronically-ill-patients#sthash

Gallup. (2016). Honesty, ethics in professions, in depth topics A-Z. Retrieved from http://www.gallup.com/poll/1654/honesty-ethics-professions.aspx

Greenberg, J., Barnett, M., Spinks, M. A., Dudley, J. C., & Frolkis, J. P. (2014). The "medical neighborhood" integrating primary and specialty care for ambulatory patients. *JAMA Internal Medicine, 174*(3), 454–457. doi:10.1001/jamainternmed

Institute of Medicine. (2001). *Crossing the quality chasm: A new health system for the 21st century.* Washington, DC: National Academy Press, pp. 1–12.

Lewin, K. (1951). *Field theory in social science.* New York: Harper & Row.

McDonald, K. M., Sundaram, V., Bravata, D. M., Lewis, R., Lin, N., Kraft, S. A., . . . Owens, D. K. (2007). *Closing the quality gap: A critical analysis of quality improvement strategies* (vol. 7). Rockville, MD: Agency for Healthcare Research and Quality. https://www.ncbi.nlm.nih.gov/books/NBK44012

Medicare. (2018). Hospital compare. Retrieved from https://www.medicare.gov/hospitalcompare/search.html

National Committee on Quality Assurance. (2018). Primary care medical home recognition. Retrieved from http://www.ncqa.org/Programs/Recognition/Practices/PatientCenteredMedicalHomePCMH.aspx, 2017

National Quality Forum. (2006). NQF endorsed definition and framework for measuring care coordination. Retrieved from http://www.qualityforum.org/projects/care_coordination.asp

National Quality Forum. (2010). *Preferred practices and performance measures for measuring and reporting care coordination: A consensus report.* Washington, DC: NQF.

National Quality Forum. (2014). Measure description display information, medication reconciliation: number of unintentional medication discrepancies per patient. Retrieved from http://www.qualityforum.org/QPS/MeasureDetails.aspx?standardID=2456&print=0&entityTypeID=1

Naylor, M., Brooten, D. A., Campbell, R. L., Maislin, G., McCauley, K. M., & Sanford, J. (2004). Transitional care of older adults hospitalized with heart failure: A randomized, controlled trial. *Journal of American Geriatric Society, 52*(5), 675–684.

Oh, J. (2012). 6 elements of a true patient safety culture. Beckers Hospital Review. Retrieved from www.beckershospitalreview.com/quality/6-elements-of-a-true-patient-safety-culture.html

Patient Centered Primary Care Collaborative. (2017). Medical neighborhood definition. Retrieved from https://www.pcpcc.org/content/medical-neighborhood

Patterson, D. (2010). Parish nursing: Reclaiming the spiritual dimensions of care. *American Nurse Today, 5*(12). https://www.americannursetoday.com/parish-nursing-reclaiming-the-spiritual-dimensions-of-care-2/

Pear, R. (2016, March 29). Shaping health policy for millions, and still treating some on the side. *New York Times,* A9. www.nytimes.com/2016/03/30/us/politics/patrick-conway-medicare-medicaid.html

Permut, S. (2016). AMA statement on VA proposed rule on advanced practice nurses. Retrieved from https://www.ama-assn.org/ama-statement-va-proposed-rule-advanced-practice-nurses

Pollack, C., Gidengil, C., & Mehrotra, A. (2010). The growth of retail clinics and the medical home: Two trends in concert or in conflict? *Health Affairs, 29*(5), 998–1003. doi:10.1377/hlthaff.2010.008

Powers, B., Milstein, A., & Jain, S. (2016). Delivery models for high-risk older patients back to the future? *Journal of the American Medical Association, 315*(1), 23–24. doi:10.1001/jama.2015.17029

Rabin, R. (2013, April 30). Health care's 'dirty little secret': No one may be coordinating care. *Kaiser Health News.*

Schumann, J. (2013). Doctors look for a way off the hamster wheel. *Shots Health News from NPR.* Retrieved from http://www.npr.org/sections/health-shots/2013/08/13/211698062/doctors-look-for-a-way-off-the-medical-hamster-wheel

Stange, K. (Ed.). (2009). The problem of fragmentation and the need for integrative solutions. *Annals of Family Medicine, 7*(2), 100–103. doi:10.1370/afm

Stremikis, K., Schoen, C., & Fryer, A.K. (2011). A call for change: The 2011 Commonwealth Fund Survey of public views of the U.S. health system. *Issue Brief,* 4–5.

CHAPTER 2

Integrated Delivery Systems—The Connected Care Ideal

CHAPTER OBJECTIVES

After completing this chapter readers will be able to:

- Define the term "integrated delivery system"
- Describe the key principles of integrated care delivery
- Identify the most common types of integrated delivery models
- Explain the strategies and tactics used in integrated delivery systems to coordinate patient care and achieve quadruple aim goals
- List integrated delivery system key measures
- Describe the roles of nurses in integrated delivery systems
- List pitfalls and obstacles in integrated delivery
- Develop an action plan for applying the tools and techniques of integrated delivery to the reader's own setting

---

▶ Introduction

Integrated delivery systems are the latest chapter in the evolution of the U.S. healthcare system. These systems are designed to combine the disparate elements of healthcare payment and delivery to provide coordinated, patient-centered care that can achieve lower costs, better clinical outcomes, and a better patient experience. When these entities are truly patient centered, and not simply profit driven, they embody the principles and practice of connected care.

Innovations in integrated care delivery are occurring all over the world, particularly in Canada and Europe. Unlike countries that have "single payer" health insurance systems, the United States has a unique and fragmented system of paying for health care that can confound attempts to integrate care delivery. For this reason, the United States, under the guidance and strong urging of the Centers for Medicare and Medicaid Services (CMS), has developed some unique integrated delivery and payment models such as accountable care organizations and primary care medical homes. These models will be explained in depth in this chapter.

Integrated delivery systems are by their nature, interdisciplinary. While most of these systems are very clearly designed to incorporate physician incentives and physician involvement in decision making, nurses also play an integral role in all aspects of integrated delivery, especially in care coordination. We will consider the role and the experience of nurses in integrated systems.

The chapter will also describe the core building blocks of integrated delivery including population health strategies and tactics, the use of data in managing care, the uniform use of evidence-based best practices, and patient engagement programs. We will discuss how readers can apply the principles and tools of integrated delivery systems to their own settings.

▸ Defining Integrated Care

Integrated care provides the philosophy and guiding principles for integrated delivery systems. The editor of the *International Journal of Integrated Care*, Dr. Nick Goodwin, describes integrated care in this way: "First, it must involve bringing together key aspects in the design and delivery of care systems that are fragmented (i.e. 'to integrate' so that parts are combined to form a whole). Second, that the concept must deliver 'care', which in this context would refer to providing attentive assistance or treatment to people in need. Integrated care, then, results when the former (integration) is required to optimise the latter (care)" (Goodwin, 2016, p. 1).

A Canadian literature review summarizes the key principle of comprehensive integrated health systems: "Integrated health systems assume the responsibility to plan for provide/purchase and coordinate all services along the continuum of care for the population served. This includes services from primary through tertiary care as well as cooperation between health and social care organizations" (Suter, Oelke, Adair, & Armitage, 2009, p. 2).

A more patient-centered definition of integrated care comes from the British National Health Service: "I can plan my care with people who work together to understand me and my carer(s), allow me control, and bring together services to achieve the outcomes important to me" (National Voices.org.uk, 2013, p. 3).

Integrated delivery systems are intentionally developed, financed, and implemented with the goal of creating a new business model for the sponsoring organization. This new model typically includes the recruitment of a network of willing and engaged providers, new care delivery structures, a value-based payment model (payment for results and not simply for volume of care delivered), more collaborative relationships between organizations and health professionals, deep and well analyzed data, and a whole new mindset for both organizations and individual providers.

Integrated delivery systems manage groups of patients with like characteristics (populations). These characteristics might include a common diagnosis or a group of patients who receive care from a specific source such as a medical practice. The integrated system manages the "white space" between providers, where patients "fall through the cracks" by building bridges between provider organizations and individual clinicians through contracts, shared data, cross-organizational work processes, and training.

🔍 CASE STUDY

Picture of an Integrated Delivery System

The Everford Hospital System senior management team and board of directors has decided that its survival depends on becoming successful at value-based payment. The hospital has affiliated primary care physicians and specialists but no contracts with insurance companies or accountable care organizations (ACOs). The hospital also has informal preferred provider arrangements with some skilled nursing facilities and home care agencies.

After prolonged negotiations, the hospital acquires a large primary care practice. Using this practice as a base, the hospital either acquires or contracts with additional primary care practices in the region. It buys sophisticated data analysis software and converts both its inpatient records and the medical group practice records to a single electronic medical record system. The hospital then engages physician leaders in redesigning the management structure for the new health system. This new structure includes a care management department to oversee care coordination and transitions. The system hires RNs to be "embedded nurse care coordinators and patient health coaches" in the medical practices. The system contracts with commercial insurers to manage some of their patient populations and it becomes part of the Medicare Shared Savings Program. These contracts stipulate that the system must achieve cost targets, target patient satisfaction scores, and meet specified clinical outcomes to achieve financial savings.

In preparation for these contracts, the new Everford ACO analyzes data about its patient population and identifies high-risk patients. RN case managers and community health workers reach out to these patients, connecting them with a primary care doctor, engaging them in better self-care and tracking, and managing their care in transitions within the continuum. While this is occurring, Everford is researching postacute preferred providers and eventually contracts with some of them.

These contracts specify how the skilled nursing facilities and home care agencies must manage the care of ACO patients. The system also gradually researches and implements clinical best practices and patient education programs for all organizations that are part of the system. As the system evolves, senior management convenes a monthly meeting of all provider groups and facilities at which population utilization, cost, and quality data are reviewed. As problems are identified, improvement teams are chartered and launched. Team training and teamwork guidelines are offered.

As the system matures it begins to require standardized processes and forms for care transitions. The system purchases an electronic patient tracking system in which providers can enter data and track their patients through the different organizations that care for them. Care managers use this tracking information to manage care and reduce costly hospital readmissions. The system hires several social workers to consult with the practices on managing the social determinants of health, treating mental health issues, and finding community benefits and entitlements for patients.

After 2 years of operation the Everford ACO is flourishing. Patient and provider satisfaction is high, quadruple aim measures have improved, and providers are reaping the rewards of shared savings.

Case Study Questions

- What structural changes did the integrated system make to build bridges between providers?
- What mechanisms were implemented to improve the flow of information between providers?
- How does the system coordinate care?
- What role does data play in creating connected care in this system?
- What elements of teamwork are present in this system?
- What are the characteristics of care transitions in this system?
- How might the newly integrated delivery system elements impact the experience of care for patients and families?

▶ Current State of Integrated Care in the United States

Integrated delivery systems are not an entirely new concept in the United States, but until recently, they had never been widely adopted. Group Health Cooperative of Puget Sound and Kaiser Permanente in California have long had both insurance and integrated delivery components. Staff model health maintenance organizations, which consisted of a multispecialty medical group and an insurance product, existed in the United States in the 1960s through the 1980s, but fell out of favor and all but disappeared in the 1990s.

In recent years, since the implementation of the Affordable Care Act (ACA), integrated care delivery systems have primarily been driven by the CMS volume-to-value shift. This is the shift from fee-for-service payment to pay for value (achieving cost, quality, and patient experience goals).

The Center for Medicare and Medicaid Innovation (CMMI) has fostered innovation in integrated delivery through large-scale national grants for testing new delivery and payment models. As grantees have gained experience and demonstrated some positive results, insurers and employers have also begun to encourage and incentivize integrated delivery. At the time of this writing, as the political system grapples with either the repeal or the modification of the ACA, the future of integrated delivery, at least in Medicare demonstration models, is uncertain. Most recently, Trump administration officials have indicated dissatisfaction with the lack of Medicare savings from one type of demonstration model—accountable care organizations. However, most analysts believe that the concept will persevere as both insurers and employers are now convinced that it can improve both healthcare cost and quality.

▶ New Integrated Delivery System Models

Out of the flurry of integrated care innovation generated by the ACA, several integrated care delivery system and payment models have become popular. It is important to note that integrated care cannot flourish without the support of value-based payment models. If clinicians and healthcare organizations are paid only for the volume of services and procedures delivered, fragmentation is inevitable, despite the best of intentions. When payment is linked to achieving quadruple aim goals, integration is much more likely to occur. Data are the glue that bind all parts of the integrated delivery system together. The four key high-level elements of integrated delivery systems in the United States are illustrated in **FIGURE 2-1**.

Integrated care comes in a variety of forms from fully integrated delivery systems that include a health plan and every part of the care continuum (hospitals, medical practices, and postacute care) to partially integrated care delivery models that address a single diagnosis or aspect of care delivery.

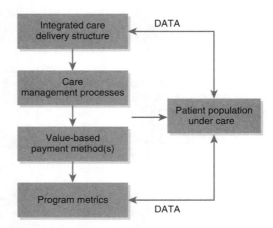

FIGURE 2-1 Integrated Delivery Systems Key Elements

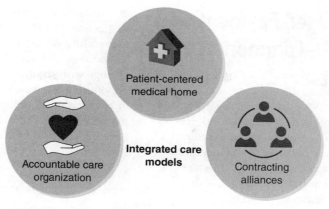

FIGURE 2-2 Integrated Delivery Models

Currently, most integrated delivery systems comprised a hospital and a group of affiliated medical group practices. Some include a health insurance plan. Some systems also own or contract with postacute providers such as skilled nursing facilities (SNFs) and home care agencies.

The most common integrated care delivery models in the United States are illustrated in **FIGURE 2-2**.

- **Accountable care organizations (ACOs)** are provider coalitions or organizations organized or owned by a hospital or large medical group. ACOs provide coordinated care to a defined population of patients and they are paid through value-based payment programs. ACOs typically include a data management and care management infrastructure. We will discuss the key features of ACOs later in this chapter.
- **Patient-centered (or primary care) medical homes (PCMHs)** are primary care medical practices with expanded capabilities, extended access to care, a commitment to quality outcomes, extensive use of evidence-based care practices, and a care coordination infrastructure. PCMHs are accredited by the National Committee on Quality Assurance (NCQA) at different levels, depending on

the sophistication of their infrastructure and care delivery systems. The highest level of accreditation is level 3. The PCMH should be the locus of the patient's care, where he or she has a regular primary care provider who organizes and coordinates care, where his or her primary medical record is kept, where all medications are reviewed and consolidated, and where all specialty care is coordinated.

PCMHs can contract directly with Medicare or insurers for value-based payment and are not required to be part of an ACO, although many choose to become affiliated with such an organization (NCQA, 2017).

- **Provider contracting coalitions** are large and often decentralized groups of physicians who band together to participate in value-based payment programs. An example is a network of orthopedic surgeons who contract to participate in the Medicare joint replacement bundling initiative. These contracting coalitions are likely to have the fewest integrated care characteristics since they are essentially physicians practicing independently and are united only by a payment model. Most of these models, however, do include a care coordination component.

▶ Value-Based Payment Models—Common Elements

Integrated care cannot exist without a payment system that incentivizes providers to link elements of care into a seamless whole, to reduce costs, and to produce quadruple aim outcomes. A variety of new payment models have been developed and tested by the CMMI. Each of these models has some common elements:

- Insurers or government payers (Medicare and Medicaid) contract with a group of providers (who practice in some type of integrated delivery model) to deliver care and to accept payment that is based on outcomes and costs, not on volume of services delivered (fee-for-service payment).
- Value-based payment methods are used to pay for care for specific patient populations. Typically, these are all the patients of a practice covered by a specific insurer or a group of patients who have a specific diagnosis or those who are undergoing a specific procedure.
- In value-based payment programs the insurer sets a target price for services based on recent claims data from the patient population or medical group.
- Quality standards are set for the payment model. These standards always include readmission and patient experience measures as well as clinical outcome measures. The provider group must meet quality standards to be eligible for value-based payments.
- A care management program and a monitoring/data collection system is developed. Provider groups sometimes purchase these services from outside organizations.
- The provider group delivers care and is paid on a fee-for-service basis.
- At the end of the care episode or after a specified amount of time, the data are analyzed

to determine if the provider group met cost targets and quality standards.
- Depending on the type of value-based payment model, the provider may share savings with the insurer, just retain the previously paid fee-for-service payment, or return a portion of the fee-for-service payment received if cost and quality targets were not achieved. (Data from McClellan, Patel, Latts, & Dang-Vu, 2015)

We will discuss the details of the most common value-based payment models later in this chapter.

Other Types of Integrated Care Clinical Models

Not all integrated care is provided by private health systems. Many other structures have evolved to address specific areas of healthcare fragmentation. Many states have also adopted elements of integrated care as they redesign their state Medicaid delivery systems. Some of these models are described in **TABLE 2-1**.

▶ Levels and Types of Care Integration

Few delivery systems are fully comprehensive and integrated. Most have pockets or sectors that are integrated as the system moves toward full integration.

Integrated Care for a Single Patient

Integration may be as simple as fully coordinated care for a single high-risk patient within a primary care medical practice. In this scenario the practice team (physician, advance practice registered nurse [APRN] or physician assistant [PA], clerical staff, medical assistant, and nurse) bands together to identify all the patient's medical and psychosocial needs, manages care transitions

TABLE 2-1 Other Clinical Models with Integrated Care Components

Type of Model	Description	Source
Hospice care	This model provides coordinated end-of-life care across disciplines and settings through an interdisciplinary team of professionals and volunteers. Hospice services are a covered benefit under Medicare and some other insurance plans.	National Hospice and Palliative Care Organization, 2012
Medical neighborhoods	This model consists of contractual arrangement between primary care physicians and specialists that ensure coordinated management of care, transition of information, and communication about shared patients.	Greenberg, Barnett, Spinks, Dudley, & Frolkis, 2014
State innovation models initiative	Many states have received CMS grants to redesign their health delivery systems to provide more connected care. Most of these models utilize the structures, tools, and techniques of integrated care.	CMS, 2017a
Accountable healthcare communities	This experimental design funded by the Center for Medicare and Medicaid Innovation, attempts to bridge the gap between medical care and the social determinants of health through screenings for unmet health-related social needs, referrals to community services, and health navigation services.	CMS, 2017a
Medicaid health homes	These are clinical practices that combine medical, behavioral health, wellness, and substance abuse services into one setting or geographic location, often in a federally qualified health center or existing behavioral health practice.	Medicaid, 2010
PACE	"The Programs of All-Inclusive Care for the Elderly (PACE) provides comprehensive medical and social services to certain frail, community-dwelling elderly individuals, most of whom are dually eligible for Medicare and Medicaid benefits. An interdisciplinary team of health professionals provides PACE participants with coordinated care. For most participants, the comprehensive service package enables them to remain in the community rather than receive care in a nursing home."	Medicaid, 2017
Community health teams	These teams are interdisciplinary groups of clinicians that support primary care medical practices by integrating clinical and community health services such as coordinating disease prevention, management of chronic diseases, and transition between healthcare providers and case management. The best-known model is the Vermont Blueprint for Health.	Association of State and Territorial Health Officials (ASTHO), 2017

by phone, coordinates referrals with specialists, reconciles medications after every transition, does comprehensive patient education and health coaching, and makes referrals to community agencies to manage social determinants of health. This type of single patient integration is most common in "concierge practices" in which patients pay a prepaid fee to have comprehensive care coordination and unlimited access to the practice physician.

Diagnostic or Service Line Integration

Integration may be organized around a specific diagnostic category or a type of service. This type of integration is often described as vertical or service line integration. For example, a hospital has aligned all of its services for cancer patients starting from an integrated referral system, an extensive online library of patient education materials, assignment of a nurse navigator to help patients through episodes of care, to linked oncology practices and highly coordinated team care and transitions at the inpatient and outpatient levels. The system has also implemented consistent clinical best practices and measures to ensure that variations in care are reduced to a minimum.

Episode-Based Integration

Integration can occur across a time span as well. This type of integration is typical for services in which care occurs in episodes with a limited time span (e.g., home health care in 60-day episodes and bundled payments for joint replacement that start with hospital discharge and end with recovery and leaving the care system). In episode integration, patients temporarily become part of a population that is receiving a specific set of services from specific providers (e.g., in a joint replacement bundling program, a coordinating organization such as an orthopedic medical group or convener [a consulting firm that takes financial risk, provides data, and coordinates care] sorts patients according to potential

risk). Payment is based on episodes of care that start at hospital discharge and include physician services, skilled nursing care facility inpatient stays, outpatient physical therapy, and home healthcare services. The medical practice that is the primary manager of the bundle uses standard protocols for performing the surgery and for postacute care.

A care coordinator provides preoperative patient education and helps coordinate care and ensure good transitions across the continuum. Once the patient is well and back to baseline function, his or her participation in integrated care delivery ends unless he or she is part of an ACO or a PCMH and is receiving integrated care in other ways (Essential Hospitals Institute, 2013).

▶ Characteristics of High-Performing Integrated Delivery Systems

The Commonwealth Fund's *Commission on High Performance Delivery Systems* describes the characteristics of an integrated care system that could solve the problems of fragmented health services delivery. Problems that must be solved by integration include lack of care coordination for patients, poor communication and lack of accountability for a patient, lack of quality improvement and clinical information, and rewarding intensive medical intervention instead of prevention, primary care, and chronic illness management.

The *Commission* identified six attributes of a high-performing, integrated care system:

1. Patient clinical information is available, in electronic form, to all providers at the time care is delivered.
2. Patient care is coordinated among multiple providers and during care transitions.
3. Clinicians of all types are accountable to each other, review each other's

work, and collaborate to deliver high-quality care.

4. Patients have access to high-quality, culturally competent care and information at multiple locations and at all hours.

5. There is clear accountability for all aspects of the patient's care.

6. There is constant innovation within the system to improve quality, value, and patient service. (Modified from Shih et al., 2008, pp. ix–x)

The key elements of high-performance integrated delivery systems very closely align with the four principles of connected care: (1) It's all about them (patients and caregivers), not just about us (health professionals). (2) We're all in this together. (3) We share relevant information to meet patient needs. (4) We do the right things right.

These delivery systems create a culture, structures, and measures that embed these principles and practices into the fabric of their organization. When integrated delivery systems function at the highest level of performance they are the most ideal example of connected care.

▶ Integrated Delivery Business Strategies

The literature on integrated delivery systems in the United States makes it clear that these systems are essentially about two goals: (1) improving market share and increasing profit, and (2) achieving quadruple aim goals through structure and care model improvements. Integrated systems with a long history of success such as Mayo Clinic, Kaiser Permanente, Geisinger Health System, Group Health of Puget Sound, and Intermountain Health Systems employ the following common strategic principles:

- **A strong brand that centers on unique types of clinical capability.** Some of these systems, such as Mayo Clinic, evolved out of elite medical practices with nationwide reputations as centers of excellence. Other systems have their own unique selling propositions for clinical excellence.

- **Accountability for integration and reducing fragmentation** that starts at the top—that is, the leadership/board level—and is deployed down to front line staff through clinical leadership.

- **Stakeholder buy-in** including engagement, involvement in decision making, and aligned incentives. In most of these systems "stakeholder" is synonymous with "physician."

- **Patient and family engagement** in self-care, wellness, and health decision making.

- **Risk management** through effective contracting arrangements, clinical management of the highest risk patients, and cost reduction through process improvement at care delivery sites.

- **Structures that support integration.** These structures usually include broad and deep networks of all types of clinical services that might be needed for effective outcomes. Integrated systems may also use team structures and co-locate providers (such as medical and behavioral health) who provide complementary services for patients.

- **Information sharing across the care continuum of the system.** This usually means adopting a shared electronic medical record (EMR) or purchasing a data platform that integrates information across multiple noncommunicating EMRs. Many systems also use shared electronic patient tracking and care coordination tools.

- **Consistency and continuity.** Integrated networks strive to achieve consistent clinical care through evidence-based best practices and highly coordinated teamwork. Consistency is not optional in these systems. A good word to describe them would be "tight." Data are used to monitor care consistency, and deviations are promptly and decisively managed by clinical leadership.

- **Continuous innovation.** These highly advanced systems have been the leaders in developing and testing new delivery innovations. Many have their own research departments or organizations. In an attempt to achieve the best outcomes these systems use data to monitor results and to test the effectiveness of innovative new methods of care (Modified from Shih et al., 2008).

▶ # How Well Do Integrated Delivery Systems Perform? Measures and Results

If theories about the connection between reducing fragmentation and improving care outcomes are correct, then integrated delivery systems should produce better results than traditional fee-for-service systems. Recent research and reporting from Medicare and other sources seems to indicate that these systems do indeed perform better on quadruple aim measures.

Integrated Delivery System Measures

An analysis of the literature on integrated delivery results found that 20 of 21 studies (dating from 2000–2011) demonstrated an association between increased integration and increased quality of care (Hwang, Chang, LaClair, & Paz, 2013). Medicare specifies standard measures for ACO integrated delivery systems in four domains:

- Patient and caregiver experience
- Care coordination/patient safety
- Preventive health
- At-risk population indicators

TABLE 2-2 provides a detailed list of Medicare-mandated ACO outcome measures.

TABLE 2-2 Measures for Use in Establishing the Quality Performance Standard That ACOs Must Meet for Shared Savings				
Aco Measure #	**Measure Title**	**NQF #**	**Measure Steward**	**Method of Data Submission**
Domain: patient/ caregiver experience ACO-1				
	CAHPS: Getting Timely care, Appointments, and Information	0005	AHRQ	Survey
ACO-2	CAHPS: How Well Your Providers Communicate	0005	AHRQ	Survey
ACO-3	CAHPS: Patients' Rating of Provider	0005	AHRQ	Survey
ACO-4	CAHPS: Access to Specialists	N/A	CMS/AHRQ	Survey
ACO-5	CAHPS: Health Promotion and Education	N/A	CMS/AHRQ	Survey

Aco Measure #	Measure Title	NQF #	Measure Steward	Method of Data Submission
ACO-6	CAHPS: Shared Decision Making	N/A	CMS/AHRQ	Survey
ACO-7	CAHPS: Health Status/Functional status	N/A	CMS/AHRQ	Survey
ACO-34	CAHPS: Stewardship of Patient Resources	N/A	CMS/AHRQ	Survey
Domain: care coordination/ patient safety ACO-8	Risk-Standardized, All Condition Readmission	1789 (adapted)	CMS	Claims
ACO-35	Skilled Nursing Facility 30-Day Readmission (SNFRM)	2510 (adapted)	CMS	Claims
ACO-36	All-Cause Unplanned Admissions for Patients with Diabetes	2887	CMS	Claims
ACO-37	All-Cause Unplanned Admissions for Patients with Heart Failure	2886	CMS	Claims
ACO-38	All-Cause Unplanned Admissions for Patients with Multiple Chronic Conditions	2888	CMS	Claims
ACO-43	Ambulatory Sensitive Condition Acute Composite (AHRQ Prevention Quality Indicator (PQI) #91)	N/A	AHRQ	Claims
ACO-11	Use of Certified EHR Technology	N/A	CMS	Quality Payment Program Data
ACO-12 (CARE-1)	Medication Reconciliation Post-Discharge	0097	CMS	Web Interface
ACO-13 (CARE-2)	Falls: Screening for Future Fall Risk	0101	NCQA	Web Interface
ACO-44	Use of Imaging Studies for Low Back Pain	0052	NCQA	Claims
Domain: Preventive Health ACO-14 (PREV-7)	Preventive Care and Screening: Influenza Immunization	0041	AMA/PCPI	Web Interface
ACO-15 (PREV-8)	Pneumonia Vaccination Status for Older Adults	0043	NCQA	Web Interface

(continues)

TABLE 2-2 Measures for Use in Establishing the Quality Performance Standard That ACOs Must Meet for Shared Savings *(continued)*

Aco Measure #	Measure Title	NQF #	Measure Steward	Method of Data Submission
ACO-16 (PREV-9)	Preventive Care and Screening: Body Mass Index (BMI) Screening and Follow-Up	0421	CMS	Web Interface
ACO-17 (PREV-10)	Preventive Care and Screening: Tobacco Use: Screening and Cessation Intervention	0028	AMA/PCPI	Web Interface
ACO-18 (PREV-12)	Preventive Care and Screening: Screening for Clinical Depression and Follow- up Plan	0418	CMS	Web Interface
ACO-19 (PREV-6)	Colorectal Cancer Screening	0034	NCQA	Web Interface
ACO-20 (PREV-5)	Breast Cancer Screening	2372	NCQA	Web Interface
ACO-42 (PREV-13)	Statin Therapy for the Prevention and Treatment of Cardiovascular Disease	N/A	CMS	Web Interface
Domain: at- risk population Depression ACO-40 (MH-1)	Depression Remission at Twelve Months	0710	MNCM	Web Interface
Diabetes ACO-27 (DM-2)	Diabetes Mellitus: Hemoglobin A1c Poor Control	0059	NCQA	Web Interface
ACO-41 (DM-7)	Diabetes: Eye Exam	0055	NCQA	Web Interface
Hypertension ACO-28 (HTN-2)	Hypertension (HTN): Controlling High Blood Pressure	0018	NCQA	Web Interface
Ischemic vascular disease ACO-30 (IVD-2)	Ischemic Vascular Disease (IVD): Use of Aspirin of Another Antiplatelet	0068	NCQA	Web Interface

Note: AHRQ = Agency for Healthcare Research and Quality, ACC = American College of Cardiology, AHA = American Heart Association, AMA = American Medical Association, CAHPS = Consumer Assessment of Healthcare Providers and Systems, MNCM = Minnesota Community Measurement, N/A = not available, NCQA = National Committee on Quality Assurance, PCPI = Physician Consortium for Performance Improvement.
https://www.cms.gov/Medicare/Medicare-Fee-for-Service-Payment/sharedsavingsprogram/Downloads/2018-reporting-year-narrative-specifications.pdf

Accountable Care Organization Results

A report from the Office of the Inspector General, U.S. Department of Health and Human Services (2017) summarized results from Medicare Shared Savings Program Accountable Care Organizations:

> Over the first 3 years of the program, 428 participating Shared Savings Program ACOs served 9.7 million beneficiaries. During that time, most of these ACOs reduced Medicare spending compared to their benchmarks, achieving a net spending reduction of nearly $1 billion. At the same time, ACOs generally improved the quality of care they provided, based on CMS data on quality measures. In the first 3 years, ACOs improved their performance on most (82 percent) of the individual quality measures. ACOs also outperformed fee-for-service providers on most (81 percent) of the quality measures. Further, a small subset of ACOs showed substantial reductions in Medicare spending while providing high-quality care.

Of the 13 health plans given the highest ranking in 2016 by NCQA, provider-run plans dominated.

Dr. Robert Pearl of the Permanente Medical Group (part of the Kaiser Permanente Health System), in his comments on earlier ACO results, said that he believes health systems and insurance plans need to be integrated to get to the level of care needed to serve complex medical conditions and to achieve quality results (Morse, 2016). These results testify to the power of integrated systems to improve care and lower costs.

▶ The Strategies and Tactics of Integrated Care

While integrated delivery systems senior managers grapple with strategy in a chaotic healthcare environment, clinicians and administrators face the daunting task of implementing structures and processes that unify and coordinate care. Even organizations that are not in a position to become part of an integrated delivery system can adopt some of these approaches to create more connected care for patients. As you read, ask yourself which of these techniques might be suitable for your organization. Literature reviews identify a series of very specific strategies that produce high-performance, integrated delivery models:

- Develop an organization with a culture aligned around integration and innovation.
- Build a comprehensive delivery system that offers excellent access to care.
- Create a professional workforce that is educated for and engaged in integrated care.
- Lower costs to be successful in value-based payment mechanisms that drive integration.
- Apply population health structures and strategies to improve care outcomes.
- Implement coordinated care, teamwork, and managed care transitions.
- Use data and analytics to drive better patient care and business outcomes.
- Support patients who need help with the "social determinants of health." (Canadian Nurses Association, Canadian Medical Association, 2013; Shih et al., 2008; Suter et al., 2009; Bogan, Calcasola, Frick-Hoff, & Orlando, 2017)

Aligning Organizational Culture Around Integrated Care Principles

Integrated systems that truly function as an interdependent whole are knit together with common goals and incentives. Work units within the delivery system are then measured on how well they achieve these goals and earn these incentives. Successful integrated delivery systems are laser focused on quadruple aim goals and they achieve these goals by providing very uniform and consistent care and service delivery.

Since the structures, mindset, and skillset for this type of system are so different from those in fee-for-service care, a highly engaged senior leadership role is necessary to effect culture change.

These engaged leaders must:

- Create a vision of integration and disseminate it down the line through effective corporate communications and training.
- Make personal connections with employees through meetings with employee groups, one-to-one conversations, and leadership mentorings to constantly provide examples and encourage behaviors that foster innovation.
- Reward clinicians and other employees who demonstrate movement toward integration.
- Create compacts that describe what clinicians and the organization expect of each other.
- Redesign structure and governance to include a clinical leadership council that oversees clinical standards, physicians, and payment mechanisms.
- Provide the tools, such as robust information systems and analytics capability, to support integration.
- Remove incentives for volume (more procedures, bed days, visits, etc.) and implement incentives for value outcomes that the organization must achieve to succeed.
- Present system level and unit level data on performance to all employees. Provide benchmarking so clinicians can see how their clinical unit is performing compared to peers. (Modified from Smith, Saunders, Stuckhardt, & McGinnis, 2013)

Organizational culture is also fostered through public positions taken by the organization. For example, Geisinger Health System literally and publically demonstrated its commitment to patient-centered care by offering a money-back guarantee to patients who were not satisfied with the services they had received (Ellison, 2015).

One of the biggest hurdles to creating a culture of integration is the "silo" mentality fostered by fee-for-service payment models. Administrators and clinicians at all levels must learn to take a systems view of their work, leave behind the narrow focus of "my service line" or "my practice," and start to "work the white space" between professions, departments, and other organizations in the network through communication and teamwork. Helping clinicians to look at their system or through the eyes of the patient can help in this effort, as can role-playing different organizational roles, spending time "on loan" to other departments, and walking through a clinical process as a patient.

Fostering Innovation in Integrated Delivery Systems

Innovation is a hallmark of highly developed integrated delivery systems and a core capability of the most successful systems. Because health care is such a complex endeavor, meeting quality goals requires continuous improvement of core work processes and incorporating newly discovered and more effective methods, technologies, and processes of care. Intermountain Healthcare in Murray, Utah, has a long-standing reputation for innovation and quality improvement. In 2013, the system launched the Healthcare Transformation Lab. Todd Dunn, director of the Transformation Lab, describes it this way: "The focus, first and foremost, is [D]oes a particular solution improve the quality and cost of healthcare?" Dunn added, the answer has to be both. The team "looks to make sure it's good for the patients and clinicians—and not just necessarily making sure that it's safe, because that's sort of a given. But is it easy for them? Does it improve their workflow? Does it make it easier for [patients] to have and receive healthcare, or for clinicians to provide care?" One project being tested by the lab is a device that can draw blood from an existing IV without sticking the patient again (Bryant, 2016).

Two other aspects of innovation in integrated delivery systems are the use of continuous quality improvement teams, which often generate unique improvement ideas and robust employee suggestion systems, and the use of new insights from data and analytics to drive improvement.

▶ Building a Comprehensive Delivery System

Integrated delivery systems are built to include the full range of services that patients might need to stay healthy or to manage serious chronic illnesses. Systems may consist of organizations that are all owned by a parent company or they may add components through affiliation and contracting. Systems that are not focused on a narrow population or a specific disease usually include primary, secondary, and tertiary care facilities.

Most systems include at least hospital inpatient services, PCMHs, and specialty practices. Hospital systems always include inpatient beds, emergency rooms, and diagnostic testing facilities such as clinical laboratories, imaging, and radiology. Integrated systems implement policies to ensure that patients receive care from within their own network. For example, medical practices within the system are strongly encouraged to refer only to diagnostic facilities and specialists within their own system. By doing this they can control costs, improve profit, ensure alignment with organizational goals, and control quality.

More comprehensive integrated delivery systems incorporate behavioral health components, postacute care such as SNFs and home care agencies, and outpatient facilities such as same-day surgery centers and outpatient physical therapy. Safety net integrated delivery systems often include a community health worker or health advocate outreach program.

Example of a Fully Integrated Delivery System

Sentara Healthcare in Virginia is an example of a large integrated delivery system with a full range of healthcare services. This nonprofit organization with roots dating back 125 years offers a wide range of services to its patients:

- 12 hospitals
- 4 medical groups
- 3,800+ provider medical staff
- 28,000+ team members
- Health plan (Optima Health)
- Outpatient campuses
- Urgent care centers
- Advanced imaging centers
- Home health and hospice
- Rehab and therapy centers
- Nursing and assisted living center
- Medical transport ambulance
- Nightingale air ambulance (Sentara Healthcare, 2017)

The service range in this system is typical of that in many large integrated systems. Some systems with more expanded capabilities also provide behavioral health and wellness services as parts of their offerings.

Access is a key issue in integrated systems. Better access to services within the health system reduces fragmentation, keeps patients (and revenue) within the system, and maintains centralized documentation in the patient's system medical record. Many systems also provide home health care or an APRN home visiting program.

Access and Primary Care Medical Homes

PCMHs within integrated delivery systems must meet accreditation requirements for expanded patient access and for on-call coverage when the office is closed. Some systems own or contract with urgent care centers so that patients can receive care quickly on evenings, weekends, or when their own practice is not available. Some systems incorporate a telemedicine program whereby patients can receive a virtual visit over the internet. The 2017 NCQA standards for patient-centered medical homes define access in some detail:

> The PCMH model expects continuity of care. Patients/families/caregivers have 24/7 access to clinical advice and appropriate care facilitated by their designated clinician/care team and supported by access to their medical record. The practice considers the needs and preferences of the patient population when establishing and updating standards for access.

Some specific access standards requirements include:

- Assesses the access needs and preferences of the patient population.
- Provides same-day appointments for routine and urgent care to meet identified patients' needs.
- Provides routine and urgent appointments outside regular business hours (generally considered 8-5) to meet identified patients' needs.
- Provides timely clinical advice by telephone. (NCQA, 2017, p. 7)

One criticism that has been leveled at large integrated delivery systems that dominate certain healthcare markets is that by becoming a monopoly and reducing choice, they drive up costs through mechanisms such as system facility fees, which are layered on top of regular healthcare costs (Hertz, 2013).

Systems do this to increase profit during a period when fee-for-service revenue may be falling while value-based payment profit has not fully materialized. This situation is an example of the types of push/pull market economics versus quality and patient-centered care imperatives that are occurring in the volume-to-value shift.

Physicians and Integrated Delivery Systems

Loosely affiliated groups of providers seldom achieve unified goals, so contractual or employment relationships, especially for physicians, are an essential element of integrated delivery systems. Most integrated delivery systems are highly and understandably physician centric, because physicians control the healthcare production system, produce the organization's revenue stream, and are the most powerful of the healthcare professions.

In most systems, PCMHs are the domain of primary care physicians and are the foundation of the integrated system. Developing integrated delivery systems spend considerable time and resources understanding physician wants and needs, engaging physicians in integrated care planning and delivery, aligning incentives to encourage physician participation, and developing governance structures that give physicians leadership roles. This is not to say that other professions, such as nursing, do not play a key role in integrated delivery, but physicians typically dominate.

Integrated delivery systems must maintain a delicate balance as they both engage and interest physicians in clinical work redesign, while maintaining control at the strategic level. For example, they must persuade clinicians to consistently adopt evidence-based best practices if they expect to achieve target cost and quality metrics. This can be a tricky proposition when best practices conflict with personal clinical preferences, and one that can determine the success or failure of the integrated delivery system. For some physicians, the quality of work life in an employment environment where there are regular hours, less on-call, and shared responsibility for complex patients is a motivator in and of itself.

Integrated delivery systems build provider networks in various ways. Some systems buy local medical practices and keep physicians and other staff on as employees of the hospital or health system. Another approach is the use of contracts to create integration. Providers who are part of an integrated delivery system are often described as the "provider network" for that system.

Nurses in Integrated Delivery Systems

While much of the integrated delivery model literature focuses on the integration of physicians, nurses are integral to the function of every facet of integrated delivery systems from the senior management suite to front line clinical care positions.

⚹ Nurses in senior management positions may be part of the governance structure of the system. Nurses are often at the core of clinical redesign work, but unless system-affiliated medical practices have a gainsharing program of some sort, they and other clinical staff seldom share in the financial savings, which typically accrue to the hospital and its affiliated physicians.⚹

Nurses in integrated delivery systems are commonly found in these types of roles:

- **Senior leadership roles** such as director of population health or vice president of operations for integrated delivery
- **APRNs** who deliver front line primary care in PCMHs or practice in system specialty offices or inpatient units
- **Nurse care coordinators** who manage care for populations of high-risk patients across the continuum of integrated delivery system partners
- **Nurse advocate/health coaches** who are often embedded in medical practices and who provide preventive health teaching and patient self-management support for practice patients
- **Quality improvement/quality assurance roles** in which nurses manage data and cross-organizational collaborations and improvement efforts
- **Front line clinicians in acute care organizations** that are part of the integrated system (American Nurses Association [ANA], 2010)

BOX 2-1 lists actual positions for nurses in ACOs found in a recent internet search and describes the role of *manager of population care management*.

🔍 CASE STUDY

A Nurse Care Coordinator in an Integrated Delivery System

Some integrated delivery systems, such as CareFirst, have created an extensive system of nurse care coordination for high-risk patients with serious chronic illness. This system, which is both a health plan and a comprehensive delivery system structured around an extensive network of primary care medical homes, makes nurses an integral part of their efforts to coordinate care for high-risk patients as described here:

> Much of the work at the local level is done by registered nurses, such as Michele Brown, who serve as local care coordinators (LCC). Supported by a regional care coordinator and a central data system, Michele is charged with identifying and then actively engaging high-need, high-cost patients by linking patients with their primary care provider and community-based services. Michele's performance as an LCC is measured by the number, type, and quality of patient and provider interactions. (National Academy for State Health Policy [NASHP], 2015)

Other Professions in Integrated Delivery Systems

Truly comprehensive and integrated systems provide a full range of services to patients. These services may include other health professionals such as pharmacists; social workers or psychologists who provide behavioral health services; nutritionists

---

BOX 2-1 Sample Nursing Positions in Accountable Care Organizations

Titles of positions in a search for "Accountable Care Organization Case Manager RN" job listings from Indeed.com:

- *Ambulatory Care Manager*
- *Manager Population Care Management*
- *RN Case Manager/Care Coordinator*
- *Nurse Navigator*
- *RN Care Coordinator*
- *RN Care Manager—Complex Care Patients*

The job description for *Manager of Population Care Management* (for an insurance company) describes the role of nurses in integrated delivery systems well:

> This position is accountable for population management within a geographic area. The knowledge and skills of an RN Case Manager are required to assist members and providers within a value based (accountable care organization and a Medicare Advantage collaborative care model) and non-value based program. This position will be required to communicate and collaborate with Value Based and non-valued based partners as well as other stakeholders to effectively manage the population. Knowledge and utilization of health analytic tools is required to identify trends and opportunities to improve satisfaction, quality, utilization and cost.

Data from Indeed.com, Accountable Care Organization Case Manager RN jobs, accessed on March 25, 2017.

---

who provide dietary assessments and consultation to clinicians; physical, occupational, and speech therapists who support patient rehabilitation and improved functional abilities; respiratory therapists who work with patients with chronic lung problems; and community outreach workers or advocates who help patients navigate the system and find help with the social determinants of health. The most cohesive integrated systems have interdisciplinary teamwork structures that support each profession in integrating its special expertise into the longitudinal patient care plan and in creating a seamless experience for patients in which each profession communicates with and collaborates with the others.

▶ Participating in Payment Models That Drive Integration

In the United States, integrated delivery systems are inextricably linked with value-based payment or pay-for-performance systems that reward outcomes instead of volume. These payment models are necessary to incent the type of collaborative behaviors that drive integrated care.

Each of these payment models directly connects the provider's actions to payment received. Medicare-sponsored, value-based payment programs allow the lead organization in the payment model to share savings with partner organizations that provide services within the program or payment bundle. The three most common value-based payment models are illustrated in **FIGURE 2-3**.

Bundling

Bundling is a single negotiated payment for all services for a specific procedure or condition. For example, Medicare makes one payment for SNFs, physicians, and home health care services to a convener or lead organization. This organization, if it meets cost and quality targets, shares savings with the insurer. If the episode of care costs more than the target or if the quality goals are not met, then payments are reduced. Typical bundles would be care for a joint replacement

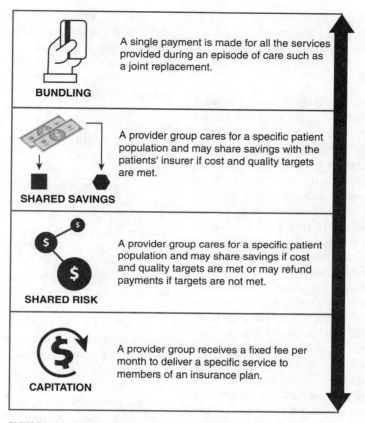

A single payment is made for all the services provided during an episode of care such as a joint replacement.

BUNDLING

A provider group cares for a specific patient population and may share savings with the patients' insurer if cost and quality targets are met.

SHARED SAVINGS

A provider group cares for a specific patient population and may share savings if cost and quality targets are met or may refund payments if targets are not met.

SHARED RISK

A provider group receives a fixed fee per month to deliver a specific service to members of an insurance plan.

CAPITATION

FIGURE 2-3 Value-Based Payment Models

episode or all postacute care for a patient with a myocardial infarction.

Shared Savings (Also Called "One-Sided Risk" or "Upside Risk")

In this model, a lead organization contracts with Medicare or an insurer to deliver care to a defined patient population for a target cost, which is usually based on retrospective claims data. Target quality metrics for clinical and patient experience outcomes are set at the start of the contract. During the episode of care providers are paid their usual fee-for-service rates. If the provider(s) in the contract deliver care at a lower cost and achieve quality targets, they keep a portion

of the savings that the insurer generates. If targets are not met, there is no penalty to the provider.

In this model, the provider does not share financial risk with the insurer. According to a survey by the Advisory Board over 90% of ACOs participating in the Medicare Shared Savings Program (MSSP) contracted for the shared savings approach (Goldman, 2016).

Shared Risk (Also Called "Two-Sided Risk" or "Downside Risk")

This model is managed in the same way as shared savings with one very important difference: If the contracted provider organization does not meet cost *and* quality targets it is required to pay back a portion of the money already earned (a penalty). In this model providers share financial risk with the insurer.

Capitation

Capitation, either partial or full, is a risk-sharing arrangement between providers and insurers. Another term for capitation is "prospective payment." It is the most extreme form of value-based payment and one that is relatively rare in American health care. The American College of Physicians describes capitation this way: "Capitation is a fixed amount of money per patient per unit of time paid in advance to the physician for the delivery of health care services. The actual amount of money paid is determined by the ranges of services that are provided, the number of patients involved, and the period of time during which the services are provided" (Alguire, 2017). Full capitation is for all services provided and is usually done only within health systems that comprise both a delivery system and an insurance company. Capitation is usually defined in per member per month (pm/pm) cost units. For example, a cardiology group would be paid x dollars per month to care for each patient who is a member of a specific insurance plan. If fewer patients need care or if the group delivers care at a lower cost, the group makes a profit. If care costs are higher than the pm/pm payment, the group experiences a financial loss.

The Impact of New Payment Models—Using Managed Care Tactics for Value-Based Payment

Participation in value-based payment models definitely shapes provider behavior through incentive change. In the early stages of value-based payment learning, the new model may motivate providers to focus on cost cutting and savings with the lead organization acting more like a managed care organization than an integrated delivery system.

In some healthcare communities facilities and providers are in the early stages of adopting value-based payment and integrated delivery models. One example is SNFs that have begun participating in bundling for patient populations with hip fractures, congestive heart failure, and acute myocardial infarction. The primary tactics used by these facilities are to reduce the length of stay in the SNF, employ a medical director and APRN who provide more intensive onsite medical care, drive referrals toward preferred provider home care agencies, discharge patients sooner (possibly before they are rehabilitated back to preadmission functional levels), do intensive phone call follow-up post discharge, and insist that the home care agencies transfer patients back to their facility rather than to the emergency room when they decompensate at home. There is considerable variation in how these SNFs employ evidence-based protocols, standardized patient teaching, and other patient self-management support techniques. The impact of these strategies is that patients are often being discharged "quicker and sicker" and families are pressured to pay privately for care at home that would previously have been part of a longer SNF stay. The home care agency is admitting sicker patients and is expected to take the primary role in teaching patients and family caregivers self-care. The SNF also expects the home care agency to send a liaison nurse to discharge planning meetings and to do onsite evaluations of patients prior to discharge.

While this approach improves care transitions, it increases costs for the home care agency and may ultimately increase the number of unnecessary care transitions. For clinicians in each part of the care continuum this approach creates pressures to reduce utilization, to push patients and families to adopt more self-care more quickly, to utilize technology such as telemonitoring rather than labor, and generally to make every minute of clinical care count.

One health system uses a novel approach called "telerehab" to reduce postacute care labor costs. This is a teaching/monitoring device for care after joint replacement, which provides a computerized "avatar" to give patients instructions on their rehab exercises. The patient fits a measurement device over the replaced joint and performs prescribed exercises while the "telerehab" unit transmits information to physical therapists at a remote location. These therapists can then coach the patients to change or improve their exercise routine. While these types of techniques force more efficiency into the system, they may sometimes result in inadequate care for high-need patients. As most lead organizations in bundling or shared savings programs do not intend to share savings with their preferred providers this may not be a sustainable model for the future.

ASK YOURSELF

- How many of these new payment models exist in your healthcare community?
- Does your organization participate in any of these payment programs?
- How have provider and patient behaviors changed as a result of these payment models?
- How have these new models impacted patient care and the patient experience?

▶ Patient Attribution and Communication in Integrated Delivery Systems

To provide integrated care, the clinical delivery system must have some formal accountability for a group of patients (the population) through insurance or by being designated as the patient's physician or provider through a signed care service agreement. Patients become part of an ACO or integrated delivery system through a process called "attribution." This means that patients who receive most of their clinical care from a group of physicians who are part of an ACO passively become part of the patient population under care.

If communication from the integrated care system is inadequate, patients may not understand that they have been "attributed" to an ACO and may not choose to engage with or stay in care with network providers.

This creates a disconnect between the integrated system—which is trying to drive patients to healthier behavior, more self-care, and utilization of lower cost health services—and the patient. The patient may have no idea of the underlying rules and motivations of the integrated delivery system and may not agree with them if he or she did understand these underlying assumptions. If the patient wants "the best care" and "more care" and the delivery system wants more "self-care" and lower utilization, patient dissatisfaction and provider frustration with "noncompliance" often follows. CMS has created a document to help patients understand what it means to be part of an ACO, but this document has not been widely disseminated (CMS, 2016).

TEST YOURSELF

Imagine that one of your patients receives a letter saying that his medical practice is now part of an ACO and that the practice may be using new care management techniques as part of this agreement.

- Your patient does not understand this letter and asks what this means to him.
- How would you explain what an ACO is and how it might affect your patient?

🔍 CASE STUDY

Patient Attribution Case Study

Holly Arundel has been a caregiver for her father, John Arundel, who is 78 years old, has chronic obstructive pulmonary disease (COPD) and congestive heart failure, and who has a recent history of hospitalizations. In the past, Mr. Arundel only interacted with his primary care doctor at regular appointments. There was little follow-up or communication between visits and his hospital care was all managed by hospitalist physicians. About 3 months ago, Mr. Arundel's doctor's practice became a patient-centered medical home and joined an ACO.

Mr. Arundel received a brief letter informing him of this change, but since he didn't understand what the letter meant, he threw it away and never showed it to his daughter. Mr. Arundel and Holly began receiving regular calls from an ACO care coordinator. After some initial suspicion, the Arundels agreed to work with the nurse care coordinator, Ally. Ally has helped the Arundels with issues such as getting home health care, ordering medical equipment, and making sure medications are reconciled. She has also exerted some pressure on the patient and his daughter to have a goals of care conversation and to consider palliative care, something that neither understands nor is comfortable with. They have resisted this discussion and have decided to talk with Mr. Arundel's primary care physician about their concerns.

ASK YOURSELF

- How well did the integrated delivery system communicate with the patient and caregiver?
- Where was the new system helpful to the patient and caregiver?
- Why was there a mismatch of expectations and resulting dissatisfaction?
- What could have been done differently?

▶ Population Health Practices in Integrated Delivery Systems

Understanding Population Health

Integrated delivery systems organize patient care at two levels, each of which informs the other. The first level is obviously individual patient care. Individual patient care in an integrated delivery system, unlike that in a fee-for-service system, is designed to be less variable and more consistent with evidence-based best practices. Standardized protocols are customized to individual patients with "thoughtful variation."

The second level is population level care. Integrated delivery systems are designed to provide comprehensive care for a very specific group of patients who have one or more like characteristics. The characteristic that links the patients in a population might be diagnosis, the medical group who cares for the patient, the patient's insurance, geography, or some other variable. **FIGURE 2-4** illustrates the concept of population health in an integrated delivery system.

Other examples of populations in integrated systems are:

- All the Medicare patients in a group practice that participates in the MSSP
- All patients of an orthopedic group that participates in a joint replacement bundling program
- All patients of a home healthcare agency who are part of a Medicare value-based payment demonstration program
- All patients of a large medical group ACO who are insured by one commercial insurance company that has contracted with the group for a shared savings program

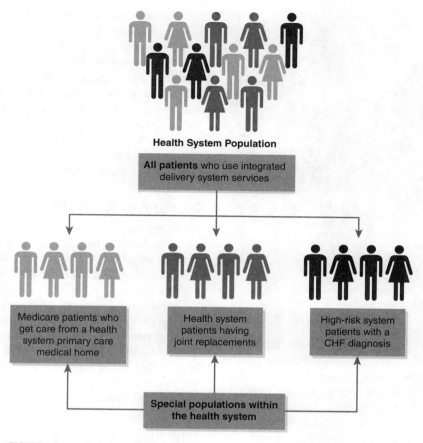

Health System Population

All patients who use integrated delivery system services

Medicare patients who get care from a health system primary care medical home

Health system patients having joint replacements

High-risk system patients with a CHF diagnosis

Special populations within the health system

FIGURE 2-4 Population Health

In integrated delivery systems, the care of these populations is managed at a systems level. One way to visualize this is to think of a group of patients (the population) as a single patient and to apply the tools and techniques of patient care: assessment, care plan development, care plan implementation, care transitions, and patient self-management support to the group rather than just to individuals.

For example, an integrated system might manage all care transitions for its patient population with a consistent process, a set of best practices, standardized patient teaching materials, patient tracking software, clinical forms, and employee training for consistent performance.

Integrated delivery systems must take actions that impact the whole patient population, especially subpopulations of patients who are high risk. This is more like public health thinking than it is like the traditional medical care—one patient, one provider thinking. **FIGURE 2-5** illustrates population health strategies used by integrated delivery systems.

Let's look at some specific ways that population health techniques are applied in integrated delivery systems.

Risk Stratification

Successful integrated delivery systems match the level of care to specific patient needs. Using sophisticated data analysis tools, integrated delivery systems obtain data from claims, from the patient medical record, or from assessment tools used in clinical encounters, and then apply algorithms that stratify or sort patients by risk level.

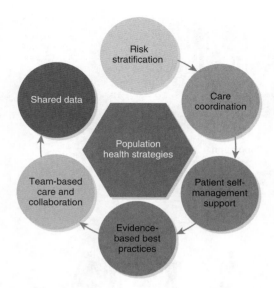

FIGURE 2-5 Population Health Strategies Used by Integrated Delivery Systems

Data used to create the risk algorithm might include the patient's diagnoses, testing and imaging results, psychosocial issues, a history of hospital readmissions, medications, level of self-activation, self-care capability assessments, and recent experience with the healthcare system. Patients are usually classified at three levels of risk.

High Risk

These patients are very high utilizers of health services. Most have many serious chronic conditions, multiple medications, psychosocial issues, and frequent hospital readmissions.

Elderly high-risk patients may be frail, they may have many deficits in activities of daily living, and a significant number may be at the end of their lives. Depression and anxiety issues are common in high-risk populations.

In some cases, these patients have concurrent mental health problems and issues with social determinants of health such as finances, access to food, transportation, and lack of caregiver support. These are the patients who are most often assigned to nurse care coordinators and managed by interdisciplinary teams.

Nurse care coordinators work to ensure that these patients have the services necessary to self-manage their medical care and have support for social determinants of health. Care coordinators try to ensure that these patients receive care in the lowest intensity, lowest cost setting and that their care transitions from one setting to another are carefully managed. If appropriate, they work with the patient and family to consider palliative care or hospice rather than continued aggressive medical treatment.

Medium or Rising Risk

These patients already have some chronic illnesses or they may have risk factors but are not yet high utilizers of the healthcare system.

These are typically middle-aged or younger patients with chronic conditions such as diabetes, hypertension, obesity, and coronary artery disease. These patients may be sedentary, may have unhealthy diets, and may have high, poorly managed stress levels. If the integrated delivery system does not engage these patients in prevention and self-management, they move into the high-risk category.

Low Risk

These patients are currently healthy and only need wellness/preventive health services and occasional urgent care. Integrated delivery systems focus on engaging with these patients (usually through patient portals or the delivery system website) and providing preventive health and health consumer education. Some systems that include an insurance component may offer low-risk patients incentives to get preventive tests, complete health risk appraisals, and attend wellness and exercise classes. The goal here is to keep patients healthy and to keep them out of the rising risk category (Bresnick, 2017).

Patient Engagement in Self-Management Support

Integrated delivery systems spend a huge amount of energy trying to engage their attributed

🔍 CASE STUDY

Population Health Case Study

The Everford Hospital system, when it was still a traditional fee-for-service system, with no incentives for quality or cost control had no special program to treat patients with heart failure (HF). These patients were treated individually and independently by various hospital-affiliated internists or cardiologists with considerable variation in the type and quality of care provided.

When Everford became an ACO, it used data to identify HF patient demographics (age, sex, home location, income, etc.) and to stratify patients by risk level. The system consulted its cardiologists and cardiac APRNs who researched and adopted evidence-based best practices for clinical care and medication management.

A team of hospital quality assurance (QA) staff interviewed patients about the issues they faced and the frustrations and failures of receiving care in the Everford system. Based on these interviews, the hospital instituted a series of online education modules, created a patient portal so patients could see their own medical records, developed an HF exercise and support program, and created an HF infusion outpatient clinic so patients could receive diuresis in a lower cost and more comfortable setting than the emergency room.

The system assigned a cardiac nurse care navigator to each high-risk patient. This navigator advocated for and helped patients with teaching, getting community resources, and through care transitions.

patients in healthy behaviors and self-care for chronic illnesses. They expend special effort on "rising risk" patients who have risk factors, but have not yet developed serious chronic illnesses.

In a fee-for-service system, there is no penalty for patients who "fall through the cracks," are readmitted multiple times, or are nonadherent to treatment. In integrated delivery there is either a loss of potential shared savings or an actual penalty for not meeting quality metrics if these patients are not engaged in self-management.

Patients are key players in these systems and cannot simply be left to their own devices if the system is to achieve its goals.

Those patients who are unengaged, who have serious issues with social determinants of health, or who are nonadherent are the ones most likely to drive up readmission rates, increase costs, and cause quality metrics to be poor. Delivery systems use various methods to engage patients including mailings, social media, community health worker outreach, and phone calls from care coordinators. For high-risk patients; physicians, APRNS, and care coordinators may employ a series of individual patient

self-management support strategies, including patient goal setting, motivational interviewing, health literacy assessment, and the use of teaching with teachback (asking the patient and/or family caregiver to describe what was learned to verify understanding).

Another method for encouraging self-care is the use of websites that offer health calculator tools, health education content and forms, and checklists that patients can use to improve their own self-care. Many health systems also offer online patient portals that allow patients to access their own medical records, make office visit appointments, or ask their health providers questions.

Health coaching for patients who want or need to lose weight, learn symptom control, or get more exercise is also common in large health systems and PCMHs. Health coaching is usually by telephone, but some systems employ face-to-face health coaches in medical practices. A fairly extreme example of patient engagement that uses very strong financial incentives is the one by the State of Connecticut for its employees (**BOX 2-2**).

BOX 2-2 The Health Enhancement Program (HEP) Description

HEP rewards state employees, select retirees, and dependents who commit to a number of responsibilities. The "ask" of beneficiaries is as follows:

- Obtain specified age- and gender-appropriate health risk assessments, evidence-based screenings, and physical and vision examinations;
- Undergo two dental cleanings per year;
- Participate in condition-appropriate chronic disease management services. Specified guideline-based clinical services are required of HEP enrollees with diabetes, high cholesterol, high blood pressure, heart disease, asthma, and chronic obstructive pulmonary disorder (COPD).

Employees who meet the requirements pay lower premiums, have deductibles waived, and pay lower copays for health insurance.

Data from Center for Value Based Insurance Design (2013).

Care Coordination Strategies in Integrated Delivery Systems

Care coordination is the vehicle that integrated delivery systems use to track high-risk patients and manage their care. Care coordinators in integrated systems are typically nurses. Coordinators may work in a central location and coordinate care for all integrated system patients or they may be embedded in delivery system medical practices or in preferred provider acute care facilities such as SNFs.

In integrated systems, high-risk or rising risk patients who have been identified through algorithms and data analysis are usually assigned to a care coordinator.

This care coordinator contacts the patient to establish a relationship, elicit patient goals, and create a plan of care that incorporates both patient goals and system goals for lower costs and improved outcomes. Based on the patient assessment and care plan, the care coordinator will identify current risk factors, deficits in patient knowledge, self-care capability, support systems, social determinants of health, and gaps in care.

The coordinator will coordinate with the primary care physician in making referrals to appropriate clinical care specialists and to community resources. A key function for care coordinators in integrated delivery systems is tracking patients through the continuum of care; ensuring

that care is delivered in the least complex, lowest cost setting; and managing care transitions. Tracking might occur through an electronic tracking system or through some other system of patient tracking and reporting.

For example, the care coordinator may be notified by a hospital that one of her patients is about to be discharged to a SNF. She would communicate with the SNF about the plan of care, confer with SNF staff about discharge plans, and then make a follow-up call to the patient to ensure that all necessary postdischarge tasks including medication reconciliation have been properly completed.

Managing the Social Determinants of Health

Another important aspect of care coordination in integrated delivery systems is managing the social determinants of health. These issues include financial resources, caregiver support systems, mental health issues, access to transportation, ability to pay for and obtain medication, and food and meal preparation. Some experts believe that these issues are just as important as physical health deficits in determining outcomes.

Integrated delivery system care coordinators or health advocates spend considerable time searching for local community resources, benefits, and entitlement programs for patients who

🔍 CASE STUDY

Ann's Story

Ann is a care coordinator with the Holly Valley ACO, which is composed of 3 hospitals, 10 medical practices, 3 SNFs, and 2 home care agencies. The ACO also works with a nonmedical home care agency that provides transport, homemakers, and personal care assistants.

Every day, Ann prints a report on the status of her caseload and reviews the list for new high-risk patients. She later contacts these patients, explains her role, and asks about their goals and current situation. She checks the ACO tracking system to see if any of her patients are currently in the hospital, in observation, in the emergency department (ED), in a SNF, or receiving care from a home healthcare agency. Ann contacts the agencies that are currently servicing these patients for a care update.

She helps resolve any problems and coordinates transfers of patients who are failing at home back to the discharging SNF. Ann also consults with or reports any actions that she has taken to the patient's primary care physician.

INTERVIEW WITH MONICA ORIS, RN, BSN, MHA, CCM, COMMUNITY NURSE MANAGER, RN SUPERVISOR, INTEGRATED CARE PARTNERS

Monica manages a group of nurses who are embedded in medical practices within an ACO that is part of the Hartford (Connecticut) Healthcare System. Monica described the role of the nurse in this setting as "trying to connect the dots for patients" and "seeing the patient holistically." One of the key functions for nurses in this system is to manage care transitions across the continuum. Monica and her team call patients after hospitalization with particular attention to the first 48 hours post discharge when patients are overwhelmed. The primary function of these calls is to ensure patients understand self-care instructions and to determine if the patient has any changes in condition.

Monica tells the story of one patient who was called during the first 48 hours after urinary tract surgery. The patient reported having an abnormally high level of pain. The nurse was able to call the urologist, explain the situation, and get an order for a urinalysis. The family assisted in getting this done, which allowed the patient to start on antibiotics for a urinary tract infection.

In more complex cases the role of the nurse in this system is to connect professionals in different parts of the care continuum for the good of the patient. System nurses are able to contact inpatient care coordinators and hospitalists and to connect their care activities with those in the outpatient setting. In one instance Monica was able to connect a hospitalist and a primary care physician who were caring for a complex patient. Each was able to tell their part of the "patient story" and to mesh their treatment plans after the conversation. Another role for ACO nurses is coordinating care with the inpatient complex care team and with its own home care agency and other preferred provider agencies.

ACO nurses are trained in motivational interviewing. They help patients articulate their own goals—say, "being able to walk to the mailbox"—and then develop a care plan based on these goals. Monica helps members of the care continuum, including inpatient and outpatient clinicians, create longitudinal care plans. The team of clinicians, which includes RNs and MSWs, is looking to conduct regular outreach with SNFs and home health agencies managing high-risk system patients to improve handoffs between levels of care. The ACO team never discharges a patient and can be a great resource as patients move between inpatient, rehab, and home health settings.

(continues)

Part of the ACO nurse role is to educate clinical staff in both the inpatient setting and the medical practices about value-based payment models and population health. One of the big challenges is to help inpatient nurses, who are overwhelmed with tasks, understand what patients face in the community when they leave the hospital and how to prepare them for better self-care. In medical practices, which have been used to working independently, the challenge is to help them see how collaboration will help them improve care for their patients. The health system has implemented some new care models, including locating behavioral health providers in medical practices that help support collaboration.

Other challenges have revolved around health information systems interoperability. Many of the medical practices continue to have their own electronic medical records that do not interface with the hospital record. The health system is working to resolve this problem with a care management platform that will provide more integrated information. Care coordinators also utilize an internal texting system that allows quick communication between providers in the system. Monica uses an example of a family caregiver who lives out of state and was able to use texting to update the care coordinator on changes in her parent's health situation.

Monica summarizes by saying, "This is really an exciting time. There are so many possibilities for improving care and reducing fragmentation with new collaboration mindset and new tools. We are really able to act as the eyes and ears for the physician and develop relationships that work to achieve the best outcomes for patients."

cannot pay for medications, have poor caregiver support, have no transportation to medical appointments, or who cannot shop or prepare meals. They also help patients apply for and use these services appropriately.

To provide solutions to the social determinant issues, the integrated system must develop a robust directory of community resources for care coordinators to access. The system must also develop either informal or contractual relationships with local mental health and social service agencies, such as Area Agencies on Aging, which administer many community programs and federal and state level entitlement programs. Some programs, such as the CareMore program, go to extraordinary lengths to help patients manage social determinants barriers.

CareMore, a highly innovative integrated system and insurance plan, goes much further than the average system in dealing with the social determinants of health. In this system, a home care intervention SWAT team of clinicians, social workers, mental health workers, and even attorneys provide support to high-risk elderly patients after a hospital discharge. "This team might help a patient with rheumatoid arthritis

to obtain non-childproof bottles, arrange for free transportation to the clinic for a socially isolated patient or intervene in family and legal matters that interfere with the patient's health" (Sinsky & Sinsky, 2015).

Consistent Use of Evidence-Based Best Practices

The paradigm in fee-for-service medicine is that all care must be customized to the individual patient and to the experience, preferences, and often profit of the clinician. In contrast, integrated systems achieve better outcomes by consistently implementing evidence-based best practices in all clinical care processes. Of all the tools and techniques of population health, this use of best practices is the one with the most potential for effecting positive results. In an article on eight high-performing integrated delivery systems, Dan Beckham (2016) describes the role of standardization in integrated care excellence:

Standardize care processes and management. Key to quality and affordability is driving out variation wherever possible. And moving beyond variation requires standardization. Quality of care, quality of leadership and quality of management all rely on a degree of standardization. It is impossible to deliver a high-quality service without the reliability and consistency that standardization delivers. (p. 4)

Given the independent nature of medical and nursing practice in the United States, standardization is difficult to implement. Systems that target high-risk patients with chronic conditions use clinical guidelines and electronic decision support tools to guide care. For example, the Mayo Clinic has a highly structured system for ensuring clinical consistency. The Mayo Clinic has clinical practice committees that are responsible for quality of care at each site. These committees disseminate expert-developed clinical protocols. A systemwide clinical practice advisory group reconciles protocols across sites and is responsible to the board of governors for overall system quality (McCarthy, Mueller, & Wrenn, 2009).

It has long been known that research findings take years to migrate into clinical practice, and in many cases, evidence-based care makes up only a portion of the care that is delivered. In integrated delivery systems, evidence-based guidelines, lists of indications for referrals and interventions, standardized order sets, operational checklists, and standardized process flows can help to standardize care and ensure the use of evidence-based best practices (Burton, 2014). Decision support tools such as templates embedded in the medical record can trigger the use of evidence-based care at the right point in care delivery. For example, a home care agency in an integrated system follows standardized clinical protocols for the care of HF patients such as an intense visit schedule at the start of care and the use of telemonitoring. A checklist template pasted into the clinical note by the intake department reminds case managers to follow these steps in the course of care.

Clinicians should be involved in reviews of relevant clinical research and in the design of practice guidelines that fit the needs of the organization.

Improvement teams can recruit champions to "sell guideline use," can conduct small tests of change to test guideline applications in the real work of clinical practice, and can develop clinician training and reference materials. Clinicians also provide advice on how to apply guidelines to the patient's unique situation. For example, HF patients should record a daily weight. Ideally, this is done via telemonitoring, but for those patients who cannot or will not use the technology, the nurse must ensure that the patient has an alternative self-monitoring system such as buying a scale, learning how to use it, and creating a paper record of daily weights.

Implementing Communication, Teamwork, and Managed Care Transitions

Communication, coordination, transitions, and teamwork are vital tactics for reducing care fragmentation and providing care integration. Establishing connections through these mechanisms is a core competency for successful integrated delivery systems. Data sharing through a common electronic medical record or data platform is a key element in connecting providers and sharing patient information within a delivery system. Teamwork techniques such as complex case conferences, clinical rounds, and team huddles are other tools for integrating care. Standardized communication techniques for quick and accurate clinical reporting such as SBAR (Situation, Background, Assessment, Recommendation) and standardized transition and referral forms can also be helpful in connecting care across the "white space" of individual professionals, departments, and organizations within the delivery system.

Some integrated systems, such as the CareMore system, use an intense team-based system of care to improve outcomes for high-risk, frail elderly persons.

Teams typically consist of 2 "extensivist" physicians who provide both hospital and outpatient care, 2 to 4 APRNs, 2 to 3 case managers, and 14 medical assistants along with a nutritionist, social worker, and pharmacist within a neighborhood of 4,000 to 5,000 covered patients (Sinsky & Sinsky, 2015).

Care Compacts for Specialty Referrals

Another method for ensuring connections between physicians in integrated systems is the "care compact." This concept is an updated version of the traditional letter sent from a referring physician to a specialist. The elements of the care compact include:

- **A preconsultation exchange** which defines the reason for the referral, the clinical findings, and the level of joint care management that will occur. For example, is the referring physician turning care over to the specialist or simply asking for a one-time consult with return information?
- **Establish management protocols for common conditions.** These protocols establish criteria for referring patients to specialty care and define what should be done before the referral. For example, specific clinical indicators and lab tests in diabetic patients trigger an endocrinology referral.
- **Set clear expectations for communication.** This process sets an expectation for

two-way "closed loop communication" in which the specialist communicates his or her findings back to the primary care physician. In addition, the primary care physician notifies the specialist if the patient's symptoms are under control and specialty visits can be stopped.

- **Establish common goals and align incentives.** When both primary care and specialty care practitioners receive incentives based on common metrics and are engaged in the same integrated care culture they are more likely to collaborate effectively (Modified from McClellan & Mostashari, 2014).

Preferred provider or network partner relationships provide better care integration for patients. Health systems may either employ or contract with postacute organizations such as SNFs and may define standards of communication through contracting. For example, SNFs in the system may expect preferred provider home healthcare agencies to employ liaison nurses who come to discharge planning meetings and conduct onsite patient assessments. The system may require the organization that received the patient to regularly report back to the referring organization on the status of patients who were sent to them. A nurse care coordinator in an SNF might prepare a monthly report for a referring hospital on patient length of stay, percent of patients who were discharged, and those who were readmitted and why.

🔍 CASE STUDY

Integrating Care in a Hospital-Based Delivery System

A small hospital integrated network consists of the hospital, a group of medical practices, and a group of preferred provider skilled nursing facilities and home care agencies. None of these organizations is owned by the hospital. The relationship is defined through contracts. All the partners are aligned around managing a population of patients in Medicare and commercial insurance shared savings plans and in Medicare bundling programs. The system is managed through the hospital and it uses a variety of techniques to integrate care and achieve quadruple aim outcomes, including:

- Population focus. Data are used to identify and track high-risk patients who are most vulnerable to fragmented care.

- Postacute providers have access to a portal into the hospital electronic medical record which they use to gather patient information when a patient is admitted to their organization.
- The system uses databases to track patients and keep high-risk patients "on the radar screen."
- Partners regularly communicate using secure email.
- The system has organizational team meetings to discuss patient status and patient care options.
- There is a structured process for care transitions between organizations.
- There is a key performance indicator system and data are shared so that all partners know both how the system as a whole works and how their own organizations are performing on quadruple aim measures.
- There are formal cross-organizational improvement teams to improve outcomes.

▶ The Use of Technology and Data in Integrated Delivery Systems

The electronic exchange of data fights fragmentation of care and fosters communication among providers who are caring for a patient or a population of patients. Integrated delivery systems use health information technology in a variety of ways:

- **Electronic health records** capture and communicate patient encounter data to clinicians in the integrated delivery system. Sophisticated EMRs may include templates, alerts, and decision support tools to support clinical best practices. An example is an alert that informs clinicians of duplicate drugs or drug interactions based on the patient medication list.
- **Patient portals** and patient EMRs obtain patient-provided data and a method for patients to obtain access to their own medical information.
- **Patient tracking systems** are tools for entering data about the patient's whereabouts in the care continuum (hospital, SNF, home care) so that care coordinators can manage care and communicate with postacute providers.
- **Health information exchanges** allow data to be shared between organizations that do not have a common EMR. For example, systems allow hospital preferred partner SNFs and home care agencies to receive patient referrals and to obtain patient hospital information through a secure portal.
- **Care management platforms** use predictive analytics to analyze patient populations, flag high-risk patients, automate care management workflows, and provide tools for communication between network partner organizations.

Tracking Performance Measures

Since integrated care delivery systems almost always participate in some form of value-based payment, strong analytical tools and expertise are key factors in the system's financial and clinical success. Integrated delivery systems invest heavily in data platforms, analytic tools, and staff such as clinical informatics experts, analysts, and statisticians with sophisticated data management skills. Many systems also educate clinicians and administrative staff on using data to drive decisions. Data are usually published in the form of dashboards, which are data summaries in graphic form. Most systems use both system level and organizational or practice level dashboard data.

A dashboard might include summaries of data on:

- **Patient population characteristics.** As mentioned, data and predictive analytics tools are used to analyze patient demographic and clinical and psychosocial data to stratify the patient population into tiers for care management purposes.

These data also allow the system to tailor clinical interventions to certain segments of the patient population. For example, education about goals of care conversations might be targeted to patients with multiple readmissions and declining health status.

- **Clinical outcomes data.** Clinical data are used by payers such as Medicare and accrediting agencies such as NCQA to provide quality ratings that are accessible to the public on the internet. Value-based payment programs use quality data for calculating shared savings and penalties. For these reasons integrated systems use considerable time, energy, and resources to proactively track and benchmark their own clinical performance. Using this data, they develop improvement projects to improve outcomes. For example, certain medical practices in an integrated system might do poorly on the ACO measure for percent of diabetics with high HbA1c measures. When the data are sorted by practice and benchmarking reports are published it is likely that the lower performing practices will be prompted to charter improvement teams or reeducate providers on system diabetic care best practices or care pathways. When data are sorted down to the clinician level findings provide opportunities for management coaching and individual improvement efforts.
- **Analysis of provider utilization and clinical activity.** These reports compare provider patient panel size, utilization of procedures, visits, and clinical activities. This data can be used to assess productivity, use of resources, and expenses per provider.
- **Tracking and analysis of performance on internal process measures** such as timeliness. An example would be tracking wait time for patient appointments. These measures are usually internally collected and reported.
- **Patient satisfaction measures.** This information is collected through surveys, such as the Medicare CAHPS program often administered by a third-party vendor.

Systems may also collect additional surveys and patient complaint data, which are aggregated into reports and benchmarked by the organization and/or team.

- **Financial analysis.** Integrated delivery systems, especially those that are partially funded by value-based payment and partially by fee-for-service contracts, must have extensive capability in estimating the costs of care by patient, by patient population, and by unit of service delivery such as the practice. Traditional financial reports that track revenue, expense, and profit margin must be part of any delivery system's metrics. For those in shared savings plans or in risk-bearing arrangements key reports analyze claims data to calculate whether the system met its target financial goals for the year and whether it incurred savings or penalties.

▶ Integrated Delivery System Pitfalls and Obstacles

To say that creating an effective integrated care system is not easy is a gross understatement. Systems require capital, highly sophisticated expertise, the will to integrate, a clear brand and marketing strategy, willing and capable clinicians, and payment mechanisms that support integration. The pitfalls are many and large, including:

- Capital and human resources to build an integrated delivery system
- Mindset, skillset, and culture gaps
- Payment obstacles
- The ability to engage physicians in the integrated system
- The ability to recruit a management team with the skills necessary to integrate care
- Regulatory hurdles
- Regional market challenges
- Unstable revenue streams and uncertain profit
- Professional and organizational silos that are resistant to collaboration and integration

Despite these hurdles the process of integration is moving forward at a rapid pace and despite numerous political and practical bumps in the road is showing no signs of stopping.

▶ Applying Integrated Care Strategies and Tools in Your Own Organization

The best way to fight care fragmentation in your own organization is to apply some or all of the tools and techniques of integrated care to produce a connected care experience for your patients. When boiled down to the essentials, there are some integrated care practices that do not require the full infrastructure of an integrated delivery system and can be applied by single organizations not part of a system. Using the checklist in **BOX 2-3**, identify integrated care strategies that your organization might be able to adopt.

▶ Chapter Summary

Integrated care delivery systems are the most complete example of connected care principles

---

BOX 2-3 How Many Integrated Care Strategies Could Your Organization Adopt?

Check off all that currently apply or that your organization could adopt.
- ❑ Identify your key patient populations and use data to understand population characteristics including demographics, diagnoses, payer mix, socioeconomic status, and other key characteristics.
- ❑ Purchase or develop an algorithm for identifying high-risk patients.
- ❑ Stratify your patient population into high-, medium-, and low-risk tiers. Develop resource allocation procedures to match the intensity of organizational resource use to patient need.
- ❑ Develop a key indicator system that measures organizational performance on quadruple aim measures including patient health outcomes, patient experience, clinician experience, and cost measures.
- ❑ Adopt evidence-based best practices to produce better outcomes for high-risk patients in your population.
- ❑ Create relationships with case managers in hospitals, insurance companies, medical practices, or home care agencies so you can collaborate on shared high-risk patients.
- ❑ Collaborate with hospitals and other providers in your medical community to develop shared longitudinal care plans for frequently readmitted patients.
- ❑ Create or purchase a system to track patients through the care continuum (emergency room visits, readmissions, discharges to SNFs, or home care agencies).
- ❑ Develop formal contracts or collaborative strategies with organizations that refer to yours or to which you refer patients after discharge.
- ❑ Formalize your care transition processes to ensure two-way communication and to avoid "throw it over the wall" transitions.
- ❑ Adopt a secure, HIPAA-compliant communication method between organizations within your care continuum (secure email, secure texting, etc.).
- ❑ Follow patients past the transition point to ensure that follow-up activities and self-care are happening as they should (i.e., check-in phone calls post discharge).
- ❑ Adopt a policy of mandatory interdisciplinary case conferencing and communication in cases in which multiple disciplines share the care of a patient.
- ❑ Conduct discharge planning meetings that include the patient and family.

(continues)

BOX 2-3 How Many Integrated Care Strategies Could Your Organization Adopt?   *(continued)*

❑ Share in or participate in sharing electronic medical records with referral sources, patients, and organizations to whom you discharge patients.

❑ Use process improvement teams to identify innovative methods for improving patient care outcomes.

❑ Use the tools and techniques of patient care collaboration such as daily huddles, complex case conferences, rounding, and nurse liaison visits to inpatients prior to discharge.

❑ Adopt technologies such as telemonitoring of high-risk patients or telemedicine visits to reduce the costs of care.

❑ Create a formal patient self-management support program that includes training and resources for both professionals and patients.

❑ Develop cross-organizational collaborative meetings and improvement projects to improve the processes of care and better integrate services across healthcare organizations.

❑ Implement a system that integrates behavioral health and medical care through co-location, offering both services onsite or through formal referral systems.

❑ Develop tools for managing the social determinants of health such as databases, relationships with community nonprofits, and roles such as health navigators to assist patients.

in action. Integrated systems are designed to reduce fragmentation and to connect information and clinical actions to achieve the best outcomes for patients. There is a worldwide movement to develop more integrated care, and extensive work on new models has been done in Europe and Canada.

In the United States integrated care has developed in a specific way because of Medicare and Medicaid interventions to achieve better clinical outcomes and patient experience at a lower cost.

These interventions, which have fostered the development of new clinical models, such as ACOs and new payment models such as bundling and shared savings, are collectively called the volume-to-value shift.

For organizations that participate in these models, reimbursement is tied to results. U.S. healthcare insurers, state and local governments, and healthcare organizations have embraced these new concepts but have found challenges in balancing fee-for-service and integrated care processes and systems. The tools and techniques of integrated care include a population health focus, the use of data to stratify risk in populations, patient engagement and self-management

support, substituting technology for labor to reduce costs, more intense use of connected care strategies such as evidence-based care transitions, teamwork, and collaboration both within and across healthcare organizations. Case management and care coordination are essential roles in integrated delivery systems and are mostly filled by nurses. Many integrated systems are highly physician centric and vest considerable control in physician leaders as physicians control the means of production and revenue generation in health care.

Managing the social determinants of health and integrating behavioral health and medical care are two other essential strategies used by integrated delivery systems to achieve better outcomes. The development of integrated delivery systems has caused significant market disruption as providers are acquired, merge, and affiliate to reach the level of capital and infrastructure necessary to achieve value-based care. In some markets, integrated delivery systems have become monopolies, driving up the local costs of care.

Clinical and administrative staff at all levels of healthcare organizations are finding it necessary to adopt a new, collaborative, and patient-centered mindset and a new, more sophisticated set of population health, collaboration, and data management skills.

Despite intense political and healthcare market turmoil, the volume-to-value shift has persisted as the nation debates the future of the Affordable Care Act, the politics of Medicaid expansion, and the future face of health care in the United States.

References

Alguire, P. (2017). Understanding capitation. American College of Physicians, www.ACPonline.org

American Nurses Association. (2010). New care delivery models in health system reform, opportunities for nurses and their patients. *ANA Issue Brief*. http://nursingworld.org/MainMenuCategories/Policy-Advocacy/Positions-and-Resolutions/Issue-Briefs/Care-Delivery-Models.pdf

Association of State and Territorial Health Officials. (2017). Community health teams issue report. http://www.astho.org/Programs/Access/Primary-Care/_Materials/Community-Health-Teams-Issue-Report/

Beckham, J. D. (2016). Eight strategic health systems: The path to integrated care, hospitals and health networks. Retrieved from hhnmag.com/articles/7531-charting-a-path-to-integrated-care

Bogan, M., Calcasola, S., Frick-Hoff, T., & Orlando, R., (2017). Driving success in bundled payments. *Institute for Healthcare Improvement*. http://app.ihi.org/FacultyDocuments/Events/Event-2930/Presentation-15672/Document-12518/Presentation_C15_Bogan.pdf

Bresnick, J. (2017). Using risk scores, stratification for population health management. HealthItAnalytics.com

Bryant, M. (2016). What's coming out of 4 healthcare innovation centers across the U.S. Healthcare Dive.com. www.healthcaredive.com/news/whats-coming-out-of-4...innovation-centers.../416355

Burton, D. (2014). The anatomy of healthcare delivery model—How a systematic approach can transform care delivery. *Health Catalyst Whitepaper*, 9.

Canadian Nurses Association, Canadian Medical Association. (2013). Health action lobby, integration, a new direction for Canadian health care. www.cna-aiic.ca/~/media/cna/files/en/cna_cma_heal_provider_summit_transformation_to_integrated_care_e.pdf?la=en

Center for Value Based Insurance Design. (2013). U. of Michigan, V-BID in action: A profile of Connecticut's Health Enhancement Program. *VPIB Center Brief*. http://www.shadac.org/sites/default/files/Old_files/shadac/publications/V-BID%20brief_CT%20HEP%20final.pdf

Centers for Medicare and Medicaid Services. (2016). Accountable care organizations and you. https://www.medicare.gov/Pubs/pdf/11588-Accountable-Care-Organizations-FAQs.pdf

Centers for Medicare and Medicaid Services. (2017a). Accountable health communities model. https://innovation.cms.gov/initiatives/ahcm/

Centers for Medicare and Medicaid Services. (2017b). Models initiative. https://innovation.cms.gov/initiatives/state-innovations/

Ellison, A. (2015). Geisinger's money-back guarantee is about more than refunds. www.beckershospitalreview.com/finance/geisinger-s-money-back-guarantee-is-about-more-than-refunds.html

Essential Hospitals Institute. (2013). Integrated health care literature review. www.essentialhospitals.org

Goldman, J. (2016). Myth busters—The path to value based care. www.advisoryboard.com

Goodwin, N. (2016). Understanding integrated care. *International Journal of Integrated Care, 16*(4), 1–6. doi:http://dx.doi.org/10.5334/ijic.253

Greenberg, J., Barnett, M., Spinks, M., Dudley, J., & Frolkis, J. (2014). The "medical neighborhood," integrating primary and specialty care for ambulatory patients. *JAMA Internal Medicine 174*(3), 454–457. doi:10.1001/jamainternmed.2013.14093

Hertz, B. T. (2013). Facility fees can change the economic equation. *Medical Economics*. http://medicaleconomics.modernmedicine.com/medical-economics/news/user-defined-tags/facility-fees/facility-fees-can-change-economic-equation

Hwang, W., Chang, J., LaClair, M., & Paz, H. (2013, May 10). Effects of integrated delivery systems on cost and quality. *American Journal of Managed Care*. http://www.ajmc.com/journals/issue/2013/2013-1-vol19-n5/effects-of-integrated-delivery-system-on-cost-and-quality

Indeed.com. (2017, March 25). Accountable care organization case manager RN jobs.

McCarthy, D., Mueller, K., & Wrenn, J. (2009). *Mayo Clinic: Multidisciplinary teamwork, physician-led governance, and patient-centered culture drive world-class health care. Case study, organized health care delivery system.* New York: The Commonwealth Fund.

McClellan, M., & Mostashari, F. (Eds.). (2014). Adopting accountable care: An implementation guide for physician practices. Engelberg Center for Health Care Reform at Brookings. www.acolearningnetwork.org

McClellan, M., Patel, K., Latts, L., & Dang-Vu, C. (2015). Implementing value-based insurance products: A collaborative approach to health care transformation. *Health Policy Issue Brief*. Washington, DC: Center for Health Policy, The Brookings Institution. www.brookings.edu

Medicaid. (2017). Program of all-inclusive care for the elderly. https://www.medicaid.gov/medicaid/ltss/pace/index.html

Medicaid. (2010). Health homes. Retrieved from https://www.medicaid.gov/medicaid/ltss/health-homes/index.html

Morse, S. (2016, September 21). Provider-run plans lead pack in NCQA health plan ratings. *Healthcare Finance News*. www.healthcarefinancenews.com/news/ncqa-releases-2016-health-insurance-plan-ratings

National Academy for State Health Policy. (2015). A day in the life of local care coordinator Michele Brown in the CareFirst Patient-Centered Medical Home Program. http://www.nashp.org/day-life-local-care-coordinator-michele-brown-carefirst-patient-centered-medical-home-program/

National Committee on Quality Assurance. (2017). Patient centered medical home recognition, 2017 standards preview. www.ncqa.org/Portals/0/Programs/Recognition/PCMH/2017%20PCMH%20Concepts%20Overview.pdf?ver=2017-03-08-220342-490

National Hospice and Palliative Care Organization. (2012). Hospice in the continuum compendium. www.nhpco.org/sites/default/files/public/communications/Hospice-in-Continuum_Compendium.pdf

National Voices.org.uk. (2013). A narrative for person centered coordinated care. Retrieved from https://www.nationalvoices.org.uk/sites/default/files/public/publications/narrative-for-person-centred-coordinated-care.pdf

Office of the Inspector General, U.S. Department of Health and Human Services. (2017). Medicare shared savings program accountable care organizations have shown potential for reducing spending and improving quality, 08-28-2017 Report (OEI-02-15-00450). Retrieved from https://oig.hhs.gov/oei/reports/oei-02-15-00450.asp

Sentara Healthcare. (2017). Sentara.com

Shih, A., Davis, K., Schoenbaum, S., Gauthier, A., Nuzum, R., & McCarthy, D. (2008). *Organizing the U.S. health care delivery system for high performance*. New York: The Commonwealth Fund.

Sinsky, C., & Sinsky, T. (2015). Lessons from CareMore: A stepping stone to stronger primary care of frail elderly patients. *American Journal of Accountable Care*.

Smith, M., Saunders, R., Stuckhardt, L., & McGinnis, J. M. (Eds.). (2013). *Best care at lower cost: The path to continuously learning health care in America. Committee on the Learning Health Care System in America*. Washington, DC: The Institute of Medicine.

Suter, E., Oelke, N. D., Adair, C. E., & Armitage, G. D. (2009). Ten key principles for successful health systems integration. *Healthcare Quarterly* (Toronto, Ont.) *13*, 16–23.

CHAPTER 3

Care Transitions—Fractured or Flowing?

CHAPTER OBJECTIVES

After completing this chapter readers will be able to:

- Identify types of care transitions
- Describe the scope and impact of high-risk care transition gaps
- List care transition consensus standards and measures
- Describe evidence-based care transition programs
- Explain key elements of effective care transitions
- Assess the effectiveness of the reader's own organizational care transitions
- Identify evidence-based transition tools and techniques for use in the reader's own organization
- List common failures in care transitions

▶ Introduction

In the course of writing this book I have spoken to many nurses and other health professionals about their perceptions of high-risk gaps and cracks in the healthcare system. One of these conversations was with a nurse population health director for a large medical practice, who dryly asked, "How many volumes will the publisher let you write?" Here, we will explore an area of care where care gaps are particularly prevalent and problematic—transitions of care from one healthcare setting to another.

In this chapter, we will explore the dimensions of care transitions and their impact on patients and the healthcare system, explore nurse care transition roles and competencies, examine evidence-based best practices, list available tools and the links for finding them, and describe measures and distill guidelines that can be applied to the reader's own practice setting.

Because care transitions are all about teamwork, we will frame this chapter with observations about care coordination from Sharon Wood, RN, MSN, the director of Population Health for Community Medical Group in New Haven, Connecticut: "I think the vast majority of people who work in health care work too independently; not in silos, but on parallel pathways towards a goal. We do not or cannot see who is to the left and right of us moving toward the same goal, so we spend too much time, too much effort and too much money trying to attain an outcome that is only achievable if we work in collaboration with one another. We in health care talk a lot about safety nets for our patients. We need to broaden that concept and think about safety nets for systems" (Wood, 2017, personal communication).

▶ Care Transitions Overview

The National Transitions of Care Coalition (NTOCC) defines care transitions as "leaving one care setting (i.e. hospital, skilled nursing facility, assisted living facility, primary care physician practice, home health care, or specialist care) and moving to another" (NTOCC, 2010a, p. 2). Care transitions are a potential care gap area and have been extensively studied and reported in the healthcare literature.

Transitions are notorious for causing patient harm and increasing costs. Transitions from acute care to home have produced the most evidence-based best practices and tools for improvement. Transitions to and from long-term care facilities, emergency rooms, and ambulatory surgery have been less studied, but they also have a significant impact on patient outcomes, especially for patients with multiple chronic illnesses and high care needs. Transitions to and from home health care have received very little research attention.

Is a Care Transition Always the Best Answer?

Before considering the types of care transitions, it is important to remember that fewer or no transitions can be the best option for patients. This point is made in a document from the American Medical Directors Association (of long-term care facilities): "[I]t is well established that transferring a patient from a familiar environment (e.g., the SNF/NF where s/he resides) to a new, unfamiliar, and potentially bewildering location like an emergency room can cause severe and sometimes permanent decompensation and lead to medical errors. Hence, avoidance of unnecessary transfers should be a primary goal, but when transfers are necessary, we support implementation of processes that optimize efficient and well-orchestrated patient transitions" (American Medical Directors Association, 2010, p. 2).

▶ Care Transition Basics

Types of Care Transitions

In the American healthcare system there are five major types of care transitions (**FIGURE 3-1**):

- **Home to acute or postacute care** (emergency room, skilled nursing facility [SNF], or acute care hospital)
- **Acute care to postacute care** (to skilled nursing, long-term acute care hospital [LTACH], inpatient rehabilitation, and home health care)
- **Ambulatory care to home** (outpatient surgery, chemotherapy, outpatient procedures such as colonoscopies to home)
- **Transitions between postacute settings** (SNF to home care, home care to SNF, LTACH to SNF, LTACH to home care, assisted living to home care)
- **Acute care directly to home** (acute care hospital, emergency room to home)

In the white space between these facilities is a "mini transition" (e.g., transport by ambulance

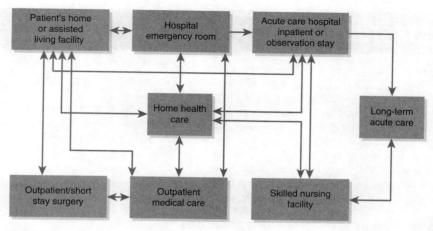

FIGURE 3-1 Types of Care Transitions

🔎 CASE STUDY

Interview with Beth Hodshon, JD, MPH, RN, Project Director of the CHIRAL Project 3—Transitions in and out of the Hospital

Yale University researchers at the Center for Healthcare Innovation, Redesign and Learning (CHIRAL), a joint partnership of the Yale Medical School and Yale New Haven Hospital, studied transitions between hospitals and SNFs. The project sites for this research included a 28-bed teaching service, a 14-bed general medicine hospitalist unit, and local SNFs. Project Director Beth Hodshon, JD, MPH, RN, shares her insights and impressions from the research.

Framing the Work of the Study

- Nationally 1:4 older hospitalized patients are discharged to an SNF and 1:4 are readmitted within 30 days.
- There is a national focus on reducing readmissions; and in 2018 SNFs and hospitals will receive readmission penalties.
- Because of the lack of SNF transition studies, one positive aspect of this project has been to "give SNFs a voice."

Impressions from Interviews and Observations

- Hospital staff lack knowledge about SNFs (when and how often a patient is seen by provider, differences in care provided by SNF vs. hospital).
- There is considerable variation in facilities in terms of their processes and the services they provide.
- There is a high volume of turnover among SNF clinicians. At various points in the study, researchers have had difficulty contacting facilities because the clinician who had originally participated in the research was no longer employed there.

(continues)

🔍 *CASE STUDY*   (continued)

- Patients discharged from SNFs are very sick, and don't look much different from hospitalized patients. Yet, SNFs are structured very differently from hospitals in terms of staffing and ability to care for patients. Capabilities vary considerably between facilities.
- SNF providers have a much different relationship with patients than do inpatient providers. Because patients often stay in SNFs longer than they do in hospitals, clinicians have a closer bond with patients and families. Some researchers wonder (this has not yet been studied) if this close bond lessens objectivity that may impact SNF staff being more willing to send patients to the hospital when the patient's condition deteriorates.
- The attitude "when in doubt send them out" often prevails at SNFs when a patient has acute changes in condition. Some SNFs are trying to change this.

Hospital Versus SNF Views of Transitions

- The process of preparing the patient for a discharge from a hospital to an SNF is a complex and time-consuming process that must be performed by hospital medical residents, nurses, and care coordinators preferably before 11 a.m.
- An effective hospital-to-SNF process requires the transfer of complex information; and follow-up on tasks begun in the hospital may need to be completed by the SNF.
- Preparation work includes:
  - Completing a discharge summary
  - Reconciling patient medications for discharge
  - Providing orders for specialty services and equipment
  - Booking follow-up appointments
  - Making a "warm handoff" from the hospital clinician to the SNF clinician
  - Arranging transportation
- Because care transition is just "part of the work" of hospital and nursing staff and not a separately defined and measured process with specific best practices, it is often sandwiched in with other responsibilities. This can lead to incomplete transfer information being provided and leaves the SNF scrambling to get the right supplies and medications when the patient is admitted. These disconnects create fertile ground for mistakes.
- On the SNF side, the process of accepting a patient from the hospital is complex and can be intense and frustrating for both hospital and SNF staff. A key driver of making a decision to accept/ not accept a patient is cost. A patient's care plan and the SNF's capacity to care for a patient may depend on the patient's insurance and/or willingness to pay for care privately. For example, patients who have been in observation and need SNF level care may not qualify for Medicare coverage in the SNF post discharge. This is a huge barrier to SNFs who are put in the position of having to accept a patient who cannot pay and potentially incurring large financial losses over time.
- On the hospital clinician side, SNF rules and constraints are not well understood. A delay in accepting a patient or a refusal to accept causes hospital clinical staff to express frustration and anger because, as they see it, after all their work, the patient is not going to get the level of service that is expected. Often refusals are seen as "unfair" and the SNF is labeled as "uncooperative" when this occurs.

Crossing the Gap Between SNFs and Hospitals

In conversation, Ms. Hodshon wonders if some future work might be done on improving communication and joint expectations between SNFs and hospital staff. Having clinicians from one facility visit the other would be ideal but not practical due to staffing constraints. Some type of videotaped interviews might be another option.

Summary

Some SNFs with a broader view of care transitions and higher level capabilities to manage complex patients are making serious attempts to reduce readmission. A high volume of staff turnover in SNFs and the lack of consistent best practices complicate the problem of effective transitions. SNF transitions can be smooth, but many of these transitions are fraught with potential errors and mistakes due to hospital staff overload and a transition process that focuses on quickly moving patients to the next setting in care. Another factor in less than ideal transitions is the difference in priorities and a lack of understanding and communication between hospital and SNF staff. In the future work of the project some improvements to address these root causes of poor transitions may be tested.

or other means). The quality and timeliness of transport between settings can be a significant factor in achieving a successful care transition.

Standards for Effective Care Transitions

A 2007 policy statement by the Transitions of Care Consensus Conference (TOCCC) tackled the daunting task of creating standards for care transitions.

This consensus group included key medical organizations such as the American College of Physicians, the Society of General Internal Medicine, the Society of Hospital Medicine, the American Geriatrics Society, and the Society for Academic Emergency Medicine. The TOCCC adopted 9 principles for effective care transitions: "1.) Accountability, 2.) Communication, 3.) Timely interchange of information, 4.) Involvement of the patient and family member, 5.) Respect the hub of coordination of care, 6.) All patients and their family/caregivers should have a medical home or coordinating clinician, 7.) At every point of transitions the patient and/or their family/caregivers need to know who is responsible for their care at that point, 8.) National standards, 9.) Standardized metrics" (Snow et al., 2009). These standards have been embedded into the evidence-based care transition programs that will be described

later in this chapter and they provide guidelines for the development of organizational level care transition efforts.

Core Care Transition Activities

A review of the literature indicates that there are a core series of specific activities that achieve the TOCCC standards for effective care transitions (American Medical Directors Association, 2010; NTOCC, 2010a; Naylor, 2008; The Joint Commission [TJC], 2012).

- A predischarge assessment of patient risk and caregiving support
- A discharge plan focused on expressed patient and family needs
- Multidisciplinary communication and collaboration
- Clinician accountability for patient support across transition points
- Patient and family engagement and self-management education
- Follow-up after a patient leaves a care setting
- Effective transfer of information between settings, preferably in electronic form

FIGURE 3-2 summarizes the essential elements of effective care transitions.

When these activities occur consistently and in concert, the patient experience is good; when one or more of these activities is faulty or

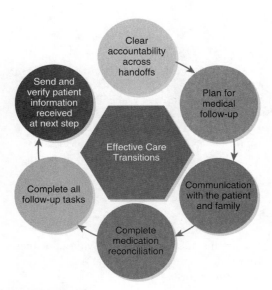

FIGURE 3-2 Essential Elements of Effective Care Transitions

missing, care transitions fail or create adverse events and poor outcomes for patients.

Care Transitions Roles and Responsibilities

The complexity of care transitions has fueled the development of a number of specific roles and responsibilities. Nurses, physicians, social workers, and support staff trained as "transition coaches" or "patient navigators" may all play a part in helping patients safely transition from one setting to another. Nursing roles dominate in care transitions, although in postacute settings, social workers also play a prominent role in discharge planning and execution. Nurses who arrange care transitions have a variety of titles (Agency for Healthcare Research and Quality [AHRQ], 2016).

Care Manager

"Care manager" is one of the most common titles, but others are "discharge planner," "care coordinator" or "transition coach." "Case manager" is a common title for nurses who organize care

transitions and discharge planning, although some experts see case management as a more long-term, intense relationship with a population of seriously ill patients and transitional care as the work of linking care across settings (Lamb, 2014). According to the Case Management Society of America (CMSA) one of the guiding principles for case managers is to "[a]ssist with navigating the health care system to achieve successful care, for example during transitions" (CMSA, 2016).

Care Coordinator

The care coordinator title is commonly used in ambulatory care settings, behavioral health, and medical offices. These positions may be responsible only for episodic coordination of care and transitions or the role may evolve into a more long-term case management.

One advertisement for a medical office nurse care coordinator describes the transition role of the care coordinator: Coordinates care across the inpatient/outpatient/community continuum to assure appropriate utilization of clinical and community resources.

Utilization Management

Utilization management is a type of care transition management that focuses on the optimal use of healthcare resources for patient care. Using standardized guidelines, utilization managers determine medical necessity, recommend the use of evidence-based clinical guidelines, and determine optimal time frames and lengths of stay for care (URAC, 2017).

Clinical Liaison Nurses in Skilled Nursing Facilities and Home Health Care

Nurses in these roles evaluate whether patients in inpatient settings are appropriate for referral to the next step in care such as the SNF or home health care. They may participate in discharge planning. They educate patients and families about the type of services they can expect in the SNF or home healthcare agency. Liaison nurses may also identify barriers and obstacles to effective transitions and communicate these to the admitting or intake staff at the SNF or home care agency.

Social Work Discharge Planners

The National Association of Social Workers (NASW) defines the social work role in SNF transitions as: "Facilitating residents' safe integration into the community through interdisciplinary discharge planning and follow-up services" (NASW, 2003, p. 15). In most SNFs, social workers collaborate with nursing and therapy staff to design a discharge plan and to facilitate both admissions and discharges from facilities.

Physician Hospitalists

Since the late 1990s physicians who specialize in inpatient care, called hospitalists, have supplanted the role of community physicians in managing patients who are admitted to acute care facilities.

Most health professionals agree that the hospitalist role has improved the quality of acute care, but many believe that it has created more complexity in care coordination. Clear accountability for patient care across the transition from hospital to home has been lost since the community physician no longer manages care in both settings. In one study, some hospitalists felt a strong responsibility to communicate their findings to community physicians through timely transmission of discharge summaries. Some go much further and contact the community physician directly. Others stated that "once the patient is out the door, they are not my responsibility" (Hongmai, Grossman, Cohen, & Bodenheimer, 2008, p. 1321). In some settings, hospitalists actually take the lead in identifying patients who are at risk for readmissions and in developing strategies for avoiding these readmissions in concert with community providers (Johnson, 2016).

Extensivists

According to a 2016 article in the online journal, *HealthLeaders Media*, yet another new specialty, "the extensivist," has been developed to address the fragmented nature of inpatient to outpatient care coordination: "Extensivists typically take their scope of practice beyond the hospital and into the home or other settings, with a focus on keeping patients healthier and reducing readmissions" (Freeman, 2016). These roles are filled by either physicians or nurse practitioners. This new role has been received with some skepticism by health professionals who wonder if it usurps the role of the primary care physician in coordinating care. Others feel that the extensivist role is ideally suited to the management of high-need, high-risk patients who may not get an adequate level of care coordination and intense medical management in a busy primary care practice.

Technology and Care Transitions

Technology often plays a role in improving care transitions. Interoperable electronic medical records are the main area of focus, but emerging technologies such as electronic tracking of patients across the continuum of care and electronic communication with patients after a transition are other aspects of technology being applied to transitions.

Healthcare professionals almost universally acknowledge that the lack of health information systems interoperability (computer systems that can exchange information) is a huge barrier to effective care transitions. While some transitions are communicated via interoperable electronic medical records (EMRs), communication is still likely to be done by fax or phone, and forms mailed and occasionally emailed via secured servers. Lack of standardized communication templates or forms and a variety of communication methods often results in care transition information being missed or misinterpreted. Even when the facility or agency that receives the patient from an acute care institution has access to the hospital EMR, information is not always condensed into a usable form.

Another problem that lacks sufficient study in the literature but is often reported in conversations with health professionals is that transition information may contain considerable clinical information but fails to "tell the patient's story." One example of this is not informing the next step in care about palliative care or hospice patient and family conversations that may have been started at the referring facility. A second example is not providing information about socioeconomic barriers to care or the patient's caregiving support situation to health professionals who provide care to the patient at the next step in the continuum.

One nursing informatics study describes a hospital-based project that did create a "patient story" portal with constantly updated patient information (Struck, 2013).

In a position paper about the use of health information technology to improve transitions of care, the NTOCC (2010b) explores the issues of barriers to effective transition communication at length. This paper identifies five significant barriers to effective care transition communication:

- **Lack of connectivity.** This issue concerns the lack of interoperability, partially due to a focus on technology as a revenue generator and not a method of improving patient care.
- **Lack of shared goals related to care transitions.** The root cause of this problem is a "silo mentality" in which each part of the care continuum focuses only on its own transition goals and tasks.
- **Misaligned incentives.** Payment for volume fosters disconnected transition communication, but pay for results fosters better communication.
- **Consumer knowledge and demand for a continuing care plan.** Low levels of health literacy and information that are not patient friendly contribute to lower levels of consumer use of healthcare information through care transitions.

- **Issues of trust.** Fears about data breaches, misunderstanding of the Health Insurance Portability and Accountability Act (HIPAA) laws, and patient fears about who can access the personal health information inhibit sharing of important clinical information between professionals and patients.

The paper goes on to propose solutions including standards, better quality measures, aligned incentives, and team-based care within and across provider groups (NTOCC, 2010b).

Electronic systems that track patients through the continuum of care are a new innovation in care transition technology. Some of these systems are internal to an organization and use the organization's EMR. For example, a home care agency used its "patient status report" capabilities to gather and document data from clinicians and families about the patient's current site of care (emergency room, observation, hospital, or SNF). By continually entering status data and running reports on patient status, clinical managers were better able to identify and manage transitions to and from home care.

An example of an external tracking system that is used by accountable care organizations (ACOs) is PatientPing. Ping is a system that "relies on feeds of admission, discharge and transfer data commonly exchanged among healthcare IT systems. PatientPing's partners provide the company with a list of their patients and the networks they use. PatientPing takes that information and connects it to those facilities' feeds. PatientPing then filters through both the list of patients and the registration system looking for matches. When a match is identified, the providers are notified" (Castellucci, 2016). The data are used in a practical way by medical groups, SNFs, and home care agencies to track the location of patients in value-based payment programs. When patients are identified as being in a different care setting, each involved provider can communicate with ACO care managers about a new transition care plan.

Middlesex Hospital in Middletown, Connecticut, uses an interactive voice response (IVR) system to communicate with patients after hospital discharge. The system calls patients within 48 hours of discharge and asks a series of questions about the patient's health status. Using a set of triage protocols and an analysis of the responses, the system provides "trigger alerts" to care managers to triage and manage the patient's changing health situation (Mackinnon & Mansfield, 2015).

Patient portals are another electronic tool that can improve the quality of care transitions. According to HealthIT.gov, "A patient portal is a secure online website that gives patients convenient 24-hour access to personal health information from anywhere with an Internet connection. Using a secure username and password, patients can view health information such as: recent doctor visits,discharge summaries, and medications" (HealthIT.gov, 2015). Patient portals are often used to provide patients with continuing access to discharge instructions. In an innovative project, one Veterans Administration hospital used a patient portal to manage postdischarge medication reconciliation with patients. The program resulted in avoiding 108 medication discrepancies and 23 potential adverse drug events, 50% of which were classified as serious (Heyworth et al., 2014).

As time goes on and these electronic systems evolve and become more widespread and more interoperable, we can expect them to make a positive impact on the quality of care transitions.

▶ Care Transition Measures

The National Quality Forum (NQF) has included a number of care transition measures in its Endorsement Summary of Care Coordination Measures (NQF, 2014). These measures include:

- **Timely initiation of home health care** within 2 days of the referral or patient discharge date
- **Medication reconciliation for older adults** (age 66 and older) within 30 days of discharge

- **Reconciled medication list received by discharged patients** or caregivers at the time of discharge
- **Transition record received by discharged patients** or caregivers at the time of discharge
- **Transition record received by the facility, primary physician, or other health professional** designated to provide follow-up care within 24 hours of discharge
- **Transition record received by patients discharged** from an emergency department

In 2014, the Care Transitions Measure (CTM-3®), a three-item question set developed by the Care Transitions Program (Coleman et al., 2002), was incorporated into the publicly reported Medicare Consumer Assessment of Healthcare Providers and Systems (CAHPS) survey. The new CAHPS measures include three new questions that assess patient perceptions of care transitions:

1. During this hospital stay, staff took my preferences and those of my family or caregiver into account in deciding what my healthcare needs would be when I left the hospital.
2. When I left the hospital, I had a good understanding of the things I was responsible for in managing my health.
3. When I left the hospital, I clearly understood the purpose for taking each of my medications. (Centers for Medicare and Medicaid Services [CMS], 2015)

The IMPACT Act of 2014 is a Medicare regulation that creates a unified measurement system across all postacute settings, including skilled nursing facilities, long-term care acute hospitals, inpatient rehabilitation facilities, and home health agencies (HHAs). The act mandates the use of several existing transition measures and it creates contracts for developing several additional care transition measures.

Within the context of the IMPACT Act, CMS Medicare Learning Network (2015) describes care transitions in this way: "Communicating and providing for the transfer of health information and care preferences of an individual when the individual transitions" (p. 9). The universal measure for care transitions across all four postacute settings is a 30-day postdischarge, all-cause readmission rate.

In 2017, CMS began soliciting comments on two new measures for care transitions (CMS, 2017):

1. Transfer of information at postacute care admission, start, or resumption of care from other providers/settings
2. Transfer of information at postacute care discharge or end of care to other providers/setting

Commonsense Care Transition Measures

While the formal measurement of care transitions is a work in progress, most health professionals and most patients and their family caregivers know a good care transition when they see one. Good care transition processes incorporate the four key elements of connected care:

- It's all about them (patients and caregivers), not just about us (health professionals).
- We're all in this together (teamwork).
- We share relevant information to meet patient needs.
- We do the right things right (work processes produce desired results with the least amount of resources).

Both groups (professionals and patients) describe good transitions in terms like these:

- "Communication was good. I knew what was happening all the time."
- "Nothing fell through the cracks. All the right supplies and equipment arrived on time."
- "The patient and family stated they knew who to call for help during the transition."
- "Somebody from the hospital called to see how I was doing."
- "The patient is taking the correct postdischarge medications."

- "The facility that sent us the referral called to give us some additional information about the 'patient story.'"
- "The doctor called me back to give me the results of my tests."

In the absence of formal measures, health professionals should be asking patients and families such questions as "How do you feel we are doing on planning your discharge?" and "Do you know who to call if your condition gets worse?"

Organizational Level Care Transition Measures

In an era of value-based payment, all programs and activities must be built to achieve quadruple aim goals (i.e., improved outcomes for populations of patients, better patient experience, lower cost of care per capita, better clinician experience). Care transition processes are no exception. Most organizational care transition programs will focus on Medicare publicly reported measures, such as 30-day readmission rates, which carry penalties for low performance, and measures that are built into value-based payment programs.

Some of the common care transition measures include:

- **Care transitions outcomes.** The overriding goal for most transition programs is a reduction in patient readmissions to the hospital. Because of Medicare readmission penalties for both hospitals, and in the near future, for SNFs, most institutions are highly motivated to improve transitions to reduce their readmission rates. Another emerging outcome measure is the rate of emergency room visits for patients who have transitioned to a new care setting.
- **Patient experience measures.** Patient satisfaction goals and measures are an essential element in monitoring effective care transitions. The care transition questions in the CAHPS survey are the most commonly used type of patient satisfaction measures. Even if the facility is not mandated by Medicare to

do a CAHPS survey, it can still incorporate these measures into its own internal patient satisfaction surveys.

- **Operational measures.** Organizations that are serious about care transitions will also dissect their internal work processes and create goals and measures to determine their effectiveness. For example, home health agencies have hospital liaison programs, in which a nurse visits hospitalized patients who are ready for discharge. The nurse educates the patient about home care services and identifies discharge "red flags" that might alert the agency to work with the SNF more intensely to create a care plan or that might result in declining a referral in the case of serious patient safety issues.

These "red flags" might include issues such as nonhealing wounds, inadequate caregiver support, financial issues, need for 24-hour care, inability to transfer safely, and need for a Hoyer lift in the home. The agency may measure effectiveness by surveying patients about how well the liaison prepared them for home care services. It may also measure the effectiveness of the liaison "red flag" screening process.

Other organizational goals and measures may be dictated by ACO or insurer guidelines. For example, SNFs that participate in value-based payment programs try to have patients who decompensate at home return back to their facility rather than sending them to the hospital. The SNF might measure what percentage of total discharges end in a return to the hospital versus a return to the SNF.

- **Cost measures.** Another key internal measure is the cost of a care transition program. Organizations will measure the cost of maintaining a department or specialized functions to manage care transitions and should also monitor the average cost of each transition and the cost of transitions that fail. For example, in an SNF, the cost of a social work discharge planner, the cost of staff time for making patient follow-up calls, and the costs of patients who are readmitted to the facility within a specific time window might all be practical cost measures. The cost of buying or licensing computer programs required to take referrals or track patients through the continuum might also be calculated as part of a care transition program cost assessment.

🔍 CASE STUDY

A Good Care Transition

Consider the case of Mr. Washington, a 77-year-old inpatient in an acute care hospital. Mr. W, who has heart failure, chronic obstructive pulmonary disease, and diabetes, lives in his own home and receives caregiving support from his 74-year-old wife and his middle-aged daughter.

Soon after admission, Mr. W's hospital primary care nurse conducted a nursing assessment and identified the patient's goals, which were to return home, continue his regular activities, and be able to walk to his mailbox every day. The nurse also identified financial barriers to obtaining needed medications after discharge. She promptly made a referral to a social worker who was able to help the patient apply for a medication discount program.

During the course of the hospital stay, the unit secretary coordinated a follow-up medical appointment with the patient's primary care doctor and the patient's family. The hospital care coordinator referred Mr. W to a home care agency for patient teaching, physical therapy, and medication management.

(continues)

🔍 CASE STUDY

(continued)

On the day prior to discharge, the home care liaison nurse visited Mr. W in the hospital to educate the patient and his wife about home care and to identify barriers to care. She also educated them about how to identify signs that Mr. W's condition was worsening and when to call the doctor. She learned that transportation to medical appointments would be a problem since the patient's adult daughter worked at the time of most appointments. She noted this in the agency medical record and made a recommendation for a social work referral after home care admission. The hospital care coordinator referred Mr. W to home care via an electronic referral system.

The home care agency was able to search the hospital EMR, retrieving the discharge summary, medication list, and social work notes for the care team.

One day after discharge, the home care nurse admitted the patient to service and conducted medication reconciliation using the hospital discharge medication list, the medications that his daughter had filled at the pharmacy, and the medications that were already in the home.

She called the physician to resolve medication discrepancies and verified that the patient would keep his follow-up medical appointment. After reading the liaison nurse's notes, she made a referral to the agency social worker who arranged for town transportation. After reviewing the hospital discharge summary, which contained information about patient goals, the home care nurse verified these goals with the patient and created a home care plan that incorporated those goals. She also reviewed the "when to call the doctor sheet" and used teach-back (having the patient repeat back what was learned) to ensure that the patient and his wife both understood when to call for help. She called the adult daughter to keep her updated on all care plan arrangements. Two days after discharge, the hospital care coordinator called both the patient and the home care nurse to ensure that the discharge had gone smoothly and to identify any problems.

By the end of the first week, the patient was taking the appropriate medications, was clear on when to call his doctors, had a follow-up appointment with the primary care physician, and had transportation to get there. He and his wife stated that they felt less stressed and more able to effectively cope with Mr. W's medical situation.

Case Study Review Question

Review the case study and identify the effective care transition activities that were used to achieve good results in this case.

▶ The Impact of Poor Care Transitions

Hospital readmissions are the most visible, measured, and costly of postacute care discharge adverse events. A 2014 report by HCUP (Healthcare Cost and Utilization Project of the AHRQ) noted that "In 2011, there were approximately 3.3 million adult 30-day all-cause hospital readmissions in the United States, and they were associated with about $41.3 billion in hospital costs" (Hines, Barret, Jiang, & Steiner, 2014, p. 1).

In 2012, in response to these huge costs, Medicare instituted a readmission reduction program that penalized hospitals for unnecessary readmissions. A recent study that analyzed data from 3,387 hospitals found that from 2007 to 2015, readmission rates for targeted conditions declined (from 21.5% to 17.8%) and rates for nontargeted conditions declined (from 15.3% to 13.1%) (Zuckerman, Sheingold, Orav, Ruhter, & Epstein, 2016). Despite this decline in readmissions, the problem continues with over half of the nation's hospitals receiving readmission penalties (Rau, 2016).

Adverse Events after Hospital Discharge

A classic older study found that nearly 20% of patients experience adverse events within 3 weeks of discharge, many of which are preventable. Some of the most common adverse events post discharge were:

- Hospital-acquired infections
- Worsening symptoms due to hospital treatment
- Procedure-related injuries
- Adverse drug events (Modified from Forster, Murff, Peterson, Gandhi, & Bates, 2003)

Post-Hospital Syndrome

Dr. Harlan Krumholtz, Yale University School of Medicine, describes the post-hospital syndrome as "an acquired, transient period of vulnerability resulting from a hospital stay" (2013, p. 100). This syndrome—which results from patients experiencing inadequate sleep, poor nutrition, the stress of change and a challenging environment, multiple new medications, and deconditioning from bed rest—produces adverse events on discharge such as falls and injuries. In practical terms, the impact of this post-hospital syndrome for patients who transition home or to a postacute setting is profound. An example is postdischarge patient functional limitations or falls that result from patient deconditioning during the hospital stay.

A hospital readmissions collaborative group attacked this issue when home health agencies complained that too many patients were being sent home unable to ambulate. This lack of functional ability was not being assessed prior to discharge or the assessment was not being communicated to the home health agency. A typical scenario described by the home health agencies was that when the home health nurse came to the patient's home to conduct the admission visit the nurse would find that the patient could not get up out of a chair. This necessitated a call to emergency services, transport to the hospital emergency room, and a subsequent hospital readmission.

A review of readmission data by both the hospital and the home health agencies revealed that this was indeed a common cause of readmissions for that hospital. A deeper analysis revealed that hospital inpatient nursing and therapy staff felt that their schedules were too busy to allow for patient ambulation and patients were spending considerable time in bed or in a bedside chair. The inpatient nursing and therapy teams subsequently worked with management to create more time and a process for patient ambulation and strengthening exercises prior to discharge.

This intervention reduced the incidence of unnecessary transfers back to the hospital due to preventable patient functional limitations.

Wasteful Spending

"Researchers have estimated that inadequate care coordination, including inadequate management of care transitions, was responsible for $25 to $45 billion in wasteful spending in 2011 through avoidable complications and unnecessary hospital readmissions" (Burton, 2012, p. 1).

Caregiver and Patient Stress and Dissatisfaction

A family caregiver, who is herself a physical therapist with extensive healthcare experience, described her frustration with her father's hospital discharge and postdischarge transition: "You leave the hospital with 5 to 10 pages of paperwork and nobody explains it. You have a bag full of meds to deal with. You get a list of appointments for doctors you have never seen and a number to call. They don't tell you the location of the office. You finally find the address and you are driving around looking for a garage or parking with a sick person in the car. You are working and trying to do this. What are you really supposed to do in this situation?" (Mary Jane Fegan, PT, DPT, Personal communication, 2018)

ASK YOURSELF

- What are the most common patient transitions in and out of your practice setting (admission, discharge, transfer between units, etc.)?
- Do you know if your patients experience adverse events when they transition out of your practice setting to home or to the next setting in the care continuum?
- If the answer to the second question is "yes," at which points in the workflow do you think things fall through the cracks?

🔍 CASE STUDY

The Pieces Don't Fit Together for a High-Risk Patient and Caregiver

A patient with a history of mental illness and sporadic homelessness who was being treated for severe arthritis, chronic obstructive lung disease, and congestive heart failure was discharged from a hospital to home health care. He was living with his wife in public housing, from which they had periodically been evicted and allowed back. Neither the patient nor his wife had been able to muster the energy or organizational skills to apply for Medicaid.

The patient was being followed by multiple specialists, but communication was poor. The patient did not have a consistent, involved primary care physician. He was taking multiple medications prescribed by a number of specialists; some of them were duplicates of others that had been previously prescribed. Many postdischarge follow-up appointments were made, but the patient came to these appointments only occasionally. He was often transported to the emergency room by ambulance after missing appointments at the congestive heart failure diuretic infusion clinic.

Ultimately, after a series of missed phone calls (due to wrong phone numbers being exchanged between social workers at the hospital and home care agency), the home care social worker was able to help the patient complete an application for a transportation service. The application had been started by the hospital social worker, but never finished. The family caregiver (the patient's wife) who was highly stressed and ill herself, received little to no attention until the home healthcare team identified her distress and provided social work counseling.

Further complicating things, the hospital palliative care team had started a goals of care discussion with the family, but the notes were not part of the discharge summary that was sent to the home care agency, so agency clinicians were left to begin the conversation again, to the bewilderment of the family. The litany of disconnects in care in this case goes on and on and could fill a short story.

Some were eventually resolved as the result of a joint hospital/home health care agency case conference; many were not. In reading both the inpatient and outpatient hospital record and the home healthcare agency notes, one consistent theme emerged: Each setting and each professional acted in a vacuum, concentrating on each discipline's focus and needs, but not attempting to tie clinical actions to patient goals and not communicating to the next step in care. Considerable time, expense, and patient and family distress could have been alleviated by a broader view and better communication.

▶ Evidence-Based Best Practices in Care Transitions

Since the start of the 21st century, there has been considerable research on best practices and tools to improve care transitions. Some of these new models have been proven to reduce patient harm, increase patient satisfaction, and improve clinical outcomes. Nurses are an integral part of many of these evidence-based care transition models. Nurses in nonspecialized care transition roles have also been able to adapt many of the care transition patient education and interdisciplinary communication tools as part of their daily practice. The most notable of the evidence-based care transition models are:

- **The Care Transition Intervention.** This approach, developed by Dr. Eric Coleman and colleagues, was tested in a large integrated delivery system in Colorado. The program utilized advanced practice nurses as "transition coaches" who coached patients on four "pillars" of self-management:
  - Medication self-management
  - Patient-centered record
  - Follow-up with patient's primary care provider
  - Identification of "red flags" that indicate a change in condition

  The program included a home visit and follow-up phone calls. The intervention reduced readmissions within 30 days by 30% (Coleman, Parry, Chalmers, & Min, 2006). Since the initial research, the Care Transitions Program has continued its research and has created new refinements such as standardized care transition measures and structured interventions for family caregivers.

- **The Transitional Care Model.** This model was tested in Philadelphia-area hospitals from 1997 to 2001 by Dr. Mary Naylor and colleagues. Advanced practice nurses provided eight home visits to high-risk patients using techniques such as risk assessment, self-management education, continuity of care, and fostering interdisciplinary communication and collaboration (Hirschman, Shaid, McCauley, Pauly, & Naylor, 2015; Naylor et al., 2004). Subsequent research revealed that this intervention resulted in a significant decrease in both cost of care and readmissions during the study period.

- **Project RED (Re-Engineered Discharge).** This intervention was conducted at the Boston Medical Center from 2003 to 2004. "A nurse discharge advocate worked with patients during their hospital stay to arrange follow-up appointments, confirm medication reconciliation, and conduct patient education with an individualized instruction booklet that was sent to their primary care provider. A clinical pharmacist called patients 2 to 4 days after discharge to reinforce the discharge plan and review medications" (Jack et al., 2009, p. 178). Participants had a lower incidence of hospital utilization after the intervention.

- **The BOOST (Society for Hospital Medicine) Program.** This program utilizes an extensive series of tools and processes to improve care transitions. Some program elements include an eight-question risk assessment, an assessment of preparedness for discharge, patient education tools, follow-up phone calls, and interprofessional rounds (Hansen et al., 2013).

- **INTERACT (Interventions to Reduce Acute Care Transfers).** This is one of the few postacute (after acute care) evidence-based care transition programs. INTERACT is a publicly available program that focuses on improving the identification, evaluation, and management of acute changes in condition of nursing home residents. The program was developed through a CMS contract to the Georgia Medical Care Foundation, the Medicare Quality Improvement Organization in Georgia. While the primary focus of the program is on identifying and taking action on resident changes in condition, there are also evidence-based best practices to improve care transitions from SNFs to and from acute care hospitals.

Three key elements of this program are a facility capabilities list, standardized transfer forms for both hospitals and SNFs, and a medication reconciliation worksheet. The capabilities list is a formal document that details the capabilities of the SNF for hospital staff. These capabilities might include such things as whether the facility is IV certified.

The capabilities list helps hospital staff understand which facilities can provide the type of care their patients need after discharge. The standardized transfer forms help emergency room staff make informed decisions about the type of care needed by SNF residents who have been sent to the emergency room.

The forms sent by the hospital to the SNF ensure that time-sensitive information necessary to deliver care in the first few days after a transfer from an acute care hospital is received. The medication reconciliation worksheet provides guidance to SNF staff about medications from the sending acute care facility. This worksheet ensures that SNF patients, especially those taking multiple medications, receive the right drugs in the right way (Ouslander, Bonner, Herndon, & Shutes, 2014).

Common Elements of Evidence-Based Care Transition Programs

Each of these care transition program models, while quite variable in length, cost, staffing, and resources required, includes common elements:

- The programs are highly focused on patient needs. They pay less attention to utilization or insurance issues, possibly because most were grant funded.
- There is one clinician or transition coach assigned to manage the transition and to act as the patient and family advocate.

- The program is designed to "close the loop" on care transitions by contacting the patient and family after the transition to ensure that all necessary tasks were completed.
- Patient education using health literacy principles is usually an integral part of the evidence-based programs.
- Patient education emphasizes practical self-management skills for the next step in care, especially about how to identify clinical warning signs and when to call for help.
- Patient education in evidence-based care transitions ensures patient mastery of key knowledge and skills by using *teach-back* (asking the patient to repeat what was taught) and *return demonstration* (actually practicing a skill that was just taught).
- The programs typically use simple, standardized forms for communication with patients and for communication with health professionals at the next step in care.
- The programs educate both the patient and his or her network of support people and family caregivers.
- The programs reestablish the patient's connection with the primary care practitioner who coordinates the patient's care.
- There is a process for identifying and managing socioeconomic barriers to care such as access to transportation to medical appointments or being able to afford needed medications. Evidence-based programs take some responsibility for managing these social determinants of health as well as managing the medical aspects of care transitions.
- There is an effective system for transmitting information from the sending to receiving provider with a means to verify that information was received.

While your organization may not have a formal evidence-based care transition program, you can and should apply the lessons learned from these programs in your own care transition program. Use the checklist in **BOX 3-1** to assess how many best practices you currently have in place and how many you need to develop.

BOX 3-1 Checklist of Evidence-Based Care Transition Best Practices

Review the list and check off all items that apply to your transition program. Fewer checkoffs indicate a weaker program.

1. ❏ The transition program balances patient needs with insurance, utilization, and value-based payment goals. Patient needs should predominate.
2. ❏ There is one clinician or transition coach accountable for managing the transition process and the patient and family know how to contact this person.
3. ❏ The accountable clinician ensures that all necessary care tasks related to the transition were completed (prescriptions were provided, equipment was ordered and delivered, test results were reported, etc.).
4. ❏ The transition team provides patient education that is based on health literacy evidence-based best practices.
5. ❏ Patient education emphasizes practical self-management skills for the next step in care, with special emphasis on "clinical red flags" and when to call for help.
6. ❏ Patient mastery of self-management skills and knowledge are verified by using teach-back and return demonstration.
7. ❏ The program uses simple, standardized forms for communication with patients and for communication with health professionals at the next step in care.
8. ❏ The accountable clinician assesses family caregiver willingness and capability for providing patient support at the next step in care.
9. ❏ Family caregivers and other patient support people are included in all transition education, communication, and support activities.
10. ❏ The program connects the patient back to the primary care practitioner who coordinates the patient's care. This is done by notifying the primary care provider of the care transition and by facilitating follow-up primary care appointments.
11. ❏ There is a process for managing financial, social, and other barriers to care such as having transportation to medical appointments or being able to afford needed medications.
12. ❏ There is an effective system for transmitting information from the sending to receiving provider with a means to verify that information was actually received.

Tools and Techniques for Care Transitions from Evidence-Based Programs

Care transition programs employ a variety of tools and techniques that can easily be adopted in other settings. These tools are both part of the evidence-based models described earlier and available from other sources. Many tools are free and most are available on the internet. The most common types of tools and forms are:

- Assessments of patient and caregiver capability and readiness for discharge or self-care
- Patient medication lists
- Patient personal health records
- Patient discharge planning checklists
- Transition information transfer checklists
- Provider communication forms

TABLE 3-1 contains a list of tools, descriptions, and sources. Many of these tools are freely available for use in your own transition program, although some require written permission or payment for use.

TABLE 3-1 Evidence-Based Care Transition Program Tools and Techniques

Tool	Description	Source	Location
After Hospital Care Plan	Patient medication, appointment, and follow-up activities forms, questions for doctor in English and Spanish	Project RED	https://www.ahrq.gov /sites/default/files /publications/files /redtoolkitforms.pdf
Personal Health Record	Patient medications, appointments, questions for doctor in English, Spanish, and Somali	Care Transitions Intervention	http://caretransitions .org
Patient Activation Assessment®	Scores patient ability to manage medications, red flags, personal health record, medical follow-up	Care Transitions Intervention	http://caretransitions .org
Patient Activation Assessment® Guidelines	Instructions for scoring the Patient Activation Assessment	Care Transitions Intervention	http://caretransitions .org
The Family Caregiver Activation in Transitions Tool©	Assessment of family caregiver transition skills; requires permission of Eric Coleman MD, for use	Care Transitions Intervention	http://caretransitions .org
Medication Discrepancy Tool (MDT)®	A form for assessing patient level and system level medication discrepancy factors and documenting resolution of these issues	Care Transitions Intervention	http://caretransitions .org
8P Risk Assessment Screening Tool	A checklist of factors that might contribute to risk of adverse events after discharge	Project BOOST	http://www .hospitalmedicine.org/
The General Assessment of Preparedness (GAP)	A checklist that helps identify patient concerns prior to transitions out of the hospital	Project BOOST	https://store.hospital medicine.org /PersonifyEbusiness /Store
BOOST Teach-back Curriculum and Video	A video and curriculum that teaches providers the patient teach-back method to improve patient understanding and adherence	Project BOOST	Available for purchase from Society of Hospital Medicine eStore

Tool	Description	Source	Location
Patient PASS: A Transition Record Patient Preparation to Address Situations (after discharge)	A simple, one-page personal medical record for tracking patient medications, questions, follow-up information, and medical tests	Project BOOST	http://www.hospital medicine.org/
Taking Care of Myself When I Leave the Hospital	An extensive patient personal medical record	Project RED	www.ahrq.gov /sites/default/files /publications/files /goinghomeguide.pdf
Interventions to Reduce Acute Care Transfers (INTERACT) Tools for Nursing Home to Hospital Communication	<ul><li>Skilled nursing facility capabilities list</li><li>SBAR (situation, assessment, background, result) communication form</li><li>Medication reconciliation worksheet</li><li>Transfer forms for use between hospitals and postacute settings</li><li>Other forms and checklists are available from the INTERACT website</li></ul>	INTERACT	Interact Implementation Guide http://www .pathway-interact.com /wp-content/uploads /2017/04/INTERACT -V4-Implementation _Guide-Dec-10.pdf
National Transitions of Care Coalition (NTOCC)	Multiple educational tools and checklists for both providers and patients; most notable is the *Transitions of Care Checklist*, which contains instruments for assessing medication management capability and continuity of care status	NTOCC	http://www.ntocc.org /Portals/0/PDF /Resources/TOC _Checklist.pdf

▶ Current Challenges and Problems in Care Transitions

While the healthcare research literature is primarily focused on transitions from hospital to home, there are a huge number of other patient care transitions in other settings, each with its own unique challenges. These challenges are especially acute for frail elderly patients, those with mental health problems, and patients with dementia.

It is important to know that unless you are functioning as a case manager with ongoing patient contact and accountability for patient care, you probably only see and manage one or two types of transitions. Patients may experience many more types of transitions. It is vital for nurses to have some understanding of care transitions in other settings so that they can educate and advocate for patients.

Observation Status and Its Aftermath

One of the most problematic transition situations for frail older adults is an inpatient stay in "observation status." The Center for Medicare Advocacy defines observation status in this way: "CMS describes the issue as outpatients receiving 'observation services.' In reality these patients are patients in hospitals who receive medical, physician and nursing care, tests, medications, overnight lodging and food, but who are called outpatients" (Center for Medicare Advocacy, 2016).

The key impact of the observation status designation is that it is not considered a real inpatient stay and thus does not meet the Medicare "two midnight" requirement (a patient requires inpatient hospitalization in an acute care hospital for at least two midnights) for coverage of an SNF rehabilitation stay. This situation results in many frail older adults, who cannot afford to pay privately for rehabilitation or temporary assisted living care, being discharged home without the functional capability for self-care. The responsibility then falls to family members and possibly a home care agency to provide intensive and expensive in-home care. In many cases it creates extreme pressure on families to hire in-home personal care assistance that would have been provided in an SNF before the observation status rules were implemented. Many professional organizations have mounted lobbying campaigns to eliminate or mitigate the observation status rules, but at the time of this writing, it remains in force.

Shorter Skilled Nursing Facility Care Transitions

With the advent of the Affordable Care Act and value-based payment programs, SNFs are under considerable pressure to both reduce lengths of stay and reduce readmissions.

Observation stays and value-based payment pressures have completely changed the nature of SNF transitions in the last few years. Patients are typically admitted to SNF short-term rehabilitation after surgery, such as joint replacement, or after an acute hospital stay for an exacerbation of a chronic condition. Previous to changes in the healthcare system, patients receiving rehabilitation services stayed in SNFs for relatively long periods of time. At the time of discharge, most of these patients had regained their previous level of function after weeks of nursing care and rehabilitation. Now, while the Medicare benefit actually allows for up to 100 days of SNF care, most patient stays are far shorter. Patients still receive nursing care, patient teaching, and therapy, but are not always rehabilitated to their previous level of function before discharge, nor are the patient or family always fully competent in self-management skills. As in the observation stay scenario, this situation has created considerable pressure on families and home care agencies to take care of much more acutely ill patients.

SNFs that participate in bundled payment programs or are ACO preferred providers have a huge financial incentive to readmit their recently discharged patients back to their own facilities rather than to an acute care facility as a readmission to acute care triggers financial penalties to the SNF. This new impetus for shorter stays and lower readmissions has led to new strategies and new partnerships between SNFs and home health care.

Some of these strategies include mutual agreement on high-risk patient discharge criteria, home care staff involvement in discharge planning meetings at SNFs, home care nurse liaison visits to SNF patients to evaluate patient capacity for functioning at home to educate patients about home care, and to identify barriers to a safe discharge. In addition, SNF staff make follow-up phone calls to determine the patient's postdischarge status and to report to the home care agency or physician if problems are occurring. Home care staff periodically meet with the SNF clinical team to report on patient readmissions and to jointly debrief the situation and identify opportunities for future improvement.

Transition from Home to Emergency Care

Transitions from home to urgent or emergency care can be problematic when they are delayed too long. One nursing study found that 93% of patients with heart failure delayed seeking treatment, in some cases up to 2 weeks after the onset of symptoms, because they did not identify that the symptoms were serious or related to their heart problems (Reeder, Ercole, Peek, & Smith, 2015). In other cases, patients report delays in seeking treatment due to "the hassles involved," wanting to try self-care first, denial that the problem is serious, and "not wanting to bother anyone." In most of the evidence-based care transition programs mentioned in this chapter, patient education about "red flags" and when to report an exacerbation of symptoms are important educational elements. Programs often use colored "stoplight" charts to indicate the seriousness of symptom clusters with green, yellow, and red stoplight graphics. This type of patient education can make the difference between a patient seeking treatment promptly and potentially lethal treatment delays.

Another potentially highly traumatic transition to an inpatient hospice facility is, unfortunately, a common last-minute, end-of-life transition (Vig, Starks, Taylor, Hopley, & Fryer-Edwards, 2010).

Medication Reconciliation—A Transition Problem That Spans All Settings

Medication reconciliation, the process of ensuring that the patient is taking all currently prescribed medications correctly, is a universal patient safety problem in care transitions across the continuum of care. An article from the Cleveland Clinic states: "As many as 70% of patients may have an unintentional medication discrepancy at hospital discharge, with many of those discrepancies having potential for harm. Indeed, during the first few weeks

after discharge, 50% of patients have a clinically important medication error, and 20% experience an adverse event, most commonly an adverse drug event" (Sponsler, Neal, & Kripalani, 2015, p. 352). These adverse events occur as a result of multiple complex variables that originate from patients, providers, and systems.

In some cases, the medication reconciliation process simply requires ensuring that prescribed drugs are available to be given to the patient. In other settings, such as in home care, where drugs have been prescribed by multiple providers the health professional must ensure that the current drug list contains no duplicates, contraindicated medications, or drug interactions. Differences in facility drug formularies may create problems by creating inconsistency in the drugs that patients receive in different settings. In the home setting, patients often have medications that were prescribed before the inpatient stay. If not told specifically to stop taking them, they may just add the old medications to the newly prescribed ones. Another problem is driven by drug costs. In home care and primary care settings, patients sometimes refuse to switch to drugs newly prescribed during an inpatient stay because they "paid for the old ones and intend to finish them."

Among the more common care transition problems are getting an accurate account of the medications that were actually prescribed at the previous step in care from referral documents or facility EMRs. Patients' inability to self-manage medications is another huge problem in transitions from inpatient care to home.

Some techniques that have proved useful to prevent medication reconciliation problems are:

- The involvement of a pharmacist in postdischarge medication reconciliation phone calls
- The use of EMR software that evaluates medication lists for duplicate or contraindicated drugs and potential drug interactions
- Patient education about medications and supporting patients to create and maintain a current medication list

- Encouraging patients to bring all their current medications to medical visits for review
- Ensuring that recently discharged patients are seen by their primary care physician within 7 days of discharge so the primary care physician can evaluate inpatient prescribed drugs and develop a current and effective drug regimen for the patient
- Ensuring that over-the-counter medications (OTCs) are listed on the patient's master drug list
- The use of prepackaged "bubble pack" medications to avoid medication errors
- The use of electronic medication dispensers for patients with cognitive impairment
- Comparing the list of drugs prescribed at discharge with the list of drugs that the patient is currently taking
- Asking patients about financial barriers to filling prescriptions and finding benefits or entitlements that can help (Data from AHRQ, 2012)

Other problematic care transitions are those that occur at the end of life, mental health–related care transitions, and transitions for people with dementia.

ASK YOURSELF

- What types of problem care transitions do your patients experience?
- What causes the problems in these transitions?
- What can be done to alleviate or compensate for these problems?
- Can your organization forge an alliance with other providers to improve the quality of care transitions for patients?

▶ Tuning Up Your Care Transitions

Every healthcare organization has work processes that include patient transitions. Some are internal, such as the transfer of a patient from the hospital emergency room to an inpatient

unit. Many others involve movement of the patient from one care setting to the other. Effective internal transfers are essential elements in patient safety since it is at these handoff points that many medical errors occur. Our focus is on transitions that occur when patients move between care settings or from a care setting back to home. A good care transition system in a healthcare organization requires three key elements:

- Goals and measures
- A structure that supports effective transitions
- Transition workflows that are efficient and effective

Building a Structure That Can Achieve Care Transition Goals

To achieve care transition goals, health organizations must pay serious attention to the structures and processes that support transition outcomes. Care transition structural elements include:

- Senior management oversight and attention to care transition processes
- Functions and roles that manage care transitions
- Resources and time allocated to care transitions
- Policies and procedures that support effective care transitions
- Computer information systems and other tools for care transitions communication
- Forms and patient education materials that foster effective care transitions
- Negotiated relationships, expectations, and contracts with other providers who send patients to the facility or agency

FIGURE 3-3 uses a fishbone diagram to detail the various elements of a care transition program structure.

Assessing Your Care Transition Structure

The effectiveness of your care transitions will be strongly influenced by how well your transition structure is built and maintained.

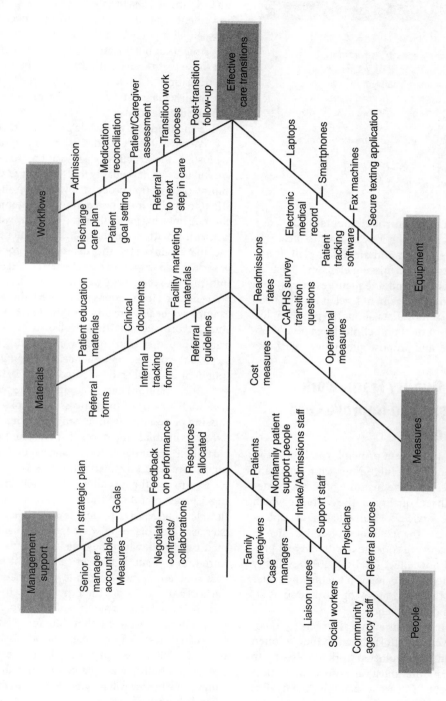

FIGURE 3-3 Fishbone Diagram—Elements of an Effective Care Transitions Program

ASK YOURSELF

After looking at the fishbone diagram:

- How many essential structural elements does your transition program have?
- Does senior management give transition programs the support they need?
- How many elements are missing or ineffective?
- Are you clear about transitions goals and measures?
- How many of these missing elements are you in a position to control?

If you can control elements of the care transitions process, it may be time to create an improvement team and an action plan. If accountability for the missing elements (such as goals, measures, and adequate resources) lies at the senior management level, it may be necessary to assemble data about the problem, list the organizational and clinical benefits of effective care, and propose alternative solutions.

Using a Quality Framework to Analyze and Improve Care Transitions

Quality improvement principles and tools can be particularly helpful in improving care transition processes. The Institute of Medicine defines healthcare quality as "the degree to which health care services for individuals and populations increase the likelihood of desired health outcomes and are consistent with current professional knowledge" (AHRQ, 2017). Quality improvement efforts focus on achieving better outcomes through improving work process efficiency and effectiveness.

Care transitions are ideal targets for quality improvement efforts because they so often involve complex, multistep work processes with multiple handoffs and a variety of communication elements. In care transitions "the devil is most definitely in the details."

Processes with this level of complexity cannot be improved just by talking about them. Improvement typically requires a formal meeting between all members of the care team—those departments or organizations that send patients and those that receive patients in the course of the transition. It is also necessary to use specific quality diagnostic and improvement tools to make the elements of the transition process visible and to identify possible gaps and cracks.

We have already used a fishbone diagram to illustrate the structure of a transition process. We will use two new quality tools to analyze and improve a transition process: flowcharting and a SIPOC (supplier input process output customer) chart. A flowchart is an illustration of the work tasks, information, handoffs, and computer entries that are linked together to produce a product or service in a work process. The AHRQ Health Information Technology website (AHRQ, 2017) offers detailed instructions for flowcharting and examples of healthcare process flowcharts. In its simplest form, flowcharting involves assembling a group of people who do the work, drawing the steps of the process in sequence, and then putting in directional arrows (Mind Tools, 2018).

Once the flowchart is complete, the team reviews the steps of the process and looks for missing pieces; problems at handoff points between individual employees, patients, and departments; redundant actions; unclear decision points; and excessive variation. It is very important to use the discipline of actually creating a paper picture of the workflow through flowcharting. Most participants in flowcharting exercises are amazed at what they learn about their own work when they see it made visible. Variation is a subtle but very important process problem. When everyone who performs parts of a process "does their own thing" in the way the work is performed, results are typically poorer because some methods are more effective than others. For example, if an admissions or intake department in a SNF or a home care agency has multiple people processing admissions, some people will inevitably perform more efficiently and effectively.

The key is to determine what the "best practice" in managing the transition should look like. An important outcome of a flowcharting process should be to create a draft "common process" for performing the transition process and testing to see if it works to produce better results.

FIGURE 3-4 provides simple instructions for creating a flowchart.

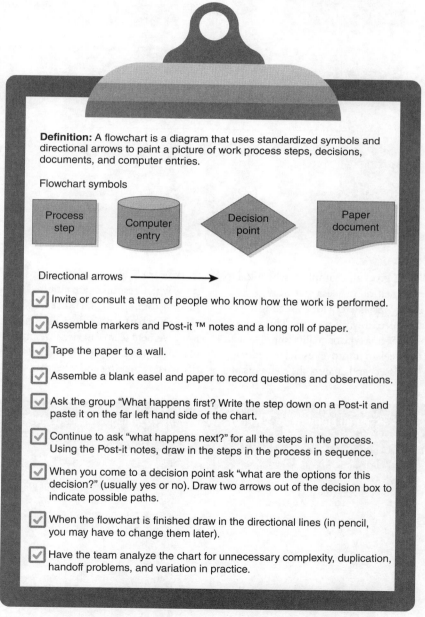

Definition: A flowchart is a diagram that uses standardized symbols and directional arrows to paint a picture of work process steps, decisions, documents, and computer entries.

Flowchart symbols

Process step   Computer entry   Decision point   Paper document

Directional arrows ⟶

☑ Invite or consult a team of people who know how the work is performed.

☑ Assemble markers and Post-it ™ notes and a long roll of paper.

☑ Tape the paper to a wall.

☑ Assemble a blank easel and paper to record questions and observations.

☑ Ask the group "What happens first? Write the step down on a Post-it and paste it on the far left hand side of the chart.

☑ Continue to ask "what happens next?" for all the steps in the process. Using the Post-it notes, draw in the steps in the process in sequence.

☑ When you come to a decision point ask "what are the options for this decision?" (usually yes or no). Draw two arrows out of the decision box to indicate possible paths.

☑ When the flowchart is finished draw in the directional lines (in pencil, you may have to change them later).

☑ Have the team analyze the chart for unnecessary complexity, duplication, handoff problems, and variation in practice.

FIGURE 3-4 Flowcharting Instructions

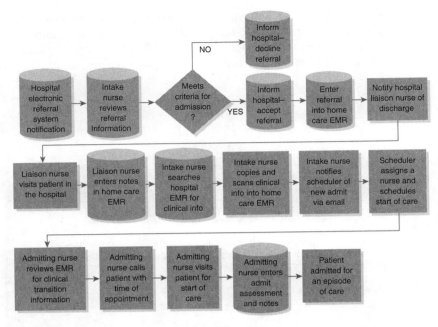

FIGURE 3-5 A Hospital to Home Health Care Transition

FIGURE 3-5 gives an example of a hospital to home care transition process workflow.

A SIPOC chart is a tool for dissecting the essential elements of a work process. This chart is used in the Six Sigma type of quality improvement projects (that seek to improve results by reducing variation) to dissect and analyze the elements of a work process, to map relationships, and to determine which resources are required and which are missing (Simon, 2018) (**TABLE 3-2**). By combining a SIPOC chart with a flowchart, members of an improvement team can visualize the key elements of a care transition process and can begin to identify what is missing and where things go wrong.

TABLE 3-2 Essential Elements of a Work Process—SIPOC Chart Definitions

Quality Term	Definition	Care Transition Example
Input	Information, tools, materials, and resources we need to do our job.	Computer programs patient information, transition guidelines, insurance authorizations, measures, forms, resource guides, etc. that are needed for care transitions.
Supplier	The people, department, or organization that provides us with the inputs we need to do our work.	Agencies or departments that refer patients to us for care. The people within the organization who do work that contributes to the care transition process.

Quality Term	Definition	Care Transition Example
Process	Linked activities that produce a product or service for a customer.	The steps in the transition process from patient assessment to checking on the results of the transition.
Customer	The people, departments, or organizations that use, regulate, or pay for the work outputs that we produce. The patient is the primary customer. Regulators, insurers, case managers, and other professionals are secondary customers.	Patients, families, insurance companies, regulatory agencies, organizations that receive patients from us.
Output	The end product or service that the customer receives and that is produced by our work processes.	The patient and his or her clinical information has been transitioned to the next step in care.
Requirements	The way the customer expects the product or service to look, feel, behave; standards for measures.	The patient and family expect a smooth transition with nothing "falling through the cracks." The next step in care expects accurate clinical information, specific requests for services, and information about the "patient's story." Regulatory agencies expect outcomes like limited readmissions.

Data from ASQ (American Society for Quality) quality glossary. https://asq.org/quality-resources/quality-glossary/o, accessed Jan 27, 2017; Baldridge Glossary, 2017.

FIGURE 3-6 shows a combined SIPOC chart and flowchart.

Here is how a SNF/home team might analyze the SIPOC chart and flowchart in Figure 3-6:

- The nursing home gets an electronic record from the patient's hospital stay when the patient is admitted to the facility. Unless we in the home care agency ask them to send us a discharge summary we won't have that information for our start of care.
- During the patient discharge planning meeting, if the patient and family are not involved, the care plan may not be realistic or reflect patient goals and needs.
- When the discharge plan is developed, if the social worker does not understand the capabilities and limitations of home care,

he or she may assume that care at home will be safe when it is not or may plan a premature discharge.

Looking at the flowchart and SIPOC chart, see if you can identify other potential care transitions problems.

ASK YOURSELF

- Would flowcharting or a SIPOC chart help my organization improve care transitions?
- If the answer is yes, try these tools and use the insights to improve your transition processes.

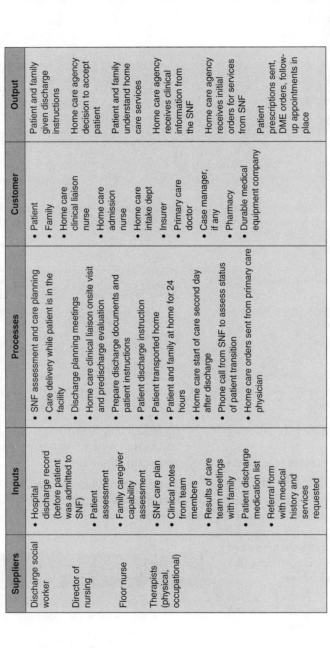

Suppliers	Inputs	Processes	Customer	Output
Discharge social worker Director of nursing Floor nurse Therapists (physical, occupational)	• Hospital discharge record (before patient was admitted to SNF) • Patient assessment • Family caregiver capability assessment • SNF care plan • Clinical notes from team members • Results of care team meetings with family • Patient discharge medication list • Referral form with medical history and services requested	• SNF assessment and care planning • Care delivery while patient is in the facility • Discharge planning meetings • Home care clinical liaison onsite visit and predischarge evaluation • Prepare discharge documents and patient instructions • Patient discharge instruction • Patient transported home • Patient and family at home for 24 hours • Home care start of care second day after discharge • Phone call from SNF to assess status of patient transition • Home care orders sent from primary care physician	• Patient • Family • Home care clinical liaison nurse • Home care admission nurse • Home care intake dept • Insurer • Primary care doctor • Case manager, if any • Pharmacy • Durable medical equipment company	• Patient and family given discharge instructions • Home care agency decision to accept patient • Patient and family understand home care services • Home care agency receives clinical information from the SNF • Home care agency receives initial orders for services from SNF • Patient prescriptions sent, DME orders, follow-up appointments in place

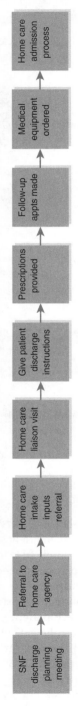

FIGURE 3-6 SIPOC/Flowchart of a Skilled Nursing Facility (SNF) to Home Care Transition

Here is a hint for looking at care transition flowcharts: Problems and gaps usually occur in the handoffs between individuals, disciplines, departments, and organizations. When results are poor, look in the "white space" between parts of the process. The tips and techniques that follow provide some potential solutions to transition workflow problems.

Tips and Techniques for Better Care Transitions

- **Analyze the types of care transitions that your organization manages** and that your patients experience in other settings.
- **Identify high-risk gaps and cracks in your care transition workflow**. Where might patients become confused or where could follow-up tests "fall through the cracks?" For example, home care agencies do not admit patients until 24 hours after inpatient discharge. During this period patients are still theoretically under the care of the discharging institution but have not yet seen a new clinician.
- **Use data to identify care transition results and opportunities for improvement**. If your organization has a patient tracking system or participates in one, find out where your patients are going. If you are getting "problem" referrals from some sources, explore the process, have a discussion with the "sending" providers, and try to improve the process.
- **List your key suppliers (places and people that send you patients) and your key customers (places and people that receive your patients)**. List their key requirements. If you don't know their requirements go to the next bullet.
- **Have a customer/supplier conversation and negotiation with your referral sources and the providers who typically receive patients from your setting**. Discuss roles, responsibilities, information needs, and accountabilities. Find out more about the capabilities and admission criteria for other healthcare organizations that you work with. Obtain brochures, marketing materials, and capabilities lists from your referral partners. When possible formulate written agreements or at least exchange emails that clarify roles and responsibilities.
- **Develop a robust network of relationships**. Organizations that have a marketing/community outreach function often develop relationships with other organizations that can be leveraged to improve care transitions. When members of the sales team attend networking functions or make sales calls, they often get to know discharge planners and clinical staff. These relationships can be very useful in negotiating workflows or resolving transition problems. In integrated delivery systems, preferred provider partners often work together in a formal way to develop joint workflows, participate in case conferences, and perform patient tracking and outcomes monitoring. These close working relationships typically result in better transition outcomes and fewer readmits.
- **Visit other care settings that send or receive patients from your facility or organization**. If you are in an SNF then go on a home visit with a home care nurse case manager. If you are in home care then tour an SNF and talk to the nurses and discharge planners. If you are in a hospital or medical office then visit an SNF, home care, or assisted living facility. Go with a visiting nurse on a home visit. This can be an eye-opening experience for inpatient clinicians who don't really know what happens to patients when they go home (e.g., all prescribed medications dumped into a single bowl, a Hoyer lift that is used only as a swing by grandchildren, no hospital or other healthcare organization literature or phone numbers to be found anywhere in the home).
- **Talk to clinical staff who perform formal care transition functions**. Ask them what obstacles they see, what questions patients ask, and where they see potential transition failures.
- **Interview patients and their families about their care transition experiences**. Focus

on what it was like when they entered your care setting and what happened when you transferred them to the next step in care.

- **Improve written and electronic communication using templates, standardized forms, and communication tools**. Using a standardized template in your medical record helps everyone understand what has occurred during a patient transition. Templates should include a checklist of standardized items such as medications, transportation, food, follow-up medical care, and knowledge of red flags.

- **Ask someone from outside your organization to read your discharge or patient transition instructions** and identify inconsistencies, unclear communications, and things they don't understand.

- **Learn from the best**. Call or visit providers who have care transition best practices in place. Learn about problems they have solved, obstacles they have overcome, and tools they have successfully used. Consider adopting an evidence-based care transition program.

- **Develop community resource lists for patients and staff**. With shorter stays, patients and families are left to their own devices to find resources after care ends. Make it easier for them and for your staff with good information about services that may be available.

▶ When Things Go Wrong—Why Care Transitions Fail

Poor care transitions can take a terrible toll in human suffering and in wasteful expenditures. Care transition failures are a problem with multiple root causes. Laurie Page, DPT, a clinician, educator, and consulting physical therapist, describes some of the factors that contribute to care transitions and connection failures:

- I find many clinicians working in one setting (hospital, SNF) have a disconnect with the reality of patients' safety in a non-clinic setting (i.e. standard use of wall grab bars for transfers in bathrooms in hospitals and SNFs).

- Patients (and their families /caregivers) would benefit from a case manager who crosses settings including the home to improve safety and reduce unnecessary rehospitalizations. Even a true case manager within settings would help.

- Many different staff instruct in many different ways in part due to their own experiences and knowledge base. (This is very confusing to patients.)

- I still see/hear/read documentation that is single discipline specific. Productivity demands, a linear hierarchy amongst disciplines, which creates barriers to true 'INTERDISCIPLINARY' care where we all respect and learn from each other." (Laurie Page, PT, DPT, 2016, personal communication)

ASK YOURSELF

- Do you really know what goes on in settings other than your own? How does your knowledge or lack of it affect the way you plan patient care transitions?
- Who is coordinating care across the continuum for your patients—the primary care physician, a case manager, the family, or nobody? If nobody, how can you help the patient achieve a safe transition?
- Are you communicating with your colleagues about how you each educate patients?
- Is your patient education consistent? Could you do more to collaborate with your colleagues on key education points, terminology, and materials to reduce patient confusion?
- Is the care you are delivering truly interdisciplinary? Are all disciplines represented in discharge planning?

Root Causes of Transition Failures

Any process that involves multiple organizations, multiple disciplines, competing expectations, and incentives is fraught with potential for failure points (Greiner, 2017). Some of the most common causes of imperfect care transitions are discussed next.

Lack of Communication or Miscommunication Between Care Providers

Health facility and provider communication is a huge root cause of poor care transition outcomes. The dimensions of this problem include:

- Little to no relevant information is transmitted to the next step in care.
- Mismatch of expectations between sending and receiving clinicians about what information is important to share.
- Lack of a common language. Each provider uses his or her own industry jargon to the confusion of other providers in the transition chain.
- No incentive to share information—the discharging provider is unaware of the next step in care or sees no reason to share information.
- Lack of standardized information checklists for postdischarge communication.

Faulty clinical data exchange between providers is one of the key reasons that transitions fail. In most cases these disconnects are honest misunderstandings of what the next step in care needs. In rare instances the communication disconnect is conscious: "If I tell the truth about this patient's insurance gaps, lack of caregiver support or functional deficits, I may not be able to get, them discharged." Situations like these require immediate conversation and issue resolution to ensure that safe care is provided to patients. **FIGURE 3-7** illustrates the difference between flowing and "throw it over the wall," care transitions.

Failure to Identify and Engage Family Caregivers

Most of the literature on care transitions addresses the engagement and education of each specific patient. Much less attention has been paid to the role of the family caregiver. In reality, successful discharges to home or between settings for seriously ill patients are often dependent on the existence and willingness of a dedicated family caregiver or other support person.

The few existing studies indicate that family caregivers often feel ignored or left out of communications and education for and about the family member they are caring for. While the healthcare system expects family caregivers to take responsibility for complex medical tasks

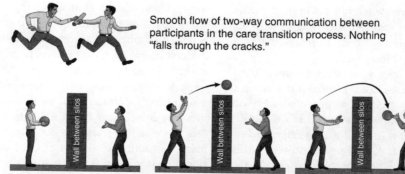

Smooth flow of two-way communication between participants in the care transition process. Nothing "falls through the cracks."

"Throw it over the wall" – one-way, disconnected care transitions communication

FIGURE 3-7 Care Transitions—Connected and Flowing or "Throw It Over the Wall"

and care coordination after discharge they typically don't receive the type of in-depth education necessary to manage these tasks (Reinhard, Levine, & Samis, 2012).

Another complicated aspect of family caregiver support is determining the roles of various family caregivers. While there is often one "lead" caregiver, other family caregivers may take responsibility for various aspects of care such as finance and insurance management and household maintenance. Without a purposeful conversation with family members, health professionals may not identify the caregiver whose role it is to manage care transitions and may mistakenly give information to the wrong person.

Another problem is the lack of availability of family caregivers to attend key patient-related meetings or to be present at discharge due to other work or family obligations. For long-distance caregivers who live away their loved one, this lack of availability can become a real barrier to good care planning.

Eric Coleman, the architect of the *Care Transitions Intervention*, described the positive impact of an enhancement to the CTI model that better incorporated the concerns of the family caregiver into transitional care. These enhancements included simulations and role-playing communication with health professionals, enhanced caregiver medication management education, and phone call follow-up specifically with the caregiver (Coleman, Roman, Halt, & Min, 2015). Even when present in the patient's life, a caregiver may not always agree with the recommendations of health professionals involved in the patient's care.

Disputes over what services are actually needed, the best place for the next step in care, the type of care that will be provided, who will be responsible for what aspects of care coordination, and how to pay for care can all be areas for conflict. A common example of this is a recommendation for 24-hour care in the home after discharge from an SNF or home health care. Health professionals, in pursuit of

a "safe discharge," will often insist on this requirement for functionally disabled patients. Families who may not have the means or the willingness to pay for such services will often either dispute the need or agree and simply not arrange for the service.

Lack of an Adequate Caregiver Support System

Of even more concern than fragmentary communication to caregivers is the lack of an adequate caregiving support system for seriously ill patients.

A Harris Poll survey of 1,000 seniors commissioned by CareMore (Caffrey, 2016) found that a third of chronically ill elderly patients stated that no one coordinated their medical care. For many nurse care coordinators, this lack of caregiving support creates a nightmare scenario for effective care transition planning. Elderly patients, especially those with mild to moderate dementia, who live alone or with an inadequate or disengaged caregiver, are at the greatest risk. Another area of high concern is a caregiver who is mentally ill, physically ill, a substance abuser, or neglecting or abusing the patient unbeknownst to the care team. Situations like these usually require intensive effort, creativity, strong knowledge of community benefits and resources, and the expertise of a cross-functional team of experts, usually including an experienced nurse care coordinator, social workers, and therapy clinicians.

Preexisting relationships with community benefit programs and agencies can make these difficult cases much easier to manage. A good example is the Interagency Council developed by an Agency on Aging in one community. This group which includes local nonprofits, community geriatric care managers, home healthcare agencies, SNFs, and hospital care managers meets bimonthly for networking and informational sessions. On months when there is no educational meeting the group holds "M" team meetings during which members bring difficult cases for discussion and get advice and support from other members.

Lack of Knowledge or Misperceptions About the Next Setting in Care

Health professionals must educate themselves about the organizations and professionals in their continuum of care—learning what these organizations do, what their capabilities are, what requirements they must meet, and what they need from the step in care before theirs.

For example, if you work in a hospital, do you know whether your patient meets the requirements for admission to an SNF, what care looks like in that setting, or what information the staff in the SNF need from you? Sometimes there is simply a failure of knowledge and imagination on the part of the sending clinician.

For example, a young, white physician or nurse from a middle-class family may have no idea of the types of problems and obstacles that an older black woman faces who has little caregiving support, is being discharged to subsidized housing, and has limited financial means for transportation, purchasing medications, and obtaining food. Clinicians who have never made a home visit or never visited an SNF may have no idea of the types of patient care capabilities and limitations that exist in these settings. As one admission liaison for an SNF commented, "Some of the residents in the hospital think that a nursing home is just like a hospital with multiple RNs available around the clock to do all the things that hospital nurses do. It isn't like that and some of the things they expect us to do after discharge aren't reasonable."

Patient Resistance to Discharge Plans

Like family caregivers, patients may not always agree with discharge plans. Many patients who have been acutely ill see a discharge as a "get out of jail free card" that enables them to escape the discomfort of the inpatient facility and return to a familiar home setting where they assume that things will go along much as they always have. These patients may not be aware of the impact of the hospitalization on their functional abilities, especially if they have some degree of dementia, have had delirium, or are simply still feeling the effects of surgical anesthesia.

A well-educated, 79-year-old man insisted on going home despite recommendations for an SNF stay because, as he put it, "I am feeling much better and I know that I will do better in my own environment." Unfortunately, his prediction was not correct and he fell at home soon after discharge and had to be readmitted.

In other circumstances, patients may refuse home health care for privacy reasons ("I don't want anybody in my house,") or because they are concerned that the home health nurse may consider the home environment unsafe and "put me in a nursing home." People with hoarding issues frequently fall into this category.

Cost is often a factor in patient and family decisions to disagree with health professional recommended discharges. While professionals may see a clear need for a short respite stay in assisted care or good reasons to hire live-in help for a period of time, patients and families who cannot afford to pay will dispute the recommendation or simply not follow it.

While patients have a clear right to follow their discharge preferences in these circumstances, and in many cases actually have no choice, these are precarious transitions that all too often end in a readmission.

Rushed Discharge Planning

When the focus is on productivity and shortening inpatient stays and not on effectiveness, discharge planning can be hurried and fragmented, leaving loose ends for both patients and providers who will care for the patient after discharge.

This is especially true in facilities that do not value effective care transitions and simply add the responsibility onto the work of an already harried clinician.

Lack of an Accountable Clinician to Oversee the Handoff of Care

This is one of the most common care transition failures, especially in settings that have an "assembly line" mentality about care and assume that once the patient leaves their setting, their care is no longer the responsibility of the sending clinician. Typically, attention is more focused on patients being admitted or coming into the setting than leaving it. All the evidence-based programs described in this chapter have a specific mechanism for closing this gap in care by having a clinician call or sending a clinician or patient advocate to visit the patient after he or she leaves the care setting to ensure that the patient is doing well or to identify problems. Families and patients experience a high level of distress when they are caught in the "white space" between two organizations without a clear idea of who to call for information or help.

Cultural Competence Barriers

Complex care transitions require clear communication to all parties involved. When language barriers and cultural misunderstandings occur, transitions can become problematic. For example, caring for a frail elder at home may be a strong value in a particular culture. A care manager's insistence on a nursing home stay for a frail elder after a hospital admission might be seen by the family as a way of questioning the family's caregiving capabilities.

Language barriers and assumptions about patient and family perceptions can create nightmare transition situations. Issues of sexual orientation and gender identity can also complicate care transition efforts if they are not properly understood by clinical staff.

⌕ CASE STUDY

Anna told the story of her mother's impending, and almost disastrous, hospital discharge. Her mother, whose native language is Spanish, had had a stroke and needed total care. She was aphasic, but could understand spoken Spanish. The family was caring for her at home and had been involved in her care, but the nurses who were coordinating her care did not seem to understand the family role. They communicated only to the patient through an interpreter. Although the patient understood what was being said, she couldn't respond. The nursing staff made arrangements for the patient to be transferred "to a facility" by ambulance, not knowing that the facility was the family home. The patient's family members were at work on the planned discharge day, so if the discharge had gone as planned. no one would have been at home to receive their mother when the ambulance arrived. Luckily, one of the patient's daughters called the hospital and was able to work with the hospital nurses on an appropriate discharge plan. The family was angered by this experience, and 5 years after their mother's death, they were still telling this story.

Patient Education Failures

Patients must leave a care setting knowing what to expect at the next stop in the care continuum and, if they are going home, how to self-manage. All too often, patient education consists of handing out a checklist or brochure and a hurried review of the items on it, without any attempt to verify patient or family understanding.

Because patients in inpatient settings are often stressed, not feeling well, and anxious to get home, patient teaching at discharge is not the ideal "teachable moment."

Teaching in this situation seldom includes "teach back" or a "return demonstration" in which the patient or family member demonstrates that he or she understands the instructions that have been given and can perform necessary self-care tasks at home.

A good example of this is outpatient cataract surgery. After surgery, patients are expected to receive several types of eye drops multiple times per day. Administering eye drops correctly actually involves a relatively high degree of manual dexterity, which many patients lack. Few facilities demonstrate the procedure and then watch the patient demonstrate proper administration. Managing the complex schedule of multiple drops requires organizational skills as well, a fact that should be checked through "teach back" by asking the caregiver or family to explain exactly how and when they plan to administer the drops. In a rushed environment, it is seldom easy to have the facility nurse incorporate this type of patient education into his or her daily routine, but doing so avoids unnecessary call backs and adverse events.

▶ Chapter Summary

Effective care transitions are an essential element in connected care. Readmissions and patient safety failures are serious consequences of poor transitions. Nurses play a key role in care transitions as care coordinators and case managers. Key measures for care transitions are 30-day readmission rates, medication reconciliation measures, costs of transitions, and CAHPS questions about patient care transition experiences. New cross-organizational measures are an integral part of the 2014 IMPACT Act implementation. There are many evidence-based best practices in care transitions, primarily for patient transitions from acute care to home.

Essential best practices for all settings include accountability across handoff points, verifying that information sent was received and understood, planing for primary care medical follow-up, completing all postdischarge follow-up tasks, and proving patient self-management support. Good transitions require an understanding of and communication with the next step in care. Technology plays a key role in communications through medical records interoperability, electronic patient tracking, and in some cases interactive voice response systems post discharge. There are significant gaps and challenges in care transitions, including insurance gaps, medication reconciliation, observation status, end-of-life transitions, and mental health–related patient discharge issues. Readers can use the tools and techniques of quality improvement including flowcharts and SIPOC charts to identify and eliminate flaws in care transitions processes.

References

Agency for Healthcare Research and Quality. (2012). Medications at Transitions and Clinical Handoffs (MATCH) Toolkit for medication reconciliation. Retrieved from https://www.ahrq.gov/sites/default /files/publications/files/match.pdf

Agency for Healthcare Research and Quality. (2016). Making care transitions safer: The pivotal role of nurses. Retrieved from https://www.ahrq.gov/news /blog/ahrqviews/pivotal-role-nurses.html

Agency for Healthcare Research and Quality. (2017). Health information technology, flowchart. Retrieved from https://healthit.ahrq.gov/health-it-tools-and -resources/workflow-assessment-health-it-toolkit /all-workflow-tools/flowchart

Understanding Quality Measurement. Content last reviewed November 2017. Agency for Healthcare Research and Quality, Rockville, MD. http://www.ahrq.gov/professionals /quality-patient-safety/quality-resources/tools/chtoolbx /understand/index.html

American Medical Directors Association. (2010). Improving transitions between the nursing facility and the acute care hospital setting. Policy Resolution H10.

American Society for Quality. (2017). Quality glossary. Retrieved from https://asq.org/quality-resources/quality -glossary/o

Baldrige Glossary. (2017). Glossary. Work processes definition. Retrieved from http://www.baldrige21.com/BALDRIGE _GLOSSARY/BN/Work_Processes.html

Burton, R. (2012, September 13). Health policy brief: Care transitions. *Health Affairs*. Retrieved from http:// healthaffairs.org/healthpolicybriefs/brief_pdfs/health policybrief_76.pdf

Caffrey, M. (2016) Poll finds major care coordination gaps among seniors. *American Journal of Managed Care*. https://www.ajmc.com/focus-of-the-week/ poll-finds-major-care-coordination-gaps-among -seniors

Case Management Society of America. (2016). *Standards of practice for case management*. Little Rock, AR: CMSA.

Castellucci, M. (2016, September 16). Innovations: PatientPing helps ACOs track patient care. *Modern Healthcare*. Retrieved from http://www.modernhealthcare.com/article/20160903/MAGAZINE/309039978

Center for Medicare Advocacy. (2016). Observation status and the NOTICE Act: Advocates not over the moon. Retrieved from medicareadvocacy.org-Observation%20Status%20and%20the%20NOTICE%20Act%20Advocates%20Not%20Over%20the%20MOON

Centers for Medicare and Medicaid Services. (2015). HCAHPS survey. Retrieved from www.hcahpsonline.org/files/HCAHPS%20V10.0%20Appendix%20A%20-%20HCAHPS%20Mail%20Survey%20Materials%20(English)%20March%202015.pdf

Centers for Medicare and Medicaid Services. (2017). IMPACT Act spotlights and announcements. Retrieved from https://www.cms.gov/medicare/quality-initiatives-patient-assessment-instruments/post-acute-care-quality-initiatives/impact-act-of-2014/spotlights-and-announcements

Coleman, E., Roman, S., Halt, K., & Min, S. (2015). Enhancing the care transitions intervention protocol to better address the needs of family caregivers. *Journal for Healthcare Quality, 37*(1), 2–11.

Coleman, E.A., Parry, C., Chalmers, S., & Min, S. (2006, September 25). The care transitions intervention results of a randomized controlled trial. *Archives of Internal Medicine, 166*, 1822–1828.

Coleman, E. A., Smith, J. D., Frank, J. C., Eilertsen, T. B., Thiare, J. N., & Kramer, A. M. (2002). Development and testing of a measure designed to assess the quality of care transitions. *International Journal of Integrated Care, 2*, e02.

Forster, A. J., Murff, H. J., Peterson, J. F., Gandhi, T. K., & Bates, D. W. (2003). The incidence and severity of adverse events affecting patients after discharge from the hospital. *Annuls of Internal Medicine, 138*(3), 161–167.

Freeman, G. (2016). 5 ways to ensure extensivists improve outcomes and cut costs. *HealthLeaders Media*.

Greiner, A. (2007). White space or black hole: What can we do to improve care transitions? Issue Brief #6. American Board of Internal Medicine Foundation.

Hansen, L. O., Greenwald, J. L., Budnitz, T., Howell, E., Halasyamani, L., Maynard, G., . . . Williams, M. V. (2013). Project BOOST: Effectiveness of a multihospital effort to reduce rehospitalization. *Journal of Hospital Medicine, 8*, 421–427. doi:10.1002/jhm.205

HealthIT.gov. (2015). What is a patient portal? Retrieved from https://www.healthit.gov/providers-professionals/faqs/what-patient-portal

Heyworth, L., Paquin, A. M., Clark, J., Kamenker, V., Stewart, M., Martin, T., & Simon, S. R. (2014). Engaging patients in medication reconciliation via a patient portal following hospital discharge. *Journal of the American Medical Informatics Association, 21*(e1), e157–e162. http://doi.org/10.1136/amiajnl-2013-001995

Hines, A., Barrett, M., Jiang, J., & Steiner, C. (2014). Conditions With the Largest Number of Adult Hospital Readmissions by Payer, 2011 - Statistical Brief #172). Retrieved from https://www.hcup-us.ahrq.gov/reports/statbriefs/sb172-Conditions-Readmissions-Payer.jsp

Hirschman, K., Shaid, E., McCauley, K., Pauly, M., & Naylor, M. (2015). Continuity of care: The transitional care model. *The Online Journal of Issues in Nursing, 20*(3), manuscript 1. doi:10.3912/OJIN.Vol20No03Man01

Hongmai, H., Grossman, J., Cohen, G., & Bodenheimer, T. (2008). Hospitalists and care transitions: The divorce of inpatient and outpatient care. *Health Affairs, 27*(5), 1315–1327. doi:10.1377/hlthaff.27.5.1315

Jack, B., Chetty V. K., Anthony, D., Greenwald, J. L., Sanchez, G. M., Johnson, A. E., . . . Culpepper, L. (2009). A reengineered hospital discharge program to decrease rehospitalization: A randomized trial. *Annals of Internal Medicine, 150*(3), 178–188. Retrieved from http://www.bu.edu/fammed/projectred/publications/AnnalsArtcile2-09.pdf

Johnson, C. (2016, February 26). The doctor is in: Hospitalists take lead role in coordinating care. UC San Diego Health Newsroom. Retrieved from health.ucsd.edu/news/features/Pages/2016-02-26-hospitalists-take-care-lead.aspx

The Joint Commission. (2012). Hot topics in health care, transitions of care, the need for a more effective approach to continuing patient care. Retrieved from https://www.jointcommission.org/assets/1/18/Hot_Topics_Transitions_of_Care.pdf

Krumholtz, H. (2013). Post-hospital syndrome—an acquired, transient condition of generalized risk. *New England Journal of Medicine, 368*, 100–102. doi:10.1056/NEJMp1212324

Lamb, G. (Ed.). (2014). *Care coordination: The game changer, how nursing is revolutionizing quality care*. Silver Spring, MD: American Nurses Association.

Mackinnon, K., & Mansfield, V. (2015). Connect4 patients ↔ CCCM ↔ primary care ↔ community. Middlesex Hospital Grand Rounds Presentation.

Medicare Learning Network. (2015). Connecting post acute care across the care continuum. Retrieved from https://www.cms.gov/Outreach-and-Education/Outreach/NPC/Downloads/2016-02-04-IMPACT-Act-Presentation.pdf

Mind Tools. (2018). Flowcharts—identify and communicate your optimal process. Retrieved from www.mindtools.com/pages/article/newTMC_97.htm

National Association of Social Workers. (2003). *Standards for social work services in long term care facilities*. Washington, DC: NASW.

National Quality Forum. (2014). NQF-endorsed measures for care coordination: Phase 3. Technical report. Retrieved from http://www.qualityforum.org/Publications/2014/12/NQF-Endorsed_Measures_for_Care_Coordination_Phase_3.aspx

National Transitions of Care Coalition. (2010a). Improving transitions of care, findings and considerations of the "Vision of the National Transitions of Care Coalition." Retrieved from http://www.ntocc.org/portals/0/pdf /resources/ntoccissuebriefs.pdf

National Transitions of Care Coalition. (2010b). Improving transitions of care with health information technology. Position Paper of the Health Information Technology Work Group for the National Transitions of Care Coalition.

Naylor, M. (2008). Transitional care: Moving patients from one care setting to another. *American Journal of Nursing, 108*(9), S58–63. doi:10.1097/01.NAJ.0000336420.34946.3a

Naylor, M. D., Brooten, D. A., Campbell, R. L., Maislin, G., McCauley, K. M., & Schwartz, J. S. (2004). Transitional care of older adults hospitalized with heart failure: A randomized, controlled trial. *Journal of the American Geriatrics Society, 52,* 675–684. Retrieved from http://www.cha.com/pdfs/Quality%5CReducing%20Hospital%20Readmissions/Related%20Articles/Transitional%20Care%20of%20Older%20Adults.pdf

Ouslander, J., Bonner, A., Herndon, L., & Shutes, J. (2014). The INTERACT quality improvement program: An overview for medical directors and primary care clinicians in long-term care. *Journal of the American Medical Directors Association, 15*(3), 162–170. doi:10.1016/j.jamda.2013.12.005

Page, L. (2016). Personal communication.

Rau, J. (2016). Medicare's readmission penalties hit new high. Kaiser Health News. Retrieved from http://khn.org/news/more-than-half-of-hospitals-to-be-penalized-for-excess-readmissions/

Reeder, K., Ercole, P., Peek, J., & Smith, C. (2015). Symptom perceptions and self-care behaviors in patients who self-manage heart failure. *Journal of Cardiovascular Nursing, 30*(1), e1–7. doi:10.1097/JCN.0000000000000117

Reinhard, S., Levine, C., & Samis, S. (2012). Home alone—family caregivers providing complex chronic care.

AARP Policy Brief. Retrieved from home-alone-family-caregivers-providing-complex-chronic-care-in-brief-AARP-ppi-health.pdf

Simon, K. (2018). SIPOC diagram. Retrieved from https://www.isixsigma.com/tools-templates/sipoc-copis/sipoc-diagram/www.isixsigma.com

Snow, V., Beck, D., Budnitz, T., Miller, D. C., Potter, J., Wears, R. L., . . . Williams, M. V. (2009). Transitions of care consensus policy statement American College of Physicians-Society of General Internal Medicine-Society of Hospital Medicine-American Geriatrics Society-American College of Emergency Physicians-Society of Academic Emergency Medicine. *Journal of General Internal Medicine, 24*(8), 971–976. doi:10.1007/s11606-009-0969-x

Sponsler, K., Neal, E., & Kripalani, S.(2015). Improving medication safety during hospital based transitions of care. *Cleveland Clinic Journal of Medicine, 82*(6), 351–360. PMID:26086494 DOI:10.3949/ccjm.82a.14025

Struck, R. (2013). Telling the patient's story with electronic health records. *Nursing Management, 44*(7), 13–15. doi:10.1097/01.NUMA.0000431433.46631.cc

URAC. (2017). Health utilization management. Retrieved from www.urac.org/accreditation-and-measurement/accreditation-programs/case-management-programs/health-utilization-management/

Vig, E. K., Starks, H., Taylor, J. S., Hopley, E. K., & Fryer-Edwards, K. (2010). Why don't patients enroll in hospice? Can we do anything about it? *Journal of General Internal Medicine, 25*(10), 1009–1019. http://doi.org/10.1007/s11606-010-1423-9

Wood, S. (2017). Personal communication.

Zuckerman, M. P. H., Sheingold, S. H., Orav, E. J., Ruhter, J., & Epstein, A. M. (2016). Readmissions, observation, and the hospital readmissions reduction program. *New England Journal of Medicine, 374,* 1543–1551. doi:10.1056/NEJMsa1513024

CHAPTER 4

Leading for Connected Care— The Senior Management Role

▶ Introduction

In our current tumultuous and challenging world, effective leadership at the senior management level is essential to the achievement of connected care. In this chapter we will explore the role of senior managers in helping organizations make the shift from fragmented to integrated and connected care. We will look at three healthcare paradigms that are driving healthcare culture change: population health, patient safety culture change, and integrated delivery systems

as well as external challenges such as the current political turmoil surrounding the Affordable Care Act. Using recent data from healthcare senior management surveys, we will look at the key challenges and opportunities that healthcare organizations face as they progress through the volume-to-value shift.

The chapter will explore how clinical leaders are gaining more organizational power and creating new and more integrated healthcare cultures in tandem with administrative leaders. We will also delve more deeply into the skills and capabilities needed by healthcare senior managers in complex environments. The chapter will describe the steps that senior managers can take to work with middle managers, front line clinicians, and support staff to connect the dots and close the gaps in care for patients, families, and health professionals. Finally, we will look at the many obstacles that leaders face as they attempt to create connected care and achieve the quadruple aim.

▶ Senior Managers Face a Storm of Change and Challenge

National Challenges Affect Senior Management

In Chapter 1 we framed the issues of fragmentation and connected care in the light of the landmark report "Crossing the Quality Chasm." In 2017, the National Academy of Medicine produced a new report, *Vital Directions for Health Care Priorities*, which provides current information on the challenges facing the healthcare system and, by extension, senior managers in healthcare organizations. This publication also proposes a clear and succinct model for new health action priorities that can also serve as guidelines for healthcare senior management teams. The paper describes the fundamental challenges facing U.S. health care as:

- Persistent inequities in health
- A rapidly aging population
- New and emerging healthcare threats such as new infectious diseases and natural disasters due to global warming
- Persisting care fragmentation and discontinuity
- Health expenditure costs and waste
- Constrained innovation due to outmoded approaches

Of the issues listed, the ones most applicable to our discussion of connected care are care fragmentation and the cost of waste. The paper describes the fragmentation issue this way: "While recent efforts on payment reform have aimed to advance coordinated care models, much of health care delivery still remains fragmented and siloed. This is particularly true for complex, high-cost patients—those with fundamentally complex medical, behavioral, and social needs" (Dzau, McClellan, & McGinnis, 2017, pp. 3–4). The paper goes on to explain that an estimated 30% of healthcare expenditures can be attributed to wasteful or excess costs, many of which are the result of missed opportunities, miscommunication, lack of follow-up, and other fragmentation issues that have been outlined in previous chapters.

In earlier chapters, we discussed the challenges of a healthcare environment that is responding to the external changes described in the *Vital Directions* report by undergoing a seismic shift from a volume-driven, fee-for-service payment model to a value-driven, pay-for-performance model.

As mentioned, we are in the middle of a transformation which many describe as "one foot on the dock and one foot in the canoe" (**FIGURE 4-1**). This means that chief executive officers (CEOs) and other senior managers must guide an organization that is partially funded under the old volume model while trying to achieve a new value model that doesn't yet yield financial gain. A particularly acute challenge is finding the revenue to build the infrastructure for value-based care while the organization is in a "revenue trough."

These revenue troughs can also disrupt collaboration and foster competition as senior managers struggle to provide resources for their areas of accountability from a shrinking revenue pool. An example of this is the drive to reduce hospital readmissions. While reduced readmissions are generally considered to be a good health outcome, they also deprive the hospital of some fee-for-service revenue from those admissions

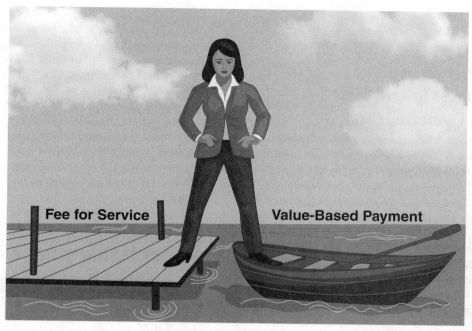

FIGURE 4-1 The Senior Management Balancing Act

that were avoided, even after readmission penalties are levied by Medicare.

Another major challenge is the mismatch of traditional senior management structures, thinking patterns, and capabilities with the needs of a value-based environment. Traditional hierarchical command and control management structures worked fairly well, at least from a financial point of view, in a volume world. In a value world that requires flexibility, innovation, collaboration, and teamwork, however, this type of structure and mindset is quite counterproductive. For organizations that persist in adhering to command thinking and silo structures, an inability to transform may actually prove to be fatal as the financial reward system changes.

With the evolution toward value comes the need to engage both patients and staff and to share power more widely. This requires senior managers to relinquish some control, to

include clinicians in the power structure, and to develop managers in the middle layer of the organization. For senior managers who relish clear boundaries and enjoy control, this can be stressful if not traumatic. This new power-sharing arrangement also requires new skills in communication, coaching, and collaboration that many senior managers do not yet possess.

Constant distraction from a chaotic healthcare political and regulatory environment, in which various provisions of the Affordable Care Act have become part of a dramatic political football game, is another serious challenge for senior managers.

It is very difficult to maintain focus on connecting the dots for patients and staff when the organization is constantly being buffeted by new regulatory, insurer, referral source and patient demands, and associated revenue shifts. As we will see later in this chapter, the ability to constructively deal with distraction is a core capability for leaders who hope to build a viable connected care organization.

Leader Views of the Progress Toward Value and Connected Care

The *2017 HealthLeaders Media Value-Based Readiness Survey* assessed healthcare organization leadership views on the level of progress that has been made in the shift from volume to value. Compared to previous years, leaders in this survey had a much more positive appraisal of their organization's level of readiness for value-based care. The survey revealed that the top three value-based care delivery competencies that respondents say their organization is committed to, or has already developed, are care coordination, access to care, and clinical integration.

- 72% of respondents indicated that their system is strong or very strong in **coordination/guiding patients to appropriate care**.
- 72% rate their organization as strong or very strong on **clinical integration**.
- 73% report they are strong or very strong on broader **access to care**.

One very low scoring area was **longitudinal care**, with 54% of respondents indicating that they are weak or very weak in this area.

ASK YOURSELF

- What types of specific challenges do senior managers in your organization face?
- What factors at the federal, state, and local levels impact your organization's drive toward population health, patient safety, value-based payment, and connected care?
- How successful has your organization been at preparing itself for the volume-to-value shift?

In this study, longitudinal care was defined as managing patient care for longer periods of time and across multiple settings. This is the issue of fragmentation raised in Chapter 1 in the case study about the patient, Mrs. Habib. As one CEO noted, "So if we don't have independent physicians aligned and we're not ready for longitudinal patient care, what we can deliver in terms of value-based care is only within our own systems and hospitals. We can do it with patients that we have full control over, but when it gets beyond us, then we're going to struggle" (Bees, 2017, p. 3).

▶ Senior Management Connected Care Strategies

For most senior managers, connected care will not be an end in itself. It will most likely emerge as a key element in the organization's efforts to make the volume-to-value shift. Three key strategic initiatives that are most likely to incorporate connected care are:

- The creation of a high reliability healthcare organization that achieves patient safety goals
- Implementation of a population health program
- Development of an integrated delivery system model for value-based payment

All of these strategic initiatives will incorporate the quadruple aim goals of improved patient population outcomes, a better patient experience, reduced per capita costs of care, and improved clinician experience.

Achievement of these strategic initiatives requires senior managers to align their organizations around a clearly defined vision and to create a culture and systems that foster this alignment. The implementation of connected care must occur at all organizational levels, as illustrated in **FIGURE 4-2**.

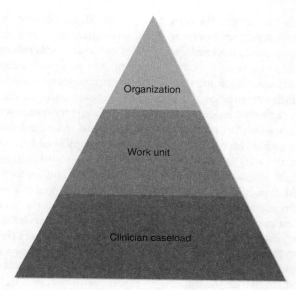

FIGURE 4-2 Connected Care at Every Level

Three Steps to Organizational Alignment

Harvard Business School professor, Amy Edmonson, in a 2017 article, detailed a simple three-part model that leaders can adopt to achieve organizational alignment. These three elements are illustrated in **FIGURE 4-3**.

Vision

The vision is a statement that clearly defines both organizational direction and the value that the

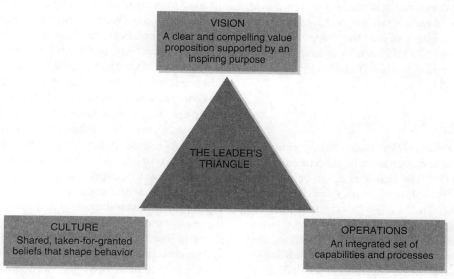

FIGURE 4-3 The Leader's Triangle

Reproduced from Edmonson, A. (2017, Feb. 21). The Leader's Triangle. Athena Insight. Retrieved from https://insight.athenahealth.com/the-leaders-triangle

organization adds to the market and the community. Editing is an important factor in creating the vision. Since no organization can be all things to all people, leaders must decide on attributes of value that will be delivered and those that will not be part of the organizational mission. The vision must be carefully considered and durable, because once set, all leaders must keep themselves relentlessly focused on it. Once the focus is clear, leaders must be vigilant about resisting the pull to expand the vision in response to internal and external demands.

For example, the organization may choose to emphasize quality outcomes but not focus on price. This does not mean that the organization will decide to exclude the cost element of the quadruple aim, but it does mean that it needs to recognize and emphasize the dimensions of performance that matter most in light of the vision. An interesting example of this type of vision in postacute care comes from Bayada Home Health Care.

This agency immediately communicates its vision on the home page of its website with a picture of a caregiver and the statements "Led by Our Hearts" and "Bayada is a career and a calling."

The website features employee stories, a letter from the owner, and numerous examples of how the "Bayada Way" is operationalized, including a history of how the vision was developed by the CEO through input from patients, families, and caregivers (Bayada Home Health Care, 2017).

Operations

Once the vision is clear, the leadership team must scrutinize and align operations, defined by Edmonson (2017) as "an integrated set of capabilities and processes through which value is delivered." Operations are the vehicle for creating organizational capability and making the vision concrete and actionable. Filtering is a key skill in aligning operations around the vision. This means that senior leaders test every operational decision against its ability to achieve the vision. Strategies and tactics that do not do this are discarded.

Workforce development and performance management are key elements of operations that can make or break organizational alignment. Key processes include workforce selection criteria, hiring, onboarding, training, and performance management. For example, an integrated delivery system with a vision of patient engagement and patient-centered care facilitated by technology would screen caregivers for their willingness to work within a culture of patient collaboration and for their ability to use technology as a key tool in care delivery.

Operations also encompass organizational structures and processes. In the previous example, structures support the use of information technology (IT) such as a robust IT clinical interface with strong clinical informatics staff and resources for the latest technology. In addition, there are enough licenses for all clinical staff to access the technology and regular meetings between information systems and clinical leadership to ensure that both groups are working together to achieve the vision.

Culture

Culture change is the least tangible, but possibly the most important, aspect of aligning the organization around the vision. Edmonson describes culture in a simple but compelling way: "An organization's culture consists of taken-for-granted assumptions about what matters, what's appropriate, how one should behave. . . . Culture tells employees how to behave in the absence of a formal rule and in the absence of oversight. It's like a 24 hour a day training program" (Edmonson, 2017, p. 8).

We will examine culture change in more depth later in this chapter, but one essential element of culture change that clearly signals alignment is role modeling. Senior managers send powerful signals about what is important to them, and to the organization, by how they behave and what they pay attention to. In the integrated delivery system example, a CEO might spend time each month talking directly to patients about how connected, collaborative, and caring their experience has been. The senior executive might share his or her findings with employees via a newsletter, email, or corporate video to clearly demonstrate the importance of a patient focus (modified from Edmonson, 2017).

▶ What Senior Managers Must Accomplish to Achieve Connected Care

Senior managers must be accountable for implementing organizational systems that produce a value-based, patient-centered healthcare system that incorporates the goals of connected care. These systems are pictured in **FIGURE 4-4**.

A review of the literature shows that more than half a decade after the implementation of the Affordable Care Act and the beginning of the transition from volume to value, there is now broad industry agreement about the type of work that senior managers must do to achieve the quadruple aim and "connect the dots" for patients. These activities incorporate all of the senior management accountabilities described in Figure 4-4:

- Create a culture that is patient centered, coordinated, collaborative, value based, and quality and safety driven.
- Maintain the financial viability of the healthcare organization so that it has the resources to deliver the best care and to support continuing innovation.
- Recruit, train, and retain the highly qualified staff who can "work to the top of their licenses."
- Develop integrated data systems that connect care providers and provide actionable clinical and operational data.
- Apply appropriate monitoring and self-management technology to patient care to reduce labor and produce better outcomes and a more integrated patient experience.
- Improve efficiency and lower the costs of care through process and productivity improvements.
- Integrate care at the structural level by developing senior management and work unit

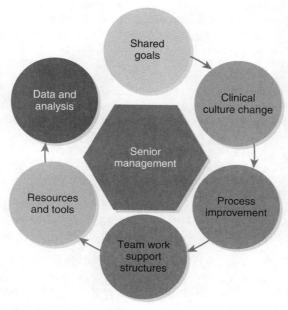

FIGURE 4-4 Senior Management Connected Care Accountabilities

structures that are both semiautonomous and collaborative.

- Engage and collaborate with the full continuum of care, both within and outside the healthcare organization, and engage with social services organizations to address the social determinants of health.

- Engage patients and families in care and develop two-way communication with health professionals.

- Foster teamwork and collaboration at all levels of the organization. (Browning, Torain, & Enright Patterson, 2011; Health Research & Educational Trust, 2014; Schyve, 2009)

INTERVIEW WITH DR. JOSEPH QUARANTA, PRESIDENT OF COMMUNITY MEDICAL GROUP (CMG)

Dr. Quaranta is the senior leader of a 1,000-provider independent practice association that is also an accountable care organization (ACO). Dr. Quaranta is responsible for all clinical, financial, and administrative functions of the organization. He still practices as an internist 2 days per week. The group is physician led and managed as a physician membership organization. The governing board is also composed of physician group members. CMG physicians and staff work together to achieve the quadruple aim: better clinical outcomes, lower costs, improved patient experience, and positive clinician experience. Dr. Quaranta describes the last goal as "maintaining the joy of practice." Dr. Quaranta feels that the independent physician plays an important role in value-based payment.

Dr. Quaranta would like to dispel the myth that more integration always results in more coordinated care. The experience of CMG is that increased complexity and more infrastructure does not equal more efficiency and a better patient experience. He uses the example of clinician communication through electronic medical records (EMRs). He says that in the previous 5 years, EMR complexity has proliferated. Where he used to get a one-page typed summary from a specialist to whom he had referred a patient, he now gets a 15-page electronic printout. This printout takes much more time to read as it contains both relevant and irrelevant information. He believes that this situation is the result of medical records being designed for coding, not for patient care—a situation that arose from misaligned incentives for providers. He calls the fragmentation of noncommunicating medical records "one of the great tragedies of the health care system because it did not create a system that worked for patients."

While Dr. Quaranta's vision is to align and integrate CMG around the quadruple aim, he finds that it is sometimes difficult to get group members refocused. One reason for this is the persistence of the fee-for-service model in which incentives are based on volume and not on value. Another issue is the lack of capital available to build a value-based program infrastructure. Despite these obstacles, the organization has hired more clinical support staff, built a robust data management system, and has begun to develop consistent best practices. Factors that have contributed to this ability to move forward on quadruple aim goals are physician ownership and group members being "closer to the benefits of quality activities." Physicians also want to "be part of something bigger than themselves" and to "do the right thing." The CMG membership practice model can also help with clinical improvements. He feels that it is easier to improve quality in this type of practice because "there is no barrier to getting a group of experts on diabetes together very quickly to create improvement around an issue like diabetes care."

In recent years, the group has added a number of nurses and other clinical support staff. There are currently 30 employees and only one physician. Dr. Quaranta says that expanding the team was necessary so that physicians and other team members can work to their highest level of skill. Physician usefulness is often diluted when the physician performs tasks that could have been done by someone else. This is a dissatisfier for physicians and has a negative impact on patient care. When the physician is engaged in too many tasks, patients don't get the attention they need. It takes a broader set of professionals to improve outcomes and make clinical processes work.

With value-based payment, each member of the team can work effectively to create a coordinated experience for the patient because the payment structure is not totally dependent on physician visits.

For example, a physician can see a diabetic patient and then have the diabetes educator do the follow-up. Some follow-up tasks can be managed through the patient portal, email, and phone calls; and some conditions, such as urinary tract infections, can be managed remotely using evidence-based protocols. For the most complex patients, such as those with congestive heart failure, the nurse might call weekly as part of the population health model.

In the old fee-for-service world, physicians would fill their schedules well in advance with appointments such as routine physicals to ensure income. This would leave urgent visits with complex patients to the mid-level practitioners, while the physician saw these patients on a less than optimal frequency. Under the value-based model, this system can be reversed with the physician seeing the more complex patients and the mid-level clinicians providing more routine care.

The practice uses two levels of support for complex patients. One is health navigators. These are support professionals who help patients manage the social determinants of health such as transportation and obtaining medications. The other level is nurse care coordinators who support the care of more complex patients. One issue with the use of care coordinators is that it creates another layer and it can feel like fragmentation to patients if the practice is not able to demonstrate the value of the care coordination to patients and integrate care coordinators into the care team. Embedding the care coordinator into a practice location helps with this integration. CMG is moving toward having the physician refer directly to the care coordinator and making the measurement of such referrals part of practice metrics.

Patient engagement is part of the work of the ACO. Because of the attribution model (attributing patients in ACO contracts to providers who see the patient most frequently for whom they are the primary care provider) most patients don't even know that they are part of an ACO. Ultimately, Dr. Quaranta believes it will be important to inform patients and to demonstrate some benefits of value-based care such as lower premium costs.

Dr. Quaranta describes the need to "inoculate" providers with the concepts of population health by using data. This is a serious challenge because the use of data requires both technical and analytical expertise. Physicians do get data from insurers, but it is very fragmented, providing a clinical picture only of the patients who have coverage through that insurer. There is also no common dataset to provide to physicians. CMG has finally found a method to aggregate data and provide physicians with a more complete picture of practice outcomes.

The process of communicating data to physicians in the practice has been an interesting one. When presented with their data, some physicians immediately say, "The data isn't right" and "My patients are the sickest." These are common reactions when data were first presented to group physicians, but they occur less frequently as the process of data sharing becomes more routine. Many physicians will argue with the data, but then immediately change their behavior. For example, at the first data presentation, one physician hotly contested the idea that his practice had a higher incidence of elderly patient falls. At the second meeting, he was still arguing that the data was wrong, but he had started a more robust fall risk screening process.

Dr. Quaranta sees data management as one of the frontiers of population health. He notes that "quality" is not yet clearly defined and that we need to demonstrate that data management will actually produce an increase in value. Patient-driven metrics will also be important but are not yet widespread.

▶ Senior Management and the Strategic Pillars of Connected Care

Connected care provides a set of cross-cutting organizational strategies or pillars for achieving patient safety, population health, and value-based payment goals. These strategies can be summarized in **FIGURE 4-5**.

The Foundation—Patient-Centered Senior Management Decision Making

Underlying the five strategic pillars is the foundational strategy—adoption of a patient-centric filter for decision making at the senior management level. In the "old days" of fee-for-service care, finance was the filter applied to most management decisions. Patient-centered concerns ran a distant second as a key concern in all but the most mission-driven organizations.

In the new world of value-based care, patient centeredness must move much higher on the priority list for senior managers who hope to successfully navigate the volume-to-value shift and achieve the quadruple aim. For the patient-centric approach to become part of the organizational fabric, its implementation must begin at the board level. Board members, as representatives of the community, are in a good position to filter organizational decisions through the patient lens.

If the board shifts from an entirely financial focus to a dual focus on finances and quality,

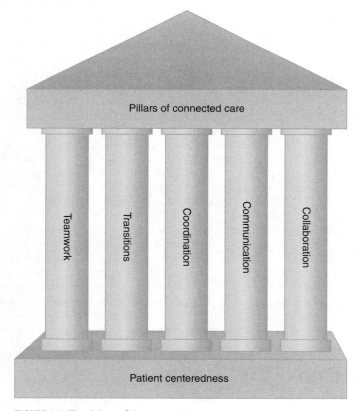

FIGURE 4-5 The Pillars of Connected Care

the organization is more likely to make headway on connected care. To truly embed the patient-centered approach, senior managers might think of the patient as an invisible presence in the room as they make decisions. Another method for giving patient concerns weight in decision making is to designate one senior manager who always represents the voice of the patient. In recent years, a new type of position, known as the chief experience officer, has been created in many organizations to fill this role. As decisions are made, the whole management team, or at the very least the designated executive, must ask questions such as, "How will this affect patients?" and "If we were the patients on the receiving end of this decision, what would it feel like?" Senior managers can also make patient and family advisory councils a more integral part of their organizations—one that is truly advisory to senior management and not simply a seldom regarded group that simply meets regulatory requirements.

An article from the Center for Creative Leadership describes this approach clearly: "Hospitals need both patient-focused business professionals and business-minded clinicians who can keep patient care top of mind. Only through education and dialogue can comprehensive solutions be reached. Alignment is created when caregivers and business leaders reach a common understanding of the clinical strategy as well as the business strategy" (Browning et al., 2011, p. 5).

ASK YOURSELF

Think of two recent major business decisions that were made by your organization.

- How did these decisions affect patients?
- What is the evidence that impacts on patients and patient concerns were taken into account?
- If patient concerns were not taken into account, how would things look if the patient view had been incorporated into the decision making?

Communication

At the most basic level, connected care for patients requires the use of two-way communication as a strategic tool at all levels of the organization. It is particularly important for communication to flow from the executive suite to the front line and the front line back up through middle management to the executive level. The healthcare organization must also be porous enough to allow two-way communication from patients, families, and partner organizations to flow freely from outside to inside the organization so that it easily reaches the people who can process and respond to it.

In his article "How CEOs Can Adopt a 21st Century Approach to Communication," Walter Montgomery (2015) paints a clear picture of the vital importance of corporate communication and the consequences of failing to do it well: "I have a particularly vivid memory of a global company, once seemingly invulnerable but quickly plunging toward near extinction. Poor communication was instrumental in exacerbating, even creating problems in execution, controls and culture" (p. 2). Montgomery makes the point that communication, while often lightly regarded, is an essential element of strategic success.

To achieve this strategic success, senior managers must model effective strategic communication. This means understanding who is likely to be affected by a decision or change (who needs to know) and thinking about specifically how they will be affected, how those groups or individuals might perceive that change, and how the message must be framed and communicated in a way that meets recipient's needs and strategic goals. Some might call this the "ripple effect" of communication. A helpful tool for planning strategic communication is a grid produced by the Rasmuson Foundation (2007) called the *Strategic Communications Plan Template*. **TABLE 4-1** provides an example of a strategic communication planning tool in a grid format.

A huge pitfall in senior management communication can be "tone deafness" or unwitting

TABLE 4-1 Strategic Communication Planning Grid Communication

Goal:_____

Who Needs to Know?	Issues/ Concerns	Key Messages	Communication Methods	Target Date	Responsible Person

blindness to the potential reactions of the recipients of the communication. These situations, in which fragmented and conflicting information is communicated, are the antithesis of connected care. There are endless examples of this type of executive behavior. One recent example is the communication by United Airlines CEO, Oscar Munoz, that seemed to blame a resistant passenger who was dragged off a plane by security guards. Videos of the event "went viral" internationally, causing a public relations nightmare that sent company stock plummeting. The antidote to this type of problem is to have a professional communication department assess major corporate communications for impact on various constituencies, especially employees, patients, families, and the press. This assessment should include "testing" the message with representatives of each constituency.

Communications professionals must then provide senior management with feedback about how to modify the message to meet the needs of recipients. A true test of the effectiveness of corporate strategic communications is the frequency of the comment, "Nobody told me." Employee surveys that include questions about communication are another way to gauge the effectiveness of the strategic communication process at the senior level. Patient experience surveys will also provide measures of healthcare organization communications.

Another communication success element is to ensure that all clinicians—including physicians and nurses, other employees, and managers—know that effective communication is a required core capability and one that will be measured and rewarded. The organization must back up this expectation with training, role models, practice, and measurement of communication effectiveness.

Providing a structure, tools, and resources for effective two-way communication is an important element of the senior management job.

🔎 CASE STUDY

Strategic Communication in a Large Home Healthcare Agency

A recent article in the *Remington Report* describes communication methods used by Joan Doyle, Executive Director of Penn Home Care and Hospice. "Doyle's leadership team sends frequent messages to all staff members about the organization's performance, and Doyle holds town hall meetings on a regular basis.

"For those meetings, staff gather at the Pennsylvania headquarters so that Doyle can explain what the current organizational vision is, and whether there have been any major changes in direction or strategy. . . . It is critical to involve everyone in changes, (Doyle says) by getting their feedback, addressing any conflicts and ensuring everyone understands why we're doing the things we're doing" (Guinto, 2017, p. 9).

For example, a home healthcare agency had relied on voicemail messages as a primary tool for communicating with field staff. This one-way communication lacked a feedback loop, produced misunderstandings, and dropped balls in patient care. Senior management decided to purchase iPhones for clinical staff and provide training and support for using them. This switch eventually resulted in a culture change that produced much more effective two-way communication.

Another key communication tactic for senior management involves resourcing and supporting a robust and healthy IT and technology infrastructure. This infrastructure must include a user-friendly electronic medical record, reporting tools, and an informatics team that helps clinical staff master and utilize the electronic medical record and other patient care technologies to their fullest.

Transitions of Care

Senior management must make effective care transitions (movement within or between healthcare organizations) a key strategic focus for three reasons:

1. Transitions are an essential element of connected care and are instrumental in reducing readmissions and improving outcomes.
2. Care transitions are also a part of the care process that poses the highest level of patient safety risk and the occurrence of adverse events.
3. Transitions are a significant element in either improving or negatively affecting the patient experience.

The National Transitions of Care Coalition (NTOCC) summarizes the ideal transitions strategic goal this way: "Improve transitions of care, increasing quality of care and patient safety while controlling costs" (NTOCC, 2008, p. 1). NTOCC recommends achieving this goal through structural changes, assignment of key accountabilities, allocation of specific resources, and alignment of measurement and reward systems around transition goals. Specific NTOCC recommendations include:

- Improving communications during transitions between providers, patients, and caregivers
- Implementing electronic medical records that include standardized medication reconciliation elements
- Establishing points of accountability for sending and receiving care
- Increasing the use of case management and professional care coordination
- Expanding the role of the pharmacist in transitions of care
- Implementing reward systems that align incentives around effective transitions
- Developing performance measures to encourage better transitions of care (modified from NTOCC, 2008)

Senior managers must work with the middle management layer of the organization to identify crucial transition points for patients. Typically these are admissions, internal patient transfers between units or departments, transfers to care in other parts of the continuum, and discharges. When senior managers are truly committed to an effective transitions strategy, they foster the implementation of evidence-based transition programs such as the Care Transitions Intervention®.

Senior management must also ensure that qualified staff (particularly those with care coordination expertise) manage transitions, that time is provided for effective transitions, that staff are well trained in transition techniques, and that the corporate dashboard contains transition effectiveness measures.

In situations in which corporate finances may dictate a less than ideal transition plan, such as when the patient has run out of coverage for a skilled nursing facility (SNF) stay, but still needs care, senior management must support staff in finding compromise solutions that keep the patient safe during the transition. Solutions may include finding a home healthcare agency to care for the patient or keeping the patient for an extra day or two until a plan can be put in place.

Care Coordination

Building and facilitating an effective care coordination model and structure is a senior management strategy that ensures that patient care activities are connected into a coherent whole. This should be done in a way that provides a seamless and comfortable patient experience. Thew's (2017) article entitled "Solidify the Nurse Leader's Role in Care Coordination" summarized key points from a panel on collaborating across the continuum to achieve mutual goals, presented at the American Organization of Nurse Executives 2016 annual conference. Panel participants clarified the role of the nurse leader in fostering care coordination.

Know How Care Is Coordinated in Your Setting

Senior managers must actually get coordination on the senior management agenda as a topic of interest and concern. The nurse leader must understand the characteristics, needs, and requirements of the patient population. One mechanism for doing this is to chart the patient journey through the organization's care processes. The nurse leader must also assess the care transitions model being used; and if there is no clearly defined model, then create one.

Define Who Coordinates Care

Senior leaders must define the roles and responsibilities of those employees who provide care coordination services. The nurse leader must identify and eliminate duplicative care coordination programs that create patient confusion and mistrust.

An example is having multiple hospital departments such as pharmacy, care coordination, and floor nurses all calling patients after discharge without coordination of the purpose and methods of follow-up.

Creating clear competency statements, providing training, and embedding care coordination competencies into performance appraisal are part of building care coordination expertise and effectiveness. Managing care coordination at the senior management level also involves negotiating lines of authority and accountability with other senior managers whose clinical staff perform some care coordination functions. Physicians, social workers, and pharmacists are clinicians who should collaborate with nurse care coordinators to create the most positive and seamless experience for patients.

Establish Relationships That Will Support Care Coordination

Nurses who perform care coordination activities must be experts in nurse-patient communication. Senior nurse leaders can foster this communication by offering communication skills training programs. One such program described in the Thew care coordination panel article is the *Communication Catalyst Program* for nurses offered by the Thomas Jefferson University Hospital (Swan & McGinley, 2016).

In addition to nurse-patient communication, nurse leaders must pull nursing out of professional isolation and foster cross-functional teamwork and complex patient care coordination.

The nurse leader should be a senior manager who negotiates with other senior leaders to create work structures and processes to support interdisciplinary communication. Finally, nurse leaders must connect themselves and their employees by participating in the larger health and human services community outside nursing. This may involve serving on nonnursing boards, becoming active in community or health and business coalitions, and interacting with healthcare leaders in other community organizations.

Understand the Value of Technology

The nurse leader must understand the technology that is being used to foster care coordination such as special care coordination software packages. He or she must integrate technology into the care coordination decision-making process.

Nurse leaders should assess the organization's current technology to determine how it affects care coordination and transitions. Leaders must also strategize with information systems about how to optimize technology and how to best use data analytics to manage care. Another aspect of the nurse leader's role is to ensure that nursing staff members are equipped with the skills, attitudes, and tools to use technology effectively. This means that the leader must assign educational resources to build technology capabilities and collaborate with information systems senior managers to develop resources such as a clinically friendly and responsive help desk, clinical informatics staff, knowledge bases of technology resource information, and "cheat sheets" that can support nurses in the most efficient use of technology.

Engage the Patient and Family

To achieve connected care, senior nursing leaders must develop a culture of patient self-management support, in which nursing staff help the patient take an active role in his or her care, are transparent about all aspects of care, and direct care according to the patient's goals and needs. Extensive culture change, led by the nurse executive, is often required to help nurses shift from a compliance to a collaborative model of care.

The nurse executive can facilitate this shift by supporting processes such as clinical conferences that include patients and by sharing data about patient perceptions of nursing care and communication strengths and gaps.

Engage All Team Members in Care Coordination

The nurse leader must reach across the boundaries of the nursing department to create alliances with other clinical leaders. Together with these other clinical leaders, the nurse executive should create opportunities for dialogue between professions and for cross-functional care coordination. It is important that the nurse leader, while fostering the role of the nurse within the power structure of the organization, does not champion nursing needs to the detriment of other professions who care for the patient. The nurse leader can also collect metrics that show the effectiveness of care coordination and transition management. This positive data can then strengthen the commitment of team members.

Teamwork

Teamwork is an essential element of connected care because no one discipline or department has the full capability to manage care for patients with complex illnesses. Effective teamwork also ensures that nothing that concerns the patient falls through the cracks. Teamwork theory, tools, and techniques are covered extensively in Chapter 8.

Senior managers foster teamwork by first modeling it themselves. A senior management team that can achieve goals jointly, manage projects together, and speak as one voice to the rest of the organization is a powerful symbol of an organization aligned around connection.

Senior managers foster teamwork at the lower levels of the organization by providing the time, space, training, and resources for teams to flourish. Incorporating teamwork effectiveness metrics into the organizational dashboard is another way of giving teamwork a high status in the organizational priority list. Senior managers must coach their direct reports on the effective use of teamwork and rate their performance in this area on annual reviews.

Collaboration

Connected care, within the context of the volume-to-value shift, requires a level of collaboration that has never been natural to the specialized and highly structured culture of American health care. Some call this "boundary spanning," others "silo busting." No matter what name is used, collaboration means developing negotiated working relationships between various parts of the healthcare organization and with other related organizations to achieve common goals. In value-based care environments, collaboration, which is often formalized with written agreements, is

essential to successful outcomes. The Health-Doers Network connects people working to improve health and health care through online tools. HealthDoers sponsored a set of interviews on collaboration with three health and community leaders in 2016. These leaders defined collaboration in various ways:

- "The public and private sectors are able to come together to develop a trusting relationship, and a shared vision and they become accountable to each other."
- "Collaborations are groups of like-minded partners who come together for a common cause. Collaboration allows organizations to leverage resources."
- "Collaboration is leading across organizations. In a collaboration you learn how to work together with organizations that are different from yours and that bring different types of value." (HealthDoers, 2016)

Senior managers foster collaboration by making contacts with other organizations, negotiating joint agreements, encouraging management staff to get involved in community or regional healthcare activities, and creating strategic alliances that foster both the interest of the organization and connected care for patients.

An example might be a regional vice president of business development for an SNF chain who negotiates preferred provider agreements with a small group of home healthcare agencies. These agreements specify how the organizations work together on providing discharge planning and care transitions, reporting data on discharged patients, and notifying each other when patients are admitted to the hospital or SNF discharge is delayed.

▶ Senior Management Structures for Connected Care

Most healthcare organizations, from small, independent nonprofits to huge integrated delivery

A NURSE LEADER INTEGRATES CARE AND SERVICES FOR RESIDENTS

Peggy Joyce, RN, MS, LNHA, is administrator of health services for Whitney Center, in Hamden, Connecticut, a life plan community with an independent living option, an assisted living program, and skilled nursing center.

Peggy's vision is focused on communication and collaboration. She has multiple director level positions reporting to her. People in these positions could easily function in "silos" without structures to support collaboration. Peggy feels that it is essential to stay in touch with work that touches Whitney Center residents. She still attends the morning report to "stay in touch with the day to day." As she puts it, "sometimes, your gut feelings aren't enough—you really need to know what is going on."

Peggy has developed a number of structures to support connected care for her residents. She jokingly says that her real title should be "meeting attender." One such meeting is with an interdisciplinary team that addresses issues of "at-risk" residents. This group includes housekeeping and dining staff who may be the first ones to notice behavior changes or health issues.

Another connecting process is meetings between the director of assisted living and the director of skilled nursing. At the meeting, these nurse directors discuss the status of their joint patients and any recent hospitalizations and exchange other relevant clinical information. Peggy joins them at this meeting. She says: "I am the person who helps pull it all together." She gives the example of a patient whose family believed she was more independent and capable than facility staff believed her to be.

Peggy worked with the two directors to have a family meeting where the clinical team was able to tactfully explain what types of issues and behaviors they had been seeing. This meeting helped bring the family along to realize the patient needed continued services.

Peggy is also working with the facility CEO to create a new service model which creates a director level role called a "liaison." The liaison is not a specialist in a particular field, but the "partner" or "go-to" person for a group of residents. In this model, the resident does not need to decide who to contact for help. Rather, the liaison works with the community resource team, which includes social work, spiritual care, a nutritionist, and an exercise physiologist. These liaisons can deal with any type of problem ranging from billing to managing things that need recycling.

Once the prototype idea was developed, the team presented it to residents through focus groups and resident "town meetings." While some residents were skeptical of the idea, now that it is a reality "they love it." One idea that was not approved by the residents was the use of the term "resident engagement." Many of them felt that they were fully engaged and such a term was not needed. Being resident oriented, the team listened and changed their language.

The liaison/community residents' team is another structure for connecting the dots for residents. The key focus is understanding the resident's story and being sure the team knows each person's likes and dislikes—truly "what matters most." These individual meetings highlight the need to balance independence with support for residents. When asked about keys to success and barriers, Peggy emphasizes having the "right people in place." Her staff must be able to collaborate, coordinate, and connect with the whole continuum of care. She says that "everyone knows the plan and the vision. Even when situations aren't clearly defined, they know how to act."

systems, have a team or council of senior managers, headed by a CEO. Each healthcare organizations is also governed by a board of directors, which is ultimately responsible for overseeing the work of the CEO, achieving the organizational mission (if it is a nonprofit), and maintaining organizational financial viability.

The structure of senior management and relationships between senior executives and between the CEO and the board have a direct effect on the organization's ability to deliver connected care. A functional and collaborative senior management team is essential to the success of connected care. The operative word here is "team."

The CEO must develop a cohesive group of senior managers who meet regularly and "speak with the same voice" about care connections at the organizational level. This unified voice is important for several reasons. First, senior managers must role model the collaboration, coordination, and good communication that are the hallmarks of connected care. Second, senior managers are the guardians and facilitators of organizational structure, resource allocation, and workforce deployment—the essential ingredients of connected care. Without senior manager cooperation and collaboration, these complex systems and processes will not align and coalesce for seamless patient care. Another key issue for senior managers in the implementation of connected care is accountability. If connected care is to flourish in an organization, either the CEO or at least one member of the senior management team must be accountable for it and must be rewarded for achieving it. Often, this is the senior manager responsible for quality activities within the organization.

Evolving Senior Management Roles and Responsibilities

Roles and responsibilities in senior management teams are evolving in response to the pressures of the volume-to-value shift. To strengthen their ability to create value-based care, many healthcare organizations are creating strategy or innovation senior leadership positions. For example, Thomas Jefferson University's Jefferson Health has a chief innovation officer and other positions such as vice presidents for decision analytics and for telehealth and urgent care, along with adding the role of chief patient experience officer (Hagwer, 2016).

Having these types of new positions allows operational managers to focus on keeping the business running, while these new executives "bring new ideas to the organization, work with the management team to implement initiatives, track and communicate performance metrics, and engage the front-line staff to identify and remove barriers to change" (Health Research & Educational Trust [HRET], 2014, p. 13).

Some of the newer titles seen on C-Suite doors include:

- Chief population health manager
- Chief clinical transformation officer
- Chief experience officer/patient engagement officer
- Head of technology innovation

Another area for innovation in senior management roles is patient satisfaction. The American Hospital Association survey of senior hospital and care system executives, described in the HRET article cited previously, revealed that 15% of survey respondents said their senior leadership team includes a patient engagement officer to ensure that innovative thinking is applied to patient service issues (HRET, 2014).

▶ Senior Management Team Structural Changes

Senior management teams are also undergoing structural changes in response to the shift toward value-based care. Matrix-type organizational reporting structures and multiple reporting relationships are another change.

In some instances, senior executives have responsibilities that cross over division lines and are responsible for standardizing practices across the entire organization.

CEOs are creating councils or committees such as an executive strategy group that includes the chief medical officer, CFO, chief nursing officer, chief information officer, and an innovation executive. These groups ensure a consistent approach to strategy across the entire organization. Health systems are consolidating or eliminating very narrowly focused roles such as chiefs of disease-specific services and replacing them with more broadly defined roles with greater spans of control. This approach is specifically designed to break down organizational silos.

Another change in executive structure is the transformation of some traditional roles such as the chief financial officer. This role, which was traditionally about financial scorekeeping and driving for fiscal responsibility and profit, is now enlarged to deal with risk, insurance, and strategic financial decisions (HRET, 2014).

The Role of Clinicians in Connected Care Leadership

A recent development in the volume-to-value evolution is the trend toward including clinician leaders on the senior management team. Many younger and midcareer clinical leaders are combining clinical education preparation with MBAs or other business degrees. In a recent article, "Clinicians in the C-Suite," Debra Beaulieu (2017) describes the drive toward clinician leadership in this way:

> Healthcare leadership is evolving in a way that must merge the silos of clinical care and administration, resulting in a growing minority of C-suite positions occupied by physicians and nurses. There are numerous industry drivers of the clinician leadership trend, not the least of which includes mounting industry emphasis on value and quality. Amid various financial pressures and a need for clinicians to help facilitate change, it behooves organizations to close the gap between providers of care and executive leadership. (p. 1)

One motivation behind this trend is to apply the filter of patient-centered care and clinical experience to balance the business side of the healthcare equation. Some clinician leaders feel that their experience at the bedside better equips them to understand and advocate for the needs of the clinical workforce.

Physicians and Nurses in Leadership Roles

In integrated delivery systems, the drive to incorporate physician leaders as equal partners in senior management decision making is a recent development that has strongly influenced healthcare organization strategic direction. The number of articles on the topic of "physician integration" in the healthcare business press has exploded in recent years as the shift to value-based payment proceeds. The source of this fervent attention to physician integration is understandable, given that physicians both drive the economic viability of healthcare organizations and control the means of clinical production. However, without some balance of power and proper attention to the contributions and needs of other professions, this physician-centric approach can have a negative impact on the organization's efforts.

Nursing, while recognized as an integral element in integrated delivery systems, is not usually accorded the same level of attention as physician integration, although there does seem to be a drive to broaden the role of nurse executives and to include them at the most senior levels of the organization. As one nurse executive noted in a recent survey of hospital executives: "It's time to get out of the nursing box and take the lead on hospital initiatives and create further relationships across the continuum of care. Nurse executives are more widely understanding of the strategies, approaches and collaboration and are beginning to be seen more as equals" (HRET, 2014, p. 13). In SNFs, rehabilitation hospitals, assisted living, and home health care, where physicians play a smaller role, the chief nursing officer is typically in a more powerful position in the senior management inner circle.

▶ Senior Management Skills and Capabilities

In a time of disruptive change, the need for new types of executive capabilities are emerging. Many of these capabilities are highly relevant to the development of connected care, as illustrated in this quote from an article in *HealthCare IT News*: "Shifts in the healthcare landscape call for

INTERVIEW WITH JANINE FAY, RN, MPH, PRESIDENT AND CEO OF VNA COMMUNITY HEALTHCARE

In the course of her career, Janine Fay has worked as a home care nurse, a hospice nurse and director, and as both the chief operating officer and CEO of a medium-sized, nonprofit home healthcare and hospice agency that also owns a nonmedical home care company and an adult day center.

Ms. Fay says that teamwork is the key to connected care in home health care. Teamwork in home care is not easy because of the autonomous nature of the work. In a home, many things can be problematic. Clinicians often try to do it all themselves and there is less of a tendency to hand off responsibility, refer to other disciplines, set boundaries, and utilize other resources. She sees one of her key roles as encouraging the use of interdisciplinary teamwork between clinicians.

The move toward patient self-management support has also been challenging for home care clinicians as many home care patients are very elderly and often have the perception that the nurse will "do things for them." Nurses often share this expectation, and sometimes try to deal with the social determinants of health by getting food for patients and helping with household chores and other nonclinical activities. While this very much connects the dots for patients, it does not do so in an efficient way.

One of the structures that VNA Community Healthcare has put into place to reduce fragmentation for patients are complex case conferences, which can be requested by any clinician and which bring together a multidisciplinary team of internal experts who help assess the patient situation and make recommendations for additional interventions.

Another technique for creating more seamless care for patients is joint scheduling in which one scheduler manages appointments for both nursing and therapy to reduce overlapping visits.

Nurse liaison visits to patients about to be discharged from hospitals or nursing homes are helpful in preparing the patient to "cross the bridge" from inpatient care back to home. They help prevent problems with things like transportation to medical visits, obtaining food, getting caregiving help, and obtaining prescribed medications.

Surprisingly, Ms. Fay also sees risk agreements as a tool that can help reduce fragmentation for patients. These agreements are usually written when a patient is not willing to adhere to the medical regimen or to get additional help that would make continued living at home safe. The agreement maps out what the patient chooses to do and not do. It also describes the repercussions of not following the medical treatment plan and clarifies the role of both the patient and clinician. The agreement is a tool that helps both clinician and patient think more creatively about what might be done to develop a plan that is medically sound as well as acceptable to the patient.

When asked how she measures success, Ms. Fay answered that it is the patient experience that counts. How connected the patients feel with their clinicians and how they feel care has improved the quality of their lives are key. A caveat to this is that many older patients have little ability to objectively judge the care they receive, so often a clinician who is "nice" is thought to have given good care. Ms. Fay feels that health literacy education is important in helping patients manage and evaluate their own care.

Ms. Fay sees home health care as being an "integrator" function. She says "the home is where the rubber meets the road. We see the reality of the patient's life and what is real for them. For example, a hospital may discharge a patient thinking that his daughter will be the primary caregiver. What the hospital care coordinator doesn't know is that the daughter is bipolar and is not reliable in helping her father." Home care is able to get data from all the other settings where the patient has received care and is able to piece together "the patient's story."

Home care patients are assigned to a "primary case manager" who can be either a nurse or a physical therapist. These clinicians see the whole picture and ensure that all the patient's doctors have the right information, family members understand how they can assist with certain responsibilities, payer requirements are followed, etc. Now home care case managers have a new job, which is to keep ACO case managers informed. As the number of case managers in different settings multiplies, Ms. Fay asks, "How many layers of care managers do we really need?"

Home care agencies are also often seen as a generic community resource. "People often walk in off the street asking for a nurse in the agency to help them figure out eldercare and health care problems." Being embedded in the community, home care agencies often have a web of relationships with community support resources that can integrate care for patients.

Ms. Fay describes her own experience of dealing with elderly parents and in-laws. She explained how as a family caregiver she helped connect the dots of care for her mother who went back and forth from Florida to Connecticut and who had a duplicate set of doctors in each place. Using her mother's medical notebook, which she calls "the bible," her mother's care was very well coordinated.

As an executive in a rapidly changing industry Ms. Fay stays abreast of industry direction by looking at the stock analysis of the largest for-profit home care companies and following what moves they are making.

She reads widely outside of home care trade journals looking at publications such as leadership and health policy blogs and articles in the *New York Times* as well as healthcare journals about technology and innovation.

Ms. Fay sees the key challenges ahead as one of greater need and fewer resources. As resources become scarce, home care continues to have workforce shortage issues, and the population continues to age, she sees a crisis developing. She feels that technology may be one answer to the problem, and while home telemonitoring is one good tool other technologies have not yet matured to the point where they can help in a substantive way.

In summary, Ms. Fay sees the two essential elements of connected care that must be fostered by senior management as teamwork and effective communication.

a new brand of healthcare leaders," wrote Invenias Partners President and CEO Curt Lucas, noting that terms such as "'innovator, risk taker and change leader' are now key to any C-suite member's skill set" (Davis, 2015, p. 2). Because of the importance of data analytics and digital connections to patients, many healthcare organizations are hiring executives with experience in the digital health arena. Other skill areas for healthcare executives that are in high demand, but not necessarily readily available, include:

- Change management
- Communications
- Patient engagement
- Strategic partnership development
- Innovation and creativity (Davis, 2015; HRET, 2014; Rubin, 2016)

Many healthcare organizations are now facing the challenge of bolstering skills for existing senior leaders, developing senior leaders from within the middle management ranks, or hiring from outside of health care, particularly from the retail industry.

The diffusion of connected care throughout the healthcare system may well depend, at least partially, on senior leaders rapidly acquiring the skills necessary for success in a value-based healthcare world.

▶ Essential Elements of Effective Senior Management Teams

A number of senior management team factors can either foster or cripple senior management success in implementing connected care. An article by Dunn (2012), "Six Characteristics of High Performing Healthcare Systems," reports the results of a Studer Group survey of over 1,000 healthcare leaders in 44 states. This survey found that effective senior leadership is an essential element in four of six factors described in the article. These leadership factors are:

- **Alignment among senior leaders.** Senior leadership must see the environment in the same way and feel a similar level of urgency about the need to adapt for the future.
- **Leadership training.** Organizations in which leaders feel well prepared for their roles do better on Hospital Consumer Assessment of Healthcare Providers and Systems (HCAHPS) scores.
- **Effective leadership evaluation systems.** Hospitals that had stronger evaluation systems that held senior leaders accountable for performance performed better.
- **Consistency of leadership.** This factor encompasses both low turnover among senior managers and alignment among leaders. (Modified from Dunn, 2012)

Of the items mentioned, the one that most commonly derails connected care is lack of alignment around a common purpose and vision. Senior management work is, by its very nature, competitive. However, when senior managers push for power and resources to achieve their own ends rather than to achieve organizational quadruple aim goals, dysfunction at all levels of the organization follows. In particular, this type of behavior encourages silo thinking, poor care transitions, and rivalries between lower level managers, eventually resulting in more fragmented care for patients.

Characteristics of High-Performing Adaptive Leadership Teams

The Boston Consulting Group Institute studied characteristics of high-performing, adaptive leadership teams. The study, in which over 100 executive members of these teams were interviewed, found that certain basic team characteristics as well as five special factors were the essential ingredients of high performance. Four "basic" teamwork factors that were present in high-performing teams were:

- **Distributed leadership**—Shared leadership at the top and development of leaders at every level
- **Optimal talent mix**—Top talent in key positions as well as the right combination of skills, backgrounds, and personalities
- **Clear charter**—The team has defined goals, roles, ground rules, and accountabilities
- **Mutual trust**—Team members can safely and openly express different views

In addition to the basics, these highly adaptive teams demonstrated some more uncommon leadership characteristics:

- **One voice**—Members of the leadership team have so thoroughly internalized the organization vision, values, and goals that they consistently describe these things in the same way.
- **Sense and respond**—The team constantly monitors the external and internal environment using multiple data sources and responds very quickly to threats and opportunities.
- **Information processing**—Highly adaptive leadership teams are able to analyze data and synthesize insights rapidly and thoroughly.
- **Freedom within a framework**—The senior team allows for bold action and the ability to take risks. It tolerates failed experiments and learns from mistakes. The team delegates considerable decision-making authority to other levels of management in the organization.

- **Boundary fluidity**—Team members are able to cross organizational boundaries to work together and typically fill in for each other as necessary. (Torres and Rimmer, 2011)

▶ A Team Effectiveness Barrier—The Gap Between Healthcare Senior and Middle Management

One area that should potentially be of concern to senior leadership, and that is largely absent from the literature on emerging healthcare leadership demands and capabilities, is the linkage between senior and middle management.

A Harvard Business Publishing article, "Danger in the Middle—Why Middle Managers Aren't Ready to Lead," describes this issue in eloquent terms (McKinney, McMahon, & Walsh, 2013): "For too long, companies have taken a 'barbell' approach to leadership development - placing heavy emphasis on training senior leaders and new managers, but giving short shrift to the middle-manager cohort. With middle managers now being asked to play ever more important roles in flatter organizational structures, continued neglect of midlevel management development carries significant risks—managerial burnout, increased turnover, and ultimately damage to the bottom line" (p. 6). This problem is particularly acute in health care where many middle managers have been promoted from the clinical ranks and have not been trained in management skills.

As dollars for education shrink, the focus in many organizations is on regulatory and technical skills leaving middle managers to achieve complex clinical culture change without the skills to be successful. As leadership teams evolve, this issue must be resolved if connected care is to be successfully implemented.

▶ Key Organizational Performance Measures for Senior Managers

Connected care performance measures for senior managers include organizational outcomes as well as specific measures of senior management performance. Measures related to patient centeredness, transitions, communication, collaboration, and coordination will be most relevant to connected care. Measures include the following:

- 30-day hospital readmission rates
- Incidence of adverse events due to communication or coordination failures
- Patient perceptions of connected care as measured by CAPHS scores
- Process measures such as timeliness and effectiveness of medication reconciliation and the number of patients who received a transition record at the time of discharge or transfer
- Measures of internal care connection processes such as consistency of nurses visiting a patient in home care, percent of cases that demonstrate interdisciplinary conferencing, communicating to a physician when the patient condition changes, and effectiveness of care handoff communication between providers and disciplines

Measures of Senior Management Effectiveness

Schyve (2009) in "Leadership in Healthcare Organizations: A Guide to Joint Commission Leadership Standards," a publication of the Joint Commission Governance Institute, describes the characteristics of effective leadership in hospitals in very specific and measurable terms.

While not all of the standards apply to postacute or ambulatory care, many are translatable. The paper defines the goal of leadership as safe, high-quality patient care. In the section "What Leaders Do," Schyve specifies what senior leaders must accomplish to achieve this goal:

- A culture that fosters safety and quality
- The planning and provision of services that meet the needs of patients
- The availability of human, financial, physical, and information resources for providing care
- A sufficient number of competent staff and other care providers
- Ongoing evaluation and improvement of performance

The Joint Commission document focuses on a specific aspect of connected care, namely achieving a patient safety culture. An example of performance standards for senior leaders is illustrated by the section on communication:

1. Communication processes foster the safety of the patient and the quality of care.
2. Leaders are able to describe how communication supports a culture of safety and quality.
3. Communication is designed to meet the needs of internal and external users.
4. Leaders provide the resources required for communication, based on the needs of patients, the community, physicians, staff, and management.
5. Communication supports safety and quality throughout the hospital.
6. When changes in the environment occur, the hospital communicates these changes effectively.
7. Leaders evaluate the effectiveness of communication methods. (Schyve, 2009, p. 25)

TABLE 4-2 provides more detailed examples of senior management connected care behaviors. It can be used as a self-assessment tool.

How Are Senior Leaders Doing?

Performance consultant Tom Olivo (2014) describes the struggles that senior executives face with maintaining performance in a highly challenging environment. Olivo's company, Success Profiles, uses a proprietary methodology to rate leadership effectiveness using a grading system:

- **A:** Leader/manager is a high achieving and talented performer who consistently exceeds expectations, brings out the best performance in others.
- **B:** Leader/manager is a good and consistent performer who consistently meets expectations, brings out a good performance in others.
- **C:** Leader/manager is an inconsistent performer who sometimes meets expectations, struggles to bring out a good performance in others.
- **D:** Leader/manager rarely meets expectations, fails to bring out good performance.

In Olivo's (2014) research, the percentage of B-level managers who were struggling to succeed had risen significantly (from 16% to 42%) over a 2-year period from 2011 to 2013. One possible reason cited for this struggle is the level of complexity of the external environment. The article quotes a hospital CEO on this topic: "The changes in healthcare's business model have surpassed the knowledge, skill and experience that many B level leader can bring to the table," says Steve Johnson, CEO of Susquehanna Health in Williamsport, PA. "And with the complexity of change hitting an exponential level, it is impossible for all but the most behaviorally astute and intellectually agile B level leaders to be successful" (p. 2). Olivo's solutions to this dilemma include systematically assessing the performance of the senior management team, developing senior manager skills and capabilities, and matching senior management strengths to assigned roles.

▶ Create a Culture of Connected Care

Earlier in this chapter we discussed Edmonson's three-factor leadership triangle. The most important and difficult of these leadership elements

TABLE 4-2   Senior Management Actions for Connected Care

Senior Management Actions	Examples
Guiding: Senior managers paint a clear picture of connected care expectations with goals, objectives, measures, and stories.	Senior managers explain the connected care strategy and vision with consistent language, specific examples, and a clear roadmap of how change will be implemented.
Resourcing: Senior managers give clinical departments the staff, materials, equipment, training, and time that is needed to achieve connected care goals.	Senior managers systematically analyze and provide the resources needed for training, electronic support systems, meeting time, consulting, new positions, and other aspects of effective connected care.
Fostering process improvement: A functional senior management quality council identifies defective work processes that impede care connections and charters and supports teams to improve these processes.	The senior management quality council meets regularly and identifies processes that interfere with seamless care such as incomplete discharge planning. The quality council charters teams with a mission statement, a facilitator, and a list of team members and would then provide time and resources for the team. The council regularly reviews team progress and provides guidance and support.
Paying attention: Senior managers pay attention to the things that are important for achieving connected care.	Connected care goals are discussed at meetings with managers and employees. Connected care anecdotes, tools, and examples are part of employee newsletters and other communication.
Measuring and communicating: Senior managers create systems for collecting data on key measures, trending results, providing measurement results to managers and staff.	Measures of connected care are placed on the organizational dashboard of key performance indicators (KPIs). These measures are circulated to clinical departments. Managers are held accountable for identifying, reporting, and resolving root causes of variances.
Recognizing and rewarding: Managers and staff who display connected care behaviors and achieve good results are publicly recognized and rewarded through performance appraisal, raises, bonuses, and promotions.	Senior managers review job descriptions and performance appraisal documents for congruence with connected care behaviors and goals. Employees who practice connected care are rewarded; those who don't are subject to performance management actions.
Structuring: Senior managers analyze the locations and sources of "disconnects" for patients within their care system. They implement structural changes to overcome these disconnects.	Senior managers create cross-functional teams, colocate related services, and insist on interdepartmental dialogue and communication. Senior managers foster collaboration among managers and discourage "suboptimization," in which some departments and professions are favored or receive more resources than others.

(continues)

TABLE 4-2 Senior Management Actions for Connected Care	*(continued)*
Senior Management Actions	**Examples**
Contracting: Senior managers develop formal working relationships with other parts of their community healthcare continuum to improve patient continuity of care.	Senior managers develop contracts and preferred provider arrangements with other organizations in the care continuum to foster smoother connected care.
Collaborating: Senior managers network and develop informal relationships with colleagues, competitors, and community organizations to provide external expertise and support for complex patients and transitions.	Senior managers venture outside the four walls of their organization and become active in professional and industry segment organizations. They also participate in education and networking with other parts of the care continuum—for example, a home care agency might attend meetings of a statewide primary care association.
Linking: Senior management invests in information systems and electronic medical records that foster connected care and information flow within the organization and with clinical partners in the continuum.	Senior managers work with local health systems or other vendors to provide secure patient tracking systems and linkages between the organization's medical records and those in other parts of the care continuum. Senior managers implement and encourage the use of patient portals.
Problem solving: Senior managers stay focused on what is working and not working in connected care development, making course corrections, mediating disputes, and redeploying resources as conditions change and the culture evolves.	Senior managers identify and acknowledge problems in internal and external connected care processes that are identified through measurements and "walking around" and talking to employees. Senior managers take action in a timely and visible way and provide feedback on any decisions about course corrections to employees.

is culture change. Organizational culture has been described as "the way we do things around here." When we dissect this seemingly simple statement we find that culture consists of highly complex and interrelated factors such as history, leadership, attitudes, values, responses to external events and crises, physical space, and external perceptions of the organization. Culture is about shared beliefs and what seems normal to employees.

In many cases, culture is so ingrained into organizational work life, and is so invisible to all those who are a part of it, that neither senior managers, middle managers, nor employees have a clear view of it. When an organization is perceived from the outside, culture is often a driving factor in its reputation. The bad news is that turning this ingrained belief and behavior system toward more integration, communication, and collaboration can be a daunting and sometimes seemingly impossible task. This is especially true if the organization has a history of provider-oriented, fragmented, and silo-type thinking. The good news is that there are many evidence-based and proven models of clinical culture change.

High Reliability Healthcare Organizations—A Model for Clinical Culture Change

Some of the best work on clinical culture change in health care has come through the patient safety and high reliability organization movement, which has been strongly promoted by the Joint Commission. This movement, which incorporates Crew Resource Management principles from the aviation industry (covered in more depth in the teamwork chapter), espouses a set of principles and practices that are closely aligned with the connected care approach. The culture of patient safety demonstrates a set of distinctive characteristics, including:

- **Multidisciplinary teamwork** and evidence-based team training
- **Use of validated tools to measure patient safety behaviors**
- **Modification of processes to address "human factors"** (such as complacency, distraction, stress, and fear) that interfere with safe patient care
- **Creation of a nonpunitive environment** in which fear and blame are reduced and constructive feedback is taught and encouraged
- **Creation of a "just culture"** in which administrative arrogance, reckless actions, bullying, and other behaviors that risk patient safety are detected, challenged, and managed by senior leaders. Appropriately assertive behavior on behalf of patient safety is recognized and rewarded. (Jarret, 2017)

By having such a clear picture of the elements of a patient safety culture, senior managers can guide culture change, create support systems, measure results, and recognize and reward behaviors that exemplify cultural values.

Senior managers must also attain this type of clarity about the principles and key elements of a connected care culture if culture change is to be successful. A recent document from the American College of Healthcare Executives (2017), *Leading a Culture of Safety, A Blueprint for Success*, provides a complete and detailed map of the steps that executives must take to achieve a culture of safety. This roadmap, which is highly specific in describing senior management leadership actions, can easily be adapted to connected care clinical culture change.

A Step-by-Step Model for Connected Care Clinical Culture Change

Shifting behaviors in a culture is no easy task given that cultures evolve over years, are "hard-wired," become the stuff of stories and organizational legends, and are usually invisible to their members. Cultural norms provide a level of familiarity that can be comforting to employees in a time of complex and sometimes chaotic external change, even when some of those norms are dysfunction and out of sync with environmental demands.

Culture change will be far more effective if senior managers follow a model, derived from both health care and business research, that can guide the change in a more coherent way. **FIGURE 4-6** illustrates a model for achieving clinical culture change.

1. Describe the "Why" and the "What" of Clinical Culture Change

This strategic vision will be the catalyst for all the change that follows. An ability to articulate this link between the "why" and the "what" of day-to-day work is essential for success. For most organizations, the strategic "why" will probably be a successful volume-to-value shift, achievement of quadruple aim goals, and development of new sources of revenue from value-based payment programs. As the culture change effort evolves, it will be necessary to link the strategic "why" to the motivation of front line clinicians and support employees.

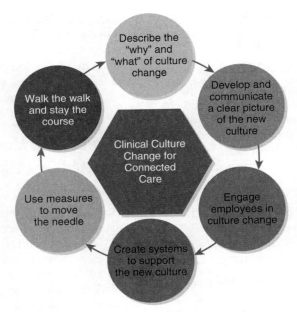

FIGURE 4-6 Clinical Culture Change for Connected Care

Senior leaders must be crystal clear about what strategic goals they hope to accomplish and the specific attitudes, behaviors, structures, and processes that must be developed to achieve these strategic goals if they are serious about "turning the organizational ship" in a different direction. If the strategy is not made visible and concrete for employees, it will be seen as empty rhetoric that can safely be ignored.

2. Paint a Picture of the New Culture

Clarity about the elements of the new culture starts with identifying what is happening now, describing deficits and problems, and painting a picture of a desirable future state. The five pillars of connected care, illustrated in Figure 4-5, and described earlier in this chapter, are a good place to start.

To develop a clear picture of the desired culture, senior managers can observe the connected care behaviors (teamwork, transitions, collaboration, communication, coordination) that are prevalent in their organization now. For example, executives in a home care agency might look at teamwork by examining the effectiveness of interdisciplinary conferencing and listening to how the staff describes, or labels, patients.

Once senior managers have assessed the current state of affairs, they can then imagine how people would act if their company were performing in the desired way. Senior managers can ask people in management positions and other stakeholders, "If we had the kind of culture we aspire to, in pursuit of the strategy we have chosen, what kinds of new behaviors would be common? And what ingrained behaviors would be gone?" Proceed to interview and observe "exemplars" or employees who already embody the values and behaviors of the desired culture. Use these examples as part of the culture change effort (Katzenbach, Steffen, & Kronley, 2012). Researching best practices models is another method for finding concrete examples of culture change strategies that can be replicated.

ASK YOURSELF

- What are the key elements of the connected care culture that you envision?
- How would people speak and act in this culture?
- How would people (inside and outside the organization) describe the level of connected care in your new organizational culture?

Another tool for painting a picture of the new culture is benchmarking. If there are organizations that embody the values and behaviors that senior managers hope to achieve, it may be possible to contact these organizations, interview their senior leaders, and gather some anecdotes and examples of connected care behaviors and structures that have worked for them. These examples can then be incorporated into the culture change effort and used to illustrate how things could work if the connected care strategy were actually realized.

3. Communicate a Clear Vision

Senior leaders must articulate a clear vision to achieve alignment around connected care goals and to develop consistent connected care behaviors. This description must resonate from the board room to the clinical manager's office and from there to clinicians and support staff. While the language may be different, the elements of the vision must be the same so that everyone involved "knows it when he/she sees it."

A white paper that summarizes research on building an integrated care organization frames it this way: "Clinical leaders must be able to articulate a clear vision about the need to improve patient care and how integrated care can produce the needed improvements, both initially when integrated care is first implemented, and on an ongoing basis" (Carter, Chalouhi, McKenna, & Richardson, 2011, p. 52).

Organizations that adopt the connected care philosophy include connected care goals in their mission, vision, and strategic plan using language such as: "The organization provides a seamless, transparent health care experience to patients." In a practical toolkit of culture change techniques, the BC Patient Safety and Quality Council (BCPSQC) notes: "At the beginning of any culture change initiative we want to talk about culture like a broken record. If we don't engage people from the beginning, it is very hard to continue with the steps that follow" (BCPSQC, 2013, p. 11).

This publication goes on to suggest that managers develop a "30 second elevator speech" that can be clearly understood by everyone. It further suggests that managers go beyond explaining the vision to engaging in a two-way dialogue with employees about how they perceive the explanation. Another excellent way of making the vision clearer is to list specific goals for achieving the vision and then describe how achievement of these goals will be measured. See **BOX 4-1** below for an example of how to explain culture change.

Utilize In-House Communication Professionals.
Utilizing the strengths of in-house communications professionals can be very helpful in this phase of vision communication. Writers in the marketing department know how to gauge the

---

BOX 4-1 An Example of Explaining Culture Change

A for-profit organization that includes a chain of nursing homes and home care agencies decided to change its culture to achieve more connected care and quadruple aim goals. Executives and managers consistently described the change this way: "Every patient care action that we take, comes from our understanding of what is important to patients and our organizational goals to achieve lower costs, better outcomes and a better patient experience. We do this by treating each other as customers, 'doing the right things right' and using data to drive decisions."

reactions of people to specific messages and in wording the messages to create the desired impact. Senior managers who have not been in the habit of engaging directly with employees should also ask these communication professionals to review planned communications so they can be vetted for potential impact. Taking this step will ensure that the message is packaged in the most effective way. It also prevents misunderstanding and anger as complex ideas are translated from the C-suite to front line employees who will filter the message through the lens of their own issues and concerns.

Before any culture change communication is implemented, it is essential to address any burning issues or grievances among the employee population. A change message will not go over well if employees have issues with working conditions, pay, communication, among others. Employee surveys provide clues to issues that need resolution before culture change can occur. **BOX 4-2** below offers an example of a culture change "elevator speech."

4. Engage Employees in Clinical Culture Change

Culture won't budge an inch without extensive and intensive employee involvement and buy-in. Employee engagement starts with understanding what employees value and ensuring that the change envisioned links to employees' core

---

TRY THIS

Write a "30 second elevator speech" explaining your vision of connected care for your own organization.

---

motivations. In a *Harvard Business Review* article, "Culture Change That Sticks," Katzenbach et al. (2012) recount the story of Aetna Insurance company's dramatic and traumatic culture change efforts. In one incident, the new CEO stood before a group of employees and was asked by an employee: "Can you tell me what it means for someone like me?" The CEO replied, "Well, I guess it is all about restoring the Aetna pride." He got a standing ovation.

The reason for this response was the CEO's reference to the traditional Aetna employee pride that stemmed from a long history of responding quickly and effectively to natural disasters dating from the Chicago Fire of 1871. In the years preceding the meeting with the new CEO, the company had changed its culture in response to the managed care movement and gained a reputation for being stingy and difficult to deal with.

"At cocktail parties," said one longtime Aetna staffer, "I really dreaded the question, 'Who do you work for?'" The CEO's answer connected the new strategy to a deeply held cultural belief about pride in helping that touched a nerve and made a link to the new cultural values for employees (Katzenbach et al., 2012).

▶ How Senior Management Engages with Employees

Effective employee engagement in culture change always includes three essential elements:

1. Visibility of top leaders
2. Two-way conversations with employees
3. Development of a cadre of committed employee champions

BOX 4-2 Connected Care—A Skilled Nursing Facility "Elevator Speech"

At ABC Skilled Nursing and Rehabilitation, we create connected and consistent care, based on patient goals that start with the first phone call to the facility and end with patient discharge. We ensure that patients experience complete and open communication about their care, smooth handoffs between clinicians, completion of any outstanding care or service tasks, and practical information on how to care for themselves after discharge.

Data from Passmore, 2012.

🔍 CASE STUDY

A small SNF which had been acquired by a larger chain was struggling to cope with an aggressive push to achieve new quadruple aim goals. Senior executives of the new company met with employees and heard stories and saw newspaper articles about the staff's "legendary" teamwork in the face of a major blizzard and anecdotes about how employees went to extreme lengths to ensure that patients were cared for and had warm food even when the power went out. These stories became part of the whole company culture change effort and helped to engage the employees of the SNF to the extent that they eventually became company leaders and champions.

ASK YOURSELF

- As you consider a culture shift toward connected care, what elements of your current culture support connected care?
- Are there stories or examples of teamwork, communication, and collaboration from the organization's past that can be tapped and communicated to help foster the new culture of deliberate connected care?

If culture change is to be successful, senior managers must abandon the comfort of the C-suite to walk around the organization and have conversations with employees on the front lines. These should be two-way conversations and should include an openness to interpreting the vision, letting employees test it, and defending it without defensiveness. Senior managers create these conversations in both formal and informal ways. Rounding (visiting clinical units to talk with staff) on each unit or with each team is one way to start this conversation.

Town hall meetings are another method for engaging employees in a dialogue. Informal methods of interaction might include sitting with employees at lunch, hallway conversations, email exchanges with employees, or mingling with employees at organizational gatherings. Of course, an open-door policy is conducive to more employee interaction.

Information gathered from this "walking around" should be taken seriously and used to modify the culture change vision to fit the realities of the organization and its employees. Giving employees feedback about what was learned and how the information will be used is one way to build trust and commitment (Katzenbach et al., 2012).

Cultivate Champions

The first stop in developing champions for change should be engaging middle managers. In most of the management literature there is a focus on the top and the front lines of the organization in culture change, but little emphasis on the role of middle managers, who are actually essential to a successful change process. Middle managers often serve as translators who help employees understand what organizational initiatives and goals mean to them. In addition to this essential translator role, middle managers keep the daily work going while change is being implemented. This managerial function makes middle managers invaluable in the process of allocating sufficient resources and creating work processes and systems that support the new vision.

Other champions for change may be the "exemplar employees" who surfaced in the vision definition phase of the culture change. These employees who already "get it" can be enlisted as teachers and mentors for the rest of the staff. A *Wall Street Journal* article on culture changes suggests appointing a "'consigliere'—a highly respected insider, who knows who is fighting you, who is supporting you, and what you need to do to build coalitions and devise strategies for change" (Murray, 2017, p. 1).

This respected insider ensures that senior managers don't become too distant from the day-to-day realities of the organization as the change effort advances (Murray, 2017). Senior executives cannot spend so much time focusing on professional clinical staff that they forget to find and support front line support staff champions. Sometimes it is the clinical secretary, the housekeeper, or the transport aide who best exemplifies positive connected care behaviors.

Create a Steering Committee

Many organizations form a steering committee or council that guides and supports the culture change effort. There may be several layers of steering councils with one at the senior management level to oversee strategy, communication, resources, and progress and another at the management/front line level to implement specific new structures, processes, and training for employees. Employees themselves should help guide culture change as part of a front line steering committee and should be part of any clinical process redesign efforts.

▶ Developing the Workforce for Connected Care

To develop a clinical and clerical support workforce that can provide connected care, senior managers must implement a full range of performance support structures and processes. Senior management, especially senior human resources executives, in collaboration with clinical leaders, creates this system. The drive toward connected care starts with hiring and orientation.

Managers are taught to screen for connected care aptitude and capabilities in employment interviews. Employees who express an interest in collaboration and who demonstrate effective communication skills are more likely to become proficient in connected care. "Lone ranger" clinicians who glory in independence and doing things "my way" are unlikely to be successful.

Onboarding is another element of effective connected care. Senior managers must invest in time for orientation, good orientation materials, online learning tools for effective training, and a strong mentoring system to teach and coach connected care skills. In a connected care culture, job descriptions contain connected care competencies, expectations are clear, training is provided, employees have access to community resources, and connected care is part of performance appraisal. Employees must become capable not only in technical skills but in clinical and personal communication, motivational interviewing, patient self-management support, teamwork, process improvement, and care management to be truly effective at connected care.

Care Coordination Roles and Responsibilities Are Clearly Defined

Connected care organizations create roles with dedicated accountability for care coordination activities. Specialty care coordination and care transitions are available and utilized to best advantage. In a medical office this may be an embedded nurse care coordinator or a health navigator. In home health care, nurse case managers are responsible for case managing a panel of patients.

In SNFs, a social worker or nurse arranges coordinated discharges. Both SNFs and home care organizations utilize liaison nurses to visit patients in hospitals, identify potential care transitions problems, and educate patients about their services. Connected care is better achieved when these specialists both practice their skills in high-risk situations and mentor other staff in the daily use of care coordination tools and techniques.

Clinical Managers Practice Connected Care

Managers monitor patient flow and potentially high-risk transitions and handoffs. For example, managers must ensure that patient care is adequately provided during low staffing times, on nights and weekends. Managers also observe employee care connection and case management skills, providing training, coaching, and if necessary discipline to achieve connected care goals.

Work Structures Support Connected Care

The connected care organization builds and maintains structures such as a patient-oriented intake system, liaison visits to referring facilities, interdisciplinary team meetings, formal care coordination roles, and patient tracking systems.

Organizational Work Processes Support Connected Care

The connected care organization ensures that high-risk intake, care transitions, care management, and discharge processes are efficient and well coordinated. Some examples of this are (1) the same clinicians are consistently assigned to a single patient, (2) professionals read charts

and don't ask patients the same questions at every encounter, (3) patient needs are followed up on, and (4) professionals give reports to the next professional or department in the patient's care continuum.

Technology Supports Connection

Connected care organizations use their electronic medical records and patient care technologies to connect the dots for patients. Medical records with longitudinal views of care activities and patient conditions, patient portals into electronic medical records, and electronic systems that track patients through the continuum of care are examples. Patient monitoring technologies like home telehealth can ensure that no condition changes or problems are left unattended.

Create Systems for Engaging Patients and Families in Connected Care

The connected care organization provides self-management support for patients and family caregivers. Using skills like motivational interviewing, employees identify patient goals, health literacy levels, and self-management skill and knowledge deficits. They then provide patient and family education with teach-back, supervised practice, information about when to call for help, electronic tools like automatic pill dispenser systems, and emotional support or counseling for dealing with the stress of illness.

Build Bridges Across Organizational Silos

Connected care organizations develop and maintain connections with external patient care resources through processes such as creating lists of community resources for patients. They invite resource people, who can help their patients, to educate their staff. They make good referrals to these resources, providing all the information needed to do a good job at the next step in care. More advanced organizations participate in local or regional care improvement collaboratives and utilize the support of care coordinators in insurance companies and medical practice to help their team with complex patient care.

Use Measures to Move the Needle on Culture Change

In an earlier part of the chapter we addressed outcome measures for connected care. In most settings, the most comprehensive measure will be 30-day readmissions. To achieve these outcome measures, senior managers must embed connected care into departmental goals, routinely ask about it, measure it, and provide resources and training to achieve it. For example, nursing consistency (having the fewest possible nurses on the case) is a key to connected care and better outcomes in SNFs and home health care. In connected care organizations, consistency becomes a regular item on the organizational dashboard and is reviewed at each management meeting.

Patient-Centered Measures

Using more fine-tuned measures of patient engagement in the organizational dashboard also demonstrates a true commitment to the patient-centered approach that is at the heart of connected care. Patient-reported outcome measures (PROs or PROMs) include health-related quality of life, symptoms (such as pain), functioning, and willingness to adhere to therapy. Interest is growing in integrating PROs into additional contexts, including adverse event reporting (National Quality Forum [NQF], 2013).

Measuring Progress in Culture Change Itself

Attaining strategic goals and achieving quadruple aim measures is the end point of culture change;

but the change effort itself must be measured to ensure that the organization's process is heading in the right direction. One way to do this is to create change milestones and examples of "I know it when I see it" that can be measured regularly and informally along with the organizational key performance indicators.

Mark Chassin and Jerod Loeb (2013), in a publication for the Joint Commission, identify four stages of high reliability culture maturity in hospitals. Each stage has distinctive characteristics that can be clearly identified. The stages are beginning, developing, advancing, and approaching. At the earliest stages of maturity, organizations move from a diffuse or absent focus on quality to making quality the highest level strategic goal in the approaching stage. This type of framework can be useful to leaders who are attempting to create a concrete picture of what elements of the organizational culture might look like as it advances toward specific connected care and quadruple aim goals (Chassin & Loeb, 2013).

In a 2005 *Harvard Business Review* article, Sirkin, Keenan, and Jackson describe a method for assessing the success of organizational change called the DICE score. This scoring system looks at four factors: duration, integrity, commitment, and effort. The system grades each item on a four-point scale with lower being better. The article describes the scoring for senior management commitment in this way:

- **Ask:** Do senior executives regularly communicate the reason for the change and the importance of its success? Is the message convincing? Is the message consistent, both across the top management team and over time? Has top management devoted enough resources to the change program?
- **Score:** If senior management has, through actions and words, clearly communicated the need for change, you must give the project 1 point. If senior executives appear to be neutral, it gets 2 or 3 points. If managers perceive senior executives to be reluctant to support the change, award the project 4 points.

▶ Overcoming Senior Management Obstacles to Connected Care

Distraction

For senior managers, clinical culture change can be both an uplifting and motivating experience and a relentless day-to-day slog that is constantly threatened by competing and distracting priorities and a myriad of unresolved problems. Starting a culture change effort and leaving it as only an ethereal vision or abandoning it part way through can be disastrous to organizational effectiveness and patient care. As mentioned earlier in this chapter, senior managers in healthcare organizations must confront challenges from both inside and outside their organizations. External regulatory, market, and financial challenges provide constant distraction as the organization moves to align around value-based connected care goals. Visible and accountable champions, regular review of measurement milestones, and problem solving around prioritizing and managing constant change are ways that senior management teams address this issue.

Sirkin and colleagues (2005) discuss why change management is hard, and recommend a review of progress toward goals every 2 weeks. They suggest that this progress be measured not in tasks completed but in milestones reached.

Resources

The ability to allocate resources to connected care is a second perplexing issue for senior managers. As government payers cut reimbursement and providers face demands to build significant value-based payment infrastructure, senior managers must constantly prioritize current needs with organizational transformation needs. One way to handle this is to take a "lean" approach to both infrastructure building and culture change. For example, teamwork is a key pillar of connected care. In an ideal world, all front line clinical employees would be thoroughly trained in all the tools and techniques of the evidence-based TeamSTEPPS program. In an organization with workforce shortages and razor-thin margins, this may not be possible.

An alternative approach is to implement "microlearning sessions" where one tool at a time is taught at a staff meeting, to use "tip of the week" text messages, online learning, and management coaching at interdisciplinary team meetings to embed teamwork principles and practices.

Senior Management Skill and Teamwork Deficiencies

A third obstacle is senior management deficits in skills and teamwork. In the old world of health care, more sophisticated skills in process improvement, collaboration building, complex data analytics, patient engagement techniques, and more sophisticated performance management tools were simply not as common in health care as they were in other industries. Now, senior managers who do not possess these skills must either go back to school or become intense self-learners. Many senior management teams in health care also have something of an aversion to structured group process, change management frameworks, and the use of structured planning tools, preferring instead to "just talk about things."

Senior management teams must build their own capabilities by incorporating these tools and frameworks to deal with far more complex systems than they have been used to. The use of an in-house organizational development person or external consultant can be helpful here.

Collaboration Challenges

The mechanics of establishing teamwork and collaborative structures with other organizations can be another big obstacle to connected care. Internally, a silo structure and mentality must be broken down by structural change, new work processes, measures, and training. Senior managers must have the will to push through the resistance that so often arises when work groups are combined and different professions are made to collaborate.

Of course, the CEO must ensure that senior managers themselves collaborate, support each other's goals, and divide resources fairly. The establishment of collaborative relationships with external organization is fraught with many potential pitfalls. One is the push/pull of collaboration versus competition. Also, collaborating organizations must weigh priorities and decide who will spend money and labor on specific parts of joint care processes. When resources are scarce, the tendency may be to say "you do it." Sometimes one organization asks for excessive access to clinicians or excessive reporting, which necessitates senior management getting involved in negotiations. Mutual respect is obviously essential to any successful collaboration.

Persistence of the Compliance Mentality

Finally, the establishment of a patient-centered culture is a huge challenge in a healthcare world in which the compliance mentality often still rules. Of all the elements of clinical culture change, this may be the hardest because it means that health professionals must let go of the idea that they are in the dominant power position and know what is best for the patient.

This transition to collaboration with patients means that many clinicians must make a paradigm shift and adopt a new worldview, something that will come hard to many and never to some.

▶ Chapter Summary

Senior managers face a healthcare world that is racked by constant change and turmoil. In this world, most organizations have one foot in the world of fee-for-service care and the other

in the value-based payment world. Implementing the elements of connected care will be an essential task for senior managers who must guide their organizations through the volume-to-value shift and toward the quadruple aim.

In organizations that hope to achieve connected care, senior managers must develop additional skills in teamwork, innovation, patient service, data analysis, and change management. Senior management teams are being restructured to include clinical leaders and are developing more flexible reporting and collaborative relationships. Measures of connected care outcomes such as readmission rates and staff consistency must become part of the organizational key indicator system. Senior managers who hope to achieve connected care must develop a clear and concrete vision and must engage employees at all levels of the organization.

They must institute clinical culture change by engaging employees in two-way conversations and incorporating positive elements of the old culture into the new. Measures of culture change success must take their place besides clinical and financial outcome measures. Senior managers must identify and further organizational structures, processes, and behaviors, such as care transitions and teamwork structures that are integral to connected care. Senior managers must develop a performance management system that ensures connected care capability beginning with hiring and ending with performance appraisal and rewards.

Finally, the senior management team must be prepared to deal with obstacles such as distraction, resource limitations, rivalries, and a compliance mentality. The senior management team must be both relentless and resourceful to achieve connected care.

References

American College of Healthcare Executives. (2017). Leading a culture of safety—A blueprint for success. Chicago, IL: Author.

Bayada Home Health Care. (2017). www.Bayada.com

BC Patient Safety and Quality Council. (2013). Health care in British Columbia, culture change toolbox. Retrieved from https://bcpsqc.ca/documents/2014/01/SQAN -Culture-Book_6x8_2013_web-FINAL.pdf

Beaulieu, D. (2017). Clinicians in the C-suite? *HealthLeaders Media*. Retrieved from www.healthleadersmedia.com /physician-leaders/clinicians-c-suite?

Bees, J. (2017). Value-based readiness. *HealthLeaders Media*. Retrieved from www.healthleadersmedia.com/finance /value-based-readiness

Browning, H., Torain, D., & Enright Patterson, T. (2011). *Collaborative health care leadership—A six-part model for adapting and thriving during a time of transformative change.* Greensboro, NC: Center for Creative Leadership.

Carter, K., Chalouhi, E., McKenna, S., & Richardson, B. (2011). *What it takes to make integrated care work.* Washington, DC: Health International, McKinsey and Co. Health Services and Practices.

Chassin, M., & Loeb, J. (2013). High reliability healthcare— Getting from here to there. Joint Commission. Retrieved from https://www.jointcommission.org/assets/1/6 /Chassin_and_Loeb_0913_final.pdf

Davis, J. (2015). Technology is changing the C-suite landscape. *Healthcare IT News*. Retrieved from http:// www.healthcareitnews.com/news/study-reveals -technology-deployment-changing-c-suite-landscape.

Dunn, L. (2012, August 17). Six characteristics of high performing healthcare systems. *Becker's Hospital Review*. Retrieved from https://www.beckershospitalreview .com/hospital-management

Dzau, V., McClellan, M., & McGinnis, J. (2017). Vital directions for health and health care priorities from a National Academy of Medicine Initiative, National Academy of Medicine. *JAMA, 317*(14), 1461–1470. doi:10.1001/jama.2017.1964

Edmonson, A. (2017). The leader's triangle. Athena Insight. Retrieved from https://insight.athenahealth.com /the-leaders-triangle

Guinto, J. (2017, May/June). What does it take to be a great change leader—The focus on culture. *The Remington Report*, pp. 8–10.

Hagwer, L. R. (2016, April 27). New structures, new roles for the future of health care. HFMA Leadership. Retrieved from http://www.hfma.org/Leadership/Archives/2016 /Spring/New_Structures,_New_Roles_for_the_Future _of_Health_Care/

HealthDoers Network. (2017). What is collaborative leadership? A conversation led by Shirley Hershberg. Retrieved from vimeo.com 155557316

Health Research & Educational Trust. (2014). Building a leadership team for the health care organization of the future. Retrieved from www.hret.org

Jarret, M. (2017). Patient safety and leadership: Do you walk the walk? *Journal of Healthcare Management, 62*(2), 88–92.

Katzenbach, J., Steffen, I., & Kronley, C. (2012, July-August). Culture change that sticks. *Harvard Business Review*.

McKinney, R., McMahon, M., & Walsh, P. (2013). Danger in the middle—Why midlevel managers aren't ready to lead. White Paper. Leadership Development Perspectives. Brighton, MA: Harvard Business Publishing. www .harvardbusiness.org/sites/default/files/17807_CL _MiddleManagers_White_Paper_March2013.pdf

Montgomery, W. (2015). How CEOS can adopt a 21st century approach to communication. *Knowledge at Wharton*. Retrieved from http://knowledge.wharton.upenn.edu /article/how-ceos-can-adopt-a-21st-century-approach -to-organizational-communication/

Murray, A. (2017). How to change your organization's culture. WSJ How-to Guides. Retrieved from http:// guides.wsj.com/management/innovation/how-to -change-your-organizations-culture/

National Quality Forum. (2013). Patient reported outcomes (PROs) in performance measurement. Expert Panel Report.

National Transitions of Care Coalition. (2008). Improving transitions of care, a vision of the National Transitions of Care Coalition. Retrieved from http://www.ntocc.org /Portals/0/PDF/Resources/PolicyPaper.pdf

Olivo, T. (2014, March 11). The profile of an effective healthcare leader. *Becker's Hospital Review*. Retrieved from http://www.beckershospitalreview.com/hospital -management-administration/the-profile-of-an-effective -healthcare-leader.html

Rasmuson Foundation. (2007). Strategic communication plan template. Retrieved from www.rasmuson.org /_attachments/SCptemplate_Oct_06_3-07.pdf

Rubin, J. (2016, April 27). Healthcare leadership skills in an era of disruptive innovation. *HFMA Leadership*. Retrieved from http://www.hfma.org/Leadership/Archives/2016 /Spring/Healthcare_Leadership_Skills_in_an_Era_of _Disruptive_Innovation/

Schyve, P. (2009). *Leadership in healthcare organizations: A guide to Joint Commission leadership standards.* San Diego, CA: The Governance Institute.

Sirkin, H., Keenan, P., & Jackson, A. (2005, October). The hard side of change management. *Harvard Business Review*. Retrieved from https://hbr.org/2005/10 /the-hard-side-of-change-management

Swan, B.A., McGinley, M.A. (2016, June). Nurse-patient communi- cation: a catalyst for improvement. *Nursing Management, 47* (6), 26–28. doi: 10.1097/01.NUMA.0000483129.93849.72

Thew, J. (2016). Solidify the nurse leader's role in care coordination. *HealthLeaders Media*. Retrieved from www.healthleadersmedia.com/nurse.../solidify -nurse-leaders-role-care-coordination

Torres, R., & Rimmer, N. (2011). What senior leaders do differently. The five traits of highly adaptive leadership teams. The Boston Consulting Group. Retrieved from www.bcgperspectives.com/content /articles/leadership_organization_design_five_traits _of_highly_adaptive_leadership_teams/What Senior Leaders Do Differently

CHAPTER 5

Middle Managers and Connected Care

▶ Introduction

The challenge of achieving quadruple aim and connected care goals ultimately falls to front line clinicians and middle managers, often clinicians themselves, who support them. In this chapter we will examine the vital, and all too frequently discounted, role of the healthcare middle manager. Middle managers must translate senior management's vision and strategic plan for clinical culture change to front line employees, who then coordinate care and manage communication and care transitions for patients. This complex work cannot be done well without clear goals, adequate skills, resources,

teamwork structures, technical tools, cooperation from other departments, external resources, personal support, and time to do the job. Providing this web of support is the essential role of middle managers.

This chapter will also focus on the middle manager's role as a "change buffer." As health care evolves from a volume to a value-based system, staff at all levels are distracted by a barrage of almost continuous change. It is at this intersection between change, the daily work of patient care, and the business of health care that middle managers implement connected care. For this implementation to be done well, managers must attempt to filter, and at least partially control, the onslaught of constant change to give clinicians time and space to focus on patients.

For clinicians, the generic term used to describe the practice of connected care is "care coordination." This term encompasses a variety of complex care techniques such as incorporating patient goals into care plans, utilizing cross-functional teamwork to achieve better outcomes, enabling seamless care transitions, maintaining constant patient and family communication, and ensuring that all patient support activities are completed without "falling through the cracks."

To achieve effective care coordination, middle managers must support clinicians in sophisticated ways by communicating performance measures, involving clinicians in the design of improved clinical processes, embedding evidence-based best practices into daily work, providing needed resources, and helping to problem solve and advocate for front line clinicians' needs and interests. A constant dialogue between clinicians and middle managers is necessary to create and maintain both technical and human systems that support connected care. Middle managers should also build internal relationships that facilitate smooth information handoffs to and from senior management. They should also ensure good communication between clinicians and support staff, such as medical secretaries, and with staff departments such as human resources (HR), quality assurance (QA), and information technology (IT) systems.

In this chapter, we will explore the roles of middle managers in achieving connected care. We will review competency statements and measures of middle manager effectiveness. The chapter will also contain information about the mindset and skillset transformation that is necessary to achieve connected care in the middle layer of the organization. We will describe managerial techniques for facilitating change such as impact analysis, strategic communication, process improvement, and performance management. We will list obstacles and issues in achieving connected care at the front lines and will discuss potential solutions.

▶ Connected Care at Every Level

Connected care requires consistent, goal-directed efforts, coordination, and integration from all levels of the organization as illustrated in **FIGURE 5-1**.

Senior managers are responsible for organizational-level connected care. Middle managers are accountable for connected care at the work unit or team level. Clinicians are responsible for the actual delivery of connected care to patients. This model assumes that managers are responsible for achieving good outcomes for two populations (groups of people who have some like characteristics): patients and employees. Interventions at both the individual patient/employee and population or group level are necessary to achieve connected care. For example, a clinical manager should develop connected care strategies for all patients who receive care from her team or unit (the patient population). To do this, the manager would analyze the demographics and clinical characteristics of the clinical unit patient population. The manager would then work with unit staff to tailor organizational connected care processes

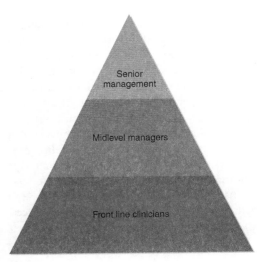

FIGURE 5-1 Who's Responsible for Connected Care?

such as admissions and care transitions to the specific needs of the unit's patient population.

For example, a clinical team that provides care to a patient population with health literacy challenges might have to simplify the standard organizational script for explaining clinical services to better meet the needs of their patient population.

The manager should consider the characteristics and performance of her own team (the employee population) in improving connected care. For example, a manager working with a team of less experienced clinicians might need to do more training in basic health coaching. The manager can analyze work unit employee group performance on connected care measures such as readmissions or effective medication reconciliation and tailor managerial interventions to improve performance. If the manager identified, through patient satisfaction survey data from the patients on her unit, that patients do not understand what to expect from the organization, who is responsible for their care, or who to call for help, she might work to coach and train clinicians who are not proficient in communication. She might also create team processes such as admission scripts and checklists, training in active listening, and patient rounds.

In this model, staff members at every level of the organization have both specific and flexible connected care roles. Senior managers are the direction setters, structure builders, and resource providers. Middle managers are the translators, integrators, process designers, facilitators, and trouble shooters. Front line staff, with support and resources from senior and middle managers, are the executors who work within an interdisciplinary team to provide care, coordinate care, offer emotional support to patients, and solve clinical problems. In effective organizations, innovation, communication, problem solving, teamwork, and continuous improvement occur at all organizational levels. Connected care is an integrating element for the organizational culture that can tie all staff together in the service of patient-centered care and achievement of the quadruple aim.

🔍 CASE STUDY

Everford Management Continuity Team Case Study

The Everford Health System senior management team decides that the key to successful outcomes, good patient experience, and more profitability is a culture that fosters collaboration and connection. To achieve this goal, senior managers charter a continuity team of middle managers, each of whom represents a sector in the Everford Continuum. Members of this group include Mary, the hospital director of care coordination; Doug, the practice manager for one of the largest Everford primary care practices; Tanya, director of nursing for the highest performing skilled nursing facility in the system; and Theresa, vice president for clinical affairs for the largest and highest performing home healthcare agency. The goal of the team is to develop methods to help system middle managers in implementing patient-centered, connected care.

The continuity team establishes a team charter, some broad measures, and boundaries. They decide that they will focus on the pillars of connected care for their work and will engage other groups or managers in other aspects of the culture change. After a meeting with the system CEO and the CEOs of each of their own organizations, the group decides to adopt a series of goals and measures that will form the basis for management connected care action. This list of goals and measures is described in **TABLE 5-1**.

The rest of the chapter will explore the various competencies that Everford middle managers will need to achieve the goals, the issues that the team will face, and managerial tools and techniques that can help achieve connected care in the Everford Health System.

The Middle Manager Role— Essential and Ambiguous

Healthcare middle managers are defined as "the first line of leadership with direct contact

TABLE 5-1 The Everford Continuity Team Connected Care Goals and Measures

Patient centeredness	■ The patient's medical record will document what is important to the patient and key patient goals for the episode of care. ■ Each chart note will demonstrate that the clinician asked the patient to describe an agenda, and concerns for that encounter.
Communication with patients and staff	■ Each system organization will meet state benchmarks for scores on patient experience survey questions about communication effectiveness. ■ Employee surveys will demonstrate a high level of satisfaction with organizational and managerial communication. ■ There will be no evidence of complaints or medical errors due to miscommunication between staff and between staff and patients.
Transitions	■ There will be a very low rate of transfers to inpatient within 48 hours of discharge from one setting to the next. ■ Chart reviews will show that risk scores and key elements of the patient's story were communicated to the organization receiving the patient in the transition. ■ Patients will receive an orientation to the next step in care and potential issues in transition to that step will be identified. ■ Discharge medication lists will be accurately transmitted to the next step in the continuum of care.
Care coordination	■ There is evidence that medication reconciliation is properly completed on admission and discharge. ■ Patient experience surveys will demonstrate scores equal to state benchmarks for questions relating to patients receiving explanations about their care and what to do after discharge. ■ Quality assurance reviews demonstrate evidence of consistent care task follow-up and do **not** find a significant incidence of missed handoffs in care that results in patient harm.
Teamwork	■ The medical record will demonstrate that there is regular interdisciplinary communication among members of the patient's care team. ■ There is medical record evidence that each profession is referring to other disciplines when appropriate. ■ For high-risk patients there will be evidence of care "huddles" or complex case conferences. Patients and families will be included in case conferences. ■ Managers periodically assess team function and review teamwork scores on employee satisfaction surveys.
Collaboration	■ Employee surveys demonstrate positive working relationships between clinical management and support departments such as IT, HR, QA, Billing, and Admissions. ■ Human Resources does **not** spend significant time mediating disputes between departments and professions. ■ The system has information on community resources and can identify individuals in each major resource to call on behalf of patients.

and supervision of frontline employees, who exercise administrative responsibilities without a clinical role" (Zjadewicz, White, Raffin Bouchal, & Reilly, 2016). The Bureau of Labor Statistics indicates that middle managers make up about 7.6% of the workforce. About 330,000 middle managers (a significant part of healthcare human resource costs) work in health care. The number of healthcare middle managers is expected to grow by 24% from 2012–2024, which is much faster than the average for all occupations (Bureau of Labor Statistics, 2016).

The literature on the role of middle managers in achieving the quadruple aim and making the volume-to-value shift is sparse. Most studies of middle managers focus on their role in innovation, quality, patient safety, and change management. First and foremost, middle managers are seen as two-way communicators who translate senior management's vision and strategies into understandable and actionable goals and activities for front line staff and then inform senior management of employees' response to proposed change. As one CEO noted in an interview: "Middle managers are the sailors in the crow's nest—sometimes they can see the icebergs and we need to rely on them to warn us and help redirect the ship through troubled waters" (Pappas, Flaherty, & Wooldridge, 2004). Middle managers "diffuse and synthesize information related to operations including the feasibility of project implementation, impact on current operations and workload" (Zjadewicz et al., 2016, p. 3). Middle managers are also "design reality testers" who transform the senior management vision into the processes, structures, training, and communications that help the organization achieve its strategic goals.

In more progressive organizations, middle managers are invited to use their knowledge of organizational culture and information from their internal social networks to participate in designing and culture change (Goldstein, 2015). In an older, but classic, 6-year study of middle managers, consultant Quy Nguyen Huy found that middle managers played four key roles in organizational change.

Entrepreneur

Middle managers are best able to restructure work to accommodate change because they are both close to the reality of the front lines and far enough away to see the "big picture." They are also close enough to patients/customers to have direct interactions with them and to understand their perspectives and issues. They are a more diverse group than senior managers and bring a broader array of perspectives and experience to the change effort. This "nuts and bolts" understanding of the work and of the proposed change allows them to recast some of the high-level, theoretical ideas of senior management into practical strategies that will work to achieve the desired goals.

Communicator

Middle managers are nexus points in communication to and from employees, patients, and external organizational partners. Middle managers use their broad and deep social networks to spread the word and get people on board. Managers may use nontraditional means of communication such as engaging employees one on one in social settings. Other managers cultivate trusted employee opinion leaders as ambassadors who can gain the support of more skeptical staff members.

Middle managers may have other methods of "selling" change that include explaining the rationale for the change, linking the change to employee benefit, and making adaptations to the change that help make it more palatable to employees.

Therapist

Since change, by its very nature, evokes anxiety and stress, middle managers have no choice but to support employees through it. They do this by providing a psychological safe space for employees, allowing them to express their concerns, providing encouragement, and giving people the tools to do the job. Managers must work through their own reservations and role model positive attitudes toward change even if they don't fully support it.

Since change brings out the best and worst in people, middle managers must encourage altruistic, supportive behavior among employees and should defuse and redirect resistance and negativity before it becomes toxic and infectious. Advocacy for employee concerns links the therapist and communicator roles. If the manager uncovers change stressors that are truly threats to employee ability to care for patients and manage their own well-being, they must communicate this back to senior management and propose more effective alternatives. One of the key stressors for employees during periods of change is a perceived lack of resources. The middle manager should assess the reality of these perceptions and lobby senior management to close legitimate resource gaps or help employees find ways to reduce waste in work and "work smarter."

Tightrope Walker

Balancing daily work and change is the essence of the healthcare manager's job. During the change process, the manager has to maintain a delicate balance between keeping the work of daily patient care going while gradually testing and implementing changes in work structures, processes, training, and technology. The manager's challenge is to hold on to core values and cultural norms while simultaneously changing how the work gets done. In essence, the manager's job is constant triage of effort, resources, and emotional energy (Huy, 2001; Zjadewicz et al., 2016).

The Negativity Perception—A Formidable Barrier to Middle Management Success

While integral to the transformation of American health care, and absolutely essential to the support of front line clinicians, middle managers are often seen in a less than favorable light. While some articles describe middle managers as

"heroic," others label them as "bureaucrats," "resistant to change," or even as "corporate concrete."

Embertson (2006) suggests that the turbulent conditions of the 1990s—which included mergers, acquisitions, cost cutting, and reengineering—contributed to negative perceptions of middle managers: "Since this trend of restructuring and reengineering, an understanding of the value of middle managers has been misplaced. Their importance in strategic formulation and implementation has largely been overlooked. They have been perceived as intermediaries that slow organizational efficiency without adding much measurable value" (p. 223).

These negative perceptions have been a barrier to achieving the full potential of middle managers in achieving connected care. Placed in ambiguous positions with limited power and support, and squeezed between senior management demands, the rigors of managing daily clinical work, constant change, and clinical staff who need structure, support, and advocacy, many middle managers find themselves becoming stressed and dissatisfied with their work. Some experts describe this situation as being "both victims and agents of change" (Braf, 2011). While managers often suffer from a lack of respect and support, actual studies of their influence prove that they are an essential element in organizational success. The challenge for many healthcare organizations is to recognize the problem and then empower and support these middle managers so they can play an essential role in achieving the quadruple aim.

ASK YOURSELF

- How are middle managers perceived in your organization?
- What key roles do middle managers play in achieving quadruple aim goals?
- How does your organization support middle managers in achieving organizational goals?
- What barriers do middle managers face?

Healthcare Middle Manager Competencies

Effective management for connected care requires a complex set of competencies, many of which are evolving in response to the radical change occurring in the healthcare system. An international consortium of 18 healthcare management organizations has created a consensus framework for health services managers under the auspices of the International Hospital Federation. This framework is illustrated in **FIGURE 5-2**.

This framework lists five competency areas for managers:

- **Communication and relationship management**—The ability to establish relationships and communicate clearly and constructively with those both inside and outside the organization
- **Leadership**—The ability to create a unified vision, to inspire organizational excellence, and to manage change to achieve organizational goals
- **Professionalism**—Aligning personal conduct with ethical and professional standards and a commitment to patients and lifelong learning

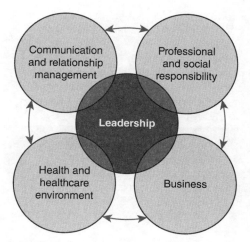

FIGURE 5-2 Leadership Competencies for Health Services Managers

Modified from International Hospital Federation. (2015). *Leadership competencies for health services managers*. Bernex, Switzerland: Author, p. 4.

- **Knowledge of the healthcare environment**—Understanding the healthcare system and environment in which the manager and the organization must function
- **Business skills and knowledge**—These competencies encompass the traditional functions of management such as financial, human resources, strategic planning, marketing, use of technology, risk management, and quality improvement (modified from International Hospital Federation, 2015, pp. 363–364)

The American Organization of Nurse Executives has created a similar framework for nurse managers. This model is divided into a three-part framework:

- **The Science**—Managing the Business
- **The Leader Within**—Creating the Leader in Yourself
- **The Art**—Leading the People

In this model, the "science" competency mirrors that of the international consensus document and lists similar skills. It does list an additional competency area, "clinical practice knowledge," which is not part of the international consensus document. The nursing management competency document emphasizes personal development, accountability, and career planning as important competency areas.

The "art" section of the nurse manager competency document emphasizes skills that are essential to achieving connected care, including human resource leadership, relationship management, influencing others, diversity, and shared decision making (American Organization of Nurse Executives, 2015).

These two frameworks encompass the whole gamut of management skills, including those key competencies necessary to achieve connected care: communication skills, change management, use of technology, systems thinking, personal competency, professionalism, and leadership. In the rest of this chapter we will explore these competencies further and give examples of how they manifest themselves in real clinical management practice.

🔍 CASE STUDY

A Nurse Manager's Connected Care Journey

Elena Mastriano, RN, MSN, has worked in various parts of the healthcare industry for 15 years. She has been in middle management positions for 10 of these 15 years. As she has progressed in her career she has evolved as a clinician and manager and has adopted the mindset and many of the skills necessary to support connected care.

Elena started her career in hospital nursing. She worked mostly on surgical floors and performed her nursing duties in a task-oriented way. Her mental paradigm in those days was: "get the work done as fast as possible so it doesn't eat you alive." She also gravitated to units where highly technical medical procedures were performed and patient stays were short. She got her job satisfaction from being part of an elite team and performing high-risk, high-tech tasks very expertly. Her interest in her patients as people was secondary. Elena was promoted to a managerial position on her unit and as she became accountable for the behavior of her staff as well as clinical outcomes, and patient experience, her view broadened and she began to think more in terms of working with systems and populations of patients and employees.

Elena eventually went back to school and got a master's degree in nursing. While in school, Elena oriented with a local home care agency and worked there as a home healthcare nurse. This experience further developed her managerial thinking as she saw how all the disconnected, task-oriented care that was delivered in various parts of the healthcare system created stress and less optimal clinical outcomes for patients and family caregivers. During this period, Elena was certified in the use of patient self-management support techniques. She became expert in health coaching and in helping patients self-manage their health in creative ways. Because of her enthusiasm and expertise she was made a preceptor for new staff.

When Elena graduated from her master's program she was promoted to nursing team manager and eventually to director of nursing at her agency. Elena had become expert in new skills such as the use of data to drive decisions, population health, the use of technology in patient care, lean process improvement, advanced communication skills, and the use of performance management and employee empowerment techniques.

Elena worked with her nurse manager team to involve staff in the redesign of care processes. She developed complex case conferences with staff nurses and involved families and primary care physicians. She created a visible measurement system so clinicians could see how they were doing on key metrics. Elena developed the habit of using data to drive decisions and she typically went beyond superficial problem solving to uncover root causes of clinical and service problems. She worked with the marketing team to develop a clinical liaison program in skilled nursing facilities and to improve care transitions. At Elena's direction, agency education staff implemented extensive training in active listening, Status Background Assessment Recommendation (SBAR), and motivational interviewing for clinical staff. Elena spent a significant portion of her time going on visits with staff, calling patients, and trying to overcome barriers to care experienced by both groups.

Partially as a result of Elena's efforts her agency received a Medicare Compare 5 star rating, the agency became the local employer of choice, and it built a reputation as an effective, patient-centered care organization. Elena currently has a very high level of job satisfaction and she has become a leader who is always learning and improving and is very well respected by patients, staff, and senior management.

▶ Measuring Healthcare Middle Manager Effectiveness

Measurement of management effectiveness in achieving connected care is currently more of an art than a science. Measures of effectiveness occur at three levels.

Achievement of Connected Care Outcomes

Middle managers are expected to help their clinical team improve its scores on quadruple aim outcome measures such as: 30-day readmissions, accurate medication reconciliation, and patient perceptions of care as measured by one of the Consumer Assessment of Healthcare Providers and Systems (CAHPS) assessment tools. Measures of adverse events, complaints, and process accuracy measures also reflect the competence of the clinical unit manager. Team or unit level measures will be most closely aligned with middle manager effectiveness. Other generic measures of management effectiveness are measures like staff turnover, achievement of unit financial goals, and successful implementation of strategic change efforts.

Organizational Assessment of Middle Manager Effectiveness

All healthcare organizations have some type of performance appraisal system that describes expectations for managers and measures how well they achieve these expectations. Middle managers typically get feedback on their performance when a higher level manager or executive conducts an annual performance appraisal and gives the manager a rating or a score. Performance appraisals usually assess how well managers have performed the skills specified in their job description, whether they have achieved specific goals that have been previously set, and their performance on organization core values. While subjective, these scores are used to drive recognition, reward, and performance development plans for middle managers. A less common, but more comprehensive approach is the use of 360-degree feedback tools in which the manager is assessed not only by his or her manager but by employees and peers. Employee surveys that ask specific questions about management support and communication are another method of assessing management effectiveness.

Personal Self-Assessment

Healthcare managers can foster their own self-development by completing a self-assessment tool and using it as a springboard for designing a personal education and development plan. One such tool, the American College of Healthcare Executives (ACHE) Competency Assessment (2017), is geared toward senior managers, although it has good assessment questions on connected care competencies such as communication, relationship building, and leadership.

▶ The New Healthcare Management

There is no clear road map for middle managers who hope to achieve connected care for their patients and employees. Senior managers are distracted by the struggle to keep their organizations moving forward through a period of political turmoil and the volume-to-value shift, in what is possibly the most tumultuous period of change for the healthcare industry in modern history. For the highest level of the organization, developing strategies that can guarantee long-term organizational survival and achievement of financial and clinical goals is paramount. This senior management distraction may mean that less time and fewer resources are spent on developing and supporting middle managers. Middle managers are also grappling with the highly stressful new reality of an unstable

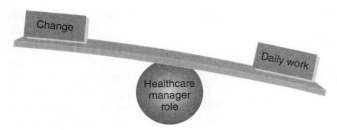

FIGURE 5-3 The Healthcare Manager Balancing Act—Daily Work and Change

healthcare regulatory and business landscape. While in previous eras managers could expect the need for change to be occasional and small scale, it is now huge and continuous. Their role in the turmoil is to keep the business going while balancing and incorporating constant change into daily work (**FIGURE 5-3**).

All levels of the organization must grapple with two types of continuous change, both of which have profound significance for reducing fragmentation and connecting the dots for patients (**TABLE 5-2**).

The first, sweeping changes in healthcare systems norms are pervasive and require organizational clinical culture change. The second, more local or limited regulatory or internal changes necessitate a planned quick response that allows the change to be assessed and absorbed

and then allows the clinical team to move on. The challenge is to allocate time, space, and resources for long-term clinical culture change while dealing with the constant distraction of frequent small-scale changes that continually disrupt daily operations.

Another area of concern for middle managers is the stress of change. For clinicians in all areas of health care, the stress of change has a huge impact as they struggle to adapt to a world of higher acuity patient care, shorter periods of patient contact, and a shift from "doing for" patients to "doing with" patients. These changes may require clinicians to relinquish deeply held beliefs and familiar ways of delivering care—something many are loathe to do. Middle managers who are themselves coping with the impact of these changes should not only transform their

TABLE 5-2 Two Types of Healthcare Change	
The Really Big Thing (Sweeping and deep—requires culture change)	**Industry Specific and Local** (Absorb into daily work and move on)
■ Political turmoil surrounding health care ■ Population health ■ New care models ■ Value-based payment ■ Industry consolidation ■ Health consumerism ■ Technology revolution ■ Population demographic shifts ■ Large employer demands	■ State regulatory demands ■ State healthcare model redesign ■ Rate cuts ■ New authorization limits ■ Insurer changes and demands ■ Industry-specific CMS regulation changes ■ Local market forces ■ Referral source changing requirements ■ Local workforce issues

own mindsets, but also help clinical staff reframe their attitudes and the way they do their daily work.

What Managers Need to Accomplish—High Level

Connected care is an integral part of the volume-to-value shift and achievement of the quadruple aim. The quadruple aim (Bodenheimer & Sinsky, 2014), which adds the vital ingredient of clinician satisfaction to the triple aim formulation, is rapidly gaining ground at a time when clinician stress and burnout are serious limiting factors for healthcare organizations seeking to be successful in the volume-to-value shift. For middle managers, achieving employee satisfaction has always been part of the job, but the emergence of the quadruple aim concept gives it new strategic significance and possibly more senior management support.

Achieving the quadruple aim and with it, connected care, requires middle managers to embark on a program of capability building both for themselves and for their operation. Middle

managers must build their own personal capability and a work operation that can withstand the impact of constant change. One way to think of this is to imagine your department as an earthquake-proof building. If it is strong and flexible enough, it will sway with change and keep everyone safe as "the next new thing" buffets and rocks the healthcare world.

Although there is no clear roadmap for the transformation of the healthcare system, there is considerable research being done, with many innovative clinical experiments, and with collaborations of the best minds working together to find the best way forward. The job of the middle manager is to search out these cutting-edge experiments and ideas and to gain energy and ideas from industry leaders and innovators (**FIGURE 5-4**).

Building Personal Capability

The new world of health care requires managers to make a radical departure from the fee-for-service paradigm of organizational silos, task-oriented work, a hyperfocus on your own profession's issues, and a patient compliance

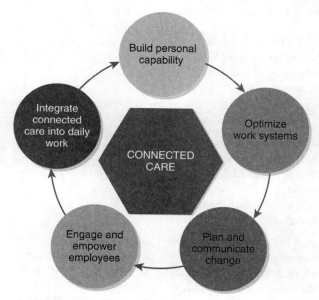

FIGURE 5-4 What Healthcare Middle Managers Need to Accomplish—High Level

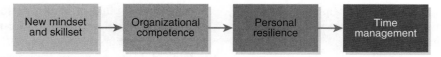

FIGURE 5-5 Four Steps to Capability and Empowerment for Healthcare Middle Managers

attitude. As a first step toward achieving connected care and quadruple aim goals, managers should try to achieve a rapid and radical improvement in capability and personal empowerment. This transformation is accomplished in the four steps illustrated in **FIGURE 5-5**.

Developing a New Mindset

Middle managers who hope to survive and thrive through the volume-to-value shift may need to change their mental paradigm. Such change is not easy, but extreme pressure from the external world and from senior management's urgency to ensure long-term organizational survival will naturally precipitate some of these changes. The more managers work with senior management on change initiatives, the more likely it is that they will develop a new, more connected care mindset.

The Institute for Healthcare Improvement, in a recent white paper on leadership, identified four mental models that are necessary for high impact healthcare leadership:

1. Individuals and families are partners in their care
2. Compete on value, with continuous reduction in operating cost
3. Reorganize services to align with new payment systems
4. Everyone is an improver (Swensen, Pugh, McMullan, & Kabcenell, 2013)

While formulated for senior leadership, these mental models are integral to middle manager success in achieving connected care. Each concept has profound implications for middle manager goals, activities, and time management.

TABLE 5-3 The New Healthcare Manager Mindset

Old	New
Task oriented	Systems oriented
Think only about the present situation	Conduct contingency planning
Make decisions with intuition and experience	Add data to the decision mix
Reactive thinking	Critical thinking
If it isn't broken don't fix it	Continuous improvement
My clinical discipline rules	It takes a cross-functional team
I am just a cog in a machine	I can take power and be accountable
Authoritarian management	Collaborative management

Once internalized, these concepts will help managers prioritize daily work and will help them triage competing change management initiatives. Middle managers can also use this list as components of culture change communications to staff. **TABLE 5-3** describes the necessary managerial mindset shift in more ordinary terms. While no manager is entirely represented by the "old mindset," most of us, if we are honest, find ourselves in a reactive, task-oriented thinking mode more often than we would like, simply from the pressures of daily demands.

Personal aspects of mindset change involve lowering personal defensiveness, being willing to accept feedback, and being open to reexamining habitual thinking patterns. One way to accomplish this is to discuss some of the ideas in this chapter with your colleagues.

Another activity that can help with mindset change is spending time with people from other healthcare disciplines or other settings in the care continuum and hearing different points of view. Reading outside your own field in the wider world of health care, scientific discovery, human resources, business literature, and other areas that are more peripherally related to your work can also help you to create the new mindset. A powerful mindset expanding activity is to ask patients and their family members how they see things. A simple question like "What has it been like to get care from our organization?" can get the conversation started. Seeing your world through the patient's eyes might be just the thing to help a manager question old assumptions and readjust mental habits.

Building the New Skillset

Connected care requires a whole new skillset for managers. **FIGURE 5-6** lists some of the essential skills that managers will need to successfully navigate the volume-to-value shift and implement connected care.

For many healthcare managers who have risen through the ranks, management training has been achieved through experience, coaching from more senior managers, and short, intermittent educational events. University programs that educate health professionals are slowly catching up to the healthcare system transformation and are creating training in areas such as population health. However, practical, non-degree educational opportunities to help middle managers who are already in the field gain the skills necessary to achieve connected care and the volume-to-value shift are scarce.

An article about building the essential skills that middle managers need to create a patient

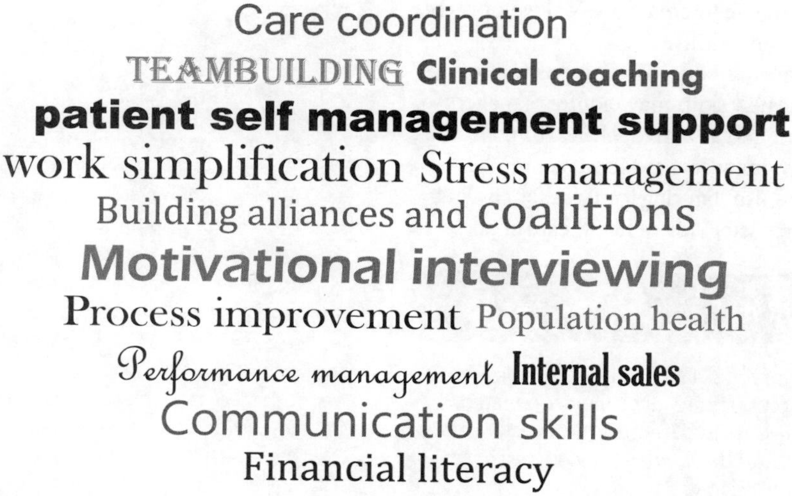

Care coordination

TEAMBUILDING Clinical coaching

patient self management support

work simplification Stress management

Building alliances and coalitions

Motivational interviewing

Process improvement Population health

Performance management **Internal sales**

Communication skills

Financial literacy

FIGURE 5-6 The New Healthcare Management Skillset

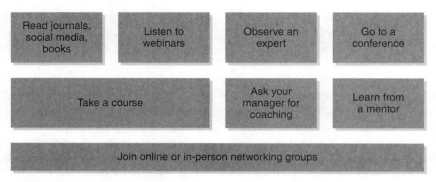

FIGURE 5-7 Methods for Developing New Skills

safety culture offers some practical suggestions for managers who need to gain higher level skills:

- Lead an improvement team with a mentor.
- Lead a project that is part of a national or regional improvement collaborative.
- Attend seminars and conferences on safety and quality improvement.
- Join an internal quality improvement group.
- Attend an in-house training program for managers.
- Use self-study or e-learning to build new skills. (Federico & Bonacum, 2010)

FIGURE 5-7 depicts some other methods that managers can use to create a self-development program for new skills.

Absent formal educational opportunities, acquiring these new skills may require managers to use persistent and assertive self-learning. In this regard, senior managers are good role models because they are also "figuring it out as they go along" on the rollercoaster ride of healthcare change.

ASK YOURSELF

- Which of the skills listed do you think are most important for achieving connected care in your organization?
- Which skills do you currently possess?
- Which skills do you need to build?
- What steps can you take to build these skills?

⌕ CASE STUDY

The Everford Continuity Team Identifies a Management Skill Gap

The Continuity Team studies the new mindset and competency standards for middle managers and concludes that many, who were promoted through the ranks without formal management training, do not have the necessary skills. Even some recent graduates of master's level population health programs have theoretical knowledge but not practical knowledge of how to apply the new tools and techniques. The team decides that improving managerial skills is outside its mission and boundaries so they enlist the aid of Human Resources, Senior Leadership, and the Clinical Management Council. A new team of individuals from these groups creates a revised list of management competencies and a performance appraisal document and works with a consulting firm to adapt its value-based payment leadership course to Everford's needs. While the Continuity Team works on the pillars of connected care, the new team is busy building middle management capability and, in some cases, replacing managers who are not interested in, or capable of meeting, the new standards.

► Middle Manager Organizational Effectiveness

To achieve connected care, middle managers must be effective at getting things done within their own organizations. Middle managers who are organizationally effective are typically those who have strong internal social networks. These networks of relationships with other managers and employees allow them to obtain information, find resources, get help with solving problems, and build an informal organizational support team.

Some managers who are content in their own department silos should make a deliberate effort to reach out and develop strong internal, collegial relationships. A good relationship with support departments like human resources, information systems, finance, and quality assurance is essential to achieving the kind of transformative change that creates connected care for patients. This network building occurs partially as a result of personal relationships, but also through deliberate actions like having conversations about what each department needs from the other, carefully reading communications from other departments, following other departments' procedures, not making unreasonable demands, negotiating interdepartmental conflicts, helping colleagues achieve their goals, and helping other managers overcome barriers and obstacles to their work.

A key element of connected care is smooth handoffs. Managers should look carefully at what happens in the "white space" between departments. This is where patient handoffs often occur and where communication and patient care tasks tend to fall through the cracks. Having a good relationship with the managers of the departments before and after yours in the clinical process flow is essential to smooth transitions for patients and for effective information transfer. Managers who "run a tight ship" are more likely to be organizationally effective, as senior managers, colleagues, and employees know that they can count on these managers to get the work done accurately and to communicate about it clearly.

Managers are organizationally effective when they get clarity from their own manager about their goals and accountabilities and when they triage their time and energy to achieve these goals. Communicating and "selling up" is another hallmark of organizational effectiveness. Managers who find that strategic goals are unrealistic as envisioned by senior managers, who have hit roadblocks, or who are underresourced must advocate for their staff to get work plans modified in a more realistic way and to obtain needed resources. The use of data and a calculation of "return on investment" can help with this.

ASK YOURSELF A VERY HARD QUESTION

If someone was to ask your colleagues and your employees how effective you are at running your department, collaborating with other departments, and getting things done ("running a tight ship"), what would they say?

► Building Resilience

The pace and impact of change in our current healthcare system is enormous and relentless. Managers sit in the epicenter of this change as they try to balance building a new clinical culture, keeping the business going, caring for patients, and supporting employees. Thriving in such an environment requires enormous resilience. Those managers who do not develop this resilience will soon find themselves on a short road to burnout. Building resilience involves two things: using stress management techniques and developing a sense of personal empowerment. The latter is especially important in our current tumultuous environment where both employees and managers feel "unmoored" from the safe and the familiar. Personal empowerment grows as managers build their new mindset, but it also involves resourcefulness and reframing.

This means reframing problems in terms of what you can do, not what you can't do. It also involves finding internal and external resources to help with the challenges you face on a daily basis. Middle managers in health care should also find resources to help them deal with overwhelming and emotionally draining clinical situations. Managers who must help staff cope with noncompliance, dying patients, patient and family discord, behavioral outbursts, and conflicts between staff need support and help themselves.

Sometimes managers need to seek out this help from their own senior manager, from quality or human resources staff, from social work or behavioral health colleagues, from their own internal collegial network, or from family, friends, or counseling professionals.

Stress Management

As the pressure mounts, it is essential for managers to evaluate and modify their current stress management routine to allow them to absorb and manage the stress of change. Classic stress management techniques such as exercise, distraction with pleasant activities, humor, and meditation are always helpful. Both at home and in the workplace it is essential to set boundaries

and negotiate or delegate activities to other family members or employees. This not only helps the manager, but also others build their personal empowerment and self-esteem.

Managing Time

How managers spend their time at work is a reflection of multiple complex factors. **FIGURE 5-8** illustrates some of the factors that compose management time.

Managers who are constantly "firefighting" and battling crises are probably dealing with either personal disorganization or some type of underlying organizational dysfunction, lack of coordination with other departments, work process failures, or staff performance deficiencies.

Use Data to Analyze Where Your Time Goes

Managers can start to gain control over their time by using data analysis. There are two methods for doing this:

1. **Use the quality improvement approach.** Review data on department performance and identify performance gaps. Localize these problems with data (staff, patients, time, type of equipment, diagnosis, type of staff, etc.). This helps you identify work systems or human problems that are

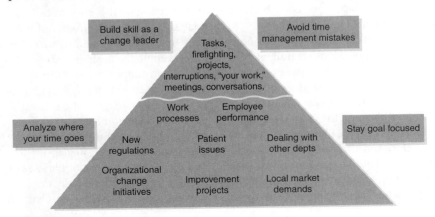

FIGURE 5-8 Take Back Your Time

consuming time in problem solving. Once you know where and when the problems are occurring, you can start to look for and eliminate root causes.

2. **Use the direct time analysis approach (the yellow sticky technique).** Set a time frame for your study. Two weeks is best. Every time you are asked to solve a problem, write it down on a sticky note. Be sure to include problems that you, yourself, have generated, such as time searching for something you can't find. Pile the notes up and at the end of the 2 weeks, sort them into piles by category. Count the number of items in each category to determine what factors are driving the time that you spend solving problems.

Once you have identified sources of problems and crises, you can put action plans into place to correct them. Some key steps in managing time are:

- Monitor the environment for upcoming changes and prepare in advance.
- Stay focused by considering how each action and task will impact achieving your key goals.
- Set small, achievable goals at the beginning of every day.
- Avoid meetings and appointments that don't have a clear purpose or focus.
- Pay extra attention to change at critical points (start up, rising resistance, maintaining change).
- Plan ahead for predictable crises (particularly scheduling issues that tend to be seasonal).
- Put staff capability building on your calendar.
- Avoiding common time management mistakes such as excessive multitasking, social media addiction, and being easily distracted.

Optimizing Work Systems

Connected care, by definition, requires smoothly flowing and effective work processes that can connect activities, tasks, and communications into a seamless whole. Given the pace of change and the complexity of healthcare systems, this is an endless and very challenging task for managers. The core skills for managers in optimizing work systems are quality improvement and work simplification tools and techniques. In more sophisticated organizations, managers may be trained to use more complex techniques such as Six Sigma or Lean management systems. Some generic techniques for optimizing work include:

1. Build staff capability, skills, confidence.
2. Engage staff in improvement.
3. Use data to localize and eliminate errors and problems.
4. Simplify work by reducing unnecessary complexity, too much checking, too many handoffs, and too much variation and inconsistency.
5. Cluster tasks and the tools and information needed to perform a task to avoid unnecessary walking or searching.
6. Work the "white space" by improving communication between disciplines, departments, and other organizations (this is where many problems and errors occur).
7. Skill up, delegate down—that is, train clinical staff to "work to the top of their license" and delegate tasks that can be performed by support staff.

Managing employees who are not performing effectively is essential to optimizing work. One common healthcare management mistake is to tolerate poor performance simply to keep a position filled for fear it will not be possible to find a replacement. Such an approach not only creates a barrier to good department performance but also demoralizes other employees who are performing well.

▶ Integrating Connected Care into Daily Work

Managers can use a variety of concrete techniques to integrate connected care into daily work. **FIGURE 5-9** lists the key steps in this process.

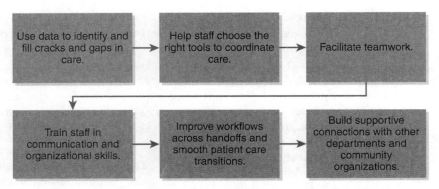

FIGURE 5-9 Integrating Connected Care into Daily Work—What Managers Need to Accomplish

Use Data to Identify and Fill Cracks and Gaps in Care

The manager should use data to monitor his or her operation and identify process problems that create fragmented, disconnected care for patients. Some of these process problems include staff inconsistency, scheduling problems, transition problem patterns, lack of interdisciplinary communication, patterns of poor follow-up, and external problems such as a pattern of patient readmissions from certain hospitals.

Much of this data can be obtained from the electronic medical record or from quality assurance data collection and studies. The key is to use data to find the gaps and then apply work simplification or clinical best practices to close them.

Help Staff Use the Right Tools to Coordinate Care

Without coaching, employees will develop their own methods for managing care and may not use the most optimal tools and techniques. The manager can help with this by coaching staff to use tools and techniques such as SBAR, when reporting to a physician, point-of-service charting, electronic medical record (EMR) tools such as sending tasks to other disciplines, online calendar tools, and organizational reference manuals or databases.

Train Staff in Communication and Organization

First, the manager herself must be an expert in communication and organization skills and should model these skills for staff. The most basic communication skills for staff are active listening, explaining, giving feedback, and reporting to other professionals. Providing some sample scripts for employees to use in common situations can be helpful in improving communication. Training clinicians who are disorganized often requires very concrete coaching and tools, such as a pre- and post-visit checklist, helping staff with more efficient charting methods, and getting help from information systems to optimize computers, smartphones, and other technical tools. It can be very helpful to observe less organized employees as they give care, so the manager can offer practical tips and tricks immediately after an issue is observed. The manager can also pair the less organized employee with one who is more efficient for some peer counseling and observational learning.

Improve Workflows Across Handoff Points

Another aspect of the clinical manager's job is to ensure that information flows smoothly between departments, disciplines, and other organizations.

For example, there should be a smooth process for the handoff between admissions/intake and the clinical work unit. This means the manager should talk to other departments about what they need and then should explain what his or her team needs from that department. If the two views of roles and responsibilities are at odds, the managers must negotiate to an acceptable compromise or miscommunication and animosity between the staff of the two departments will certainly ensue.

Monitor Common Disconnect Situations

Certain situations and processes are more prone to producing care fragmentation than others. It pays to focus attention in these areas to prevent disconnected care. Some common examples of high-risk disconnect situations are:

- Combining a high-risk patient with a low-performing clinician

- Admissions or start of care when things are busy and rushed and important tasks are missed
- Reporting and responding to patient changes in conditions when many staff members or different work shifts are involved in patient care
- During the implementation of new procedures when processes and accountabilities are not entirely clear
- When a patient is being moved from one location to another
- Uncontrolled variation in which each staff person performs a clinical process differently, thus creating fuzzy expectations, accountability, and communication
- When a group of clinicians is caring for a patient, but no one is in charge and the "team" is not communicating

Debriefing the root causes of clinical errors due to disconnects or miscommunications will often uncover one of the situations listed as a root cause.

INTERVIEW WITH ALEXANDRA CHIN, GENESIS HEALTH CARE

Ms. Chin has been the director of nursing at a rehabilitation and long-term care skilled nursing facility for 2 years. She oversees all nursing staff, certified nursing assistants, and medical records staff. Ms. Chin had worked in a hospital and had been a floor nurse and a unit manager prior to her current position. Each floor of the facility is staffed with a charge nurse who oversees resident care plans and administers medications and treatments. Certified nursing assistants provide personal care to residents and help them with activities of daily living.

Ms. Chin describes the long-term side of the building as the resident's home. The care is very personalized and coordinated and the facility provides recreation, social work, psychologist services for those with psychiatric diagnoses, as well as physical, occupational, and speech therapy. The nursing staff takes time to talk with residents at length, understand what matters to them, and create a very individualized care plan which is updated at least quarterly.

In this setting; staff, family members, and patients become "members of a family." Residents are given as much choice as possible, such as the ability to choose food from a restaurant-like menu. The facility is very patient centered and tries to foster resident decision making. There is a resident council. Members of the council are very involved and often have strong opinions. The facility tries to accommodate council decisions. Families are an important part of integrating care for facility residents. They are very involved in care planning and are invited to care planning meetings. Families are always called when a resident experiences a change in condition.

(continues)

The facility uses a number of strategies to create a positive and connected experience for each resident. The facility team works together to create a customized care plan and schedule that incorporates patient preferences. The recreation department assesses resident preference for things like the type of bathing that the resident wants and asks the resident how late he or she wants to sleep. The facility also tries to create a cohesive experience for residents through periodic interdisciplinary team meetings which involve both the patient and family. Nurses are highly involved in these meetings.

On the short-term unit, home care agencies that will follow the patient after discharge come to discharge planning meetings to facilitate more coordinated discharges. The facility liaison goes into the hospital and meets patients who have been referred to the facility prior to discharge to help them understand what to expect and to facilitate discharge and transition communication.

Ms. Chin believes that teamwork is an important part of avoiding fragmented care for residents. The organizational culture fosters a teamwork mentality. Each employee, no matter what their rank or status, is expected to pitch in and help residents as needed. Ms. Chin coaches aides to help each other with resident personal care tasks and not to "go it alone." If a patient light is on, each and every staff member knows that they are responsible for answering it, even administrative staff. All staff also help with meals and with passing out trays. A member of the staff who is certified in the Heimlich maneuver is always on duty during meals. Someone must be with the residents at all times when they are eating, so even office staff take their turns at covering the dining room.

Ms. Chin's facility works hard to help the certified nursing assistants (CNAs) understand that they are very important and that they see situations with residents that no one else sees. The facility uses INTERACT communication tools such as the STOP and WATCH tool (a one-page tool that helps CNAs know when to report a resident change) to identify resident changes in condition. The form is printed in hot pink so it catches staff attention.

All clinical staff are also instructed to use the SBAR method of reporting for a resident condition change. The facility uses the INTERACT template for reporting when a patient is transitioned to an inpatient facility.

A section of the EMR is used to monitor unplanned patient transfers. Ms. Chin regularly meets with the medical director to review unplanned admissions. She then educates the staff about root causes and talks with individual clinicians who were involved in the patient transfer. Ms. Chin tries to call the hospital when a patient is transferred, but does not always find that hospital staff are interested in transition reporting.

The facility uses standardized, commercially printed teaching materials. The nurses have access to this material online. Facility nurses also teach patients and families self-care using a "stoplight" tool, which labels various symptoms as "red," "yellow," or "green" to signify the level of symptom severity. Nurses use teach-back, asking the patient to repeat what was taught.

The facility has been able to reduce care fragmentation due to patient hospital transfers by improving its medical capabilities. Staff are now IV certified, and can do procedures such as peritoneal dialysis, total parenteral nutrition (TPN), and wound vacs. They can provide IV push Lasix to avoid transfers for congestive heart failure (CHF) patients who are retaining fluid.

Ms. Chin summarizes by saying that there are many misconceptions about skilled nursing facilities. Many people think of them as mini-hospitals. In the skilled nursing facility, there is access to a team but not as many medical resources as in a hospital. "You have to be a better nurse in this setting and use quick critical thinking." Working in this setting has given Ms. Chin a newfound respect for skilled nursing facility nurses.

▶ Applying the Pillars of Connected Care in Middle Management

As mentioned previously, the core elements of connected care are called "pillars." These pillars are the key characteristics of a culture of connected care. The foundation of connected care is patient-centered care. The pillars are teamwork, transitions, coordination, communication, and collaboration. To achieve connected care, each level of the organization must play its part. Senior managers incorporate the pillars of connected care into the organizational vision and strategic plan. **Middle managers create the structures and processes that support performance**. Frontline clinical staff apply connected care principles, tools, and techniques to actual patient care. Professionals in staff positions support managers in achieving culture change, particularly in the areas of quality improvement projects, team building, and data management. In the rest of this chapter, we will examine specific managerial tactics that can be used to build the pillars of a connected care system.

Implementing connected care requires a mindset shift from task-oriented to patient-centered care, an improved skillset, and the constant application of critical thinking to patient care.

To help employees evolve and make this transformation, managers must employ more sophisticated training and coaching techniques than are usually used in health care. Most of all, the connected care transformation requires managers to put aside sometimes pressing tasks to provide the meaningful engagement and coaching that employees need to transform their practice.

▶ Middle Managers and Patient-Centered Care

Patient centeredness is THE core element of a connected care culture. The manager's job in developing patient centeredness is to focus, direct, and support clinicians to put patient needs ahead of their own. To accomplish connected care, professionals need their own level of support, but in a patient-centered culture the patient's needs come before all others.

Making Connected Care Matter to Clinicians

Clinical staff, especially those steeped in a compliance mentality, may not be inclined to adopt a patient-centered attitude and behavior unless the organization makes it matter. The organization can get clinicians' attention on the issue of connected care by embedding it into job descriptions, through clinical coaching, and in the performance appraisal process. Employees should also be offered training on practical techniques for collaborative patient care such as patient self-management support tools and techniques.

The new Medicare Conditions of Participation (COPS) for Home Health Care and Skilled Nursing Facilities contains provisions that mandate more patient-centered care and care delivery through teamwork. These new regulatory requirements can be used as leverage to get employees to accept connected care. The organization should integrate connected care competency testing into new clinician orientation and the annual clinician competency assessment process. An example may be to role-play a patient situation and to see if the nurse uses active listening techniques. Another approach may be to have the nurse read a patient case study and create a patient-centered care plan. Managers should consistently monitor clinical employee's use of patient-centered behaviors during case reviews, huddles, and case conferences and provide on-the-spot coaching to turn behavior in a more patient-centered direction.

Those employees who do not consistently demonstrate collaborative patient care attitudes and action will require clinical coaching, possibly combined with motivational interviewing techniques by the manager. Ultimately, clinicians and support staff should be evaluated on their patient-centered care attitudes and actions. This occurs both during coaching and performance appraisal and should be tied to annual salary increases.

Connecting Patient-Centered Care to Health Professional Job Satisfaction

Paradoxically, a focus on patient needs can only be accomplished if staff feel valued and supported. The Institute for Healthcare Improvement in a paper on "Joy in Work" describes this aspect of the middle manager role: "Primary responsibilities of core leaders are utilizing participative management; developing camaraderie and teamwork; leading and encouraging daily improvement, including real-time measurement; and promoting wellness and resiliency through attention to daily practices. Core leaders have the pivotal role of improving joy in work every day at the point of service. They work with their teams through the process of identifying what matters, addressing impediments through performance improvement in daily work. They analyze what is and is not working well, developing strategies, co-creating solutions with team members, advancing system-wide issues to senior executive champions, and working across departments or sites for joint solutions. This practice of participative management combined with collaborative process improvement makes it possible to meet fundamental human needs." (Perlo et al., 2017, p. 20).

Techniques for Building a Patient Centered Care Culture

The balance between staff and patient needs is no easy task, as managers are confronted with clinician needs on a minute-by-minute basis, while they may be somewhat more distant from interactions with patients. Helping clinicians shed the compliance mindset for a patient collaboration mindset requires the manager to first examine his or her own feelings about "compliance" issues and

clearly articulate a vision of what patient-centered care looks like. The stark reality is that patient nonadherence to medical recommendations creates discomfort, lower outcome scores, and considerable inconvenience and frustration for staff. The other stark reality is that try as we might, we cannot control patients and their caregivers to achieve the results we want.

We can only help patients find their own motivation to change or set limits through approaches such as risk contracting that specify the actions health professionals will take as a consequence of patient and family choices. Spending more time asking patients what is important to them and asking how well your clinical team is doing on providing these important elements of care is a good way to continually adjust personal clinician attitudes.

Another way to revise attitudes about patient-centered care is to ask clinicians to visualize themselves being lectured by a health professional about the need to change behavior "for your own good" and then being scolded if they don't change. Maybe you have had such an experience and can bring it to mind when you are tempted to reinforce a heavy-handed clinician approach to achieving compliance. Shedding the compliance mindset also requires managers to coach clinicians about the limits of their power to "fix patient's lives" and to accept that adults who are mentally competent have the right to make "bad decisions" (or at least decisions we as health professionals do not agree with). Helping staff spend more time talking to patients about their lives and the challenges they face may also help with this issue. Encouraging clinicians who are more expert in patient-centered care to share success stories is another way to help other staff visualize what patient-centered care looks like in daily practices.

One good way to help staff stay in touch with the patient viewpoint is to encourage them to visit the Patient's View Institute (2018) website (gopvi.org) and read some of the stories that patients have told about what has worked both well and poorly in their experiences with the healthcare system and health professionals. The manager can then facilitate a discussion about some of these stories at staff meetings. As the stories illustrate, the more acute the setting, and the more compromised the patients, the more important it is to make an extraordinary effort to treat patients with respect and to give them what little control they are able to use.

Another method for fostering patient centeredness is to encourage the use of patient-centered language and ban the use of derogatory labels such as "train wreck." Modeling respectful discussion about patients, after acknowledging staff concerns, helps to counteract negative feelings that clinicians may have about difficult patients. "I know that this has been a difficult case for you to manage. Mrs. Jones seems to have a very challenging life situation without much support. It must be very difficult for someone with her personality to not be in control of her life and her health. How could we look at it from her point of view?"

Managerial Tools for Developing Patient-Centered Staff Behavior

While managers may be tempted to become defensive and automatically take the side of staff in misunderstandings with patients, it is essential that the manager remain balanced and look at the problem from both the staff and patient points of view. Luckily, while the challenge of achieving patient centeredness is great, the tools to achieve it are many. Some tools that managers can employ include:

- **Expectation setting.** If senior management has aligned the organizational culture around patient-centered connected care, middle managers, when they interpret organizational vision and goals, must turn the senior management message into clear actions and accountabilities. Before creating this communication, the manager should clearly visualize what a good job would look like and how she would know it if she saw it.

  The manager must fight the urge to communicate expectations in platitudes and generalities, neither of which is effective in changing employee behavior.

For example, "We as an organization are committed to better care transitions and care coordination. This means that each individual clinician is responsible for not allowing any tasks, information, or follow-up to fall through the cracks. It is the job of support staff to help clinicians in dealing with the follow-up details such as ordering supplies."

- **Adopt a patient-centered filter for management decisions.** This technique is a matter of awareness. To do it, ask yourself: "Who will this decision benefit and how will it impact patients?" If you decide to change scheduling practices, will it result in more clinician continuity for patients or more fragmentation?

- **Motivational interviewing.** This is an advanced communication technique that builds on active listening skills and can be used to help people find their own motivation to change. It works well as a tool to help staff in changing their attitudes toward patient care. We will discuss this technique more in the section on communication.

- **Clinical coaching.** Managers help to embed patient centeredness into the clinician's day-to-day work by reviewing cases with clinicians, asking questions about the patient's goals and the use of self-management support strategies, acknowledging frustration with adherence issues but focusing on constructive problem solving. Managers should try to elicit suggestions from staff themselves and use active listening, but offer resources or ideas if none are forthcoming.

- **Involving patients in staff teaching and in clinical conferences.** Hearing directly from patients is the best way to achieve patient centeredness. If the clinical unit does complex patient conferences or daily huddles, invite patients and their families to participate.

  If you are doing training on care coordination, communication, or patient teaching, ask a patient to attend and to play a part or to give feedback. Creating a patient/family advisory committee and heeding their recommendations is also a powerful way to demonstrate commitment to patient-centered care.

- **Share patient comments from CAHPS surveys, complaints, and compliments.** Patients often provide both positive and negative comments about their experiences of care when they answer surveys or when they write letters to the organization. Reading from these comments at each staff meeting is another way to bring the patient voice into the world of clinicians.
- **Support staff in providing patient-centered care.** As mentioned, providing patient-centered care, especially when patients are very ill or nonadherent, can be stressful and frustrating for staff. Sometimes the manager should intervene and become the buffer between clinical staff and patients/family members who are particularly hostile or who have overwhelming problems. The healthcare manager can help staff deal with

stress through techniques such as active listening, acknowledging frustration, finding community resources, advocacy on behalf of staff, problem solving and simple nurturing through creating a lower stress environment, giving praise, and thanking staff for their efforts. Even bringing in a plate of cookies occasionally can go a long way to nurturing in a highly stressful clinical environment. If staff are particularly frustrated with certain situations or if morale is very low, it may be time to seek help from a senior manager or from human resources staff.

BOX 5-1 describes an exercise that can be used to encourage clinician patient-centered care thinking and actions.

The Planetree organization (Planetree.org, 2016) provides managers with a simple self-assessment tool called Person-Centered Leadership Self Reflection Questions. The quiz is available to download at https://planetree.org/wp-content/uploads/2017/04/20.-Person-Centered-Leadership-Self-Reflection-Questions.pdf.

BOX 5-1 Acknowledge Team Blind Spots

Katie Owens, vice president of Healthstream Engagement Institute, describes an exercise that managers can conduct at staff meetings to help their team renew their commitment to patient-centered care excellence:

1. "Perform a fill-in-the-blank exercise with your team to identify the following:
   - It is hard to feel empathy for patients who_____
   - It is easy to feel empathy for patients who_____
   - It is hard to prioritize patients when_____
2. Discuss your answers frankly and purposefully.
3. Acknowledge some of your common stereotypes or labels.
4. Address common vulnerabilities that can trip you up when attempting to eradicate patient labeling.
5. Communicate openly with the understanding that a nonnegotiable expectation is that you will practice patient-centered behaviors with every single patient, every interaction.
6. Get help and support from your senior leadership team and others who are stakeholders and champions of the culture you are trying to create" (Owens, 2017, p. 5).

INTERVIEW WITH KRISTIN LAGANA, RN

Kristin Lagana, RN, is a clinical quality specialist with Genesis Health Care, a holding company with subsidiaries that operate skilled nursing facilities. Kristin provides consultation services to directors of nursing in the 10 rehabilitation centers that she supports. These 10 centers primarily provide long-term care, but some provide more intensive services such as caring for patients with left ventricular assist devices (LVADs) and serious cardiac disease. Kristin has an online calendar that centers can access and request assistance as needed.

Kristin helps facility administrators and directors of nursing "build a team and supports everyone working to the top of their license." She acts as a role model and coach. Kristin helps centers develop quality assurance/quality improvement (QAPI) programs. Kristin monitors facility quality through environmental rounds, infection control monitoring, chart reviews, an assessment of best practices use, survey preparedness, and an analysis of reportable events. Kristin assists the center leadership in identifying trends in quality indicator data, which generate improvement projects. She checks to ensure that action plans have been initiated for quality issues.

In addition to helping centers identify trends in quality data, she helps teams investigate and test improvements. Kristin says, "People feel they are alone in dealing with some of these problems. I provide them with help." Kristin feels that an important part of improving care is her role modeling behavior for staff. She tries to create a no-blame atmosphere in which center staff can ask for help more than once. They can develop and implement a plan and then come back for help.

Kristin consults with line staff, nurse managers, clinical liaison, and sometimes families. She is most likely to interact with families in times of difficult situations or poor outcomes and the family "needs to hear from someone else. People see me as an outside regional person." Often, people just need to feel that there is someone who cares and with whom they can establish a relationship. Kristin may get involved with complaints. She spends a lot of time listening and is able to prevent situations from escalating.

Kristin helps provide more connected care for patients by facilitating monthly regional meetings in which nurse executives can share ideas for improving care. Connected care in Kristin's view is "all about communication." Another area important to connected care is medication reconciliation when a patient is admitted to the facility after a hospital discharge. Providing consistent staff, especially certified nursing assistants, to each patient is another important aspect of "connecting the dots" for patients. Finances for the patient and the patient's family are an area of stress and sometimes create fragmented care for patients. Within a few days of admission, center staff meet with the patient and/or patient's representative regarding financial planning for the admission with the hope to put their minds at ease and give them the information they may need.

The patient care plan is another aspect of connected care in Kristin's view. The care plan is intended to be personalized to the patient and includes attention to diagnoses, behavior, and quality of life. Patient preferences are an integral part of the care plan.

▶ **Communication**

Communication is possibly the most essential pillar of connected care. Consider the huge amount of harm that occurs when two-way communication about patient information is not communicated across the continuum. Managers have a vital role to play in ensuring that all members of the team receive accurate and updated information both about organizational issues and about the care of their current patients. They must also ensure that patients receive clear, accurate, and constantly updated information about their condition and the care they are receiving.

Effective communication in health care is a risk management tool, as many incidents relating to patient harm and subsequent malpractice suits result from miscommunication. In a 2015 study, Crico Strategies, a risk management firm, evaluated 7,100 malpractice cases in which miscommunication was a key root cause of patient harm, much of it serious. The study found that 57% of cases involved poor provider-to-provider communication and 55% involved provider-to-patient communication with a 12% overlap (Ruoff, 2015).

Common problems included miscommunication about the patient's condition, poor documentation, not reading the medical record, inadequate informed consent, and an unsympathetic response to patient complaints. Every single one of these disconnection issues can be addressed by focusing management attention on clinical culture change for better communication. Managers accomplish this by using a set of core principles that are illustrated in **FIGURE 5-10**.

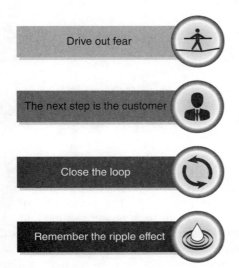

FIGURE 5-10 Communication Key Principles for Managers

Key Communication Principles for Middle Managers

- **Drive out fear.** In health care this is necessary because of the often painful and difficult information that must be conveyed and because of the power differentials and status differences between patients and professionals and within professional hierarchies that can create fear and blame. Creating an open, blame-free environment has been an important element in the patient safety culture movement. Managers drive out fear by not reacting negatively or defensively to hearing messages from staff and patients that may not be welcome. They also advocate for staff who tell the truth about difficult clinical situations and buffer employees from powerful clinicians or managers who may prefer that they stay silent. Managers should also lower the threat level for patients by ensuring that they have time, privacy, and a sympathetic person to whom they can tell their story.

- **The next step is the customer.** In the concept of "throw it over the wall" transitions there is one-way communication without feedback. This is diametrically opposed to what should happen in a connected care environment. In connected care, each profession and department has a basic understanding of what the next person or function in the workflow needs to know to care for the patient. The "supplier" department or worker provides that information in a form that is usable and complete. By treating the next step in the continuum as the customer, staff ensure that the right information gets to the right person at the right time. Managers implement this principle by monitoring communication, identifying root causes of miscommunication, and coaching staff to think about internal customer service when doing care planning.

- **Close the loop.** In closed loop communication, information is sent to a listener or receiver who then verifies receipt of it. In high-risk situations such as when orders are transmitted in an emergency, the receiver may repeat back what he or she heard: "The order is for 50 milligrams of Benadryl." In other situations, the receiver simply replies to indicate that the information was received: "Got it."

Managers foster closed loop communication by modeling it. One way they do this is to acknowledge and return phone calls and emails from staff and peers. The second step in closing the loop is taking time to read, understand, and respond to the message that has been delivered. Another way to foster closed loop communication is to immediately address situations in which staff used only one-way communication, such as leaving a message about a patient's condition change but not ensuring that the clinician at the other end received it.

- **Remember the ripple effect.** Every organizational action, decision, or change affects multiple staff and their patients. However, communication is often incomplete or misses some of the people who need the change information. Managers can ensure that they get important information to key people by using strategic communication tools and techniques and by not forgetting people who work per diem, part time, or in lower level support jobs. Every major managerial communication should be preceded by the question, "Who needs to know?" One failure in communication is leaving out part-time, per diem, remote, or off-shift employees. Managers should be vigilant about ensuring that these employees are included in important communications.

How Managers Facilitate Communication

- **Modeling.** Managers also achieve effective communication by modeling the key interpersonal communication techniques such as active listening, negotiation, motivational interviewing and assertiveness, and training and coaching staff to use them as well.
- **Using strategic communication** to ensure that information about organizational issues gets to the right people in a form that they can understand and use. One way to facilitate strategic communication is to create a simple list or spreadsheet that identifies who is impacted by a decision or change and how best to communicate with them. The strategic communication grid in Chapter 4 can be used for this purpose. This is a formal tool for answering the key question, "Who needs to know?"
- **Providing access to formal communication skills training.** Organizations such as the Institute for Healthcare Communications (http://healthcarecomm.org) provide intensive in-person courses. Other programs are available from the Academy for Communication in Healthcare (http://www.achonline.org).
- **Providing accessible and understandable information** about policies, procedures, and organizational changes through email, written communication, or formal presentations.
- **Implementing training, processes, and tools that foster the use of evidence-based clinical communication techniques** such as SBAR reporting or structured care communications about changes in condition such as the STOP and Watch Tool from the Interact Program (Pathway Health, 2017).
- **Creating processes that support effective communication** to patients and between members of the clinical team. An example is implementing standards and specific mechanisms for interdisciplinary communication exchanges, and monitoring to ensure that this communication occurs. An example from home care would be to set a standard that interdisciplinary conferencing must occur every 2 weeks and working with staff to develop a template that can be used for communication between nursing, therapy, and social work.

- **Providing support in the use of communication technologies** such as email, secure mail, texting, use of specialized software, portals, and patient tracking systems.
- **Giving constructive feedback** to employees, peers, and in certain circumstances, senior managers when a problem arises.

Practical Communication Improvement Practices

A white paper from the company Healthstream identifies 10 best practices that managers can apply to improve communication in the healthcare workplace. This paper provides a series of step-by-step guidelines for improving both employee communication skills with patients and managerial communication. One technique suggested in this paper is "Words that Work" (SM). This approach helps healthcare professionals analyze a typical patient experience situation and brainstorm a list of words or phrases that can be used to communicate a consistent message to patients in a friendly way. Another term for this approach is "scripting." See an example of this technique in **BOX 5-2**.

The paper suggests that managers embed the Words that Work (SM) concept into daily work by including staff in the development of the scripts, posting the key words in a prominent place where staff can see them, recognizing and rewarding staff who use the scripts, coaching staff who are struggling to use the "words at work concept," and continuing to develop and refine scripts at staff meetings. The paper recommends a series of managerial communication support techniques, including teaching step-by-step formulas for patient communication, regular rounding (meeting) with both patients and employees to get feedback on how things are going and to identify potential problems, creating department communication boards with data about department performance, and relaying compliments and information about new procedures (Healthstream, n.d.).

BOX 5-2 Words That Work (SM) Example

Issue Addressed: **Staff Responsiveness** (use this during admission rounding)
Example: "Let me explain how to use your call button. Our team responds to the call button immediately at the nurses' station. It may take x (determine call light response time) minutes before your nurse can be with you in your room; however, we will treat your request with urgency" (Healthstream, n.d., p. 6).

🔍 CASE STUDY

Clinical Managers Tackle Communication Challenges

A group of home healthcare clinical managers from the Everford Health System decided to develop a process improvement team to improve employee and patient communication. This project was launched because employee surveys identified concerns about fragmented communication, and patient experience scores showed that clinician communication with patients was less than ideal.

Based on data from focus groups and individual interviews with both staff and patients, the team decided to adopt a set of management communication best practices that included closed loop communication between clinicians, managing out-of-office voicemails and email messages, reducing email overload for clinicians, and ensuring that anyone affected by a clinical issue gets notified.

The managers also decided to create a system of "radical transparency" in which they would help employees to better understand the agency's business environment, goals, and strategies for achieving the quadruple aim. The group created a weekly email newsletter update that included agency procedure changes, compliments, key metrics, and new programs of interest to clinicians. They also instituted a "letters to the management" section so employees could communicate back with ideas and issues. The managers reduced the amount of employee email overload by using a set of standardized subject headings in emails so staff could triage those emails that needed to be opened first. They reinstated regular staff meetings and dedicated a period of time for employee suggestions and input into workflow changes, procedures, or other issues. The managers adopted a standard form for strategic communications that cued them to think through the issue of "who needs to know." Working with employees, they then devised an agency-wide process for interdisciplinary communication that incorporated the idea of "closing the loop" or always responding to patient-related communication.

The clinical managers asked the organization to provide them with some intensive interactive training in clinical interviewing and motivational interviewing. They then restated communication expectations for staff, instituted a series of education programs on communication, made communication skills part of the annual competency evaluation, and incorporated more stringent communication requirements into performance appraisals.

Managers modeled communication skills, went on visits to observe employees, and coached employees to improve these skills. The team also worked with clinical employees to develop scripts for specific steps in the care process such as the start of care and discharge. After 6 months of intensive work on communication, a second employee survey revealed significant improvement. The agency's next HCAHPS (CMS publicly reported survey, Home Health Consumer Assessment of Healthcare Providers and Systems) survey also showed improvement in outcome scores.

Anecdotal data suggested that complaints and care transition problems had dropped significantly as a result of better communication. Eventually the Everford Continuity Team adopted the communication best practices developed by the home health agency for all entities in the system.

▶ Middle Managers and Care Coordination

Care coordination, one of the most essential of the pillars of connected care, requires special clinical skills and expertise and considerable support from management to achieve the best outcomes for patients. Within the care coordination function, nurses or other clinicians organize the elements of information, health services, and resources that patients need for recovery and self-care and transition to the next step in the care continuum.

Managers support the complex process of care coordination through employee selection, training, assembling resources, and helping clinicians with organization and complex patient problem solving.

In specialized care coordination departments, the manager him or herself will be an experienced care coordinator who is responsible not only for supervising and managing care coordinators but for overseeing and managing care coordination policy, processes and structures. In other settings, such as in ambulatory care or home health care, care coordination may be only a part of the clinician's and manager's jobs. Several methods that can help the manager support clinicians who perform care coordination functions are:

- **Review and analysis of clinician caseload data and tracking of the highest risk patients** with clinicians.
- **Clinical coaching** to help clinicians manage the more challenging patients in their caseload.
- **Debriefing of the root causes of faulty care coordination** such as transitions that resulted in transfers to inpatient, emergency room, or a higher level of care.
- **Facilitating interdisciplinary meetings, such as complex case conferences**, to help

support clinicians in coordinating care for complex patients.

■ **Providing education and training in new care coordination techniques and resources.**

■ **Acting as an advocate and intermediary with other employees such as the organization compliance officer** for clinicians who are dealing with risk management

situations or when external agencies such as a protective services agency is involved.

■ **Providing advice, support, and community resources** or higher level medical resources in cases in which the clinician and/or the team doesn't have all the skills or knowledge to deal with a high-risk/high-need patient.

PROVIDING CONNECTED CARE IN A LONG-TERM ACUTE CARE HOSPITAL

Interview with Kathy Reilly, RN, Director of Care Management, Gaylord Hospital; Deb Kaye, RN, Care Manager, Gaylord Hospital

Gaylord Hospital is a long-term acute care hospital (LTACH). This type of facility provides hospital level care for complex patients. Patients usually have a longer length of stay (3–4 weeks) than inpatients in acute care hospitals. Typical patients who are admitted to this setting include those who have complex wounds, must be weaned off ventilators, have respiratory failure, or have traumatic brain or spinal cord injuries. Gaylord also provides a rehabilitation component for patients with problems such as strokes who also have other severe comorbidities or unstable medical conditions. Patients in this setting are typically admitted from an acute care hospital.

Case management is an integral part of the services provided by the LTACH. These services begin with a regional clinical liaison nurse who visits potential patients in acute care hospitals. The liaison nurse conducts a thorough clinical assessment, reviews the medical record, and visits the patient and family. The liaison decides whether the patient meets the criteria for LTACH admission and whether LTACH is the appropriate level of care.

If Gaylord agrees to admit the patient, the liaison explains the services to the patient and family and describes what to expect. Ms. Reilly notes that a referral to an LTACH is usually quite acceptable to patients as they feel safe in an environment that provides a hospital level of care and in which they are seen by a doctor every day. The LTACH setting also provides much more intensive levels of nursing care than a skilled nursing facility with nurse-to-patient ratios of one RN to six to eight patients. A big issue for the facility is that patients do not want to leave when it is time for discharge. The LTACH goal is not to completely return patients to full function but to help them transition to the next and most appropriate level of care, which may be a discharge home or a skilled nursing facility.

Every patient admitted to Gaylord is assigned to a nurse case manager. The case manager starts to plan the patient discharge from the admission. Starting with information provided by the hospital liaison nurse, the case manager assesses patient clinical needs, finances, insurance coverage, family support, psychosocial issues, and patient goals and wants. While direct care clinical staff mostly coordinate care when the patient is an inpatient, the case manager may intervene to ensure the services essential to the discharge plan, such as occupational therapy, are brought into the patient's case.

Gaylord has weekly interdisciplinary team rounds in which case managers participate. These are "walking around" rounds in which the team goes to the patient's room to discuss care, family members are included, and the plan and target dates for discharge are discussed. If the patient or family members cannot attend the team meeting, the case manager will share the team's discussion with them later.

(continues)

The case manager will work with the inpatient nursing staff to prepare the patient and family for discharge. For example, if the patient has a complex wound or needs a technical procedure to be done at home, the case manager will create a communication sheet that outlines necessary patient teaching.

Gaylord sees postacute and medical equipment providers as colleagues and has an open-door policy that allows these agencies to send in a clinical liaison to meet the patient, evaluate the case, and possibly create a teaching plan that can be started on the Gaylord inpatient unit. For example, a company that provides enteral nutrition may develop a patient teaching plan for the inpatient nurse unit staff.

Case managers do a thorough assessment of potential barriers to discharge—for example, considering how to arrange the home for a patient who has had a leg amputation but who lives on the second floor. Case managers also consider the patient's caregiving support network and may refer to community agencies to close the gaps. In recent years, case managers have found housing to be a big barrier for lower income patients. While case managers do not actually arrange for housing they will try to find a social services agency in the community that can help.

Care management staff continue to follow patients after discharge from Gaylord by calling the patient 3 to 5 days after the discharge to clarify medication orders, ensure that supplies and equipment have arrived, and check on the status of medical follow-up appointments, postacute services, and problems. For those patients who are discharged without services, the case manager will schedule a postdischarge appointment with the patient's primary care doctor.

Creating discharge plans for patients with highly complex and resource intensive needs is a constant challenge for Gaylord case managers. For example, few skilled nursing facilities want to accept ventilator-dependent patients. Finding resources for patients who need long-term, complex wound care or daily physical occupational or speech therapy can be very difficult. In many cases, these patients may need to be placed in facilities far from their homes, sometimes in another state.

Another challenge is finding a primary care physician who will accept these complex patients. Regulations surrounding reimbursement are other issues for LTACH case managers.

Ms. Reilly and Ms. Kaye state that as highly challenging as this work is, it is rewarding in the same measure. In some ways it is a pure form of nursing where there is intense engagement with patients and families and the satisfaction of knowing that front line clinical staff and case managers make a big difference in patient's lives.

When asked about the case they are most proud of, both case managers tell about a man who was a patient at Gaylord. He had had a cardiac arrest and was revived, but suffered anoxic brain damage. He had a tracheostomy, a feeding tube, and was ventilator dependent. He was also on renal dialysis. Through intensive research the case manager was able to find a company that would do home renal dialysis. The wife, who had been an emergency medical technician (EMT) at one time, was so desperate to take her husband home that she agreed to learn all the complex high-tech procedures that he would need. The dialysis company also helped to train the wife in their procedures. After 9 months as an inpatient, the patient went home. Ms. Kaye says "there wasn't a dry eye in the hospital when they left." Unfortunately, the home stay was short lived as the patient contracted a respiratory infection and subsequently died. The wife was so grateful for the time she had at home with her husband that she continues to return to the hospital for visits and to express her gratitude for the extraordinary efforts that the Gaylord team made.

Employee Selection and Training for Care Coordination

Managers who hire clinicians for jobs that contain a care coordination component should expect candidates to have excellent basic clinical skills in assessment, patient teaching, and the performance of clinical procedures. Managers should also assess job applicants for highly developed organizational skills and advanced communication, negotiation, and health coaching skills.

A 2013 article in the journal *Nursing Economics* describes the range of competencies necessary to effectively perform care coordination (Haas, Swan, & Haynes, 2013). Because care coordination usually involves coordinating multiple resources for patients, potential employees should be well versed in the role of other health professions and in the use of community resources. One method for assessing potential care coordination capability is to provide candidates with some typical patient case studies and ask them to describe how they would approach care coordination for this patient.

Use of Data and Population Health Tactics

Care coordination is by nature a population health effort. The clinician manages a caseload or population of patients, each of whom is at a different level of risk for decompensation or a return to acute care. The manager in turn oversees the caseloads of the whole team or unit. More sophisticated organizations apply evidence-based best practices to patient populations at different levels of risk. The manager should understand how to use data to identify the levels of risk and to apply these best practices. For example, a home care agency may apply frailty best practices to patients who are in the medium risk category.

The manager must support clinicians in constantly triaging their patient population using clinical assessment and caseload data. **FIGURE 5-11** provides an example of a "commonsense" risk triage system for nurse case managers.

In a primary care medical home setting, the manager may assess population risk by automatically receiving risk scores from the practice electronic medical record or from information received on referral. The manager must help clinicians stay focused on high-risk situations within their caseload such as a patient newly returned home after an acute care transfer.

Helping Employees Prioritize Care Coordination Tasks

Using data, the manager can help employees prioritize care coordination tasks and determine the level of care intensity needed by specific patients. Often this involves discussion with clinicians about the use of time and scheduling. For

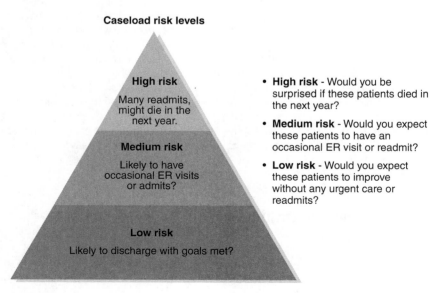

Caseload risk levels

High risk

Many readmits, might die in the next year.

Medium risk

Likely to have occasional ER visits or admits?

Low risk

Likely to discharge with goals met?

- **High risk** - Would you be surprised if these patients died in the next year?
- **Medium risk** - Would you expect these patients to have an occasional ER visit or readmit?
- **Low risk** - Would you expect these patients to improve without any urgent care or readmits?

FIGURE 5-11 Case Manager Population Risk Assessment Guide

example, in the early stages of a home health-care episode, care is "frontloaded" for high-risk patients (such as a patient recently discharged from the hospital after an exacerbation of heart failure), meaning that the employee must have time to make extra visits and phone calls. The manager should help keep caseloads balanced, so no one clinician is overloaded with the highest risk, most intense cases. The manager can help coach and train employees in time management and efficiency techniques such as point-of-service charting using the nurse's laptop computer in the patient's home.

Facilitating Referrals and Case Sharing

High-risk, high-need patients with many issues related to the social determinants of health will need help from community resources.

The middle manager should ensure that clinical staff does not simply work in isolation, focusing on their own professional responsibilities while ignoring factors such as food, transportation, mental illness, or substance abuse that might completely derail any medical care plan.

To help staff utilize community resources, the manager may need to work with the organization's community outreach, social work, or marketing department to create resource guides or listings for community resources, and other community care coordination resources programs, such as those in medical offices and insurance plans. Through reading and networking, the manager should get to know other managers in local community organizations, learn what these resources are capable of providing, and encourage staff to make good referrals and sometimes to coordinate care with these other entities. In more complex cases when multiple agencies are involved, or in cases in which the care coordinator goes into a residential facility to provide services (such as a home care nurse seeing patients in an assisted living facility), there may need to be case sharing or some type of formal agreements about clinician roles and responsibilities.

🔍 CASE STUDY

Hanna, a regional clinical care director for the local Everford skilled nursing facilities that specialize in short-term rehabilitation, found that many patients were being discharged without adequate care support at home and often without referrals to home health care. These patients were being readmitted to the hospital at a high rate. Hanna contacted Tanya, the skilled nursing facility representative to the continuity team, to help her with this problem. Together they researched insurance company and Medicaid care coordination programs and developed relationships with these care coordinators so social workers could refer high-risk patients to them on discharge.

Tanya and Hanna also worked with the Everford Continuity Team to develop a clinical liaison and referral program with the system home health agencies. Hanna created a resource directory of community organizations that could help patients with social determinants of health and Tanya researched the availability of MSW services from within the health system.

Using these resources, both nursing and social work staff were able to create much better transitions for patients and subsequently a lower readmission rate for Hanna's facilities.

Care Coordination Helping and Hindering Forces

A study reported in the *Journal of the American Board of Family Medicine* looked at the factors that both help and hinder good care coordination (Friedman et al., 2016). The results of the study can guide middle managers in their efforts to build both human and technical systems for good care coordination. The study used an online social learning collaborative with 25 care coordinators in primary care medical homes to identify the factors that facilitate and hinder their effectiveness.

The study found that facilitating and hindering forces for care coordination fell into three categories: organizational/system, interpersonal, and individual. Specific factors are discussed next.

Providing Resources for Care Coordination Effectiveness

Caseload and Workload. Coordinators stated that having too many patients on their caseload (one person had 300 patients) diluted the bond between patient and coordinator, making a workable relationship difficult. Patients who had many problems with mental health and socioeconomic issues required a greater time commitment from the care coordinator but these factors were not always taken into account when assigning work. Another issue was the requirement that coordinators both deliver care coordination and conduct patient tracking activities, functions that the care coordinators felt were incompatible with success.

Time and volume of work is a resource-related factor that is controlled by managers. The manager may determine how many new patients the unit or the team can take, how many patients should be on a caseload, and how many care transitions or care coordination activities each staff person can reasonably handle. Managers should assign tasks and workload by truly understanding the care coordination tasks that their employees are performing, the intensity of the work, and the characteristics of the patient population.

Providing Good Quality Clinical Information Technology

Clinical technology that is not functional for care coordination purposes was a big complaint of study participants. In particular, the inability to run reports by patient population was a frustration. Coordinators reported running multiple reports and then cobbling them together manually. Another frustration was lack of interoperability

between hospitals, specialists, and the practice. Some coordinators created work arounds by developing relationships with other facilities and having information faxed to them. This an area where a manager with good organizational effectiveness skills can make a difference. Since many managers do not have the skill or the knowledge to address these issues directly, good relationships with internal departments such as information systems, quality assurance, or marketing/community outreach can be leveraged to get employees the help they need. By working with their information systems department to create integrated reports, by advocating for the purchase of interoperable systems (which allow outside agencies to look at hospital electronic records), and by building information exchange relationships with partner organizations in the care continuum, managers help employees better perform care coordination.

The Availability of Community Resources

Care coordinators found searching for community resources to address issues such as transportation, medication delivery, mental health services, and low-cost dental care to be essential to their success. Coordinators indicated that having a good community resource directory was invaluable in creating better patient care plans. Managers can help with this problem by finding community resource directories, advocating for their organization to develop their own directory, and inviting representatives of community agencies to come into their facility to explain how their agencies can help patients.

Interactions with Clinicians and Other Healthcare Facilities

Coordinators in the study who practiced in primary care medical homes report that getting "buy-in" for care coordination and collaboration from physicians and other care team members was a big obstacle to success. Likewise, some coordinators complained of the difficulty of getting cooperation from other healthcare organizations, while still others found relationships with health professionals in hospitals or other practices to be invaluable. For managers, working with senior managers, physicians, and other managers to understand and support the care coordination role can be a key success factor for employees.

The manager should be able to explain the benefits of the care coordination function, be able to back up any claims with data, and act as an advocate for those who are performing the difficult task of coordinating care for high-risk patients.

Interactions with Patients

Coordinators often found patient's lack of health literacy, unwillingness to engage in self-care, and distrust of the care coordinator to be barriers to working effectively. One solution that worked for some coordinators was to become an expert at motivational interviewing even to the point of creating an "MI club" where coordinators met monthly to discuss strategies for dealing with patients who are struggling with effective self-care. As noted in the section on communication, managers can impact this problem by role modeling excellent communication skills, spending time with very demanding or angry patients to relieve staff of stress, teach and coach communication skills, and provide scripts for common situations.

The Coordinator's Own Self-Care Practices

Many care coordinators struggled with high stress levels and in some cases difficulties setting boundaries with patients. Without support from managers in the form of coaching, respite breaks, forums for expressing concerns, and coaching about self-care, employees who perform care coordination functions are vulnerable to burnout (Friedman et al., 2016).

Creating Structures and Processes for Better Care Coordination

Providing a clinical work structure that produces the best outcomes for patients is a key role for managers. This is particularly important in care coordination, where either a lack of structure or overly rigid organizational or professional structures can result in fragmentation, patient safety issues, and poor outcomes. The key structures and processes for care coordination are those that involve admitting patients, transmitting information, transferring patients, or situations in which staff must work cooperatively for the good of the patient. Some of the processes that are most prone to fragmentation and errors in all settings are:

- Patient admissions or starts of care
- Scheduling multiple services for patients
- Identifying patient changes in condition, reporting, and taking action
- Processes for ordering supplies and equipment for patients
- Patient movement between different organizational entities or to other facilities
- Transmittal of patient information between departments
- Reassessing patients when they have returned from a more acute level of care

Each of these key processes works best when the manager works with staff to create a standardized workflow, applies work simplification techniques, uses consistent forms or computerized templates for transmitting information, schedules staff in a consistent way so there is continuity of care for patients, and develops a system for monitoring whether the process was completed properly.

Middle Managers and Collaboration

Rarely can one clinician provide all the services necessary to care for a patient. The manager should help clinicians identify internal and external resources for patients and provide coaching on how to use these resources appropriately. Managers must encourage clinicians who are coordinating care to learn about the scope of practice and types of support that other professionals can provide to patients.

They should also monitor internal referrals to ensure that their staff are referring appropriately and frequently enough. For example, nurses may not understand the types of assessment and support that physical, occupational, and speech therapy can offer patients. They may not even truly understand the differences between these professions. It is up to the middle manager to educate nursing staff about how the therapies can help and how they function differently from nursing. Social work is another profession that is often poorly understood by nurses who may perceive it as simply finding benefits and entitlements and not understand the type of emotional support and help with social determinants of health that a social worker can provide. In settings that have pharmacy consultants as members of the team, clinicians should learn how to utilize the pharmacist's special knowledge to help with medication management, drug interactions, and medication reconciliation.

The manager should work with other professional managers to facilitate joint training and dialogue between the professions to build respect and teamwork. Managers must also develop collaborative arrangements with other organizational professionals and departments to support the work of connected care. An example is a nurse manager and physical therapy manager who realized, through feedback from their respective staffs, that there was considerable misunderstanding and even distrust between the professions. Each profession had its own philosophy of patient care with therapy being very goal focused and nursing being focused on patient emotional needs and care tasks.

The managers of the two functions organized a "get to know you" session with a facilitator. After some group icebreakers, the facilitator was able to do a series of exercises that helped the two professions better understand each other.

Middle Managers and Care Transitions

Patient and information transitions are the most crucial aspects of connected care. Care transitions are often invisible and elusive for managers since they involve managing the "white space" between professions, departments, and other providers in the care continuum.

Managers should understand how their department's finished work impacts the next step in care. For example, in acute care facilities and in home care, the next step in the continuum is often a discharge to home and a handoff of information and responsibility to the primary care physician. Managers must have a sense of what the patient, the family, and the physician need to know and need to do to make the transition successful. For example, if the nurse has been managing medications for the patient, what strategies will be used to prepare medications in the home once the professional is out of the picture? To achieve care transition goals, middle managers should pay serious attention to the structures and processes that support transition outcomes. Care transition structural elements include:

- Senior management oversight and attention to care transitions.
- The adoption of evidence-based care transition models.
- Clear functions and roles for managing care transitions such as admission and discharge management responsibilities.
- Resources and time allocated to care transitions.
- Policies and procedures that support effective care transitions.
- Computer information systems and other tools for care transition communication.
- Forms and patient education materials that foster effective care transitions.
- Negotiated relationships, expectations, and contracts with other providers who send patients to the facility or agency. This is particularly important in value-based payment relationships when clinician behavior (i.e., a home care nurse sending all patients with

a decline in condition to the emergency room) can create financial penalties for partner organizations.

Middle Managers and Teamwork

Teamwork in clinical care is highly dependent on management support. Without clear direction, individual clinicians and support staff may perform their work in a way that suits them and does not necessarily contribute to better team outcomes. Managers support teamwork by ensuring that team members know that it is an important expectation for everyone. Managers should provide a clear message about the goals of the team and explain how each employee's job, and performance, contributes to the work of the team. Managers should also clarify expectations about mutual respect between team members, meeting behaviors, supporting other team members and team communications. Data about team outcomes and performance can help keep everyone focused on improving clinical results.

Other managerial actions that support teamwork are giving staff time to do interdisciplinary conferencing, scheduling high-risk case conferences and team huddles, giving staff a voice at meetings, and listening for care coordination, communication, and care transition barriers. Managers should encourage teamwork and mutual staff support outside team meetings.

▶ Performance Management—A Key Tool in Achieving Connected Care

Effective management of employee performance is absolutely essential to achieving connected care. The process of performance management does not start with orientation and end with a yearly performance appraisal. It is a continuous process of setting expectations, providing

resources, coaching, giving feedback, and helping employees make course corrections. **TABLE 5-4** describes examples of specific performance management techniques that can be used to achieve connected care.

▶ Clinicians and the Performance Continuum

Managers can apply performance management techniques to support and encourage good employee connected care performance and to improve low performance. Managing lower levels of performance is often a big part of the healthcare middle manager's job, especially in areas where workforce shortages create a smaller pool of well-qualified clinicians.

This focus on lower levels of performance can divert manager attention away from steady and reliable staff and high-performing clinicians who, if nurtured, can become role models, mentors, and champions of connected care innovation and improvement. Reliable and high-performing employees need regular attention. To sustain and encourage these clinicians, managers give specific feedback on what they are doing right, encourage and support attempts at improvement, even if they fail, provide public recognition for good performance and offer opportunities for new skill development or participation on committees or change projects.

Each department has its share (hopefully small) of staff who do not perform up to standards. Chronic low performance produces less than optimal patient care, and often creates complaints, resentment from other staff, and time pulled away from the manager's clinical culture change work. Looking at performance as a systems issue can help managers improve the performance of their whole employee population.

Low performance is not only a matter of employee attitude and commitment. It can often be traced back to system failures in performance management including: rushed or

TABLE 5-4 Performance Management Techniques for Achieving Connected Care

Action	Examples
Set expectations	<ul><li>Explain, in very specific ways, what is expected and offer examples.</li><li>Tell stories that illustrate the expectation.</li><li>Show videos that provide examples.</li><li>Share patient comments that illustrate how clinician behaviors affected the patient experience.</li></ul>
Offering training and job aids	<ul><li>Provide training in the tools and techniques of patient-centered, connected care.</li><li>Direct employees to outside webinars, lectures, conferences, and training.</li><li>Help each employee conduct a self-assessment of skill gaps and create a plan to close the gaps.</li></ul>
Build competence with supervised practice	<ul><li>Offer classroom opportunities for practice.</li><li>Use teach-back and return demonstration to verify learning.</li><li>Have employees observe and give each other feedback.</li><li>Provide an opportunity for the employee to work with and observe an expert in action.</li><li>Test skills at competency fairs.</li><li>Find and show video models of connected care techniques in action.</li></ul>
Provide the resources to do the job	<ul><li>Provide access to needed technology.</li><li>Give clinicians time to do the job.</li><li>Provide continuous access to needed supplies and equipment.</li><li>Provide support staff help as appropriate.</li></ul>
Offer tools to support performance	<ul><li>Add scripts, templates in the electronic medical record to cue connected care activities as well as forms, email, and text reminders.</li></ul>
Give feedback and coach for improved performance	<ul><li>Tell employees, in very specific ways, how they are doing: "Mrs Jones responded well when you asked her what was really important to her. It might have been helpful to allow her to talk a bit more afterward."</li><li>Coach employees to identify improved behaviors.</li><li>Use motivational interviewing techniques to help employees find their own motivation to change.</li></ul>
Praise good work	<ul><li>Give positive feedback, naming specific actions that the employee has performed: "Your documentation clearly shows that you have been helping patients set smart goals. Every one of your records achieved the goal."</li></ul>
Incorporate new expectations into workflows	<ul><li>Get employee input on how to examine and improve work processes to accommodate new requirements.</li><li>Ask groups of employees to a meeting to discuss and flowchart a modified patient encounter that uses patient-centered care techniques.</li><li>Engage employees in patient-centered care process improvement projects.</li></ul>

Data from Mager and Pipe, 1997.

inadequate orientation, lack of clear expectations, inadequate training, no opportunity for practice, not enough time and resources to do the job, limited feedback on performance, and perverse rewards such as getting smaller work assignments because of poor performance. After diagnosing the problem, the manager, sometimes with the help of human resources, should take direct accountability for daily monitoring, coaching, feedback, and counseling or discipline if the poor performance does not resolve itself. Simply tolerating low performance in the vain hope that things will change of their own accord creates both a risk management situation and imposes a less than adequate practitioner on sick patients.

Measuring Front Line Clinician-Connected Care Performance

Managers need methods for evaluating clinician-connected care competence and effectiveness. These methods can include observation of patient care, clinician self-assessments, peer assessments, supervisory performance appraisal, and individual clinician outcome measures. The QSEN Institute website provides a variety of evidence-based tools to assess mastery of the QSEN competencies (QSEN Institute, 2017). These methods could possibly be used in periodic nurse competency testing, although they tend to be laborious to administer and may be more useful in an academic environment.

In organizations that have a quadruple aim key indicator system, and that publish regular performance reports, measurement is easier because goals are clear and managers understand connected care key indicators for their organization and their own team. Visible measurement, in which care teams get frequent updates on their own performance, can be a highly motivating strategy for staff. In some settings, managers can provide clinical staff with data on their own outcome measures, such as readmissions of patients on their caseload, and help

them compare their performance to team and organization benchmarks. While each setting will have its own key indicators, core care coordination measures that are key to measuring connected care are:

- Hospital readmission rates
- Patients who received a transition record at the time of discharge
- Medication reconciliation accuracy
- Patient experience of care coordination using the Consumer Assessment of Healthcare Providers and Systems (CAHPS) survey

Another key measure of connected care is adverse events that result from miscommunication and lack of care coordination.

The data are likely to be measured and communicated by the organization quality assurance function. For example, missed visits and adverse events can occur in home care when a nurse case manager goes on vacation and does not adequately report on her patient caseload care needs to her supervisor or to the per diem nurses who will be covering her patients.

Outcome Measures and Individual Accountability

While organizations may be tempted to use outcome measures as a true reflection of clinician effectiveness, this approach must be taken with caution. There should be a careful evaluation of the link between the outcome and the influence that clinician behavior has on achieving it.

For example, effective medication reconciliation is a key outcome measure. Individual clinicians are usually responsible for this process, so it may be an appropriate measure of individual clinician effectiveness. However, other organizational, patient, and external factors may play as much a role in outcomes as individual clinician work. A nurse may report medication discrepancies, but she cannot reconcile them without physician response and involvement. Readmissions, while influenced by clinician behavior, may have a number of other root causes that are outside the control of the individual clinician. For example, a nurse may identify a weight gain and increased shortness of breath in a patient with heart failure. If she notifies the physician and suggests an additional trial dose of a diuretic, she has reached the limit of her ability to control the situation. It is then up to the physician to concur with the nurse's recommendation or to send the patient to the emergency room. Organizational workflows can also strongly influence individual clinician outcomes. However, a pattern of patient readmissions from a nurse who refuses to use best practices consistently is probably a true performance problem.

Connected Care Self-Auditing

Another type of connected care measurement is self-audit or peer audit. Clinicians periodically review their own work or that of their peers if that is the organizational process. They then become aware of gaps and cracks in their own practice and identify patterns in their work processes that create a fragmented experience for patients. Clinicians can then strive to eliminate these disconnected care habits. For example, a nurse may not regularly check her cell phone voicemail and may miss important calls from patients or colleagues. Self-audits identify situations in which patient care tasks have "fallen through the cracks."

In many cases, these situations do not necessarily result in an adverse event if the clinician or another staff person has quickly "picked up the pieces." For example, a busy nurse is receiving patient care questions from aides or medical assistants and is not responding in a timely fashion. Once the nurse reviews her own work, or gets complaints from the aides or their supervisor, and becomes aware of this problem, she can build in time to communicate with aides and close that particular gap.

Chart Audits and Supervisory Monitoring

These are the most commonly used tools for evaluating clinician connected care competence

and effectiveness. As noted earlier, embedding connected care responsibilities and competencies into job descriptions and performance appraisal makes the criteria for performance clear. Quality assurance staff check adherence to these performance standards through focused chart audits on processes such as medication reconciliation, the consistent use of clinical best practices, the quality of patient care transitions, and documented evidence that the clinician has worked with the patient to set goals. Managers should make opportunities to observe employees delivering clinical care.

Discussing cases with clinical staff on a daily basis can help the manager determine whether the tools and techniques of connected care are being used. By monitoring comments and complaints from patients and families, managers can get a sense of whether there are issues with lack of follow-up or miscommunication that originate with clinical employees. Once quality assurance data have been collected, the data can be reviewed with groups of staff to get input on possible root causes and to identify solutions that staff feel they "own."

Monitoring Connected Care by Talking to Patients

One important measure of how well connected care is working on a clinical unit or team is patient and family perceptions of care connection or fragmentation. While formal surveys like CAPHS scores provide semiquantitative measures of the patient experience, the data from these surveys are typically stripped of nuances and emotion. When managers speak with patients about their experiences they get the details and much more information about the impact of staff behaviors and unit work processes on the patient experience. One way to gather data on patient perceptions of unit connected care is to periodically call or visit patients who have experienced a transition—into or out of the clinical unit—or who have had a decline in condition or some intensive care experience.

These conversations can be as simple as "What was it like for you when you were admitted to our service or unit?" The manager can consolidate information from these conversations into themes and anecdotes and bring it to staff meetings for discussion.

Managers and Obstacles to Connected Care

Managers face a variety of hurdles in working with their employees to achieve connected care for patients. Organizational systems with rigid boundaries that discourage teamwork are a barrier to collaboration and smooth transitions. Senior managers who disparage or are not supportive of the work of middle managers can be an insurmountable barrier to the type of fluid and collaborative work needed to achieve connected care.

Another major issue for managers is what some describe as "being the meat in the sandwich," in which the manager is caught between unrealistic demands from both senior management and employees. A large volume of required administrative tasks and paperwork can become a barrier for managers who do not have time to observe, coach, and interact with employees; a situation that allows performance problems and staff discontent to take root

Mergers, acquisitions, downsizings, and reorganizations are fertile breeding grounds for disconnects, fragmented care, and medical errors. These situations are especially problematic if management staff are being moved around, laid off, or put in different positions, thus damaging continuity of support for employees.

Distraction from constant regulatory and business changes, even when there are no major organizational upheavals, keeps both managers and employees off balance as they struggle to perform the daily work of patient care while absorbing new requirements, forms, procedures, and tasks.

If not managed well, these changes not only contribute to fragmented care for patients, but may actually cause medical errors if unfamiliar procedures disrupt routine clinical practice. Finally, manager burnout is a very real obstacle to connected care. If managers are left to juggle too many demands without adequate resources to do the job and without positive reinforcement and support, they become disillusioned, stressed, and ultimately unable to maintain empathy for staff or patients.

The Everford Continuity Team Tackles Connected Care Implementation

The Everford Continuity Team wants to be sure that they are deploying the connected care vision of senior management. To do this, they decide to go back to their mission statement and to review documents developed by senior management to describe their part in the effort. The team finds that senior managers at the beginning of the connected care culture change (about 8 months ago) had planned to implement clinical culture change in several areas:

- Develop the workforce for connected care
- Clearly define connected care coordination roles and responsibilities
- Clinical managers practice connected care
- Work structures support connected care
- Organizational work processes support connected care
- Technology supports connection
- Create systems for engaging patients and families in connected care

In the intervening time, the senior management team had been challenged by a number of market forces, new regulations, and turnover in key positions at the senior management level. While some of the planned activities had been implemented, some were still "on the back burner."

The continuity team decides to convene a focus group of middle managers to get their perceptions of how far connected care clinical culture change has progressed, how they see their roles, and obstacles they face. The focus group reveals that middle managers are not fully clear on what is expected of them. They have been given some direction on areas that need connected care improvement such as patient transfers between facilities and discharges to home. They have not received training in process improvement or performance improvement as promised. They have become embroiled in managing constant change and feel that senior management has downplayed their concerns and been reluctant to provide resources for the connected care effort. The continuity team relays these issues to senior management and a joint working session between senior management and key middle managers results in an action plan that includes the following:

- Senior managers clarify middle manager expectations and accountabilities.
- Training for managers will occur and will be provided by a local consulting firm.
- There will be regular meetings between the two groups to monitor progress and troubleshoot obstacles.
- Senior management will charter a "Change Management Group" of staff from HR, QA, marketing, and senior leadership who will monitor external changes and do a better job of managing the impact on middle managers and the clinical workforce.
- Senior managers will be more open to recommendations on process improvement and structural changes to support connected care. One senior management meeting per quarter will be devoted to this topic.
- Both groups agree to take a snapshot of quadruple aim measure scores and to use those scores to monitor progress of the connected care effort.

Energized by more support from senior management the middle manager team creates its own action plan around the pillars of connected care:

- Each manager reviews and revises job descriptions to incorporate connected care competencies.

- At the request of the team, HR modifies the performance appraisal system to reflect the importance of connected care accountabilities.
- Middle managers work with QA to identify the elements of patient-centered care and to integrate it into the quality assurance monitoring processes.
- Middle managers start to implement connected care by creating and implementing a patient-centered care communication and training plan for staff. Part of this training focuses on: "What does a good job of patient-centered care look like?" and "How will I know it when I see it?"
- Middle managers conduct an audit of how well the pillars of connected care are being implemented in their own facilities.
- Based on the audit findings, managers institute a series of customer/supplier conversations between front line staff and support departments.
- Managers set up "get to know you" sessions between professional groups such as nursing and social work to talk about differing viewpoints and patient care goals.
- Managers adopt a set of communication best practices including the adoption of closed loop communication for all clinical communications.
- Whenever there is a new staff communication, managers create a "who needs to know" grid and check off each group/individual as they send communication.
- Managers identify "cracks and gaps" in work processes, especially around care transitions and discharges. They ask the senior management team to charter a cross-organizational improvement team to improve these processes.
- Managers study team-building techniques, adopt teamwork tools, and work on getting more employee input and team building within their own departments.
- Each manager agrees to incorporate connected care principles into interdisciplinary team

meetings and individual coaching sessions with employees.

- Middle managers meet with the continuity team on a regular basis to discuss progress and to provide mutual support in overcoming obstacles.

Over a 6-month period, the Everford system, while still buffeted by constant change and distraction, had made significant progress on connected care. CAHPS scores had improved and readmissions had declined. An employee satisfaction survey revealed improved satisfaction, although some staff, who were not comfortable with the level of patient centeredness and collaboration, had decided to leave. The middle management team had gained more respect from senior management and was now being included in discussions about innovation and implementation of the new strategic direction.

BOX 5-3 lists expectations for managers, developed by the Everford Continuity Team.

▶ Chapter Summary

Middle managers are the vital link between senior management strategic goals and the front line staff who deliver connected care. Middle managers play the role of translator, facilitator, and therapist for clinical staff. In stressful or problematic situations, middle managers act as the face of the healthcare organization for patients and families and function as buffers between staff and problematic situations. Middle managers walk a tightrope between high-level strategic plans and the realities of implementation in the day-to-day clinical world. Middle managers implement change while keeping their own clinical operations running smoothly.

The middle manager's job is to communicate both to senior managers above and to the front line staff below her. Sometimes this requires middle managers to provide senior management with a "reality check" about the practicality of

---

BOX 5-3 Manager Connected Care Checklist

- ❑ Managers are clear on their accountability for connected care.
- ❑ Achievement of connected care is part of manager performance appraisal.
- ❑ Managers have been trained and receive coaching in the principles and practices of connected care.
- ❑ Managers create a personal self-development plan that includes both mindset and skillset changes needed to implement connected care.
- ❑ Managers communicate connected care principles and expectations to staff.
- ❑ Managers consistently use the principles of effective communication.
- ❑ Managers foster teamwork and run effective team meetings and interdisciplinary case conferences.
- ❑ Managers foster understanding and cooperation between disciplines.
- ❑ Managers collaborate with other internal departments to clarify customer/supplier requirements and to gain support for their team.
- ❑ Managers provide internal and community resource information to staff.
- ❑ Managers set clear expectations for connected care performance.
- ❑ Managers ensure that staff are trained in patient-centered care, teamwork, communication, collaboration, care coordination, and effective care transitions.
- ❑ Managers audit charts for evidence of connected care activities.
- ❑ Managers monitor work processes for handoff failures and implement improvements.
- ❑ Managers advocate for the resources necessary to implement connected care.
- ❑ Managers assess organizational changes for their potential impact on connected care and try to align change with connected care goals where possible.

some strategic level plans. Middle managers are also process engineers who must turn organization policies and procedures into practical workflows and handoffs between individuals and departments.

Managers must assess employee requirements for information, technical tools, administrative support, and time. They must then provide these resources within existing organizational constraints. In the day-to-day world of care delivery, middle managers must coach and facilitate implementation of the pillars of connected care, particularly communication, teamwork, collaboration, and care transitions. Care transitions, in particular, require the manager's attention because they involve activities that must be coordinated outside the boundaries of the organization. Transitions require managers to foster collaboration with other healthcare organizations, families, and community resources.

Managing through the volume-to-value shift requires middle managers to achieve a higher level of competency in areas such as communication, higher level clinical expertise, driving decisions with data, the use of technology, and process improvement strategies. Clinical middle managers must also make a shift from a task-oriented to a goal-oriented, value-based mindset. Managers require additional and more sophisticated training to function effectively through the volume-to-value shift. Effective training opportunities may be scarce in an environment where education lags behind the realities of a rapidly changing healthcare system. Given the challenges of their role, middle managers should build both organizational effectiveness and personal resilience skills. These skills include time management and the ability to create functional internal support networks of colleagues and support staff.

Organizations assess middle managers on team-level quadruple aim outcomes and through more subjective performance appraisal by a more senior manager. Middle managers do not always get the recognition or support their vital role demands. Many suffer from a misplaced and negative senior management perception about their value and effectiveness. Managers are often perceived as rigid or obstacles to change, and in some cases are seen as readily dispensible. This is an issue that can contribute to burnout and turnover in the middle management ranks.

Middle managers integrate the pillars of connected care into daily work through staff performance management and support. Managers must extricate themselves from firefighting and a mountain of administrative work to set clear expectations, train, coach, monitor, and give feedback to staff. Managers use the key principles of communication to drive out fear, treat the next step in care as a customer, and ensure that everyone affected by a patient care issue or decision uses closed loop communication ensure that patient care messages are acknowledged and managed. Managers use chart audits, peer chart reviews, clinical case conference, and employee coaching sessions to assess levels of care coordination, communication, and teamwork. Middle managers play a vital role in implementing connected care. Building their skills, and supporting and recognizing their efforts, must be essential elements of any connected care organizational implementation.

References

American College of Healthcare Executives. (2017). American College of Healthcare Executives competency assessment tool. Chicago, IL: Author.

American Organization of Nurse Executives. (2015). AONE nurse manager competencies. Retrieved from www.aone.org/resources/nurse-leader-competencies.shtml

Bodenheimer, T., & Sinsky, C. (2014). From triple to quadruple aim: Care of the patient requires care of the provider. *Annals of Family Medicine, 12*(6), 573–576.

Braf, P. (2011). The role of middle management in change management programmes. A case study of Telesur. Thesis Paper. The Netherlands: Maastricht School of Management. Retrieved from www.fhrinstitute.org

Bureau of Labor Statistics. (2016). *Occupational outlook handbook* (17th ed). Washington, DC: U. S. Department of Labor. Medical and Health Services Managers. Retrieved from www.bls.gov/ooh/management/medical-and-health-services-managers.htm

Embertson, M. K. (2006). The importance of middle managers in healthcare organizations. *Journal of Healthcare Management, 51*(4), 223–232.

Federico, F., & Bonacum, D. (2010). Strengthening the core. *Healthcare Executive, 25*(1), 68–70. Retrieved from www.ACHE.org

Friedman, A., Howard, J., Shaw, E. K., Cohen, D. J., Shahidi, L., & Ferrante, J. M. (2016). Medical homes (PCMHs) from coordinators' perspectives. *Journal of the American Board of Family Medicine, 29*(1), 90–101. doi:10.3122/jabfm.2016.01.150175

Goldstein N. (2015). Clinical managers—Ignored yet critical to innovation success. *I Procurement 1*(1), e15. doi:10.2196/iproc.470 (Conference Paper presented at Connected Care Conference, Boston, 2015.)

Haas, S., Swan, B. A., & Haynes, T. (2013). Developing ambulatory care registered nurse competencies for care coordination and transition management. *Nursing Economics, 31*(1), 44–47.

HealthStream. (n.d.). Ten best practices for improving communication. Retrieved from www.Healthstream.com

Huy, Q. N. (2001). In praise of middle managers. *Harvard Business Review, 79*(8), 72–79, 160.

International Hospital Federation. (2015). *Leadership competencies for health services managers.* Bernex, Switzerland: Author.

Owens, K. (2017). Reconnecting your team to patient centered excellence. White Paper. Healthstream. Retrieved from http://www.healthstream.com/docs/default-source/white-papers/white-paper-reconnecting-your-team-to-patient-centered-excellence.pdf

Pappas, J.M., Flaherty, K.E., & Wooldridge, B. (2004). Tapping into hospital champions: Strategic middle managers. *Health Care Management Review, 29*(1), 8–16.

Pathway Health. (2017). Interact 4.0 tools. Retrieved from www.Pathway-interact.com

Patient's View Institute. (2018). About pvi. Retrieved from www.gopvi.org

Planetree. (2016). The role of leadership in creating a culture of patient and family centered care. Patient centered leadership self-reflection quiz. Retrieved from www.planetree.org

Perlo J, Balik B, Swensen S, Kabcenell A, Landsman J, & Feeley D. (2017). IHI framework for improving joy in work. Cambridge, MA: Institute for Healthcare Improvement.

QSEN Institute. (2017). www.qsen.org/competencies

Ruoff, G. (Ed.). (2015). Malpractice risks in communication failures, 2015 benchmarking report. Boston, MA: Crico Strategies, A Division of The Risk Management Foundation of the Harvard Medical Institutions Incorporated. Retrieved from www.rfmstrategies.com

Swensen, S., Pugh, M., McMullan, C., & Kabcenell, A. (2013). *High-impact leadership: Improve care, improve the health of populations, and reduce costs.* Boston, MA: Institute for Healthcare Improvement.

Zjadewicz, K., White, D., Raffin Bouchal, S., & Reilly, S. (2016). Middle managers' role in quality improvement project implementation, are we all on the same page? A review of current literature. *Safety in Health, 2*, 8. doi:10.1186/s40886-016-0018-5

Care Coordination and Communication on the Front Lines—The Clinician Role

CHAPTER OBJECTIVES

After completing this chapter readers will be able to:

- Describe the role of front line clinicians, particularly nurses, in using care coordination and communication to achieve connected care
- List core connected care competencies for clinicians
- Identify methods for helping clinicians develop a connected care skillset
- Describe methods for measuring the effectiveness of clinician connected care activities
- Describe the application of the specific tools and processes of connected care to daily work

▶ Introduction

The work of individual clinicians and support staff in delivering care to patients is where "the rubber meets the road" in achieving connected care. Clinicians must build a repertoire of techniques for applying the foundation (patient centeredness) and five pillars of connected care (communication, coordination, collaboration, transitions, and teamwork) in their daily work. Clinicians must also become adept at utilizing processes of connected care such as interdisciplinary conferencing, structured care transitions, and complex case conferences to achieve better connected care for their patient caseload. The complex challenge of connecting care further requires front line clinicians to develop expertise in the use of clinical and communication technologies such as patient tracking systems, telemonitoring, videoconferencing, and communication through patient portals in the electronic medical record (EMR).

To successfully implement connected care in daily practice, clinicians must develop a new, more expansive mindset and a repertoire of new skills in communication, health coaching, organization, technology use, higher level clinical expertise, and teamwork. An essential element of this "will/skill" transformation is the need to move from a "compliance" mentality to a collaborative patient care mindset. This can be the biggest hurdle for practicing clinicians who have long worked in traditional, hierarchical, clinical care structures (Bishop, 2016).

Transforming attitudes and acquiring new skills while delivering care in a busy clinical setting can be challenging for both healthcare organizations and clinicians.

Another new, and required, competence for all clinicians is business literacy. Clinicians must understand the principles and practice of population health and the finances of value-based care.

Part of this understanding includes knowing their organization's current state of development in the volume-to-value shift, the market challenges that the clinician's organization faces, key organizational goals, organizational measures, and expectations for the clinician's personal practice. Finally, clinicians must become organizationally effective, recognizing opportunities for improvement of clinical and administrative processes, participating in organizational improvement efforts, and selling their ideas upward.

▶ New Medicare Rules Foster Connected Care at the Front Lines

In recent years, Medicare, through the implementation of new Conditions of Participation for skilled nursing facilities (SNFs) and home health care, has made a determined effort to foster more patient-centered and connected care. As these new regulations are implemented, they will force clinicians to adopt more value-based connected care behaviors.

The National Association for Home Care and Hospice describes the principles of the new Home Health Care Conditions of Participation, which are being phased in through 2018:

- Develop a more continuous, integrated care process across all aspects of home health services, based on a patient-centered assessment, care planning, service delivery, and quality assessment and performance improvement.

- Use a patient-centered, interdisciplinary approach that recognizes the contributions of various skilled professionals and their interactions with each other to meet the patient's needs. Stress quality improvements by incorporating an outcome-oriented, data-driven quality assessment and performance improvement program specific to each home health agency (HHA).

- Eliminate the focus on administrative process requirements that lack adequate consensus or evidence that they are predictive of either achieving clinically relevant outcomes for patients or preventing harmful outcomes for patients. (National Association for Home Care and Hospice, 2017)

The new skilled nursing facility Medicare Conditions of Participation, also known as the "SNF Megarule," details a new set of principles for the management of care in nursing homes:

- Ensuring that long-term care facility staff members are properly trained on caring for residents with dementia and in preventing elder abuse
- Ensuring that long-term care facilities take into consideration the health of residents when making decisions on the kinds and levels of staffing a facility needs to properly take care of its residents

- Ensuring that staff members have the skills and competencies to provide person-centered care to residents; the care plans developed for residents will take into consideration their goals of care and preferences
- Improving care planning, including discharge planning, for all residents with involvement of the facility's interdisciplinary team and consideration of the caregiver's capacity, giving residents information they need for follow-up after discharge, and ensuring that instructions are transmitted to any receiving facilities or service (Centers for Medicare and Medicaid, 2016)

Implementation of these requirements will provide the impetus for a much broader application of connected care, at least in the postacute care continuum.

▶ Connected Care Core Competencies

Competency statements help to define the knowledge and skill necessary to achieve connected care. Connected care competencies are usually a subset of the competencies necessary to achieve value-based, quadruple aim goals. Most health professions have a role in connected care, but nursing may be one of the most important, simply by virtue of the size and reach of the nursing profession. With more than 3 million members, nurses compose the largest portion of the clinician population in the U.S. healthcare system.

A major national initiative called "The Future of Nursing," from the Robert Wood Johnson Foundation and the Institute of Medicine (2011), provides a comprehensive national roadmap for the transformation of the nursing profession in the new world of health care. According to this report, nurses play a vital role in achieving the quadruple aim, but are faced with numerous barriers to success.

The report provides a series of recommendations for overcoming these barriers which are also relevant to the practice of connected care. These recommendations are:

- Nurses should practice to the full extent of their training and education.
- Nurses should achieve higher levels of education through a system of seamless academic progression.
- Nurses should be full partners in redesigning the U.S. healthcare system.

The report also defines three key roles for nurses:

- Provide direct patient care, teach and counsel patients
- Coordinate care and advocate for patients
- Research and evaluate more effective ways of caring for patients (modified from Institute of Medicine, 2011)

Each of these roles is key to the achievement of connected care and will be explored later in this chapter.

Nursing Connected Care Competencies

In response to the Institute of Medicine (2011) report on nursing and the Future of Nursing initiative, a group of respected nurse educators has developed a set of core competency statements for practicing nurses. While not specific to connected care, these statements describe the knowledge, skills, and attitudes that form the foundation of a connected care practice. This project, known as "Quality and Safety Education for Nurses" (QSEN), lists the key competencies areas as follows:

- Patient-centered care
- Teamwork and collaboration
- Evidence-based practice
- Quality improvement
- Safety
- Informatics

QSEN references specific connected care knowledge, skills, and attitudes using phrases such as

"Values seeing health care situations through patients' eyes," "Communicate care provided and needed at each transition in care," and "Clarify roles and accountabilities under conditions of potential overlap in team-member functioning" (Cronenwett et al., 2007, pp. 123–129).

A presentation from Banner Health, an integrated delivery system in the Southwest, lists some more specific population health skills needed by nurses (Calhoun & Harris, 2017):

- Managed care 101
- Population health competencies
- Continuum focus
- Leveraging cognitive expertise using technological tools
- Coaching skills
- Value-based care
- Motivational interviewing techniques
- Coordination of multidisciplinary teams
- Pattern recognition
- Moving from novice to expert in nonlinear ways

In the rest of this chapter we will explore the practical implementation of these competencies in daily clinical practice.

As the volume-to-value shift proceeds, so does the transformation of nursing and other clinical professions within the healthcare system. One part of this transformation includes the effort to have professionals "skill up and delegate down." This means that professionals and support staff use every aspect of their skills for patient care.

One fragmenting issue related to professional roles and responsibilities is competition between professional groups for status and control. In these situations, individual professions lobby state legislatures to increase their profession's scope of practice while limiting the scope of other professional practice. Only unified goals, advocacy from patients themselves, and a determined focus on patient-centered care can overcome these destructive rivalries. A more positive transformation is the move toward interdisciplinary teamwork in every corner of health care. As the complexity of patient

care escalates, such a move is inevitable and positive for patient care outcomes.

Connected Care Competencies for Other Professions

Other professions, including medicine and social work, have defined competencies for achievement of quadruple aim goals. Many of these overlap with the QSEN competency statements.

For example, Combes and Arespacochaga (2012) explain the need for new clinician competencies: "All care providers will need new skills and knowledge to reach this triple aim. As health care financing moves from volume-based to value-based payments, clinicians will be required to work in inter-professional teams, coordinate care across settings, utilize evidence-based practices to improve quality and patient safety, and promote greater efficiency in care delivery" (p. 401). Some specific connected care competencies for physicians include (1) improve patient care practices, (2) work effectively with the healthcare team, and (3) coordinate with other providers.

The Interprofessional Education Council—comprising health professional training schools for disciplines that include dentistry, nursing, medicine, osteopathic medicine, optometry, pharmacy, physical therapy, social work, and public health—has defined competencies that cross professional boundaries. The group has defined four competency areas for interdisciplinary practice that are clearly relevant to the achievement of connected care:

1. Work with individuals from other professions to maintain a climate of mutual respect and shared values.

2. Use the knowledge of one's own role and those of other professions to appropriately assess and address the healthcare needs of patients and to promote and advance the health of populations.

3. Communicate with patients, families, communities, and professionals in

health and other fields in a responsive and responsible manner that supports a team approach to the promotion and maintenance of health and the prevention and treatment of disease.

4. Apply relationship-building values and the principles of team dynamics to perform effectively in different team roles to plan, deliver, and evaluate patient/population-centered care and population health programs and policies that are safe, timely, efficient, effective, and equitable. (Interprofessional Education Collaborative, 2016, p. 10)

Building Connected Care Skills

Value-based connected care requires a wider skillset than most employed clinicians currently have. Health professional undergraduate and graduate programs are beginning to teach skills such as health coaching, patient self-management support, the use of data in decision making, and interdisciplinary teamwork, but this type of training has not been widely available to practicing clinicians. For these clinicians, the options for learning population health and connected care have primarily been through internal organization education or through webinars and online learning from nursing and other organizations. An example is the four-part, free online population health program offered by the Connecticut League for Nursing. The content covered in this program includes:

1. Introduction to Population Health
2. Identifying Outcomes Representing Achievement of a Healthy Population
3. Population Health and the Affordable Care Act
4. Evaluating Practice at the Population Level and Future Policy Trends (Connecticut League for Nursing, 2017)

Commercial vendors of online education also provide webinars and written material on topics related to connected care. For example,

Relias Learning.com (2017), an online education provider for health and human services professionals, offers courses such as Person Centered Planning and Principles of Shared Decision Making. Another example of online professional continuing education is a program developed by Arizona State University called "Care Coordination in Interprofessional Primary Care Practice" (Lamb, 2017).

Modules in this program include:

- Defining care coordination
- Optimizing teamwork
- Strategies and tools
- High-risk patients
- Interprofessional collaborative practice

Many of these continuing education materials are comprehensive and useful, but they must be coordinated with the real work of daily clinical practice. While some front line clinicians are avid self-learners, many others are consumed by the demands of the job and their own lives and will not access these learning tools without organizational encouragement. Education specialists in healthcare organizations can foster learning about population health and patient-centered care through required internal education programs and online learning resources. The best use of these types of resources is as a catalyst for discussion about how the techniques presented in the training program can be adopted to the clinician's own patient care practice. For example, after a presentation on population health and risk stratification, a facilitator might ask clinicians to consider how they can risk stratify and triage their own patient caseload needs.

▶ Connected Care at the Front Lines— What Does a Good Job Look Like?

Front line clinicians are at the receiving end of the work begun at the senior management and board levels of the organization. While organizational transformation plans are being crafted at the higher levels of the organization, and managers are trying to turn these plans into viable work structures and processes, front line clinicians are often consumed with, and overwhelmed by, the sheer volume of patient care tasks; documentation; finding needed equipment, supplies, and information; and coping with patient changes and crises.

In an ideal world, organizations that want to achieve connected care would paint a very practical and concrete picture of how organizational quadruple aim goals and the pillars of connected care translate into daily workplace actions. After painting this picture, the organization would support clinicians in achieving it through training, empowerment, and processes that support connection. Quadruple aim goals and connected care activities can sometimes seem very theoretical and impractical to front line clinicians. For example, what does care coordination really look like to a unit nurse in a long-term care acute hospital, to a social worker in a SNF, or to a home care nurse in the field? When the average clinician plans his or her daily work, is the plan about accomplishing tasks, accomplishing goals, or is there no plan at all but simply frenzied activity? Is the clinician always thinking of one individual patient at a time or triaging the needs of a caseload or population of patients?

Before embarking on culture change to achieve connected care, senior leaders and managers must very purposefully clear time and space for clinicians and empower them to analyze and change their own practice methods.

To achieve connected care at the front lines, employees at every level of the organization must be allowed to step away from the fray and spend a little time considering how organizational goals relate to them and ultimately creating and internalizing a personal picture of "what a good job looks like." This is particularly difficult for front line clinicians who have to achieve both outcomes and productivity goals to maintain a

financially viable healthcare organization and who have very little time or energy for creative thinking. To achieve connected care, clinicians, with the help of their clinical manager, can follow the practical steps outlined here:

- Understand what the organization is trying to accomplish in measuring success.
- Use self-learning and organization resources to find the information and build the skill necessary to achieve connected care.
- Understand connected care expectations for the clinician's own job.
- Translate expectations into daily practice activities that work for the clinician.
- Think about: "What does connected care mean to me? Why is it good for me and my patients?"
- Talk to patients about their expectations of connected care.
- Ask: "What barriers keep me from achieving connected care and how can I get help to overcome them?"

A simple way to start, and one that doesn't require too much deep thinking, is for clinicians to ask themselves: "What can I do in my daily work to make the pieces of care fit together for a better patient experience?" Another approach is for clinical managers to discuss these issues at team meetings where employees have time to share ideas, pose examples, and express concerns. In the next section, we will give some examples of real, daily clinical work activities that provide connected care for patients.

Translating Organizational Goals into Clinical Activities

In the messy, real world of clinical care, clinical culture change is seldom precisely orchestrated or communicated in the ways recommended by experts. It may not always be easy for clinical staff to understand and internalize the connected care goals that are formulated in the "C-suite" and the boardroom. As senior managers and their middle managers struggle to deal with external healthcare system changes, they may not always offer fully formed goals, measures, and action plans to front line clinicians and support staff.

In the best reality, culture change is a constant, iterative process in which the big goals are clear and operationalizing them occurs through small steps during discussions between management, front line staff, and patients. This type of culture change almost always involves some missteps and frequent course corrections.

In situations in which goals and performance expectations are not clearly defined, clinicians can be empowered to be part of the transformation process by being proactive in asking about,

and trying to flesh out, quadruple aim and connected care goals and expectations. Instead of waiting passively for direction while continuing to deliver task-oriented and fragmented fee-for-service care, clinicians can talk among themselves about issues such as, "How can we accomplish our clinical goals while working with patients who aren't taking care of themselves or who have serious psychosocial problems?" or "How can we better connect the dots for patients so they don't feel confused and overwhelmed?" Clinicians can also approach their own managers to start a discussion about how they can positively impact team results, goals, and work processes to improve care.

TABLE 6-1 provides some examples of how goals can be translated into specific connected care activities at the front line.

TABLE 6-1 What Does a Good Job Look Like? From Goals to Clinician Actions

Organizational Goals	Clinician Actions to Achieve Goals
Improve quadruple aim outcomes. ■ Reduce readmission rates below the national average. ■ Improve performance on clinical outcome measures. ■ Achieve 4-star ratings on CAHPS scores. ■ Reduce the cost per episode of care.	■ Monitor and report changes in condition using the SBAR method. ■ Consistently use organization mandated clinical best practices in your daily work. ■ Use active listening and two-way communication in conversations with patients. ■ Become aware of and eliminate waste in your own work (too much walking, wasting supplies, time spent correcting errors you made, etc.).
Utilize patient-centered care practices so that care activities are filtered through patient wants and needs.	■ Perform a patient assessment that incorporates questions such as, "What is important to you?" and "What do you want to be different as a result of your care?" (goals). ■ Collaborate with patients on behavior change using methods such as motivational interviewing. ■ Avoid arguing with, pleading with, or cajoling patients to do what is good for them. Instead ask, "what might work for you?" ■ Chart progress toward patient goals, not just clinician goals.

(continues)

TABLE 6-1 What Does a Good Job Look Like? From Goals to Clinician Actions   *(continued)*

Organizational Goals	Clinician Actions to Achieve Goals
Ensure that care transitions are timely, smooth, and complete.	■ Treat the next step in care as the "customer." ■ Know what information the next step in the continuum needs and provide it the way the patient wants it. ■ Ask patients about their wants and needs during a transition.
Communication—The patient and everyone on his or her care team is heard and properly informed about care activities.	■ Use active listening in every interaction with patients and colleagues. ■ Always verify that verbal and electronic communication was received and understood. ■ Consider the "ripple effect" of every action you take and communicate to all those affected.
Coordination—Ensure that all care activities are smooth, unduplicated, and finished.	■ Coordinate your schedule and care actions with other members of the patient's care team. ■ Finish all patient care follow-up tasks. ■ Find and refer to resources that can help the patient in and outside your organization.
Collaborate with other individuals and departments to achieve connected care and quadruple aim goals.	■ Have conversations with professionals from other disciplines who regularly interact with your patients to understand their roles and priorities. ■ Follow guidelines set by other departments for how best to work with them to achieve good patient care. For example, does the IT department function better if you call the IT helpline and not ask individual computer techs for personal help?
Teamwork—Work with other members of the care team to achieve better outcomes and satisfaction for patients and teammates.	■ Take personal responsibility for regular conferencing with other members of the patient's care team. ■ Regularly attend high-risk patient interdisciplinary care conferences. ■ Identify other team members who need help and offer to provide it.
Use technology to improve outcomes and reduce labor.	■ Use the electronic medical record correctly. ■ Learn and correctly use every tool the system has to offer to document, track, and organize patient care. ■ Explain care technology in a way that patients can understand and accept.

Note: HCAHPS, Hospital Assessment of Healthcare Providers and Systems; IT, information technology; SBAR, situation-background-assessment-recommendation.

🔍 CASE STUDY

Understanding "What a Good Job Looks Like"

A nurse in a medical practice has attended educational sessions about the quadruple aim and value-based care. She has talked with her manager about her role in achieving practice goals. The nurse understands that, for her, a goal of "reducing patient hospital readmissions" translates into tracking hospitalized practice patients, calling patients after discharge to check on their status, making postdischarge appointments for patients, and calling skilled nursing facilities or home care agencies that are servicing the patient to track progress and coordinate the transition to the next step in care. A practice clinical secretary has been told that she is responsible for maintaining the patient tracking database, making reminder calls, and monitoring whether patients actually come to appointments. When she makes reminder calls, she asks patients if they have transportation to appointments. A practice community outreach worker might be sent to the patient's home to engage him or her in care if the patient consistently does not come for appointments. Each of these employees periodically gets feedback on performance and gets reports on how well the practice and their team in particular is doing on reducing hospital readmissions.

▶ Supporting Clinicians in Delivering Patient-Centered, Connected Care

Organizational Support

A key factor in the achievement of patient-centered care is organizational support for the professional clinician and support staff. Overburdened, stressed, and unsupported staff will have a difficult time focusing outward on patient wants and needs, especially when those wants and needs interfere with the smooth flow of work and take up a disproportionate amount of clinician time. Providing support for staff in these circumstances is clearly the job of both senior and middle management. This organizational support takes several forms:

- A management team that takes personal accountability for creating working conditions that support the achievement of quadruple aim goals

- Creating work processes that flow smoothly and contain roles and responsibilities that are clearly defined and ensuring that everyone who does the work has needed resources

- Communication about organizational goals, changes, and new resources

- Clinician work scheduling practices and support staff help clinicians to deliver care efficiently and without excess stress

- Empowerment and advocacy, in that management ensures that work is fairly distributed, that aggressive employees do not take advantage of less assertive employees, and that employees have a voice in decision making and can speak up when things are not going well

Care for the Professional Caregiver

Shaller (2007) in an article for the Commonwealth Fund, entitled "Patient-Centered Care: What Does It Take?" describes the issue of care for the caregiver this way: "Erie Chapman, president and CEO of the Nashville-based Baptist Healing Trust, suggests that the 'single biggest responsibility of caregivers is to take care of people that take care of people.' He describes a 'wave theory' of behavior that can contribute to a positive work culture, based on the premise that the majority of people in an organization or on a team model their own behavior in accordance with those around them. Positive behavior modeled by team leaders will encourage similar behavior in other team members, which will in turn contribute to the ability of the entire team to provide responsive, service-oriented care to patients and their families" (p. 11).

Clinician Self-Care—A Prerequisite for Connected Care

As noted, clinicians cannot be patient centered if they are overburdened, stressed, and on the verge of burnout. While healthcare organizations certainly have a responsibility to manage this issue through clinician support, training, workload assignments, shared governance, and control of aggressive behaviors in the workplace, clinicians must also take personal responsibility for managing their own well-being. The full range of these self-care activities is beyond the scope of this discussion, but may include:

- Effective personal efficiency and time management techniques
- Thoughtful setting of boundaries with patients and colleagues by defining what you can and can't do for and with them
- Personal stress management and building resilience
- Improving skill in active listening and giving feedback
- Incorporating exercise and other healthy behaviors into daily routines
- Paying attention to work-life balance
- Soliciting feedback from colleagues on "How am I coming across?" to assess how you are perceived by others

An excellent set of strategies for achieving clinician well-being and avoiding burnout are outlined in the slide presentation from the University of Wisconsin entitled, "Whole Health: Change the Conversation; Advancing Skills in the Delivery of Personalized, Proactive, Patient-Driven, Clinician Self Care" (Integrative Medicine Program, 2018). Access this practical toolkit at http://projects.hsl.wisc.edu/SERVICE/modules/13/M13_EO_Clinician_Self_Care.pdf.

Lora Polowczuk, a health professional turned coach, provides this advice: "Health care professionals serve as role models to their patients. To best assess and treat patients, they must bring a positive attitude, a vibrancy to their step, and a sense of resilience." Polowczuk, a Certified High Performance Coach®, who recovered from burnout, calls this the Verve Factor in her Movement Paradox™ Framework. She coaches stressed out and overwhelmed high achievers who are passionate about helping others: "We can't serve greatly when we're tired and exhausted. Self-care is not a yearly vacation when you don't unwind until the last day. Self-care must be an uncompromised daily ritual filled with mind clearing exercises, regular breaks, gratitude, body movement, and healthy eating habits" (2017, personal communication).

Empowering Healthcare Employees

Some organizations go well beyond employee communication and support to empowerment and engagement in improving the patient experience and solving organizational problems. A "Solution Brief" from the Experience Innovation Network (2014) defines employee empowerment as "a key driver of cultural strength and resilience. It results when employees have the competence and confidence to make key decisions about their work, without constant recourse to leadership. This results both in lower management overhead for trivial operational decisions, and higher likelihood that employees will make decisions that align with organizational goals and values because they have embraced them as their own" (p. 3). The paper further defines four leadership strategies that empower employees:

1. Inspire employees to embrace the mission or change process by linking the effort to improving patient care.
2. Listen to the voices of the employees and understand their goals and the barriers they face. Engage them in crafting solutions.
3. Enable front line employees to implement change by giving needed resources and removing obstacles.
4. Reward success and provide opportunities for front line leaders to have more influence.

A concrete example of this is "The No Excuses Team" at Twin Rivers Regional Medical Center, empowered to identify and fix workplace and workflow inefficiencies. The team achieved 116 "quick wins" such as decluttering the nurse's station, getting clocks in patient rooms, and creating employee-of-the-month parking. Their efforts improved patient satisfaction by 117% (Experience Innovation Network, 2014).

Design Thinking—A New Strategy for Clinician Empowerment and Work Improvement

Design thinking is a newer concept that originated in industry as a way to quickly design, prototype, and test new products. It is an approach that is now being used to engage front line clinicians in intensive and innovative improvement of clinical processes. One example cited by the *New York Times* is an innovation developed by a hospital design team: having the lead clinician on a trauma team in the emergency room wear an orange vest so everyone on the team can immediately see who is in charge (Kalaichandran, 2017).

An article in the *Harvard Business Review* describes design thinking: "One of the most promising approaches for understanding patients' experiences has been design thinking, a creative, human-centered problem-solving approach that leverages empathy, collective idea generation, rapid prototyping, and continuous testing to tackle complex challenges" (Kim, Myers, & Allen, 2017, p. 2).

In practice, design thinking starts with a healthcare organization identifying a problem such as no-shows for medical appointments. The organization creates a multidisciplinary team that studies the problem from all angles, with special emphasis on capturing the patient or employee view through focus groups, interviews, or surveys. The team then tries to take a fresh look at the real cause of the problem. Once the real cause has been identified the team develops redesign ideas often with patients' participation. The redesigned process is mapped out using flowcharts, diagrams, stories, skits, or other methods that create a picture of what the new design would look like. The next step is rapid trialing of the idea on a small scale and then collecting data on the impact. If the new design idea is successful, it becomes part of clinical operations. If the trial is not successful, the team performs another round of design and testing (Kim et al., 2017, p. 3).

A full implementation of design thinking is not something that the average health professional can accomplish alone. Clinicians can, however, read about design thinking and share articles like the ones cited here with their manager and suggest that the organization consider adopting the design thinking approach. If a clinical process problem is within the scope of a single clinical team or work unit, clinicians can learn about design thinking techniques and, working with their own manager, can use elements of this creative approach to design a new and improved process that solves the problem.

▶ Incorporating the Pillars of Connected Care into Clinical Practice

Connected care is composed of a foundation—that is, patient centeredness, and the five

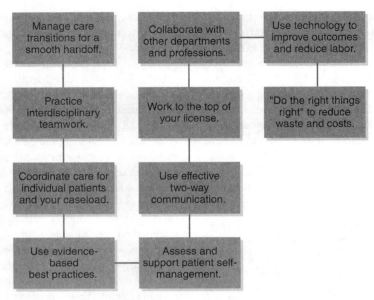

FIGURE 6-1 Connected Care—What Clinicians and Support Staff Need to Accomplish

pillars: communication, coordination, collaboration, transitions, and teamwork.

To achieve the quadruple aim using connected care, front line clinicians must actually understand, accept, and embed connected care activities into their daily work life. In the rest of this chapter we will explore the specifics of how clinicians implement patient centeredness and the five pillars of connected care into the busy and challenging world of daily clinical practice. **FIGURE 6-1** summarizes the actions that clinicians must take to implement connected care.

▶ Connected Care Pillar 1: *Care Coordination* for Front Line Clinicians

Once the healthcare organization has identified connected care competencies, and provided training and support for clinician mindset change and skill development, it must bolster

the processes of care that connect the dots for patients. Achieving connected care at the front lines of patient care is a complex process of resource management, changing workflows, personal attitude transformation, and acquisition of a new set of skills. Many of the connected care activities performed by front line staff can be grouped under the broad heading of "care coordination."

The Structure of Care Coordination

Care coordination for both individuals and for clinician caseloads (the clinician's patient population) is the cornerstone of connected care. The Agency for Healthcare Research and Quality (AHRQ) defines care coordination in this way: "Care coordination involves deliberately organizing patient care activities and sharing information among all of the participants concerned with a patient's care to achieve safer and more effective care. This means that the patient's needs and preferences are known ahead of time and communicated at the right time to the right people, and that this information is used to provide safe, appropriate, and effective care to the patient" (AHRQ, 2016, p. 1).

Care coordination is either a specific job for a clinician or part of the clinician's role. There is considerable overlap among the terms used to describe the function of helping patients with organizing and sequencing their care. Care coordination, care management, and case management are sometimes used interchangeably, but in practice they have different characteristics.

Care coordination activities can be seen as a continuum, ranging from very simple and episodic organization of a specific patient care task to long-term, intensive management of all aspects of the patient's health care and health insurance benefits.

Hospitals, insurers, accountable care organizations, long-term acute care facilities, and medical practices hire nurses, and occasionally other types of clinicians, to practice full-time care coordination with a population of patients. In other settings—such as in SNFs, outpatient surgery, and home health care—clinicians both provide direct care to patients and coordinate care within their own organization and for patient care transitions.

Care Coordination Functions and Activities

The Care Coordination section of the AHRQ website lists activities of care coordination:

- Establishing accountability and agreeing on responsibility
- Communicating/sharing knowledge (interpersonal communication and sharing patient information)
- Helping with transitions of care
- Assessing patient needs and goals
- Creating a proactive care plan
- Monitoring and follow-up, including responding to changes in patients' needs
- Supporting patients' self-management goals

- Linking to community resources
- Working to align resources with patient and population needs (AHRQ, 2016)

In addition, care coordinators must ensure that all patient care and follow-up tasks have been assigned and completed in a timely manner. Of all the care coordination activities, this is probably the one that has the most impact on the patient experience.

Case management is a broader role than care coordination. The Case Management Society of America (2017) lists the functions of a case manager as:

- **Assessment:** identifying health conditions, patient needs, abilities, and preferences
- **Care planning** involves helping individuals identify goals and developing strategies to help them achieve goals and move toward more self-care
- **Alignment:** coordinating the "moving parts" of care for a more cohesive experience
- **Evaluation/outcomes measurement** which tells the individual and case manager what's working, what's not working, and how much progress has been made toward achieving goals
- **Promotes client self-determination:** the individual learns the skills necessary to take control of his or her care with confidence (modified from Case Management Society of America, 2017)

The Spectrum of Care Coordination and Case Management Functions

Care coordination and case management can be either episodic or long term and continuous, depending on the setting and patient situation. In such settings as acute care hospitals, outpatient surgery, rehabilitation units of SNFs, and home health care, care coordination is temporary and linked to a specific procedure or episode of care.

For nurses or social workers who coordinate care in a medical practice, a case management agency, or an insurance company, care coordination relationships, especially with high-needs patients, are likely to be long term and more complex, moving more into the realm of case management. In a blog post on Researchgate.net, researcher Ellen Schultz (2017) of Stanford Medicine describes the differences in this way:

> Care coordination is a process to try to bridge the gaps in patients' care as they move through the healthcare system. It's about logistics, like getting information from one provider/location to another, but it's also about making sure that patients' needs are assessed and that someone is trying to help meet those needs. Not just medical needs, but also social needs for how the patient can cope with their medical condition . . . Case management usually refers to a model of assigning a particular person, a care manager (or care coordinator - title isn't as important as the actions), to help make sure a patient gets the care they need. It can involve lots of coordination activities, like making

appointments and calling patients to check-up on them, but also often involves helping arrange for services or connecting patients to community resources, like finding a nursing home and getting the patient accepted into it.

FIGURE 6-2 illustrates the spectrum of care coordination and case management.

Care Coordination— What Works?

In the book *Care Coordination: The Game Changer*, Lamb (2014) describes a set of care coordination best practices distilled from a care coordination and chronic disease management program (MCCD) administered by Medicare.

Only a few of the sites in the project reduced hospitalizations for high-risk patients, but those that did implemented a core set of care coordination processes, including:

- **Targeting.** Identifying patients with a history of hospital readmissions for care coordination interventions

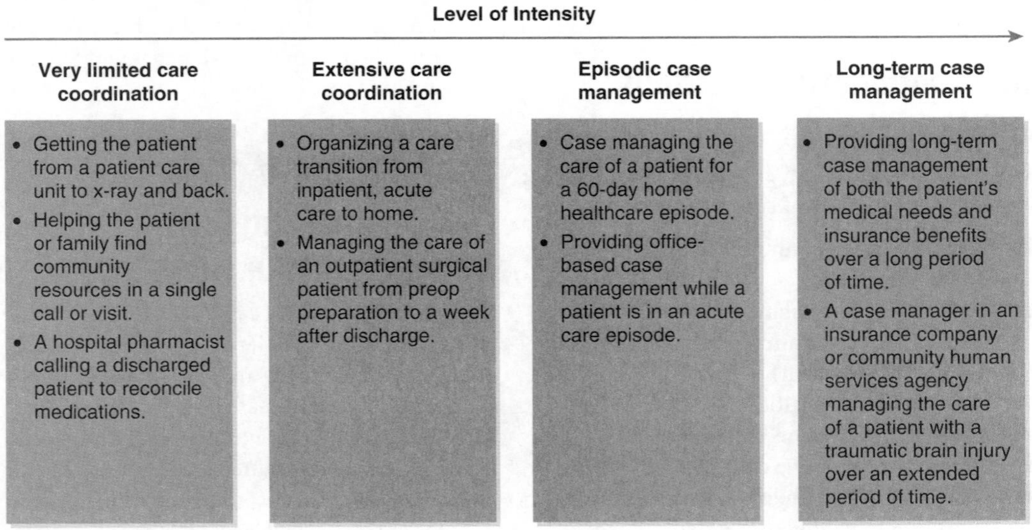

Level of Intensity

Very limited care coordination	Extensive care coordination	Episodic case management	Long-term case management
• Getting the patient from a patient care unit to x-ray and back. • Helping the patient or family find community resources in a single call or visit. • A hospital pharmacist calling a discharged patient to reconcile medications.	• Organizing a care transition from inpatient, acute care to home. • Managing the care of an outpatient surgical patient from preop preparation to a week after discharge.	• Case managing the care of a patient for a 60-day home healthcare episode. • Providing office-based case management while a patient is in an acute care episode.	• Providing long-term case management of both the patient's medical needs and insurance benefits over a long period of time. • A case manager in an insurance company or community human services agency managing the care of a patient with a traumatic brain injury over an extended period of time.

FIGURE 6-2 Continuum of Care Coordination and Case Management Functions

INTERVIEW WITH JOAN PITEO AND ANGELIQUE MORALES

Joan Piteo, RN, is the manager of care management and Angelique Morales is the manager of the Patient Navigation Program at Community Medical Group (CMG), a medical group and accountable care organization comprising 1,000 physicians who practice in their own private offices. Joan and Angelique work in the CMG office in New Haven, Connecticut.

CMG supports patients who are discharged from acute care facilities and also engages high-risk patients in health coaching. The practice uses data and an algorithm to identify high-risk patients. The practice has two outreach teams for these patients. One team, the patient navigators, focuses on the social determinants of health. The other team, nurse care coordinators, focuses on the more medical aspects of care. The RN care coordinators tend to focus more on helping patients with chronic disease self-management.

The two teams use a decision tree to decide which team is primarily responsible for coordinating care for a particular patient. The two teams often "trade the patient back and forth," depending on the type of problem they need to solve. The team makes three attempts to engage high-risk patients in health coaching and then, if the patient does not agree to participate, they stop. Team members may try to engage the patient again at a later point

The five patient navigators, who are not medical professionals but who have training in health advocacy and community resources, focus on helping patients with the social determinants of health. The practice maintains a database of resources for all staff such as diabetic information, healthy recipes, cooling centers for patients who don't have air conditioning, among others. The navigators often email specific resource information to patients or provide it over the phone. The patient navigators may also find resources for patients who have problems such as malfunctioning medical equipment. One example is a glucometer that does not work. They have done things such as obtaining special shoes for a diabetic patient.

Patient navigators and RN care coordinators reach out to patients who are discharged from a hospital or a rehabilitation facility. They help patients understand discharge instructions. They also help patients obtain needed medications. A navigator reviews the discharge medication list with the patient on the phone to ensure that the patient has gotten and is taking currently prescribed medications. If there is a problem with a medication, or the patient has a specific medication question, the navigators refer the patient to an RN care coordinator or the primary care physician.

The patient navigators also help patients obtain durable medical equipment, make appointments for follow-up medical care, and find transportation to those appointments. The navigators use prede-signed scripts for outreach calls. The navigation department follows and supports patients for 30 days after discharge.

The navigators may also work with care coordinators in insurance companies to find patients additional resources in specialty areas such as behavioral health or oncology. If home care has been ordered for a patient, they coordinate care with the home care nurse. This can sometimes become problematic if the patient is confused about who is calling—the nurse in the home or the patient navigator. Patients frequently cannot remember which agency they are getting care from or who their nurse is; this makes the navigator's job more difficult.

The RN care coordinators and the patient navigators work together closely. Both teams have their own group meetings and they sometimes have case conferences about specific patients. The practice uses spreadsheets and an internal database to track high-risk patients longitudinally.

CMG has a manager of clinical quality initiatives who works on quality improvement auditing and improvement. The practice focuses on identifying care gaps. Since not all practices have electronic medical records, the clinical quality coordinators go to the individual practice site and audit paper charts to find health outcome gaps. The gap analysis looks at metrics such as the percentage of

(continues)

INTERVIEW WITH JOAN PITEO AND ANGELIQUE MORALES *(continued)*

patients in a practice who have had a HbA1c (a measure of blood sugar levels over time). The practice also has two coders who help practice physicians better document the care that they give.

CMG uses evidence-based best practices to guide care and a health coaching model to help patients change health behaviors. Clinical best practices are derived from authoritative resources such as the American Diabetes Association. CMG also uses standardized patient education tools, some of which are from other sources and some of which have been created internally. An example is the American Lung Association "Stoplight" tool which is used to teach patients how to respond to changes in condition.

CMG uses the "Transtheoretical Model" of the stages of change to guide health coaching efforts. This model begins with helping patients identify what they want and then coaching them to set health goals. The team monitors where patients are in the stages of change as they (hopefully) move toward their goal.

- **Staffing.** Use of multidisciplinary teams with an RN delivering the majority of the interventions
- **Primary care provider collaboration.** Keeping the physician informed and involved
- **Information technology.** Using electronic charting, tracking of patients between care settings, and electronic communication between team members

- **Training and feedback.** Team members are trained in care coordination and individual care teams get feedback on outcomes for their patients (modified from Lamb, 2014, pp. 62–63)

Care coordination usually proceeds in a sequence that incorporates all of the elements of care coordination identified in competency statements.

The reality of care coordination becomes clearer when illustrated with an example. **BOX 6-1**

BOX 6-1 Care Coordination Activities During an Episode of Home Health Care

- Nurse case manager conducts an assessment and evaluation of patient needs, strengths, and deficits.
- If appropriate, conduct medication reconciliation with the patient and physicians.
- Elicit patient goals and preferences.
- Develop a care plan with the patient, physician, and family.
- Identify the need for help from other disciplines and make appropriate referrals.
- Deliver patient-centered care, conducting patient teaching, monitoring patient status and progress.
- Identify, report, and manage patient changes in condition.
- If the nurse observes a change in condition or is called about one, she assesses the situation and uses SBAR reporting to report to the physician and suggest alternatives.
- Manage supplies, equipment, appointments, insurance, medications, and authorizations.
- Give and obtain information from physicians, family caregivers; coordinate the care plan.
- Participate in team huddles, complex case conferences, rounds, and supervisory coaching sessions.
- Regularly communicate with the patient's physicians.
- Identify and manage care transitions past the transition point using two-way communication to the next step in care.
- Check in with the patient and family about their level of satisfaction or concerns.
- As she cares for a single patient, the nurse case manager must also constantly monitor her full caseload and triage patients whose condition has declined and who need more care. As she does this, she must keep her schedule organized and leave time for new admissions.

describes the sequence of care coordination activities during a home care episode of care.

Patient Assessment and Care Planning

Care coordination starts with a comprehensive assessment of a patient's strengths, needs, and desires. An AHRQ white paper on coordinating care for adults with complex needs defines the elements of a comprehensive assessment: "Care coordination for complex patients starts with a comprehensive assessment of each individual's need for health and social supports. This involves much more than a standard medical history and complete physical examination. In addition to evaluation of medical diagnoses and the traditional family and social history, a comprehensive assessment should note how individuals function in their daily lives and with their family and other social supports. This assessment should also clarify the patient's preferences" (Rich, Lipson, Libersky, & Parchman, 2012, p. 11). **BOX 6-2** describes a simple tool that can be used for care coordination assessment.

In many cases, the specific setting in which care coordination occurs will dictate the type of assessment tool used. For example, home health care uses the Medicare OASIS dataset; SNFs use the MDS system. Home- and community-based services use other standardized tools. Many commercial care management firms use proprietary software care coordination assessment tools.

The Connected Care Plan

After completing the patient assessment, the clinician must develop a care plan that outlines the tasks that must be completed to achieve patient goals, develop self-care skills, and produce the best clinical outcomes. The best care plans revolve around whatever is most important to the patient and patient goals. Each clinical activity, communication, coordinating task, and referral to other disciplines should be filtered through the patient focus.

Care plan formats depend on the setting and clinical discipline, but most include assessment, diagnosis, medications, an assessment of mental health status, a social history, identification of social determinants of health, planned

---

BOX 6-2 A Day in the Life—Understanding the Patient's Story

A simple tool for assessing patient strengths, deficits, and desires is called "A Day in the Life." In this approach, the clinician asks the patient to describe a typical day from the time he or she gets up until bedtime: "Can you tell me about a typical day for you, starting with when you get up and ending with your going to bed?" The clinician uses active listening to help the patient express his or her thoughts. While the patient is talking, the clinician is listening for:

- What is important to the patient—What does the patient want to be able to do?
- What activities the patient can and cannot do
- What strengths, resilience, and vulnerability the patient describes
- What emotions are expressed in the course of the story

At the end of the patient's story the clinician summarizes what she thinks was expressed and asks the patient to give feedback on the accuracy of the summary. This information can now go into the medical record as the basis for the "patient's story" so that all clinicians on the team can better understand the patient and personalize care to his or her needs.

clinical activities, and a planned schedule for clinician visits or tasks. Patients should certainly have input into the care plan and ideally should be given a copy of the relevant parts of the care plan for their personal medical records.

Clinicians must also design the care plan within the limits of insurance coverage and authorization or private pay resources. For example, Medicare Advantage plans often authorize very limited, short-term postacute services for their members. The same holds true for Medicaid coverage in many states.

As resources become more scarce, clinicians must maximize each interaction with the patient, start planning for discharge from the time of admission, bolster family caregiver skill and self-confidence, and quickly find community support resources.

In an ideal world, patient care plans would be shared and coordinated across the continuum of care and between disciplines. This type of care plan sharing is much more likely to happen if clinicians use a shared electronic medical record or are part of an integrated delivery system.

Organizing Coordinated Care— Some Tools and Techniques

The healthcare literature is heavy on articles about professional views of care coordination and light on studies about patient views of the effectiveness of care coordination strategies. Information from clinical practice suggests that patients are most concerned about the coordinating or aligning element of care coordination and communication about the care plan.

These are the actions that nurses and other care coordinators take to orchestrate all the elements of care for the patient so that no clinical tasks are left undone, no supplies or equipment go missing, and the patient is not left wondering who is in charge and what is going on. For patients, this is often the essence of connected care.

This coordinating function involves knowing who is actually in charge of the patient's care, ongoing communication, scheduling, ensuring

that medical equipment and supplies are available to the patient when needed, and smooth and cohesive interactions between the patient's many professional caregivers.

This is the function that requires clinicians to be the most organized, connected, and communicative. It also often requires communication and coordination with a network of support personnel including front desk receptionist or medical secretary, schedulers, insurance coordinators, and clinical support staff such as certified nursing assistants. This intense level of clinician organization requires a large arsenal of tools and techniques which are illustrated in **TABLE 6-2**.

Home healthcare coordination and case management are good examples of the connected care tools and techniques in action. Because home care is delivered in an uncontrolled, nonmedical setting, it is one of the more challenging frontiers of connected care. Connecting the dots for patients in this environment involves multiple interactions and negotiations with patients, families, technology vendors, equipment suppliers, pharmacists, hospitals, other providers of care, physicians, and community agencies. **FIGURE 6-3** illustrates the complexity of these interactions for a nurse with a typical home care caseload of 25 to 30 patients.

"Working to the Top of Your License"—A Care Coordination Efficiency Strategy

The example of home healthcare nurse case management illustrates how all the pillars of connected care can be aligned within the role of one clinician. Of special note is the need for the clinician to carefully juggle and coordinate scores of detailed follow-up tasks to achieve connected care for the patient. In the current intense and cost-conscious healthcare environment, it is virtually impossible for one person to do this alone.

Hence the need to master the highest level of professional skill and competency possible

TABLE 6-2 Connected Care Tools

Interpersonal Communication	Written/Electronic Communication	Team Tools	Coordinating Tools and Techniques
Active listening	Emails, texts, phone calls	Visible measurement	Liaison visits
Scripting	Templates and forms	Interdisciplinary conferencing	Case management
SBAR reporting	Shared electronic medical records	High-risk patient huddles	Joint care plans
Motivational interviewing (MI)	"Cheat sheets" for patients/staff	Complex case conferences	Calendars, tracking databases or spreadsheets
Use HCAHPS language in teaching	Patient portals	Shared schedules	Procedures flowcharts

HCAHPS, Hospital Assessment of Healthcare Providers and Systems; SBAR, situation-background-assessment-recommendation.
Data from BK Health Care Consulting.

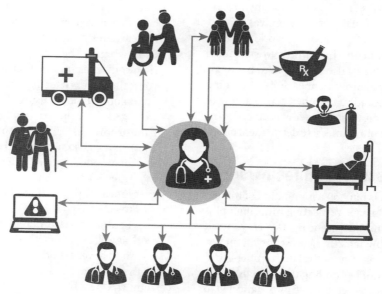

FIGURE 6-3 Home Care Case Manager Care Connections

and then to delegate tasks that do not require professional expertise. Some examples are delegating patient tracking and tracking of medical orders to medical secretaries. Another example is occupational therapists teaching home health aides to cue and instruct patients toward more self-care in activities of daily living. Medical assistants in medical offices frequently take an initial medical history and obtain and enter an updated medication list from the patient.

▶ Connected Care Pillar 2: *Teamwork*

Multiple studies have identified the value of teamwork in achieving patient/professional satisfaction and better outcomes and reducing medical errors and adverse events. Since health care is a highly complex endeavor, the expertise of multiple professionals and support staff working together is essential for success. The complexity and emotional intensity of health care also puts a great burden on health professionals—one that can be alleviated by mutual aid and support within a team structure. However, with the press of tasks and deadlines, many professionals unintentionally find themselves going it alone. The core of teamwork is working effectively with your own department work team.

Clinicians may also be invited to be members of quality improvement or project planning teams. Collaboration, another connected care pillar, and a somewhat broader concept, is teamwork outside your immediate department circle.

Mutual Respect and Teamwork

All teamwork is built on a foundation of mutual respect. This means respecting differing opinions and cultural differences between yourself and other clinicians. It also means maintaining an open mind about team members who you feel may not be "pulling their weight." One way to remain respectful in this situation is to be curious about why the person is not doing

what you think he or she should be doing and finding a way to address the issue face to face.

Behaviors for Effective Teamwork

An article in the career advice blog Allhealthcare (2010), from Monster.com (the online employment site), provides some practical teamwork reminders for front line clinicians:

- **Communicate.** Talk about the work that you do together and if you see a problem with boundaries or with someone not doing his or her part, use positive assertiveness to find out why and to discuss how it impacts you and what you would like to see done differently. If you do this, be prepared to get the same type of feedback.
- **Support and encourage.** If you see a team member struggling and can't actually help, you can always acknowledge that the person is having a hard time and sympathize. Just getting some support may be enough to help that coworker go on.
- **Use constructive suggestions instead of complaints.** If a clinician sees that work processes or patient care is not flowing smoothly, he or she can formulate suggestions to management and make things better rather than simply complaining.
- **Lend a hand.** The strongest expression of teamwork is helping out. Even if you are busy yourself, helping a team member will both build goodwill and ensure that important work gets done properly and on time.
- **Compromise.** Health care, because of its complexity, absolutely requires teamwork to achieve good patient outcomes. In certain cases, such as the use of best practices, everyone really must do things in a similar way to achieve goals.

In other cases, different methods may work as well as your method. Clinicians who are good at teamwork learn that "my way or the highway" is a path to isolation and conflict. One way to be better at compromise is be curious, observe other team members' work methods, and potentially learn other and perhaps better ways of doing things.

- **Mentor.** Team players are observant about other employees who may be struggling with how to do a task, how to use some piece of technology, or how the steps in a process work. Seasoned clinicians can be particularly helpful to new employees who need some guidance and support. With more experienced employees it can be helpful to ask permission before offering support.

- **Keep an open mind.** In a healthcare world that is constantly changing, and in which new research is constantly providing new and better methods of care, rigidity is not only the enemy of success, but also can be destructive. When clinicians decide that new policies, procedures, or techniques do not apply to them, the whole team suffers the consequences. Clinicians who are open to new methods and changes can influence other team members to think through and better adapt to change.

- **Ask questions.** If clinicians are honest about their own level of expertise and their own limits, they will know that they sometimes have to seek advice. Asking other team members for ideas and suggestions demonstrates mutual respect, provides the clinician with valuable new information, and creates a stronger bond with the team member who is giving help and advice.

- **Squash gossip.** A team can quickly turn toxic if team members allow negative gossip to flourish. Always applying the principle of mutual respect, getting the facts about rumors, and directly asking the people involved about their point of view are good ways to keep rumors and misinformation at bay (Data from Allhealthcare, 2010). (ata from Allhealthcare, 2010)

Improving Teamwork Skills

Front line clinicians can improve their teamwork skills by attending training sessions and doing some personal research about being a more effective team player. Clinicians who participate in process improvement teams have a great opportunity to learn techniques of team communication, compromise, and team decision making. Another way to be a positive team player is to participate in team meetings in a helpful way, by asking questions, offering suggestions, and helping to keep the discussion focused.

▶ Connected Care Pillar 3: *Collaboration*

Collaboration is a close but more broadly defined relative of teamwork. Sullivan, Kiovsky, Mason, Hill, and Dukes (2015), in an *American Journal of Nursing* article on interprofessional collaboration, describe it this way: "Inter-professional collaboration is based on the premise that when providers and patients communicate and consider each other's unique perspective, they can better address the multiple factors that influence the health of individuals, families, and communities. No one provider can do all of this alone" (p. 47).

Larson (2013) in an article on hospitalist/nurse collaboration describes a culture that fosters collaboration: "Trina Seals, MS, RN, credits the successful collaboration between hospitalists and nurses in her hospital, Forsyth Medical Center, to a culture that encourages them to work 'hand in hand.' Forsyth is part of Novant Health, a nonprofit health care system with facilities in Virginia, North Carolina and South Carolina that has hospitalists in its 13 hospitals. 'It's more than pulling people together,' said Seals, the nurse manager on her hospital's 30-bed innovation unit. 'It's creating that atmosphere where it's expected that you're going to communicate and connect'" (pp. 1–2).

Understanding Other Professions

Collaboration starts with an understanding of the different roles and functions of other health professionals and of other organizational functions that support the clinician. For example, some nurses do not have a good understanding of the roles, scope of practice, type of expertise, and professional culture that social workers and therapists (physical, occupational, speech) bring to the clinical team. Physician-nurse communication about roles and responsibilities is a vast and evolving topic and one that is made more complex by a history of power struggles and misunderstandings.

One way to develop a better understanding of other professionals is simply to ask colleagues from other professions how they would approach a specific patient care situation, what their priorities are, and what patient care skills they provide. Another method is to ask management to develop joint meetings with other professional groups and to have someone with group dynamics skills facilitate a discussion about differing professional assumptions and viewpoints. Some important questions to ask:

- When you care for a patient, what are your priorities?
- What do you wish other professionals understood about the work you do?
- What types of patient care activities do you do?
- What does a good job look like in your profession?
- What are some of the challenges that you face?
- What are some of the misconceptions that other people have about your profession?
- What would you like to know about your profession?

Learning from Each Other

In the most open and collaborative settings, professionals gain new insights and learn "tips and tricks" from each other. This can only happen when there is mutual respect, openness to learning, and time to communicate. A good example of this is a monthly meeting of a hospital staff and the multiple postacute providers that service their patients, including SNFs, home care, assisted living, ambulance, pharmacy, and other groups. As group members became more comfortable with each other, people from different organizations and disciplines routinely began asking each other for advice, collaborated on cases, and invited each other to do educational program presentations at their facilities. At a more basic level, a nurse might ask a social worker for tips on boundary setting or how to deal with a depressed patient. A physical therapist might learn more about the effect of medications on falls from nurse colleagues.

Negotiation as a Connected Care Strategy

Once professionals understand each other's viewpoint, and sometimes even if they have not had an opportunity to do this, relationships may have to be negotiated. An example of this is ensuring that nurses can get access to a physician when a patient's condition changes. Another example is primary care medical practices creating formal relationships with specialty groups to receive feedback from consultants and information about treatment that the specialist may initiate.

Sometimes, negotiation must occur between professionals in the same discipline but different specialties. For example, internists are typically expected to reconcile medications for elderly patients. These patients may be on multiple medications and may have been prescribed drugs by other physicians that are contraindicated for the elderly. The primary care physician may need to negotiate with his or her peers to reduce the number of medications and alleviate the problem of polypharmacy.

Interdisciplinary negotiations or those that cross organizational boundaries require clear statements of what each organization or profession needs from the other, discussion about what each will and will not do, processes for resolution of disputes or conflicts, agreement on process steps for collaboration, and a written memo, contract, or document that clearly delineates roles and responsibilities. These are collaboration support systems that must be developed by organizational managers.

Mechanisms for Collaboration

Interdisciplinary collaboration should be both formal and informal. Informal communication occurs when two professionals are involved in a patient's care and they need to ask each other questions or coordinate their activities. This type of informal collaboration is typically accomplished through phone calls, texting, or email. Formal interdisciplinary communication should occur at specific points in the care process.

- **Referrals to other professionals.** Referrals must provide information about what the other profession is being asked to do and they must contain clinical information needed by that profession. If a standardized referral form is being used, it is up to the sending clinician to fill out completely. The receiving clinician has an obligation to "close the loop" and respond with the results of his or her interaction with the patient.
- **Reporting on changes in condition and taking action to resolve them.** This step in care requires clinicians to evaluate which other discipline might need to be called to help or to intervene to facilitate good patient care. For example, a nurse in an SNF or home care setting might need to contact an advanced practice registered nurse (APRN) to see a heart failure patient to further evaluate and treat increasing shortness of breath. A home care physical therapist might contact the patient's nurse to evaluate a potential medication side effect. All clinicians must use short and focused reporting to contact a physician to report changes in condition and suggest possible actions or alternatives.
- **Reporting care transitions.** When patients move between settings, say from home to the hospital, each organization in the continuum has a responsibility to notify a contact person at the next step in care. This is particularly important in value-based payment, in which the care setting has a large impact on payment. For example, if a home care nurse identifies a change in decline in patient functional ability she may be able to coordinate a return to an SNF rather than a hospital admission. By communicating and collaborating with the next step in care, the clinician ensures that no information, medication changes, or care plan changes are missed.
- **Care conferencing to coordinate care planning.** Regular case conferencing or team huddles between clinicians who share the care of a single patient are essential to creating a coordinated experience for patients. These meetings allow clinicians to share information, to identify and resolve problems, and to ensure that they are each maintaining a patient-centered focus.
- **Complex case conferences to problem solve patient care problems.** Complex patients often require the expertise of the whole continuum of care. Complex case conferences, which can be requested by the clinician or required by management, bring together experts from all disciplines. At these meetings, the patient record and care plan are reviewed and members of the team can advise the clinician on additional patient care strategies and resources.
- **Using internal experts.** Many healthcare organizations have specialty trained and certified staff who can assist clinicians in coordinating care for the most complex patients. An example is consulting a certified wound care nurse. By utilizing this type of help, clinicians can more easily connect the dots for patients by finding the most effective and efficient methods of care and, sometimes, additional resources.

Collaboration Between Organizational Functions

Another form of collaboration that helps connect the dots for patients occurs internally between front line clinicians and nonclinical departments and support staff. Many of the issues that create uncoordinated care occur in this realm. For example, clinicians in settings such as outpatient surgery, medical practice, and home health care are heavily dependent on the people who schedule visits or procedure times. Without a good mutual understanding of patient care goals, distribution of resources, and triage principles, appointment overlaps or gaps can occur causing chaos for patients and conflict among professionals.

Another area where internal collaboration is essential is the relationship between clinicians and information systems staff. When staff are fully trained in the use of the electronic medical record, telephone systems, and communication tools such as texting and videoconferencing, care and communication flow more smoothly. When the information systems staff provide helpful consultation, technical problems are more easily solved and care can be delivered properly and on time. Clinical staff must also understand the capabilities and limitations of the information systems staff who support them. In many cases, this ideal situation does not occur. Let's look at a case study to better understand this problem.

○ *CASE STUDY*

An Internal Collaboration Problem

A group of home health agency clinician managers met weekly to improve the processes of care and to achieve better outcomes and lower readmission rates. The team identified a series of barriers to achieving these goals and found that a less than ideal relationship between clinicians and information technology (IT) systems was one of them. Nurses in the field were identifying significant problems with the use of the electronic medical record (EMR) and synchronizing data with the agency server.

A frequently mentioned scenario was one in which a nurse angrily marched into the IT department, interrupting the first person he or she saw, then dropping the offending computer on that employee's desk saying, "You have to fix this, right now so I can get back to work." Naturally the response from the IT staff person was not too cordial. At first, the team wanted to call in the chief information officer (CIO) and barrage this person with a list of all the problems in her department, but cooler heads prevailed. The group switched gears and first considered whether they themselves had fostered the problem.

In subsequent discussion, it was revealed that new nurses had an EMR orientation but little ongoing education. There were "cheat sheets" in the shared drive of the EMR but most were inaccurate and out of date. Managers themselves did not use the EMR on a day-to-day basis and did not have the skills to coach their own employees. Information systems staff had become frustrated, labeling many clinicians as incompetent and developing a nonservice-oriented attitude in which the first line of defense was always "user error." The managerial team spoke with nursing staff, engaged the help of the clinical informatics nurse to do "catch-up" training, updated the cheat sheets, and developed their own expertise. They then engaged the CIO in a conversation about service standards and customer service.

Since the clinical team had taken responsibility for their own part in the problem, the CIO was much more willing to collaborate, manage customer service on her team, and agree to service standards. The result was vastly improved nursing skill in the use of the EMR, improved nursing and IT staff satisfaction, and subsequent more efficient and effective patient care.

External Collaborations

Clinicians in the current tumultuous healthcare environment are facing the issue of very sick and frail patients being moved from acute care to postacute and ambulatory care. This change has ratcheted up the level of care complexity for all levels of clinicians. One solution to effective care in these situations is collaboration with outside experts such as care coordinators at insurance companies, Medicaid managed care organizations, or accountable care organizations. Front line clinicians can sometimes reach out to these care coordinators, who have access to additional resources, and possibly more time, to help coordinate complex care tasks.

Another set of resources for fostering patient self-care is finding community organizations and support systems to help with social isolation and the social determinants of health. An example is the "village" movement. Villages are membership networks of seniors who band together to provide volunteer help to each other, to access vetted businesses that provide member discounts, and to create a social support network through group social activities. Some villages create partnerships with healthcare organizations such as visiting nurse associations. Most provide some sort of centralized coordination to help members find services. A good place to find information about these organizations is the Village to Village Network (http://www.vtvnetwork.org).

One example is Shoreline Village, Connecticut, which offers social events such as theater trips, provides volunteer services such as transportation, and offers personal health assessments and wellness programs through VNA Community Healthcare, a local home care and wellness agency. A coordinator is available to help members find volunteer help or community services (shorelinevillagect.org).

▶ Connected Care Pillar 4: *Communication*

Of all the connected care strategies, communication may be the most important in ensuring safe, seamless, patient-centered and team-based care. It is probably no exaggeration to say that communication is the lifeblood of connected care. Patient dissatisfaction, patient harm, and malpractice suits that result from poor clinical communication take a huge financial and emotional toll on patients, families, and health professionals. We will start the discussion on healthcare communication by looking at the most widely used objective data from the HCAHPS survey section of the online Medicare Hospital Compare hospital rating website (Medicare.gov, 2017) (**TABLE 6-3**).

While not terrible, these ratings clearly indicate room for improvement, particularly in the area of patient preparation for self-care at home, a key element of connected care transition management. Organizations that are required to participate in one of the CAHPS surveys (Medicare mandated patient experience surveys) can use their publicly reported results as a way to monitor organizational progress in improving communication.

Those organizations that are not covered by CAHPS can use their own patient satisfaction data, trended over time, to do the same thing.

TABLE 6-3 Hospital Compare Patient Survey National Benchmarks

HCAHPS Question	National Average
Patients who reported that their nurses "Always" communicated well	80%
Patients who reported that their doctors "Always" communicated well	82%
Patients who reported that YES, they were given information about what to do during their recovery at home	87%
Patients who "Strongly Agree" they understood their care when they left the hospital	52%

www.Medicare.gov/hospital-compare, accessed August 25, 2017.

Applying the Connected Care Communication Model

Most of the literature on communication uses a common model that was first developed by Bell Lab scientists Shannon and Weaver in the 1940s. While this model was designed to illustrate radio communication, it has been widely applied to interpersonal and electronic communication in health care and other industries. **FIGURE 6-4** illustrates this model.

In the universal communication model a **sender** (the person sending a message) encodes or packages the message in words, symbols and gestures, body language, and voice tone if the communication is in person. The sender uses a specific channel (communication method) to send the message—in person, by phone, or electronically. During the sending phase of the communication, "noise" or interference can occur. Noise might include technical problems that interrupt electronic communication, distraction, language barriers, negative body language, or a voice tone that distorts the message. The receiver (the recipient of the message) gets the message and decodes it to understand its meaning.

Ideally, the receiver responds to the message, using feedback to relay his or her own understanding of it to the sender. Noise can also interfere with sending this feedback message. If the communication is effective, the receiver has gotten the message that the sender intended and the sender knows that the communication loop is closed. This model is the basic foundation for all verbal and electronic communication in health care (Communication.org, 2017).

Communication Model Checklist

When health professionals communicate with patients and with each other, they should ensure that all elements of their communication are in working order.

When someone makes a request, when a patient needs to learn a new self-care skill, when clinical team members are working together to complete a medical procedure, when other health professionals need to know about a change in the care plan, and when a change in the patient's condition needs to be reported, everyone involved should be following the steps. Using these steps becomes habit only through training and frequent self-reminders.

Communication Model Checklist

✓ Who needs to know (message receivers)?
✓ What information does the recipient want and need (the message)?
✓ How should the information best be packaged so the recipient can understand it (encoding)?
✓ What are the potential pitfalls or problems in this communication (noise)?

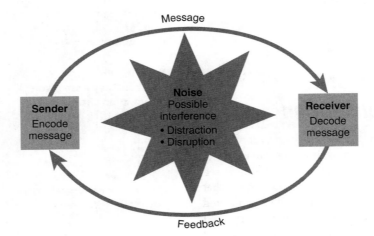

FIGURE 6-4 The Communication Model

✓ How will you overcome these potential communication problems?

✓ How will you know that the communication was received (feedback)?

Another interesting example of communication noise is the recent trend toward electronic check-ins. Theoretically, this method should produce more accurate and timely communication and reduce the labor required to check patients in. In a recent example observed by the author in an outpatient surgery center, many of the patients, particularly the elderly, were completely confused by the electronic check-in device and would not even try it. Some solicited the help of other patients sitting in the waiting room, while others simply went to the registration desk and insisted

🔍 CASE STUDY

Practicing Good Communication

A patient admission or start of care is a part of the care process that requires consistent and disciplined communication between multiple senders and receivers.

The first sender might be the patient who checks in at the front desk, communicates his or her name, and completes a registration form. The patient encodes his or her information in words and in writing and uses both a verbal and a written channel to communicate. In this process the patient sends a message about being present at the appointed time, his or her demographic and insurance information, and possibly the reason for the visit

The receptionist is the receiver of the communication. He or she verifies that the patient has an appointment at that time (feedback). He or she checks the registration form for completeness and asks for clarification or additional information (feedback).

Once the registration is complete, the receptionist may send a verbal message to the patient about how long the wait for the medical visit might be. Noise in this example would be a registration form that is not easy to understand and that requires the patient to keep coming back to the receptionist for help.

on getting assistance. This is a good example of noise (the use of a device that is not understood by patients) interfering with good communication.

▶ Interpersonal Communication in Health Care

Although electronic patient communication is becoming more common, health care is first and foremost a face-to-face business in which clinician and patient communicate directly and personally. This communication can range from the delivery of simple factual information, such as the time of a follow-up appointment, to the complex and emotionally laden process of telling a patient that he or she has a fatal disease. The effectiveness of this communication depends heavily on the clinician's and, to a lesser extent, the patient's communication skills.

The core communication skills for clinicians are active listening and clinical interviewing. Other important skills include clinical reporting, teaching, negotiating, giving constructive feedback, assertiveness, and conflict resolution. Health coaching and motivational interviewing are more advanced skills that are used to help patients find their own internal motivation to change. The delivery of bad news and discussion of palliative care and hospice options are another type of specialized and challenging communication skills.

Interpersonal communication includes both verbal and nonverbal components. The verbal component is words and voice tone. Body language and expressions are nonverbal components of communication, and research indicates that nonverbal behaviors actually get more attention than words. Attitude is the invisible component of communication that drives words, voice tone, body language, and gestures. Even clinicians who are not particularly articulate can be good communicators if their presence is attentive and relays a caring and listening approach. Either natural aptitude or repetitive training makes positive communication a reflex for health professionals. In the book *Smith's Patient-Centered Interviewing*,

Fortin and colleagues (2012) describe a defined set of relationship-building skills.

Emotion Seeking Skills

Because emotions are such an important part of the patient experience, clinicians must use communication skills to elicit and address patient emotions. These skills include:

- **Direct inquiry:** Asking a specific question such as "How did that make you feel?"
- **Indirect inquiry:** Learning about emotions by asking about impact, using self-disclosure, asking about what the patient believes caused the medical problems, and asking about triggers (why the patient sought care at this particular time).

Empathy Skills

Empathy skills are used to communicate that you have heard the patient and result in the patient feeling cared for. Clinicians can remember the empathy skills by using the initials NURS, as a memory device (an easy one for nurses):

- **Naming** is repeating an emotion expressed by the patient: "You say you feel depressed" or simply stating an observation: "You look a little anxious."
- **Understanding** implies using statements that validate the patient's expressions or concerns: "I can see how that must have been very frightening."
- **Respecting** is an explicit expression of respect or praise that reinforces positive behaviors: "You have been through so much and yet you keep moving forward."
- **Supporting** statements indicate the clinician's willingness to work as a member of the patient's team: "I am here to work with you to get this illness under control." (Modified from Fortin, Dwamena, Frankel and Smith, 2012)

Active Listening

Most communication skills in health care build on the technique of active listening. This approach utilizes a specific set of questions and steps to ensure that the person sending the message has been understood by the listener. In brief, the technique follows these steps:

- **Use open-ended questions to encourage the speaker to talk.** These are questions that cannot be answered with a "yes" or "no" answer: "Can you tell me what has happened since you got out of the hospital?"
- **Use reflection to give feedback on the message and to ensure that you have understood the speaker correctly.** Reflection can involve simply repeating what you have heard or paraphrasing what you think you heard in your own words: "You were in the CCU for 5 days, and your heart stopped, but they were able to bring you back. You feel very shaken by that experience."
- **Use probing questions to explore an issue further.** "So you felt that you weren't getting good medical treatment in the hospital. Can you tell me what made you think that?"
- **Use closed-ended questions to verify that you have heard correctly.** "You are willing to take the blood pressure and cholesterol meds that were prescribed but you want to find a different cardiologist. Is that right?"
- **Summarize key points.** "Let me be sure that I have the story right. You had a heart attack and went right in for cardiac bypass surgery. The surgery was successful but you had a cardiac arrest while you were in CCU. You came back but were very sick and frightened and still are. You are not too sure about the quality of the cardiology care that you got because all the doctors disagreed with each other in front of you. You are willing to take the meds they prescribed, but you want to find a new cardiologist. Is that correct?"

Connected Care Key Communication Principles for Front Line Clinicians

Managers apply connected care communication principles and best practices to work systems and processes as well as to interpersonal communication. We will now look at how these principles should be applied by clinicians on the front lines of care.

The Next Step Is the Customer

This concept, which comes from the field of quality improvement, says that any action that a worker takes affects the next worker in the process chain or the patient. High-quality work is done with the needs of the next step in mind. The clearest example of this in health care is care transitions.

When a nurse discharges a patient, he or she must consider the information needs of the facility or agency to whom the patient is being referred.

If the patient is being discharged home, the nurse must envision the information that the patient will need to function safely such as a medication list, a phone number to call, and a follow-up appointment. Internal examples are shift changes, where the next shift to come on duty, needs clinical information about patient status and what happened during the current shift.

The key is for each person to communicate what the next step wants and needs to know, not what the clinician wants to tell them. In practice this means having discussions with people and departments that are in the process chain before and after the work that you do. The people before you in the process chain need to know your information needs and you need to understand what the information needs are of the people after you in the chain.

Remember the Ripple Effect

Since health care consists of complex work processes performed by multiple individuals on the care team, actions taken by a clinician will affect others on the team as well as the patient and family. Glance back at Figure 6-3 to get a sense of this issue. For effective communication, the clinician must communicate with those people who are impacted by his or her actions.

For example, if a care coordinator in a medical practice is going to be away on vacation, she needs to contact the front desk, medical secretaries, physicians and APRNS, and families who depend on her for help with coordinating care. She will need to hand off unfinished tasks to a back-up person to ensure that nothing is lost. She will also need to change her phone and email message to ensure that anyone who contacts her knows she is away. When clinicians who are good at connected care take an action that affects others, they get in the habit of doing a quick mental checklist of all the people who will be affected, and then communicate to each person or function on the list.

Creating email groups for common recurrent communications to people who have joint responsibility for a work process or function can be helpful in this regard.

Close the Loop

Of all the communication skills, this one is the most important in connecting care, reducing medical errors, and improving the patient experience. Closed loop communication means that the clinician must ensure that the information that he or she provided was actually received and understood by the next person in the process chain or the next step in care.

This two-way communication is vital in care planning, communicating patient information during shift changes or care transitions, and in reporting changes in condition. A therapy manager described it this way: "Interdisciplinary communication is a web that supports the patient. When one piece of the web breaks, the patient can fall through the cracks." Two-way communication means that clinicians actually talk to fellow team members and don't just leave messages, agree upon care plan activities, and resolve problems jointly. This two-way communication can sometimes take extra work especially when dealing with busy physicians who may not always respond to messages in a timely fashion.

For example, an SNF or home care nurse, who does not have access to a physician onsite and who is reporting a change in condition, cannot just wait indefinitely for a return call. He or she must describe the urgency of the problem, ask for a call back, and keep trying until a response comes or an alternative action is required. The core of closed loop communication is that receivers of information repeat what they think they heard from the message sender: "Let me be sure I have this correctly. You want me to increase the dose of Lasix from 20 to 40 mg for the next 2 days only, monitor the patient's condition, and call you back with a status report?"

Closed loop communication should also occur when communication is electronic or telephonic. For example, if a clinician receives an email, text, or phone call from another team member about some aspect of patient care, he or she is obligated to email, text, or call back with a response. This is particularly important when dealing with information requests from support employees such as certified nursing assistants. In many cases busy clinicians may triage these calls to the bottom of the task pile, creating not only resentment but misinformation and potential patient care problems.

Follow Organizational Communication Best Practices

When communication structures and processes such as daily huddles, required interdisciplinary conferences, complex case conferences, and transition templates exist, front line clinicians must consistently participate and use them as intended. For example, if the organization requires biweekly interdisciplinary conferencing, it should routinely be put on the clinician's schedule. If nurses are supposed to attend complex case conferences, they must make every effort to be there, despite a busy schedule. If the organization requires a nurse who is out sick to call in and report on planned patient care, then she should do so if at all possible.

These organizational norms apply to communication processes such as email, use of texting, leaving voice messages, and setting out-of-office notifications on both phones and computers. The use of these structured techniques will build up

a web of good communication, will reduce the level of chaos and confusion in the workplace, and will contribute to a better employee and patient experience.

Drive Out Fear

Fear and intimidation in the clinical workplace that inhibits communication is certainly a managerial issue, but clinicians also play a role in combatting it.

Obviously, overtly aggressive and disrespectful behavior, as well as consistent patterns of ignoring communication and responding in a negative manner by other clinicians, must be reported to management. Clinicians themselves can learn and practice assertive communication techniques to resist aggression, being ignored or becoming the recipient of other clinicians' impatience or annoyance.

A training program on assertive communication for health professionals, entitled "Assertive Communication, Making Yourself Heard on a Clinical Team," provides some practical suggestions for health professionals who are confronted with disrespectful or aggressive behavior (Edith Cowan University [ECU], 2017):

- Appears self-confident and composed
- Maintains eye contact
- Uses clear, concise speech
- Speaks firmly and positively
- Speaks genuinely, without sarcasm
- Is nonapologetic

Other suggestions are be clear, concise, and factual; remain calm; and avoid blame. Use "I" statements instead of blaming and accusatory statements that start with "You did. . .," "You must. . .," or "You have to. . ." that generate defensiveness (modified from ECU, 2017).

The DESC assertive communication technique can be effective in these situations. See **BOX 6-3** for an example of how DESC works.

A communication skills program from Johns Hopkins Medicine (2016) describes a technique called the "Two Attempt Rule" in which a patient safety concern is being expressed by

BOX 6-3 DESC Model of Communication

Describe the specific situation:

I have tried to case conference with you about three of our joint patients in the last few weeks. In each case you have not gotten back to me to discuss these cases.

Express your concerns about the action:

I am concerned about this situation because we have an agency policy that we have to case conference every 2 weeks and we are not doing it. I think the care of these patients is more disjointed because we are not working together. I am worried that you might ignore me if I call you to go out and check on a patient if there is condition change.

Suggest other alternatives:

Would it help if we set up a regular time in the schedule to have a conference call or a meeting to discuss our joint patients? Is there anything else we can do to get our case conferencing on track?

Describe consequences that will occur if things improve or if they don't improve:

This will continue to be frustrating for both of us and it is not helping patient outcomes. I will be forced to report the situation to my supervisor if things don't change right away.

a member of the clinical team but is not being heard (**FIGURE 6-5**). In this scenario, the person recognizes the problem using clear and concise language to express the concern and then, if the concern is not acknowledged, the person takes it to the next level of organizational authority for a resolution. This technique is sometimes called the "Two Challenge Rule."

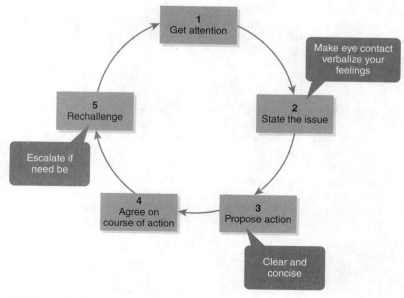

FIGURE 6-5 The Two Attempt Rule

▶ # When Healthcare Communication Fails

Far too often, the steps in the communication model are not followed and communication fails. We will start this discussion of communication failures and remedies with a story told from the viewpoint of a family caregiver.

MacDonald (2015) suggests that healthcare providers can avoid this type of less than optimal patient and family experience by following three simple steps:

1. **Communicate every step of the way.** Assign one person to communicate to the family in the ER setting.
2. **Use the teach-back method when relaying information.** MacDonald

found that family members often relayed erroneous information because they didn't really understand what the health professional was telling them.

3. **Don't forget that the patient is a person, not a case.** Patients, even though they may not be able to communicate their fear and pain, still feel them. It is up to the professional to demonstrate respect for patients and find a way to communicate with them. (Modified from MacDonald, 2015)

Miscommunication in Health Care—Some Root Causes

Communication seems simple on the surface—everyone taking care of the patient should share information through personal communication, written reports, or electronic documents in a timely, accurate, and patient-centered way.

🔍 CASE STUDY

When Clinical Communication Fails

In a 2015 article in *Fierce Healthcare*, Ilene MacDonald describes a harrowing experience in a hospital emergency room with a relative who is mentally challenged and who often communicates with sign language. MacDonald describes a series of disconnects with medical providers: restraining the patient who talks with his hands so he won't pull out an IV, nurses uninformed about the patient's status after a shift change, a multitude of doctors attending the patient but no clear information about who is in charge, and little consistent ongoing communication about the patient's status.

MacDonald (2015) sums it up this way: "We seemed to get conflicting reports on his condition and discharge plans every day. Although one member of our family is a registered nurse and I write about healthcare, we often felt lost in the system, confused by what seemed to be a lack of communication among clinicians about his care plan."

ASK YOURSELF

- Read the article at http://www.fierce healthcare.com/healthcare/3-ways-to -improve-communication-and-care -coordination-from-patient-and -family-s.
- After reading the summary of Ilene MacDonald's article, how well do you think the hospital practiced patient-centered care?
- For whom were the hospital systems designed—the patients who received care or the health professionals who delivered it?
- Who could or should have been in charge of coordinating this patient's inpatient experience? (There was a care coordinator who managed discharge plans.)
- Does any part of this story sound like something that could happen in your organization?

But if communication is so simple, why does healthcare communication frequently go so badly, even to the extent of causing adverse events and patient deaths?

Structure and Processes of Care

One reason for healthcare miscommunication is the structure and process of healthcare delivery. Since care is typically organized around specialty units, procedures, or health professions, it is usually not designed with the patient in mind. Typical communication fosters communication within the clinical unit or profession, but not outside its boundaries. To patients, there are no such artificial boundaries. They experience interactions, often disjointed, with all the members of the healthcare team.

Lack of Standards and Consistent Methods

When a healthcare organization has no clear standards or methods of fostering communication, health professionals are unlikely to take their communication responsibilities seriously. Another reason is that interpersonal communication is a behavior. Behaviors are ingrained and highly resistant to change. In an article in *Becker's Hospital Review* (Gooch, 2016), nurse executive Martie Moore, RN, cites the example of a health professional who brings dysfunctional communication behaviors to work: "For instance, an individual who grew up learning that throwing a tantrum, pouting and withholding information was a way of effective communication may bring aspects of those behaviors into the workplace."

Skill Gaps

A lack of skill is another root cause of communication failures in health care. Many health professionals receive basic training in communication during their prelicensure education.

Communication skills training is often embedded in, and closely linked with, behavioral health courses and clinical rotations. This results in many practitioners not internalizing or generalizing these skills to their current daily work.

A real-life example of this is the author's own experience in teaching motivational interviewing (an advanced communication skills technique that helps patients with behavior change). The author and other program instructors had made the assumption that course participants (primarily nurses, physical and occupational therapists) had basic skills in active listening techniques, which is the foundation of all interpersonal communication in health care. This proved not to be the case. Many participants struggled to practice relatively simple techniques such as open-ended questioning, reflection, and summarizing—the essential skills of communication. When the instructors finally realized that this was a problem, they asked participants about their educational preparation in communication. A number of participants stated that they did not ever remember being trained in communication skills. This same instance held true across similar training programs in a home care agency, medical practice, and community health center. If this experience is generalizable, it means that while many new practitioners may be learning these skills in their basic nursing and medical education, many who are already in the clinical workforce do not have such skills and need organizational help to gain them.

Distraction and Multitasking

The daily work of a clinician who is caring for multiple patients is complex and challenging. Trying to juggle patient schedules, medication administration, diagnostic tests, patient teaching, medical procedures, and rounding can completely absorb the clinician and create constant distraction. This distraction is the "noise" illustrated in the communication model. It is the source of many of the serious or even deadly communication gaps that occur in health care. There is really no magic answer to the issue of distraction, but one approach is to develop the habit of quick, focused attention. When using this method, you must build a space around the communication by waving off distraction: "I will be with you soon, but for the next few minutes, I need to give Dr. Atar my complete attention." You then take a mental deep breath, consciously block out distractions, and focus on the verbal interchange between yourself and the other person, using active listening techniques.

Limited Feedback

Unless health professionals receive feedback on the effectiveness of their communication, they are unlikely to improve it. Most people, in the absence of evidence to the contrary, assume that their communication is effective, clear, and understood by recipients. Only data from patient surveys, supervisory observation, and information from other clinicians who interact with the professional can provide more objective evidence of the clinician's communication competence level. Packaging and delivering this feedback is the responsibility of the clinician's clinical manager.

Fear and Intimidation

The patient safety literature provides numerous examples of the dampening effect that fear and intimidation have on effective communication. In a 2008 Sentinel Event Alert, the Joint Commission clearly defined this problem: "Intimidating and disruptive behaviors are often manifested by health care professionals in positions of power. Such behaviors include reluctance or refusal to answer questions, return phone calls or pages; condescending language or voice intonation; and impatience with questions. Overt and passive behaviors undermine team effectiveness and can compromise the safety of patients. All intimidating and disruptive behaviors are unprofessional and should not be tolerated" (p. 1).

A 2013 survey of over 4,800 health professionals, including nurses, pharmacists, and some physicians, by the Institute for Safe Medication Practices (ISMP), described disturbing findings about the impact of intimidation on medication safety: "At least once during the year, 33% of respondents had concerns but assumed an order was correct rather than interact with an intimidating prescriber. More than one-third asked another professional to talk to a disrespectful prescriber about an order. Eleven percent reported a medication error that occurred primarily due to intimidation" (ISMP, 2013). The survey also showed a drop in clinician confidence that their organization would support them in the face of intimidation. While 70% of respondents in a 2003 survey felt their organization would support them, only 52% in the 2013 survey felt that this would happen. Senior managers and clinical leaders are clearly accountable for resolving the issue of poor communication related to clinician intimidation.

▶ Connected Care Pillar 5: *Care Transitions*

Evidence-based transition processes and techniques can be adopted by clinicians who are not care coordination specialists for a more coordinated patient experience and fewer medical errors due to missed handoffs.

It is important to note that the most problematic care transitions are often those that occur during shift changes, between weekday and weekend staff, between per diem or float and regular staff, and when patient care is delivered by part-time or temporary staff for vacations or sick time coverage. Another common type of internal transition is integrating a new clinical staff member into a case.

Some transition techniques that are applicable to any care transition, even those within a facility or department, include the following:

- One person is responsible for completing the transition or ensuring that it is completed by another clinician.
- Information needed by the department or shift that is receiving the patient is complete and provided in a usable and user friendly form.
- Patients are educated, in advance, about what will happen during the transition and are asked about any concerns.
- Clinical staff use closed loop communication and written communication for high-risk internal transitions such as shift changes, weekend and nighttime transitions, and communication to temporary or per diem staff.
- Staff check with the patient and family to ensure that all transition tasks were completed.
- There are templates or written forms to document care transitions in the medical record.

An example is the assignment of a home health aide to a home care case. The aide must receive a written care plan that details the tasks that he or she is supposed to perform that is based on the case manager's care plan. The aide must be verbally oriented to the case by the case manager.

In preparation for the aide coming into the case, the case manager must educate the patient and family about why the aide was ordered and what he or she can or cannot do.

FIGURE 6-6 summarizes key clinician activities that are needed to achieve connected care.

Overcoming Obstacles to Connected Care on the Front Lines

Good connected care in clinical practice is a combination of organizational and individual clinician effectiveness. Both are absolutely necessary for the dots to connect. Some of the common barriers to connected care are:

- **Fuzzy goals and lack of vision.** When senior management does not create a clear set of goals and a vision and middle management does not clearly communicate it to front line clinicians, in words that they can understand, clinical staff are not sure what to do and cannot modify their work to provide connected care.
- **Persistence of a professionally focused, task-oriented care mentality.** Clinicians who fail to make the mental shift to patient-centered care will never be able to provide coordinated

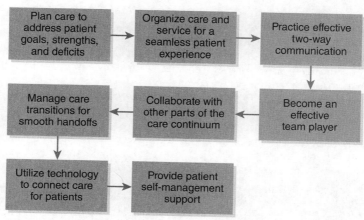

FIGURE 6-6 Front Line Clinician Connected Care Essentials

INTERVIEW WITH KERRI OKUNEWICZ, RN, HOME CARE NURSE CASE MANAGER

Kerri Okunewicz is a home care nurse case manager who works for VNA Community Healthcare. In answer to the question, "What factors help or hinder connected care for your patients?" Ms. Okunewicz answers, "The social determinants of health—demographics, education, finances—cause the most disconnects." She finds that patients with more socioeconomic issues have the biggest problems with self-determination and nonadherence. Having family support is a factor in making care more connected.

She finds that it takes considerable case management work to coordinate care for people who lack an adequate support system. One issue for her patients is obtaining and managing their own medications. Medications that are prepackaged by the pharmacy can be helpful with this problem. She frequently refers to social work to help patients find benefit or entitlement programs that can help get medications paid for. For example, some of her patients have never signed up for Medicare Part D (the Medicare prescription drug coverage program). Ms. Okunewicz notes that sometimes her patients want help and sometimes they don't.

Ms. Okunewicz says that she never takes patient nonadherence personally, although it can be frustrating. Earlier in her career having patients who didn't care for themselves made her feel inadequate. "It's your soul, what you were made to do. When it doesn't work, it can make you feel empty." Over the years she has learned to "provide/assist as much as I can" and allow patients to make their own choices.

"I use all my networks to help my patients." She cites the example of a patient who had a catheter that didn't fit right and was leaking urine. She called a drug rep who she knew from a former job and he found free supplies and shipped them to her patient. With his help, she finally found a catheter that worked.

Ms. Okunewicz notes that she frequently refers to the agency caregiver support network. This program provides a caregiver counselor who will advise and support family caregivers on their own issues and concerns and helps them manage stress. She says that about 50% of the caregivers who she refers take advantage of the program.

In dealing with people with low health literacy, Ms. Okunewicz "gets down to their level by listening to their concerns and issues." For the first few visits she listens much more than she talks. After that she starts self-care teaching, because by then she better knows what the patient needs. She works with patients to set goals by asking, "Can you tell me what I can do for you?" and "What are the things that are important to you and how might I help?" She tries to relate patient goals to medical things. If the patient says, "I don't want to have this sore on my leg anymore," Ms. Okunewicz might say, "How do you think we can work together on this? Let's try to find a wound care strategy that works for you."

Ms. Okunewicz describes the essence of case management as "communication and organization." She does not wait until the morning to look at her schedule, but rather checks it the night before and calls patients to be sure things are working for them. She feels that this approach is respectful of their time and allows them to make changes if they need to.

Another aspect of organization is setting boundaries on the work: "I don't treat my home as an office. I organize my work so I can start at 7:30 and end around 4:30." Experience helps her manage her day more efficiently. A good case manager must be "determined, caring and focused." Good organization helps a case manager "maximize coordination and efficiency." She finds that case management also involves learning how other providers, such as physicians, prefer to be contacted. Some want a phone call, some want a fax. Providers tend to respond better to their preferred method of communication.

Ms. Okunewicz finds that having a home visiting APRN available is a valuable tool in creating connected care for her patients. For patients who can't easily get out of the house to a medical appointment, having the APRN come reduces the need for a difficult care transition.

"My networks are my team," Ms. Okunewicz says. There is "continual interactive communication" with her agency interdisciplinary team including social work, occupational therapy, speech therapy, and other nurses. Much of the communication is by telephone or by text. For complex patients who are vulnerable to readmission, the team works together, and if there is a problem, someone always goes out the same day or next day.

Other tools that Kerri uses to manage complex patient cases are risk agreements with nonadherent patients and complex case conferences. She often requests case conferences for high-risk patients. The goal is to "regroup everybody and avoid a readmission." She tries to frontload (add) disciplines when the patient is in a difficult situation.

When asked about challenges, Ms. Okunewicz identifies "changes in health care": "These very complicated patients get a 15-minute appointment slot with the doctor. It isn't enough. The patients don't feel they are getting one on one attention and sometimes feel that the doctor doesn't care." Many patients who don't have family support go to their medical visits alone. She tries to help them write down questions, but the patients often don't always ask them.

Ms. Okunewicz feels that the electronic way of documentation will be "mandatory and time efficient" for home care nurses, but there is "still some growing to do" with electronic documentation systems. She does not always bring her laptop into the home and finds that many patients dislike her "typing during the visit." She tends to complete her documentation in the office or at home.

Ms. Okunewicz says, "We will see a different breed of nurse in the next 15 to 20 years. Less 'hands on' and more 'tech savy'. This is just the way things are being driven by economics." She summarizes by saying, "Some people are born to a vocation. This (nursing) is a vocation. If you don't have it in your heart, you won't be good at it."

care for patients because it is not a priority for them. As the volume-to-value shift proceeds, changing incentives may reduce the incidence of this problem.

- **Inadequate connected care structures.** When the organization does not carve out time and space for interdisciplinary conferencing, huddles, quality improvement teams, and complex case conferences, clinical staff have no good mechanisms to support the teamwork, collaboration, and communication necessary to achieve connected care.

- **Faulty systems and processes.** Clinical work processes that were built for an era of fee-for-service silos will not support connected care. Unimproved processes typically include narrow roles, work designed for department convenience, faulty handoffs, and unnecessary complexity. Process improvement is necessary to link care and service activities across departmental and organizational boundaries. All these must be addressed through managerial action or process improvement teams. For example, an organization that does not insist on closed loop communications across all handoffs and care transitions will experience consistent care disconnects.

- **Front line clinicians are not engaged in connected care.** Organizations that still use a top-down hierarchical system of management will be unlikely to engage clinicians in connected care. At the very least, clinicians should be asked for their opinions about improving care at staff meetings and management rounds. In the best case scenario, clinicians would be deeply involved in process improvement and clinical work redesign.

Another antidote to disengaged clinicians is the development of champions and mentors who can role model connected care and coach other clinicians.

- **Perverse incentives.** If the organization says that it wants to achieve the quadruple aim through connected care but if it uses only a productivity-oriented monitoring and reward system for individual clinicians, behavior will naturally gravitate toward volume, not value. Organizations must build in measures of patient-centered, collaborative, connected care behaviors; use these measures in performance appraisal; and reward clinicians who demonstrate these behaviors.
- **Lack of support and recognition for clinicians.** If clinical staff are not valued, nurtured, and empowered, they are unlikely to practice connected care. Organizations must think long and hard about what they are asking clinicians to do and what support they are providing for them to do it. One particular area of concern is the proliferation of "more everything": more regulations, more best practice, more internal process changes. One rule to consider is, "When you add something, take away something." This can be done by using work simplification procedures, automation and training, and empowerment of support staff. It is also essential to provide support for overstressed and troubled clinicians through mechanisms such as employee assistance programs.
- **Accountability gaps.** When employees at all levels of the organization don't take personal responsibility for connected care, it doesn't happen. Too often in the hectic world of health care it is easy to adopt a victim mentality and to blame external circumstances or organizational dysfunction for clinical disconnects. Clinicians can avoid adopting a victim mentality and waiting for the healthcare organization to "fix itself." They can provide constructive ideas, adopt a self-learning program, and trial new and possibly improved methods of care.
- **Lone rangers.** Some clinicians who have very good clinical skills, who take pride in their work and in "saving lives" or "going the extra mile," can foster a lone ranger mentality in which their own interactions with "their" patients are all that matter to them. These clinicians may be dismissive of best practices, thinking that "their way" is better. This type of approach is a barrier in a connected care environment. Performance management interventions may be necessary to both retain the proven expertise of this type of employee but to uproot some of their deep-seated individualistic behavior.

Clinicians as well as managers must become organizationally effective, abandoning a narrow focus on their own personal and professional needs for more of a patient, team, and organization focus.

Another key element in the mindset/skillset transformation for connected care is becoming more willing to train and delegate support staff to perform tasks that were formerly only done by clinicians. This is both an efficiency and an effectiveness technique.

- **Skill and resource gaps** play into disconnected care. As mentioned, skills in both communication and teamwork are essential to connected care. Organizations that invest only in technical training will end up with a workforce that is technically competent but deficient in soft skills essential to value-based connected care.

Another barrier to connected care is resource gaps. When there are not enough pieces of clinical equipment or enough supplies, gaps in care can occur.

For example, if a home care agency does not have enough telemonitors or INR machines, more handoffs will be required, care may be delayed, and more time may be taken up in driving back to the office or transferring machines between staff in the field. Of course, in these situations managers must balance convenience and efficiency for staff and cost issues for the organization.

▶ Chapter Summary

The work of individual clinicians is where connected care theory and the achievement of quadruple aim goals becomes a reality—or not. The work of individual clinicians is influenced by a complex set of forces that includes individual clinician accountability, managerial account-ability, and organizational processes and systems that support connected care.

In this chapter, we have reviewed new competencies that are needed for nurses and other professionals to achieve connected care goals. We have also seen that educational programs for new clinicians may be starting to build the skills necessary to attain these competencies. In real health care, organizational life training in regulatory and technical competencies predominate.

Currently employed professionals have limited access to the types of training necessary to achieve connected care competency. This means that organizations must somewhat alter their focus to provide "soft skills" training and more business literacy education for clinicians.

Care coordination and communication are two front line clinician skills that are essential for the achievement of connected care. Case management/care coordination is a specialty role for some nurses and a piece of the job for other nurses. These functions require the nurse to assess the complete range of patient needs and to either provide services directly or refer and coordinate needed services. Ensuring that all patient-related activities and tasks are completed and that the patient has been communicated with are key elements of effective care coordination.

Teamwork and collaboration are two other essential ingredients of good front line clinical connected care. Health professionals must be adept at working in teams, in understanding how their actions impact shared goals, and in utilizing team behaviors such as supporting teammates. Interdisciplinary collaboration and working across internal organizational department lines is another essential element of effective front line connected care. Each of the health professions must learn to understand and respect the others and to use each other for maximum advantage to the patient. Collaboration with internal healthcare organization departments such as information systems, human

resources, and quality improvement is essential to achieving lean and effective work processes that achieve patient requirements.

Good interpersonal communication is the most basic element of connected care. Health professionals must understand and use techniques such as active listening, closed loop communication, assertiveness, and motivational interviewing to ensure patient safety and to ensure that no patient-directed activities are fragmented.

Unfortunately, in many organizations, not all clinicians have mastered these skills and those who have mastered them are not always able to practice them due to obstacles such as lack of time, skill gaps, and pressure to multitask. It is the job of the organization to ensure that the workplace climate is free of fear and that effective communication is taught and rewarded.

The best way for organizations to achieve connected clinical care is to listen to the voice of the clinician, empower clinicians to have more control over clinical work processes, and empower managers to identify and remove obstacles to connected care for clinicians.

References

Agency for Healthcare Research and Quality. (2016). *Care coordination*. Rockville, MD: AHRQ. http://www.ahrq.gov/professionals/prevention-chronic-care/improve/coordination/index.html

Allhealthcare. (2010). Ten ways you can be a team player. Retrieved from http://allhealthcare.monster.com/benefits/articles/4065-10-ways-you-can-be-a-team-player

Bishop, M. (2016). Patient compliance vs collaboration: Highlight from patients as partners. Pulse. Panel discussion on LinkedIn. Retrieved from https://www.linkedin.com/pulse/patient-compliance-vs-collaboration-highlight-from-patients-bishop

Calhoun, B., & Harris, K. (2017). The promise of nursing in population health (Slide share presentation). The Experience of Banner Health, University of Arizona.

Case Management Society of America. (2017). What kind of work does a case manager do? www.cmsa.com

Centers for Medicare and Medicaid. (2016). CMS finalizes improvements in care, safety, and consumer protections for long-term care facility residents. Retrieved from https://www.cms.gov/Newsroom/MediaReleaseDatabase/Press-releases/2016-Press-releases-items/2016-09-28.html

Combes, J. R., & Arespacochaga, E. (2012). Physician competencies for a 21st century health care system. *Journal of Graduate Medical Education, 4*(3), 401–405. http://doi.org/10.4300/JGME-04-03-33

Communication.org. (2017). Shannon and Weaver communication model. Retrieved from www.Communication.org

Connecticut League for Nursing. (2007). Population health course. Retrieved from www.ctleaguefornursing.org/event/introduction-to-population-health-new-free-course

Cronenwett, L., Sherwood, G., Barnsteiner, J., Disch, J., Johnson, J., . . . Warren, J. (2007). Quality and safety education for nurses. *Nursing Outlook, 55*(3), 122–131.

Edith Cowan University. (2017). Interprofessional ambulatory care unit, making yourself heard on a clinical team. Retrieved from http://www.ecu.edu.au/community-engagement/health-advancement/interprofessional-ambulatory-care-program/interprofessional-learning/ipl-through-simulation/assertive-communication

Experience Innovation Network. (2014). Solution brief—Empowered employees, empowering frontline staff to solve problems. Retrieved from https://www.vocera.com/experience-innovation-network

Fortin, A. H., Dwamena, V. I., Frankel, F. C., & Smith, R. (Eds.). (2012). *Smith's patient-centered interviewing: An evidence-based method* (3rd ed.). New York, NY: McGraw-Hill.

Gooch, K. (2016, March 21). The chronic problem of communication: Why it's a patient safety issue, and how hospitals can address it. *Becker's Hospital Review.* Retrieved from www.beckershospitalreview.com/quality/the-chronic-problem-of-communication-why-it-s-a-patient-safety-issue-and-how-hospitals-can-address-it.html

Institute for Safe Medication Practices. (2013). Intimidation still a problem in hospital workplace, ISMP survey shows. Retrieved from www.ismp.org

Institute of Medicine. (2011). *The future of nursing: Leading change, advancing health.* Washington, DC: The National Academies Press. doi:10.17226/1296

Integrative Medicine Program, Department of Family Medicine and Community Health, University of Wisconsin-Madison School of Medicine and Public Health. (2018). Whole health – Change the conversation, power of the mind. Retrieved from bhttp://projects.hsl.wisc.edu/SERVICE/modules/1/M1_CT_How_a_WH_Visit_Can_Be_Different.pdf

Interprofessional Education Collaborative. (2016). *Core competencies for interprofessional collaborative practice: 2016 update.* Washington, DC: Interprofessional Education Collaborative.

Johns Hopkins Medicine. (2016). JHM teamwork & communication program (slide presentation). Retrieved from http://www.k-hen.com/Portals/16/Documents/PSCTCommunicationsLab

The Joint Commission. (2008). Sentinel Event Alert. Behaviors that undermine a culture of safety. Retrieved from https://www.jointcommission.org/assets/1/18/SEA_40.PDF

Kalaichandran, A. (2017, August 3). Design thinking for doctors and nurses. *nytimes.com, New York Times.* Retrieved from https://www.nytimes.com/2017/08/03/well/live/design-thinking-for-doctors-and-nurses.html

Kim, S., Myers, C., & Allen, L. (2017, August 31) Health care providers can use design thinking to improve patient experiences. *Harvard Business Review.* Retrieved from https://hbr.org/2017/08/health-care-providers-can-use-design-thinking-to-improve-patient-experiences

Lamb, G. (2014). *Care coordination: The game changer.* Silver Spring, MD: American Nurses Association.

Lamb, G. (2017). *Care coordination in interprofessional primary care practice* (interactive video module). Phoenix, AZ: Center for Advancing Interprofessional Practice, Education & Research, Arizona State University.

Larson, J. (2013). Interdisciplinary collaboration: Helping hospitalists and nurses work together. AMN Healthcare News. Retrieved from https://www.amnhealthcare.com/latest-healthcare-news/interdisciplinary-collaboration-helping-hospitalists-nurses-work-together/

MacDonald, I. (2015, July 31). 3 ways to improve communication and care coordination—from the patient and family's perspective. Retrieved from www.FierceHealthcare.com

Medicare.gov. (2017). Hospital compare. Retrieved from www.medicare.gov/hospitalcompare/search.html

National Association for Home Care and Hospice. (2017). CMS issues new rule for home health COPS. Retrieved from http://www.nahc.org/NAHCReport/nr170109_3/

Passmore. J. (2012). Motivational Interviewing techniques, Typical day. *The Coaching Psychologist, 8*(1),50–52.

Relias Learning. (2017). Patient centered care. Retrieved from www.reliaslearning.com

Rich, E., Lipson, D., Liebersky, J., & Parchman, M. (2012). *Coordinating care for patients with complex needs.* Publication No. 12-001. Washington, DC: Agency for Healthcare Research and Quality.

Schultz, E. (2017). Is there a fundamental difference between case management, patient care coordination and population care coordination? Retrieved from https://www.researchgate.net/post/Is_there_a_fundamental_difference_between_case_management_patient_care_coordination_and_population_care_coordination2

Shaller, D. (2007). *Patient-centered care: what does it take?* Publication 1067. New York, NY: The Commonwealth Fund.

Sullivan, M., Kiovsky, R. D., Mason, D. J., Hill, C. D., & Dukes, C. (2015). Interprofessional collaboration and education. *American Journal of Nursing, 115*(3), 47–54. doi:10.1097/01.naj.0000461822.40440.58

CHAPTER 7

Experiencing Connected Care—The Patient Role

▶ Introduction

Connected care, at its most basic, is about connecting the wants, needs, and preferences of the patient with health services that are designed to meet those needs. The worst disconnect for patients is care that is extensive and expensive, but does not deliver what they hope for and desire.

As health care evolves toward more value-based models, the wants and needs of patients and family caregivers have taken center stage in research and in practice. Recent research on patient requirements and on satisfaction with the patient experience has taken three very different viewpoints: patient as consumer, patients as individuals experiencing the healthcare system, and a population health view in which big data are used to segment patients into groups with like characteristics. Patient experience research relevant to connected care focuses on access issues, perceptions of care coordination, patient expectations of health professional communication, patient's requirements for transitions of care, and information handoffs between health professionals. By reviewing this research, we can learn more about how patients themselves define connected care, what patients see as the most important dimensions of connected care, and their views of healthcare fragmentation.

Measures of the patient experience are essential elements of connected care measurement. The Centers for Medicare and Medicaid Services (CMS) Consumer Assessment of Healthcare Providers and Systems (CAHPS) family of surveys (which differ slightly by healthcare setting) are the most frequently used experience measures. Patient-reported outcomes (PROs) are an emerging field in health care and one we will consider as very relevant to the issue of connected care.

We will begin to explore how well the healthcare system performs in meeting patient requirements and where the experience of health care fails to match the expectations of patients.

We will also discuss issues of motivation and compliance from both the professional and patient viewpoints and look at ways to equalize the power differential between patients and providers.

The chapter will describe methods that can be used by professionals, and by patients themselves, to create a more connected care experience. We will describe tools and techniques used to help patients gain more control over their health such as health literacy assessment, self-management support, goal settings, motivational interviewing, and teaching techniques such as "Ask, Tell, Ask." The chapter will provide case studies about patient engagement and self-management. We will explore the issues of burden of treatment and shared decision making. Finally, we will provide a self-management support assessment tool for healthcare organizations.

▶ What Do Patients Want from Health Care? A Research Overview

To provide patient-centered connected care, we must understand how patients and individuals who never or infrequently use the healthcare system view the issue of care integration and connection. It is only by fully understanding the patient point of view and altering our (health professional's) interventions to meet patient requirements that we will truly provide connected care. For individual clinicians, this research is fairly simple and consists of asking patients, "What is important to you?" and "How can I best help you?" Population level research on "what patients want" in contrast to the simplicity of assessing single patient requirements is wide ranging and variable, with results depending on the perspective and sometimes the incentives of the researchers who are assessing patient requirements. For example, companies that sell digital engagement products and conduct research on the topic may have an understandable bias toward overestimating the number of patients with an interest in digital tools. Academic researchers, if they have no financial stake in a product or service, may take a more generic and objective view.

Patient as Consumer

One type of research on patient requirements takes the perspective of patient as consumer. This research tends to focus on concrete issues of access, provider selection, customer service at health facilities, and the costs of care. Other research segments patients into groups by diagnoses, geographic location, or insurance coverage status and then explores the issue of care fragmentation and connection depending on the viewpoint of the selected patient population. Another type of study explores patient perceptions of the various dimensions of connected care, including patient-centeredness, communication, professional collaboration, and transitions. The last type of research, which is based on "big data" (a large volume of structured and unstructured data that are difficult to process with usual methods), analyzes the opinions and behaviors of large populations of patients. Psychographic analysis segments consumers into groups by personality traits, values, attitudes, and interests. Using data on these factors, researchers attempt to group patients into types and use data to predict consumer/patient behavior. This type of research is most often used for marketing/branding purposes but is starting to be explored for clinical implications.

Healthcare Consumer Requirements

The **consumerism approach** characterizes patients as customers of the healthcare system who want certain types of value and service for their insurance or out-of-pocket payments. These types of surveys are heavily weighted toward questions about primary care, the doctor/patient relationship, and new forms of healthcare delivery such as retail clinics and telemedicine.

A 2016 poll of healthcare consumers in seven states conducted by National Public Radio, Robert Wood Johnson Foundation, and Harvard T.H. Chan School of Public Health focused on respondents' perceptions of care quality, cost, barriers to accessing care, and experiences of care at different types of healthcare sites such as doctor's offices, urgent care centers, and retail clinics. Several questions in the survey asked for respondent perceptions of quality, both in the United States as a whole and in their personal health care. The concept of quality was not defined, so responses are entirely subjective. As a whole, respondents had mixed feelings about their health care. Few respondents rated their care as excellent, but few rated it as poor, either. Financial barriers

to care, a key issue in achieving connected care, were thoroughly explored in the survey.

The final report states: "Survey results also indicate that health care costs cause serious financial problems for more than a quarter of Americans, more than forty percent of whom report spending all or most of their personal savings on large medical bills" (National Public Radio, RWJ Foundation, Harvard School of Public Health, 2016, p. 11). Prescription drug costs are the source of another serious gap in care. The survey found that 19% of respondents do not fill prescriptions and one in eight cut pills in half or skipped doses to save money. In terms of access to care, most respondents felt they would be able to get care if they needed it, but one in seven reported that they had not been able to access the care they needed in the last year. Of these people, 25% stated that they had been turned away from a doctor or hospital because of an inability to pay (National Public Radio, RWJ Foundation, Harvard T.H. Chan School of Public Health, 2016).

A 2016 survey by the consulting firm Deloitte used focus groups and a survey of over 1,700 health plan members to determine what was most important to participants as consumers of health care.

The research found that respondents identified their priority needs in descending rank order as:

1. Personalized care from providers (doctors, hospitals, and other healthcare providers)
2. Economically rational coverage and care choices
3. Convenience-driven access and use of care
4. Digitally connected to manage health care

A *personalized experience with providers* was clearly the top priority for consumers in the survey: "Consumers want to be heard, understood, and given clear directions through a personalized health care experience" (Deloitte, 2016, p. 4).

Dimensions of this personalization dimension of care included:

- "Doctors or other health care providers who spend time with me and do not rush me
- Doctors or other health care providers who listen and show they care about me
- Doctors or other health care providers who clearly explain what they are doing and what I need to do later
- Clear, helpful information about my diagnoses and conditions" (Deloitte, 2016, p. 16)

Consumers in the survey also wanted personalized care in the postvisit period, describing a need for providers to communicate with each other after care is done.

The second priority for consumers in this survey was *economically rational coverage and care choices.* Since respondents in this survey were health plan members, all had some degree of insurance coverage and access to care. For this population of patients, connected care from a health plan meant having their own doctors in the plan network, knowing when a service will not be covered or covered at higher out-of-network rates, and price transparency. Each of these issues influences the consumer's ability to access connected care by receiving service from current physicians and being able to obtain needed care through insurance coverage. The prior authorization process (getting health plan authorization before receiving a service) was mentioned as a factor that might create more disconnected care for consumers.

The third factor that was important to health plan consumers in the survey was *convenience-driven access and use of care.* This factor addresses issues such as help in finding and accessing a provider (important to occasional users of the health system) and finding a doctor who takes new patients. Surprisingly, when consumers were asked about the relative importance of quality versus convenience, convenience won out, perhaps because it is so difficult for consumers to identify what "good quality care" actually looks like.

Patient Perceptions of Quality and Provider Communication

A 2017 study by Public Agenda surveyed a nationally representative sample of 1,200 people who had received care for diabetes, had a joint replacement, or had maternity care. The study attempted to explore patient perceptions of the importance of care quality as well as care provider communication. Participants in the survey said that both clinical and provider interpersonal qualities were important for high-quality health care. The most important interpersonal quality that respondents from all three groups identified was "the doctor makes time for the patient's questions and concerns."

While many people in the survey spent time researching the care they needed, few researched the quality of doctors or hospitals who delivered the care. A few of the questions about interpersonal quality used in the study directly touch on patient perceptions of connected care. As noted, making time for patient questions ranked as the top desired interpersonal quality (81% to 93%). Respectful and helpful staff was the second most desired quality (70% to 85%). After that, patients rated doctor responses to calls and emails (70% to 74%), communicating with the patient's other doctors (66% to 80%), and doctors asking for patient expectations and preferences for care (60% to 74%) as somewhat important (Schleifer, Silliman, Rinehart, & Diep, 2017).

Patient-Centered Care Requirements

Another strong body of evidence about patient requirements comes from the patient-centered care movement and from the emerging field of integrated care. Some of the earliest research on patient-centered care was conducted by the Picker Institute in the United Kingdom. Since the late 1980s, Picker surveys have been used with thousands of patients in the United States, Canada, and Europe to measure patient requirements and experiences with care. This research, which is summarized in the book *Through the Patient's Eyes* (Gerteis, Edgman-Levitan, Daley, Delbanco, & Picker/Commonwealth Program for Patient-Centered Care, 1993), culminated in the development of a factor model of patient-centered care. These factors include:

- Respect for patient values, perceptions, and needs
- Coordination and integration of care across services
- Information, communication, and education on illness status, prognosis, and processes of care
- Emotional support and alleviation of anxiety.
- Involvement of family and friends in decision making
- Transition and continuity between patient encounters with the healthcare system
- Access to care and waiting time

Patient Perceptions of Care Integration

The Patient Perceptions of Integrated Care (PPIC) survey is a validated instrument developed to measure the integration of care as perceived by the patient. In initial research, the instrument, which was administered to 527 patients, identified a six-dimension model of integration. The tool was specifically designed to measure whether new models of care integration such as primary care medical homes actually achieve better integrated care for patients.

The dimensions of integration found in the study included three dimensions that relate to communication and care coordination and are labeled "information flow." The study looked at information flow to the patient's own doctor, to specialists, and to other providers in the medical office. Physician coordination with home and community resources was a fourth factor. The fifth factor, patient-centeredness, included items about the responsiveness of the medical system to the patient's ideas and suggestions. The results

of this initial study of the PPIC instrument revealed that while most patients rated their care integration as good, there were some serious perceived gaps—one gap being low scores on the dimension of coordination with home and community resources. The question used to assess this dimension stated: "Question 12. *In the past 6 months, did your doctor or staff in your doctor's office ever ask if you need help at home in managing your health conditions?*" (Singer, Friedberg, Kiang, Dunn, & Kuhn, 2012).

ASK YOURSELF

The PPIC survey is a reliable and valid measure of care integration as defined by patients. Could your organization adopt questions from the PPIC survey to assess the level of care integration and connected care in your organization?

Access the survey here: https://www.hsph.harvard.edu/ppic/ppic-resources/the-survey/

In another study of care integration, University of California researchers (Walker et al., 2013), in a series of focus groups with 44 patients conducted in both Spanish and English, explored patient views of the concept of "integrated care." The researchers' own definition of integrated care was adopted from the PPIC study: "[P]atient care that is coordinated across professionals, facilities, and support systems; continuous over time and between visits; tailored to the patients' needs and preferences; and based on shared responsibility between patient and caregivers for optimizing health" (p. 2).

Patients in the California study were confused by the term "integrated care," but understood the concept very well. Patient's own "definitions pertained to collaboration, information sharing, coordinated care, and a medical home, thus capturing the essence of integrated care. In the words of one patient, 'To me it means that all parties involved are working as a whole as everything that goes on is shared with everyone.'

Another patient wrote that integrated care is 'a system that has components working together'" (Walker et al., 2013, p. 4).

The study identified several themes that characterized integrated care in patient's minds: **coordination** within the care team, across the care team, and between care teams and community resources. This coordination consisted of providers knowing the patients' medical history and not asking them to constantly repeat it, their clinical information being shared between providers and care sites, and providers creating connections with community resources to help with social determinants of health.

Another theme was **continuous familiarity with the patient over time**. This concept included the idea of seeing the same provider, and also that other providers who see the patient know his or her medical history, care plan, medication, and lab test results.

Continuous proactive and responsive action between visits included patient requirements for getting appointments, follow-up, receiving test results, and getting answers to insurance questions without serious delays or barriers. Patients expected these activities to be conducted by phone, email, or through an electronic medical record patient portal. As one patient in the study stated, "For me, email is just fine . . . but a phone call every now and then . . . that was a good way for her to let me know that she was on top of things" (Walker et al., 2013, p. 5). Patients described patient-centered care as being able to get information about their health and care according to their personal preferences.

The last dimension of integrated care described by patients was **shared responsibility**. Focus group participants described this concept as changes in the care plan discussed between the patient and providers. Interestingly patients saw ultimate responsibility as resting with three stakeholders: the patient, the provider, and the insurance company (financial responsibility). Patients in the study acknowledged their role as a member of the healthcare team but many described an excessive burden of responsibility for having to coordinate their own care and share their medical information among many providers.

Care Transitions

Patient requirements for care transitions, in which the patient moves from one setting to the other, is an area that has also been studied by researchers. In a study entitled "The Patient Circle, a Descriptive Framework for Understanding Care Transitions," Lee and colleagues (2013) describe a series of care transition themes that emerged from focus group interviews with general medicine patients who had been readmitted to the hospital and with health professionals at both the hospital and in home healthcare agencies who cared for these patients.

Lee et al. (2013) created a framework for successful transitions called the "Patient Care Circle," which they describe as "a multidisciplinary, collaborative and coordinated support network integral to effective care transitions." (p. 2). The patient care circle consists of the network of patient health professionals, family, and friends who provide healthcare treatment and support. When participants in the study were asked to identify modifiable reasons for the readmission, they uniformly identified lack of communication and collaboration between patient circle team members. The study identified five themes that can influence care transitions:

- **Teamwork.** Effective collaboration and communication are driven by a common purpose and shared incentives. Fragmented care resulted from poor teamwork, notably between specialists in the hospital and between the hospital staff and home care nurses.
- **Health systems navigation and management.** Hospital and community healthcare systems priorities and hours of operation thwarted the achievement of this requirement. As one hospital nurse noted, "Educat[ing] people and empower[ing] them about their health . . . it's kind of lost . . . when we have so many [tasks] that we're responsible for, the patient gets lost in all of these things . . ." (Lee et al., p. 5).

- **Illness severity and health needs.** Patients' ability to cope was influenced by health literacy, the number of comorbidities, and mental health status. Those patients with higher level needs, in particular, needed more help from a cohesive patient care circle.
- **Psychosocial stability.** The need for a psychological adjustment to an illness, the ability to cope with anxiety, and social determinants of health influenced readmissions. Engaging seemingly capable but resistant patients in their own care was a source of frustration to professionals in the study.
- **Medications.** The complex issue of medication management required effort on the part of the patient circle team. Issues identified included patients not understanding medication instructions due to pain or stress, and home health nurses finding that medication instructions given at discharge were not always realistic.

Patient-Reported Outcome Measures

There is a huge volume of data on the issue of patient requirements and satisfaction with health care. The vast majority of these measures have been designed by professionals who inform their measure design and choices through focus groups, surveys, and other methods of eliciting the patient perspective. A more rigorous type of patient-centered measure is patient-reported outcomes (PROs). The National Quality Forum (NQF) offers this definition: "any report of the status of a patient's (or person's) health condition, health behavior, or experience with healthcare that comes directly from the patient, without interpretation of the patient's response by a clinician or anyone else" (NQF, 2013, p. 1).

Patient-reported outcome measures (PROMs) are the actual instruments, such as surveys, that measure the achievement of the PRO requirements. The logic behind the development of PROMs is that patients who are engaged in their care tend to achieve better health outcomes and often choose more cost-effective treatment after participating in shared decision making. Patients are arguably the most accurate and meaningful source of which outcomes are meaningful and work best for them. Thus, when care is designed to achieve outcome measures that strictly adhere to the patient's definition of success, it is more likely to be both patient centered and effective (NQF, 2013). PROMs require intense engagement with patients to elicit very specific ideas about what matters to them. PROM research is still in its infancy and has not yet had a widespread impact on the healthcare delivery system, but clearly has promise for improving connected care.

PROM Examples

A 2017 U.K. conference on PROM research explored patient perceptions of outcomes in many areas, including cancer, mental health, varicose veins, and diabetes. One study sought to use existing qualitative research to identify which domains were most important in patient experiences and their impact on quality of life for patients with varicose veins. The study identified five overarching themes: physical impact, psychological impact, social impact, adapting to varicose veins, and reasons for seeking treatment. A study of PROs for patients with breast cancer revealed three main themes: normality, dependency, and reciprocity (giving back by supporting other women with cancer or supporting research efforts). Cost of treatment and quality of life were two patient reported measures of importance to patients with Parkinson's disease (Proceedings of Patient Reported Outcome Measures (PROMs) Conference, Oxford, 2017).

One overall impression from the wide range of PROM research presented at this conference is that, for patients, one size outcomes research does not fit all. Clearly, the patient's condition or situation dictates what is important to him or her in both care and cure of the illness. This suggests that even when PROMs are not available, individual clinicians must ask individual patients what is important to them to achieve true patient-centered care.

Patient Requirements Research and Connected Care

Each of the studies described in the first part of this chapter identify patient requirements for connected or integrated care. Taken as a whole, the research verifies that the themes described in the pillars of connected care are indeed important to patients. The research, especially the PICC survey studies (Singer et al., 2012; Walker et al., 2013), clearly delineate what patients perceive as a "good job" in integrated or connected care. **FIGURE 7-1** illustrates the key themes from recent patient requirements research.

Communication with providers, and having the provider take the time to listen and answer questions, was an almost universal theme in each of the studies. Communication is also one of the key pillars of connected care. An added and vital patient requirement is **access**. There is no way to connect the elements of care for patients into a coherent whole if money, insurance coverage, eligibility, location, or inadequate distribution of healthcare facilities acts as an initial hurdle to getting any care at all.

Patient-centeredness, which several studies defined in terms of health professionals responding to patient care preference and including patients in care decisions, is a key underpinning of connected care. The need for, and lack of, smooth transfers of information between providers and follow-up between visits is part of the **care coordination** and **care transition** theme

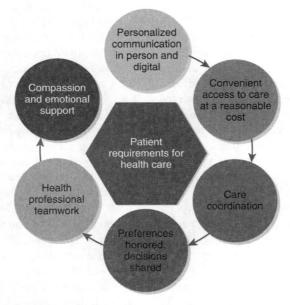

FIGURE 7-1 What Patients Want—Some Key Themes from the Literature

Data from National Public Radio, RWJ Foundation, Harvard School of Public Health, 2016; Deloitte, 2016; Schleifer et al., 2017; Singer et al., 2012; Walker et al., 2013.

of connected care. Two other themes related to the pillars of connected care, **teamwork among providers** in the same facility and **collaboration** between providers in different parts of the continuum, emerged from several studies.

Not surprisingly, teamwork and collaboration were often seen as problem areas by patients and providers, especially when there is a need for providers to work "the white space" between care settings. Some study findings identify clear discrepancies in the ways providers in different settings view each other's responsibilities and performance—a potentially serious barrier to collaboration.

An area that received some attention in the studies was the issue of patient engagement and focus: engaging patients in their own care, shared responsibility for health decision making, and in modifying care in response to patient preferences. One patient described the theme this way: "The surgeon thought I just needed radiation after surgery and the oncologist said no, she thought I needed chemo. So after they discussed it, I made the decision myself.... The decision was up to me. Healthcare providers: They all will help you out.... They have been careful as to not overstep any boundaries or take it upon themselves to assume.... I'm going to be the doctor" (Walker et al., 2013, p. 5).

How Well Are We Meeting Patient Requirements?

Patient requirements research describes what patients want (requirements). Patient satisfaction surveys and research studies identify how well healthcare organizations and providers are meeting patient requirements for care integration and where gaps exist.

Wolf (2017), from the Beryl Institute, in the publication *The State of Patient Experience 2017: A Return to Purpose*, describes the methods that U.S. hospitals are using to evaluate the patient experience in their institutions. The top method is government-mandated surveys such as CAHPS. The second most common

evaluation approach is the use of patient satisfaction surveys that are purchased or customized for the organization. A third commonly used method for measuring the patient experience is postdischarge calls. Hospitals also used focus groups, patient/family advisory groups, and bedside surveys to monitor the patient experience (Wolf, 2017).

Measuring Care Integration

One series of studies that evaluated care integration effectiveness was commissioned by the Council of Accountable Care Physicians in conjunction with Nielsen's Strategic Health Perspectives survey (Fegraus, Taylor, Colamonico, Morrison, & Pearl, 2016). Accountable care, as defined in this research, has five dimensions:

- Care/team coordination
- 24/7 access to care
- Treatment based on proof
- Robust health information technology
- Preventive primary care

Much of the reported data was compiled from an online survey of 30,000 U.S. consumers and 626 physicians done by Nielsen in March 2016.

For the purposes of connected care, we will consider survey results on the topics of care coordination and access. The study found that about half the time patient information is not shared across providers. Patients and providers both said that about 60% of the time, physicians are able to access hospital records. About half (49%) of both providers and patients agreed with the statement: "My doctors are now able to share information about my health and know my history before I get to the appointment."

Physician follow-up was rated as poor by patients in this survey. Only 30% of patients said their doctor followed up if they missed an appointment or did not fill a prescription; and 37% of patients said the medical office had a nurse or care coordinator to help them stay on track or comply with treatment instructions. Of the respondents, 30% said they received a call from a doctor within 2 weeks of an appointment to review treatment instructions and find out how they were doing.

Access was another issue for which patient expectations and the reality of medical practice were at odds. Only 34% of patients said their doctor's office has evening and weekend hours; 38% said their medical office had a phone line that offered treatment advice. A very discouraging finding of the survey was that patients with complex chronic conditions get no better care coordination than the general population of patients (Fegraus et al., 2016).

CAHPS Survey Results

The Consumer Assessment of Healthcare Providers and Systems (CAHPS) survey is the standard for Medicare patient experience assessment. This survey is used in many industry segments, most notably hospitals and home health care.

Several CAHPS questions are relevant to connected care. A CMS Hospital Compare online survey accessed in October 2017 illustrates key connected care questions and national benchmark results on key questions (**TABLE 7-1**).

The discrepancy between patients who strongly agreed that they were given information about what to do during home recovery and those who strongly agreed that they understood their care when they left the hospital is striking and is consistent with the results of the PPIC survey that showed this to be a highly problematic area of care integration.

AHRQ Healthcare Quality and Disparities Report

The 2016 National Healthcare Quality and Disparities report from the Agency for Healthcare Research and Quality (AHRQ) provides data on the state of healthcare quality in the United States and trends in various quality indicators. Trends in patient-centered care, which the report defines as patients achieving their

TABLE 7-1 Sample Questions from Hospital Consumer Assessment of Healthcare Providers and Systems (HCAHPS)

Question	National Benchmark Score
Patients who report that nurses "always" communicated well	80%
Patients who reported that doctors "always" communicated well	82%
Patients who reported that staff "always" explained about medicines before giving it to them	65%
Patients who reported that "YES," they were given information about what to do during their recovery at home	87%
Patients who strongly agree they understood their care when they left the hospital	52%
Patients who gave their hospital a rating of 9 or 10 on a scale from 0 (the lowest) to 10 (highest)	73%

Data from Medicare.gov/hospitalcompare website, January 2,2018.

desired outcomes, were positive with 80% of patient-centered care measures improving overall. Most access measures did not show significant change over time (2004–2014). The AHRQ (2017) report describes the issue of care coordination: "Coordinating basic patient information among providers is essential so that important information is not ignored, lost, or never communicated. About one quarter of all measures of care coordination, such as avoidable readmissions, had worsened over time" (p. 17). On most of the measures, low socioeconomic status contributed to greater health disparities.

Capturing the Patient Voice

A roundtable group convened by NEJM Catalyst (2017a), called *Measuring What Matters and Capturing the Patient Voice,* addressed the complex issue of patient-centered care. Panelists discussed how terms such as *patient engagement, patient experience,* and *patient satisfaction* relate to each other.

The panel also discussed issues such as patient-centered design and PROMs. The discussion was framed in the context of results from an opinion leader survey from the NEJM Catalyst Insights Council. Although two-thirds of survey respondents said that improving the patient experience was a high priority for their organizations, 42% stated that their attempts to incorporate patient feedback were ineffective (NEJM Catalyst, 2017a).

When Standard Measures Don't Capture the Patient Voice

One issue tackled by the group was the problem of "one size fits all" measures, such as CAHPS, that drive care, rewards, and reimbursement for providers, but do not drill down far enough into individual patient requirements to be truly patient centered. Providers who do try to elicit patient's personal wants and needs may find themselves at a disadvantage when standard measures of outcomes conflict with what patients want. An example would be a diabetic patient who values quality of life and less burden of care more highly than a very positive outcome and chooses not to go on an injectable medication. This patient may make alternative treatment choices, despite the organization's defined best practices and target outcome measures, such as driving down HbA1c results.

Another area of disconnect in using the patient voice to design care is not listening to patients carefully enough to uncover specific areas of concern that do not surface in generic patient experience measures.

An example is the terrible fear of care disconnects that cancer patients and their families experience when their care is transitioned from a highly specialized care facility, which provides very focused treatment and attention, to a community provider who may be less expert in their particular diagnosis and have less time and resources for customized care. Getting input from patient and family councils is a method for uncovering these special aspects of the patient voice.

Making sense of the sheer volume of patient experience data is another barrier to incorporating the patient voice into care. Some panelists suggested that technology in the form of apps that allow patients to input their own data at various points in the care journey, artificial intelligence, machine learning, and the ability to capture patient preferences electronically may help to embed the patient voice into the daily practice of care. Panelists in this roundtable made a valiant attempt to sort through ways that the patient voice can be incorporated into the care process. **TABLE 7-2** describes the results of their discussion.

Hearing the Patient Voice Through Patient Stories

Today's health care is so much about evidence-based practices, well-tested measures, and quantifiable data. Amidst all this evidence, we have to remember that patients' universal

TABLE 7-2 Taxonomy of the Patient Voice

The patient's voice is critical to health care. Here are the ways it can be included.

In the *Design* of care	As an *Input* to care	As the *Outcome* of care
Patient-centered design (system design)	Patient goals, values, and preferences	PROMs
■ Patient and Family Advocacy Council (PFAC)	Patient engagement ® activation	■ Symptoms
		■ Physical function
		■ Mental/social health
	Biometric data/sensors	■ Quality of life
Co-production of care (individualized design)	Patient-reported outcome measures (PROMs)	Patient experience
		■ Confidence/trust
	Patient needs:	■ Peace of mind
	■ Health-related social needs	Patient satisfaction
	■ Informational needs (language, preferred communication, health literacy, knowledge)	■ How did the process of care compare to my expectations?
	■ Social isolation	

NEJM Catalyst. (2017). Measuring what matters and capturing the patient voice. Roundtable report. www.Catalyst.nejm.org

connected care requirement is to be listened to and heard. Listening to patient stories is a way to capture the richness of the patient experience and to uncover specific themes and issues that are not obvious from standardized surveys and measures.

The Patient's View Institute (PVI) (2017) is a nonprofit organization that is "committed to organizing and amplifying the patient voice so patients can have an impact on the quality of care they receive."

The website for this organization solicits patients' stories and shares them. In some cases, patients receive cash prizes for stories through contests. Some of the recent stories posted on the website are titled:

■ "For my daughter, compassion made all the difference"
■ "Have you ridden the antibiotic roller coaster?"
■ "Childhood trauma brings on adult illness—it happens to many of us"

■ "Losing My Husband Changed My View of Medical Care": A Conversation with Sue Hassmiller of the Robert Wood Johnson Foundation

Through stories, the PVI has identified a series of patient requirements that can guide care, including safety, empowerment, respect, information, affordability, and accountability. The PVI website explores each of these issues in depth, providing an excellent outline of the attributes of patient-centered, connected care.

The PVI (2017) also addresses the issue of patient responsibility for care in "MY PLEDGE: I understand I am responsible for my health, too. I'll keep my appointments, share as much health information as possible (including changes in my condition), follow through on treatment I've agreed to, and prepare an advance care directive that I expect you to follow (a written statement of what I want to happen if and when I get too sick to decide for myself)."

Patient-Centered Care—Linking Patient Requirements and Practice

If healthcare organizations and individual professionals adopt the philosophy and methods of patient-centered care, patient requirements will be met and connected care can be achieved. Patient-centered care is a concept that encompasses, and even extends beyond, connected care. The healthcare industry, under intense pressure from the CMS to adopt value-based payment models and to implement new CMS conditions of participation (particularly for skilled nursing facilities and home health care), has been more rapidly adopting patient-centered care as part of the volume-to-value shift. It remains to be seen whether the changes implemented by the Trump administration will foster or hinder this healthcare culture change.

A blog post on the NEJM Catalyst website provides a clear, workable definition of patient-centered care: "In patient-centered care, an individual's specific health needs and desired health outcomes are the driving force behind all health care decisions and quality measurements. Patients are partners with their health care providers, and providers treat patients not only from a clinical perspective, but also from

an emotional, mental, spiritual, social, and financial perspective" (2017b, p. 1).

Patient-centered care has also been described as "care that honors patient's needs, value and goals and forges a strong partnership between patient and clinician" (Greene, Tuzzio, & Cherkin, 2012, p. 49).

In *Health Affairs Blog*, Rickert (2012) describes patient-centered care as improving not only outcomes as perceived by the patient, but also lowering costs because of good communication between physician and patient about potential treatment choices, their costs, and possible results. Rickert describes three essential elements of patient-centered care:

- Patients must be asked to rate or judge their care.
- The relationship between patient and provider must be personal and it must include both good communication and empathy.
- Providers who practice patient-centered care have systems in place to measure patient perceptions.

This type of care, Rickert asserts, produces better outcomes, a much better patient experience, and less overprescribing of medical tests and treatments that are actually a substitute for a good doctor/patient relationship.

Making Patient-Centered Care Concrete

Patient-centered care has been well studied and has begun to be implemented on a widespread basis due to vigorous advocacy from a number of patient-centered care organizations and patient advocacy groups. Until recently, work on patient-centered care has focused on individual patient/provider relationships. In the recent period of rapid evolution in the healthcare industry, work on patient-centered care has broadened to include systemic issues such as care environments, the use of digital tools, more sophisticated interpersonal communication and behavior change techniques, shared decision-making systems, and resources for health consumerism.

Patient-centered care is a core element in population health strategies. Greene, Tuzzio, & Cherkin (2012) describe research on patient-centered care conducted at Group Health of Puget Sound. This research sorts patient-centered care systems into three categories:

■ **Interpersonal dimension,** which includes listening, clear and empathic communication, knowing the patient, and the importance of teams.
■ **Clinical dimension,** which includes clinical decision support and self-management support, coordination and continuity through care transitions, coordination with community resources, and types of encounters which include accommodating virtual as well as office visits and a reimbursement structure that supports patient-centered care.
■ **Structural dimension,** which includes the physical environment that makes "way-finding easy" and is calm, welcoming, and patient friendly; access to care which includes reduced waiting time, easy payment procedures, and information technology which supports clinicians and patients, tracks patient preferences, and provides patients with good self-care information.

TABLE 7-3 lists actions taken by Group Health to improve its level of patient-centered care.

TABLE 7-3 Patient-Centered Changes Made at Group Health Cooperative	
Patient-Centered Feature	**Related Dimension**
Online self-management program introduced to accommodate growing demand for peer-support workshop for individuals who could not attend in-person version of workshop	Clinical
Previsit outreach to patients by medical assistants to ensure that the encounter focuses on the most important problem, and that patients bring relevant history and medications to visits	Clinical
Direct access to specialty care clinicians	Clinical
Secure email access to clinician for virtual visits	Clinical
Smartphone app to give patients mobile access to their medical record, ability to reach their clinician or 24/7 nurse service, find locations check symptoms, and view wait times for laboratory and pharmacy services	Clinical
Regular surveys of patient experience, with feedback to individual clinicians and comparative data across facilities	Interpersonal
Communication training for new clinicians, and retraining as needed on the basis of patient ratings of clinician communication	Interpersonal
Patient-centeredness training for nurses caring for complex, chronically ill patients	Interpersonal

Patient-Centered Feature	Related Dimension
Electronic medical record tracks patient preference for "what I'd like to be called"	Structural
Integrated electronic medical record and participation in regional "Care Everywhere" program to promote continuity and coordination within and outside of Group Health system	Structural
Way-finding signs and maps improved following ethnographic study of how patients see and interpret signage in facilities	Structural
New clinic designed with input from patients to improve flow, decrease wait times, and co-locate services that are frequently used together.	Structural
Billing statements modified following input from patients about unclear elements	Structural
Design of new clinics included patients as part of the team with clinicians, nurses, technicians, and architects to collaboratively address "the ideal patient experience"	Structural

Reproduced from Greene, S., Tuzzio, L., & Cherkin, D. (2012). A framework for making patient-centered care front and center. *The Permanente Journal, 16*(3).

🔍 CASE STUDY

Patient-Centered Care—What Does a Good Job Look Like?

A group of managers in the Everford Health System preferred provider home healthcare agency, Value Home Health, undertook the task of making patient-centered care specific and actionable by defining "what a good job looks like."

The group decided to follow a typical clinician workflow to identify specific clinical interventions that can be incorporated into the daily work of home care nurse case managers and therapists. The managers defined the attributes of patient-centered care for this home healthcare agency:

- Interactive, caring relationship between patient and care team
- Interdisciplinary approach with development of patient goals and plan of care
- Consider the whole patient—their physical, emotional, social, economic, and spiritual needs
- Consider the patient's response to the illness and the effect the illness has on the patient
- Assess and promote the patient's ability to self-manage
- Involve the patient in the development of his or her plan of care
- Encourage the patient's active participation in the plan of care
- Customize care to reflect patient's needs and values
- Offer strategies and choices for treatment and ongoing care
- If a patient is averse to following the medical plan of care, attempt to understand by asking why five times

The clinical manager team then brainstormed a list of specific expectations and tips for clinical staff to use when implementing patient-centered care as described in **TABLE 7-4**.

TABLE 7-4 Home Health Agency Patient-Centered Care Expectations and Ideas for Clinical Staff

Goal setting with patients	When creating the patient care plan	When charting patient-centered care	When a clinician presents a patient case at a complex case conference
When setting goals with the patient at the start of the home care episode: Use the "Day in the Life" technique and have the patient tell about a typical day in her life and what during that day is important to her. **Ask**: "What are the things that are important to you at this point in time?" **Ask**: "What are some of the things you would like to achieve as a result of my work with you?" **Ask**: "When you have a good day, what are the things that make it good?" At the end of the visit, recap by asking the patient what he/she thinks was accomplished. The clinician then summarizes what he/she did during the visit and asks what the patient would like to address at the next visit.	Develop the care plan in the home with the patient. Give the patient a written copy of the jointly developed care plan. Consider health literacy when giving written documents to patients such as care plans. Revisit the care plan each visit and ask the patient how satisfied she is with progress toward meeting goals.	Be specific on the plan portion of the SOAP note including patient goals and ideas on how to achieve them. Be specific in the plan portion of the note about what needs to be done to work toward patient goal. Write a statement about the focus of the visit. Document abnormal findings with a plan to follow up, right next to the findings to encourage linking. Set up templates to prompt clinicians to think about providing patient-centered care.	Prepare the presentation to focus on patient-centered goals, progress, and obstacles to achieving. Clinician uses a patient-oriented SBAR format for the presentation. Managers who run the conference use coaching and motivational interviewing to reinforce patient-centered care practice. When the clinician falls back into talking about his or her goals for the patient, a manager uses prompts like: "What is important to this patient?" and "How do you think your instructions came across to the patient?" Ask clinicians to discuss barriers and their frustrations in providing patient-centered care.

ASK YOURSELF

Now that the managerial group has an idea of what patient-centered care looks like in their setting, what actions would you suggest that they take to explain and operationalize these expectations for their staff?

by innovation and a willingness to tolerate and learn from mistakes. A learning culture maximizes individual potential and understands the relationship between team and system processes. The **physical environment** needs to act in concert with the culture to create patient-centered care. The patient-centered environment is not stark and sterile with a nurse's station dominating the physical space for the convenience of the staff (McCormack et al., 2011).

Embedding Patient-Centeredness into Daily Practice

A group of nursing researchers in the United Kingdom have explored the issue of embedding patient-centered care into daily practice (McCormack, Dewing, & McCance, 2011). They describe the reality of daily nursing practice as the experience of "patient-centered moments" when things seem to come together for a satisfying and rewarding outcome. They describe these moments as a meaningful connection with a patient, a comment of support from a colleague, or a letter of thanks from a grateful family. "Why," they ask, "can't it be like this all the time?" They pose the idea of linking these patient-centered moments into patient-centered cultures where feelings of involvement, satisfaction, and well-being are commonplace. In their work, the authors extend the concept of patient centered to beyond patients to include all persons engaged in caring relationships, including colleagues and families.

The authors suggest that three practice contexts must be managed to achieve true day-to-day patient-centered care in practice: workplace culture, learning culture, and physical environment. This culture change—which is much more than just slogans, logo branded clothing, and language—encompasses shared values, teamwork, transformational leadership, and a commitment to continuous improvement. A **learning culture** is one characterized

When Design Supports Patient-Centered Care

The Planetree organization is an international leader in implementing patient-centered environments and cultures. Planetree has actually implemented many of the elements of patient-centered care identified in McCormack et al. (2011) in various healthcare facilities. Founded in 1978 by a patient who had experienced personal trauma within the healthcare system, Planetree pioneered the concept of creating a healing environment within a traditional hospital, allowing open visitation for family and open access to medical records.

In an article in *Health Care Design*, Planetree Executive Director Susan Frampton describes the key elements of a healing environment: "We look at environments and the extent to which they help to facilitate compassionate and dignified human interactions. For instance, when the door of the treatment room opens, where is the patient situated in that room? Are they right there on full display for anybody who is walking by in the corridor or has there been thought given to the way that the room is set up so that their privacy is ensured?" (DiNardo, 2015).

Ms. Frampton goes on to describe environments that support transparency and access to clinical information such as having computers with clinical information readily accessible not only to clinicians but to patients and families as well.

▶ The Compliance Conundrum

Are Patients Our Hostages?

In the context of this discussion, patient-centered care and partnerships with patients seem like an obvious and acceptable approach to care. This is certainly not always true in the average healthcare organization. While the idea of partnerships with patients is gaining ground, large power differentials between patient and professional widely persist among health professionals. A truly horrifying article from the Mayo Clinic, called "Why Patients and Families Feel Like Hostages to Health Care," describes the terrible consequences of putting the patient in a subservient situation: "Patients are often reluctant to assert their interests in the presence of clinicians, whom they see as experts. The higher the stakes of a health decision, the more entrenched the socially sanctioned roles of patient and clinician can become. As a result, many patients are susceptible to 'hostage bargaining syndrome' (HBS), whereby they behave as if negotiating for their health from a position of fear and confusion. It may manifest as understating a concern, asking for less than what is desired or needed, or even remaining silent against one's better judgment. When HBS persists and escalates, a patient may succumb to learned helplessness, making his or her authentic involvement in shared decision making almost impossible" (Berry, Danaher, Beckham, Awdish, & Mate, 2017, p. 1373). One of the authors, a physician, describes her experience of having major abdominal surgery and being described as a "difficult patient."

She says: "In that bed, in pain, I felt terribly, frighteningly vulnerable, dependent on strangers for my most basic needs in addition to their complex care. I felt powerless in a way that is impossible to imagine when one is in a privileged position of wholeness and well-being. I know this because . . . I pathetically tried to ingratiate myself to the care team" (Berry et al., 2017, p. 1377).

ASK YOURSELF

- Have you ever observed a very ill patient or a family caregiver act subservient and try to ingratiate himself with the care team to get the patient's needs met?
- Under what circumstances have you seen this type of behavior occur?
- What could have been done to prevent the situation?

The Nuances of "Compliance"

Despite articles like the one on "hostage bargaining syndrome," "noncompliance" is a term that is very commonly and comfortably used by health professionals. The term *adherence* has begun to replace *compliance* as the preferred term for patient's following medical advice, although many feel that both terms imply a level of coercion that is not appropriate for describing professional patient interactions.

"Noncompliance" continues to be viewed primarily as a patient problem. As evidenced by the thousands of articles written on the topic, patients often seem to adhere to medical treatment recommendations either imperfectly or not at all. A comprehensive review of the topic, "Why Are So Many Patients Noncompliant?", was published in the online journal *Medscape* (Chesanow, 2014). It is interesting to note that as recently as 2014, the article still used the term "noncompliant" in its title.

Whatever the problem is called, it is huge: "In the United States, some 3.8 billion prescriptions are written every year, yet over 50% of them are taken incorrectly or not at all" (Chesanow, 2014, p. 1). The article goes on to describe noncompliance as "an unbelievably complicated problem."

Reasons for noncompliance include forgetfulness; lack of knowledge about the medication and its use; cultural, health, and/or religious beliefs about the medication; denial or ambivalence regarding the state of their health; financial challenges; lack of health literacy; and lack of social support. Other factors were lack of education by health professionals and overly complex and impractical treatment regimens.

In an interesting article in the *Boston Globe*, internist Dr. Suzanne Koven (2013) explores her own feelings about noncompliance and asks one of her patients about his reasons for choosing not to follow her advice. Koven describes her feelings about the patient this way: "When faced with a patient who stubbornly refuses to do what's so obviously right—i.e. what I tell him or her to do!—I find myself slipping into that military mentality. Why isn't the patient following my orders? Is he or she questioning my authority? Have I failed to communicate my orders effectively? Is it the patient's fault, or mine?" (p. 4).

The patient in Koven's (2013) story, who ultimately made his own decision to take his medication and change his lifestyle, explained his original point of view: "Hi Dr. Koven: Here's my best take at what was behind my resistance:

1. For some reason, taking a pill every day to solve a health problem feels like a defeat, while solving the problem through behavior/diet modification feels like a success.
2. A basic mistrust is triggered in me every time I witness a large marketing effort trying to push a drug on me. It goes back to the fact that somewhere along the line I developed a mistrust of the pharmaceutical companies.
3. I have a spontaneous, creative streak. It feels confining and defeating to have a regimented routine. Putting 1, 2, and 3 together, you end up with a huge resistance" (pp. 5–6).

The complexity of factors such as these argues for an approach more sophisticated than that employed in the course of the average medical encounter: ask about symptoms; use history, examination, and diagnostic tests to make a diagnosis; prescribe a treatment plan; ask if the patient has any questions; and end the interview. This approach, which eliminates the patient's participation other than to agree to the instructions and ask a question or two, may partially contribute to patients rejecting the advice given and subsequent nonadherence.

Since the traditional "compliance" method works imperfectly, especially for patients with complex illnesses, psychosocial issues, and financial barriers, a new way forward is necessary. The various tools and techniques of patient-centered self-management support eliminate many of the barriers of the compliance approach. These tools and techniques offer a way for clinicians to develop a partnership with patients that produces a jointly developed care plan that both patient and clinician can accept and work with.

Patient Self-Management and Health Professional Needs

For many clinicians, patient self-management and self-determination, while theoretically obvious and desirable, is an area fraught with ambiguity, confusion, and concerns. In the chapter on individual clinicians, we explored the issue of patient unwillingness to "comply" with treatment plans, clinician accountability, and perceived risk. In an era of value-based payment, patients who won't "play ball" with professional directives and best practices may not only create more work and anxiety for clinicians, but actually put the organization and the clinician's income at risk. The professional, like the patient, brings a complex set of attitudes, skill, resource needs, and wants to the table.

Successful patient-centered, connected care requires meshing the patient's wants and needs with the requirements and resources of the health professional—a circumstance that occurs all too rarely.

To some professionals, the idea of patient-centered care, shared decision making, and self-management support seems like a positive and natural way to practice. To others, such an approach may conflict with deeply held personal beliefs and professional needs. The review of the research on patient requirements described in the previous section clarifies what patients want from health professionals.

The flip side of the coin is the health professional's requirements for his or her patients. Observations from practice indicate that for many health professionals, achieving good outcomes and having a positive, caring, and satisfying relationship with patients is enough. For others the practice of health care is a way to satisfy their own strong personal needs. At the extremes, these needs, especially if unconscious and unmanaged, can be a huge barrier to meeting patient requirements and achieving connected care. Conflicting needs and priorities can also create tension and often outright conflict between professionals and patients.

Health professionals with a strong compliance mindset, for example, expect patients to take personal responsibility for their health, respect the professional's expertise, comply with medical treatment plans, and take medications as prescribed. Very passive patients may readily accept this approach, but those who feel more empowered will not.

For compliance-minded professionals, repetitively dealing with patients who "won't do what is good for them" can be a form of torture and may contribute to burnout.

Professionals may also see their role in a way that works against patient interests and goals.

For example, a minority of physicians refuse to refer patients to hospice care, even though the patient may prefer symptom relief to ongoing treatment, because the physician is so driven by the need to cure.

At the other extreme are those professionals who become overinvolved with their patient's lives and care "for" the patient rather than "with" the patient. This is another form of control that can meet the needs of patients who are very dependent or disabled, but does not work well for those patients who want to manage their own care. This type of problem is often more common among nurses who see their role as providing hands-on help instead of finding resources and fostering independence. An example is the home care nurse who makes meals for patients and does errands for them rather than trying to find resources for ongoing personal care support.

Despite all the conflicting personal needs and priorities inherent in healthcare relationships, patient-centered care can be a highly positive experience for clinicians. At its best, the patient-centered care approach can provide a return to purpose and an antidote to burnout for clinicians who are suffering from disconnection and are overwhelmed with the administrative and regulatory demands of their jobs. **FIGURE 7-2**

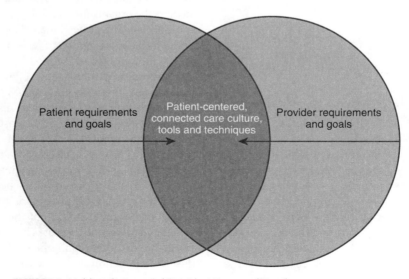

FIGURE 7-2 Melding Patient and Provider Wants and Needs

illustrates how patient-centered connected care can meld the wants and needs of both patients and professionals.

In high-risk situations, when patient and clinician cannot reach agreement, clear behavioral contracts with patients, such as risk agreements (signed contracts that define what both the healthcare organization and the patient agree to do as part of the care plan, and the consequences of failing to follow the agreement), define what both parties are responsible for and when the care relationship can end, helping to put an end to the need and expectation mismatch that is so frustrating to both patients and providers.

▶ The Ultimate Partnership—Shared Decision Making

A 2017 paper from the National Academy of Medicine (Frampton et al., 2017) describes a concept of patient and family engaged care (PFEC) as "care planned, delivered, managed, and continuously improved in active partnership with patients and their families (or care partners as defined by the patient) to ensure integration of their health and health care goals, preferences, and values. It includes explicit and partnered determination of goals and care options, and it requires ongoing assessment of the care match with patient goals. Shared decision making is a method of ensuring that patient goals and care options are appropriately matched" (p. 1).

Shared decision making between patients and providers is succinctly expressed in a simple phrase: "Nothing about me without me." Barry and Edgman-Levitan (2012), in a *New England Journal of Medicine* article, "Shared Decision Making—The Pinnacle of Patient-Centered Care," describe shared decision making this way: "In shared decision making, both parties share information: the clinician offers options and describes their risks and benefits, and the patient expresses his or her preferences and

values. Each participant is thus armed with a better understanding of the relevant factors and shares responsibility in the decision about how to proceed" (p. 781).

Steps in Shared Decision Making

The *Informed Medical Decisions Foundation* (Wexler, 2012) offers six steps to shared decision making:

1. **Invite patient to participate:** *We have several different options for how to manage your care. I would like to make this decision with you, not for you. Knowing your goals and preferences will help us make the best choice together.*

2. **Present options:** Describe each of the care options. Be sure to include information about the level of self-care effort required of the patient for each option.

3. **Provide information on benefits and risks:** Describe risks and potential benefits clearly. Describe the likelihood each risk and benefit. Give information in numbers rather than words if possible. Patients often underestimate the risks of a treatment. Use teach-back to determine what the patient has heard and understood. *We have talked about several different options. Let's stop here for a minute and have you tell me what you heard about these different options?* Clarify any misunderstandings now.

4. **Assist the patient in evaluating options based on his or her goals and concerns:** *As we go through the choices it is important to decide what is most important to you in choosing a treatment. What do you feel is most important in your situation?* (Use open-ended questions to probe for preferences such as lifestyle, level of effort, pain, ability to do regular activities, etc.)

5. **Facilitate deliberation and decision making:** Try to elicit what the patient has decided, what additional information he needs, and who else needs to be part of the decision. *Are you ready to make a decision at this point? What other information do you need? Who else do you need to speak with or bring in to speak with me?*

6. **Assist with implementation:** *Let's talk about next steps and when and how we will communicate after this visit.*

ASK YOURSELF

How could you incorporate the techniques of shared decision making into your practice?

Using Decision Support Aids

Another set of essential tools for shared decision making are decision support aids. These are educational materials such as pamphlets, videos, or web-based tools that describe the decision, explain the options, and help people think about the options from a personal view (e.g., How important are possible benefits and harms?).

A review by Cochrane (Stacey et al., 2017) listed 105 studies involving 3,000 patients who used decision support aids in shared decision making. The review found: "When people use decision aids, they improve their knowledge of the options (high-quality evidence) and feel better informed and more clear about what matters most to them (high-quality evidence). They probably have more accurate expectations of benefits and harms of options (moderate-quality evidence) and probably participate more in decision making (moderate-quality evidence). People who use decision aids may achieve decisions that are consistent with their informed values." See **FIGURE 7-3** for an example of a decision support aid.

While much of the shared decision-making literature centers on patients sharing decision making about treatment options with physicians, other health professionals can also apply the concept.

Nurses, health coaches, and care coordinators may have more time to spend with the patient and may be able to elicit additional patient preferences and issues because patients may perceive talking with them as less threatening than talking with a physician. An article in *Nursing 2013* provides a nice summary of how nurses can use decision aids (George, 2013). The article provides a succinct example of a nurse using shared decision making to help a patient choose a contraceptive method. The article also provides a good list of references for examples of decision aids.

ASK YOURSELF

- Do any of your organization's health education materials provide information about patient options and the pros and cons of different care choices?
- If the answer is no, could you incorporate some of these elements into your materials to create a decision support aid?
- If you do have some decision support aids, how frequently and how well are they used by clinical staff?

Shared Decision Making and the Burden of Treatment

An emerging body of work from the Mayo Clinic, specifically from the work of Dr. Victor Montori, has explored the issue of the burden of treatment for patients (Leppin, Montori, & Fionfriddo, 2015). The techniques used for this type of shared decision-making approach are called "minimally disruptive medicine (MDM)," which is described as "a theory-based, patient-centered, and context-sensitive approach to care that focuses on achieving patient goals for life and health while imposing the smallest possible treatment burden on patients' lives" (p. 50).

What are the downsides to the medication?

Directions
Bisphosphonates must be taken
- Once a week
- On an empty stomach in the morning
- With 8 oz of water
- While upright (sitting or standing for 30 min)
- 30 minutes before eating

Possible Harms

Abdominal Problems
About 1 in 4 people will have heartburn, nausea, or belly pain. However, it may not be from the medication. If the medication is the cause, the problem will go away if you stop taking it.

Osteonecrosis of the Jaw
If 10,000 patients are treated, we would expect fewer than 1 to have bone sores of the jaw that may be painful or need surgery.

For comparison, if 10,000 patients who have a tooth extracted are treated, we would expect fewer than 30 to have bone sores of the jaw that may be painful or need surgery.

Out of Pocket Cost
$10 with or without insurance

What is my risk of breaking a bone?

As you get older, your risk of breaking a bone, often through a fall, increases. This increased risk may be due to weakened bones or *osteoporosis*.

Your risk is estimated primarily by:
Your age: _____
Your Bone Mineral Density (T score): _____

It is also affected by:
- ☐ If you have had a fracture
- ☐ If a parent had a fracture
- ☐ If you currently smoke
- ☐ If you have taken prescription steroid medications
- ☐ If you have rheumatoid arthritis
- ☐ If you have a disorder strongly associated with osteoporosis
- ☐ If you drink 3 or more glasses of alcohol per day
- ☐ Your body mass index (BMI)

Based on these risk factors, we estimate your risk is _____ % over the next 10 years.

Your fracture risk can be lowered with medications called *bisphosphonates*, which work to reduce bone loss. This decision aid will walk you through the benefits and downsides of bisphosphonates, so that we can make an informed choice about whether or not they are right for you.

Prepared for: _____

©2009 Mayo Foundation for Medical Education and Research. All Rights Reserved.

What does my risk number mean?

Your risk number means that if 100 people with that same number, people like you, choose not to take medication for their osteoporosis, over the next 10 years....

_____ will not break a bone.   _____ will break a bone.

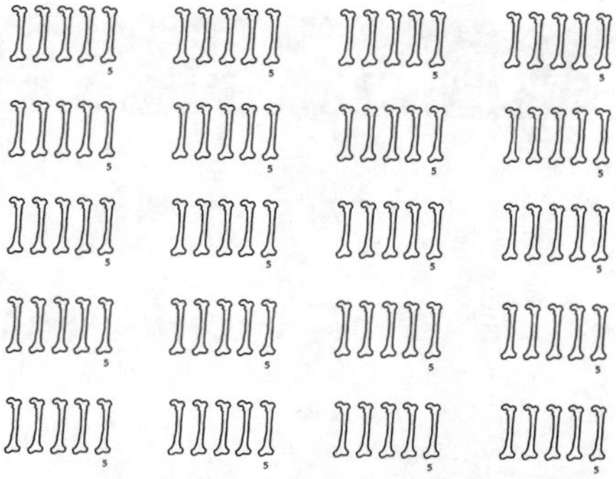

Each bone represents a person like you. There are 100 bones.

How can the medication help?

If those same 100 people, people like you with your risk number, choose to take medication for their osteoporosis, over the next 10 years....

_____ will not break a bone.   _____ will break a bone.

_____ will avoid breaking a bone because of the medication.

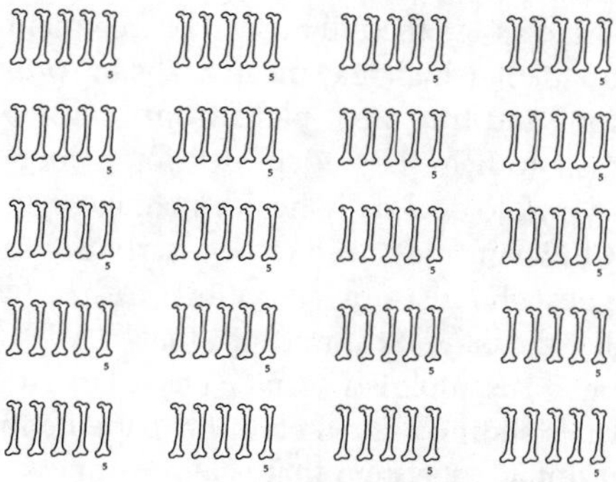

Each bone represents a person like you. There are 100 bones.

FIGURE 7-3 Example of a Decision Support Aid

Reproduced from LeBlanc, A., Wang, A. T., Wyatt, K., Branda, M. E., Shah, N. D., Houten, H. V., . . . Montori, V. M. (2015). Encounter Decision Aid vs. Clinical Decision Support or Usual Care to Support Patient-Centered Treatment Decisions in Osteoporosis: The Osteoporosis Choice Randomized Trial II. *PLOS ONE 10*(5): e0128063. https://doi.org/10.1371/journal.pone.0128063

The Mayo Clinic Center for Innovation (2015) blog gives some startling insights about the burden of treatment:

- "A patient with type 2 diabetes could spend a little over two hours a day on average following all doctors' recommendations."
- "About 45% of the population has at least one chronic condition. In addition to the burden of illness, patients are affected by the burden of treatment, defined as the impact of the 'work of being a patient' on functioning and well-being. This work includes medication management, self-monitoring, visits to the doctor, laboratory tests, lifestyle changes, etc. Coping with all these healthcare tasks requires a significant amount of time, effort, and cognitive work from patients and caregivers."

The techniques for reducing the burden of illness in shared decision making are many and complex. The most obvious is to help patients make choices from among multiple treatment options using decision support tools. Another is to develop the simplest treatment regimen that will achieve desired results. Clinicians can also help patients with organizational techniques such as the use of calendars, cell phone alarms, and pill dispensers.

It is very important for a single accountable clinician to assess the full burden of treatment for the patient, which may mean analyzing prescriptions and treatment plans from multiple specialists to help the patient develop a coordinated and logical daily health management plan. Clinicians may need to be assertive with colleagues who insist on an optimal treatment plan that the patient cannot sustain.

A good example is a hospital physician who prescribes sliding scale insulin for patients to take at home—a system that is almost impossible for most people to manage on their own. It is important to incorporate the concept of burden of treatment into patient teaching, goal setting, and action planning with patients. One way to do this is to ask patients questions about the practicality of their treatment plan: "How do you think this plan is going to fit into your daily routine?" and "What will you have to do differently to make it work?" and "Are there things we need to change to make this work for you?"

If clinicians simply advise patients to follow "best practices" and offer "canned" health education prescriptions without regard to practicality, cost, and willingness to assume the burden of treatment, positive outcomes will not occur. This issue is especially important to family caregivers who are frequently forced to assume responsibility for highly technical home medical support (such as wound care) for a family member without the benefit of consent or sufficient education or support. We will explore this issue in a future chapter.

Shared Decision-Making Resources

Dartmouth Hitchcock Health System offers an online Center for Shared Decision Making that provides education, tools, and techniques for practitioners at https://med.dartmouth-hitchcock.org/csdm_toolkits.html. Mayo Clinic also offers a website for clinicians called Mayo Shared Decision Making National Resource Center at https://shareddecisions.mayoclinic.org/ (Ridgeway et al., 2014).

ASK YOURSELF

- When providing patient education or discussing care options with a patient, do you ever explore the issue of "burden of treatment"?
- Do you use questions such as, "How is this treatment or care plan going to affect your life?"
- "How easy or hard will it be for you to start doing this (recommended health action)?"

Considering Patients' Hidden Healthcare System

Clinicians often perceive patient self-care as something that they must engineer for patients or do for them. In reality, patients are truly "driving the bus" on what they will and won't do to an extent that most clinicians don't totally fathom.

Nothing compels patients to do what they are told once they leave the office. For example, a patient who nods and says "yes" in a clinical encounter may walk out the door and throw the prescription that was provided into the trash. Patients almost always have their own methods, tools, and support systems for achieving health goals that are largely invisible to health professionals. Health professionals (other than home care clinicians who actually see what happens outside the healthcare setting) are bounded by their perception of what happens when the patient is with them. They often have no idea what happens once the patient gets home; starts talking to family, friends, and coworkers; watches television; and goes on social media for health advice. Recognizing this, and feeling humility in the face of it, is key to a sane relationship with patients and to more effectively providing patient self-management support. It is possible to ask the patient about the likelihood of his or her following the recommended treatment plan: "How willing are you to do what I have recommended? Do we need to make changes in the plan so it will work better for you?"

🔍 CASE STUDY

A Health Professional Learns About the "Hidden Healthcare System"

As a clinician, health educator, and manager, I have been interested in the concept of patient self-care and self-management since my days as a nursing student. After being trained and certified as an advanced practice registered nurse (APRN) in the late 1970s, I found the concept of self-management support difficult to implement in the community health center and hospital outpatient clinic environment where I worked. Visits were task oriented, and the preferred solution, for both patients and providers, to problems of social determinants of health (we called them poverty and mental illness in those days) was often a tranquilizer prescription.

My watershed experience with self-care support came after leaving clinical practice to work as a health educator with a Kellogg Foundation community self-care grant, based at the Yale University School of Public Health. Working in a community hospital in a blue-collar, multiethnic neighborhood, my job was to teach members of the community medical self-care and wellness tools and techniques. I was a somewhat naïve young practitioner who was used to having patients defer to my medical "expertise."

Working in a community setting was a rude awakening. I was the only health professional among a large group of laypeople.

Without my stethoscope and white coat, and outside the tightly controlled surroundings of a healthcare setting, I was in the minority and was not always well respected. I often taught classes to church groups, or in finished basements of private homes, to my best customers—participants in a weight-loss group that was sponsored by a vitamin and supplement company.

Under these humbling circumstances, I learned the truth—that what health professionals tell people to do has very little to do with patients' actual beliefs and actions. Most of those who I encountered took professional healthcare advice "with a grain of salt." They consulted family, friends, books, magazines, and alternative health practitioners (this was before the internet) and then made their own decisions.

An oral history project conducted as part of the project revealed that many folk remedies and beliefs such as charms against the "evil eye" were alive and well within the community population and

(continues)

🔍 CASE STUDY   (continued)

had a profound impact on how people cared for themselves and family members. Other people who were suspicious of the financial motivations of health professionals treated themselves with vitamins, supplements, and home remedies. I also found that when people were treated with empathy and respect and received practical and helpful advice from health professionals, they would make it a part (but not the only part) of their self-care plan.

A profound lesson learned was that the world of the patient and health professional overlap, but often are not fully known to either party. The practitioner who ignores the force of the patient's "hidden world" of health beliefs and actions or who does not respect it is doomed to frustration in helping patients care for themselves.

ASK YOURSELF

- In the "hidden world" of self-care practiced by your family and friends, how big a role does medical advice play?
- How much do people do their own research and make their own treatment decisions, outside the boundaries of interactions with health professionals?

Patient Needs and Willingness to Engage in Care Partnerships

The literature of health coaching and patient self-management support sometimes makes it seem that most patients are ready, willing, and able to partner with health professionals to make shared decisions and to improve their own health. As the case study illustrates, and as every health professional knows, this is

not quite true. Patients themselves have a wide range of tolerance or intolerance for adherence to professional recommendations and engagement in self-management support partnerships with professionals, regardless of their healthcare needs. **TABLE 7-5**, while certainly not representative of all patient situations, illustrates some of the combinations of patient need and willingness to engage in partnered self-care support.

Everford Health System has a patient population of over 70,000 patients in its accountable care organization (ACO) and Medicare Shared Savings programs, as well as many patients who are not part of a value-based payment program. These are patients who simply use Everford's physicians and other services.

Three patients illustrate the spectrum of challenges and opportunities that the system and its clinicians face in providing patient-centered care and engaging patients in shared decision making and self-management support.

TABLE 7-5 Patient Needs and Engagement Preferences

High Need—Low Engagement (Serious health needs and resistance to engagement with the healthcare system) The danger zone	**High Need—High Engagement** (Serious health needs and a high level of engagement with the healthcare system)
Low Need—High Engagement (Worried well patients seeking reassurance)	**Low Need—Low Engagement** (Minor or intermittent health issues, patient directs and manages self-care)

🔍 CASE STUDY

Supporting Everford Patients in Self-Management

Martina Allmore: "I'll Do it My Way, Thank You"

Martina Allmore is a 41-year-old woman. She is basically healthy, but has low-grade hypertension and a borderline blood sugar and HbA1c, which is the result of a pregnancy in which she developed diabetes. Martina is an ambitious and driven worker in the high-tech industry and one who has little interest in, or time for, engagement with the healthcare system. She is part of the ACO only because her insurer has a contract with Everford. She has been attributed to a primary care doctor who she seldom sees. Martina's primary healthcare requirements are access and convenience. Martina does her own internet research on hypertension and prediabetes, often using the Everford health information website portal. She relies on her own findings and seldom seeks advice from Everford clinicians. Martina uses her insurer's gym discount to join a gym and she does vigorous exercise three times per week to keep her blood pressure and blood sugar under control. She does get lab work at her annual physical. During the physical, her physician, Dr. Vasan, tries to engage her in some collaborative work on her risk factors, but she politely declines and states that she can handle things on her own.

Martina sometimes drops into the Everford home care agency screening clinic to get her A1c checked. Martina is contacted by the Everford population health coordinator but again declines to become involved in the health coaching program. When Martina has an episodic illness, such as a respiratory infection, she goes outside the Everford system to a local walk-in clinic which has hours that are convenient for her.

She occasionally uses the telemedicine virtual visit program offered by her company, which has no connection with the Everford system and does not send records back to her primary care physician. Martina is highly engaged in her own self-care but she chooses not to become heavily engaged with the Everford system and has little to no relationship with its clinical staff. As a result she has a somewhat fragmented healthcare experience, by her own choice, and remains outside the orbit of the Everford ACO and its programs. To date, her efforts to manage her own health by herself have been effective, if frustrating, to Everford ACO staff.

Carl Haddad: Ambivalence and Chronic Disease Self-Management

Carl Haddad is a 55-year-old man who works in a factory and has some health risk factors. Carl is part of the ACO through a direct contract between the Everford ACO and his employer. He has a strong family history of heart disease. Carl is not much interested in health issues, but he has some low-grade anxiety about his own potential for a heart attack. Carl has had one "false alarm" in the last year, during which he had chest pain, called 911, and went to the emergency room (ER). He was eventually diagnosed with anxiety, but the ER discharge coordinator suggested that he see his primary care provider for some help in reducing his risks. Carl reluctantly comes for his annual physical with the practice APRN, John. He is not anxious to think about or deal with any potential "heart issues." Prior to the visit, John has accessed the integrated medical record and seen the note from the ER discharge planner about Carl's chest pain episode.

Using the techniques of patient-centered clinical interviewing, John asks open-ended questions and finds that Carl, a smoker with hypertension and high cholesterol, is really very worried about having a heart attack. He is not happy with his level of endurance and wants to have more energy.

Using open-ended questions and the "Day in the Life" technique, John helps Carl explore these issues and eventually helps him set a goal for reducing his risk factors and starting an exercise program

(continues)

to improve his endurance. He is not ready to quit smoking and John respects his resistance on this issue. John refers Carl (with his permission) to the practice nurse health coach, Evette, for ongoing follow-up.

Evette reviews the goals that Carl and John had agreed upon. Carl starts the first session by explaining how much he enjoys sitting and watching TV with a beer and snacks, and how much he hates exercise. Evette uses motivational interviewing at each encounter to help Carl explore his ambivalence about change, to rate his own change readiness, and to find strategies that will work for him.

Carl takes one step forward and two steps back as he works through his own ambivalence: "It's just too much work. I might have a heart attack on the treadmill" with "I'll be there for my kids" and "I can take less medication." Gradually, Carl's own motivation to change overcomes his ambivalence and he begins to take small action steps, exercising 5 minutes a day to start and then gradually increasing to 20 minutes per day. By the end of the coaching sessions, Carl has purchased a personal fitness tracker, set up a small reward system for every gain made, and found that his blood pressure and cholesterol are lower. He has now made exercise a part of his life and he feels more empowered, healthier, and sure of his ability to make change when necessary—possibly even to quit smoking.

Cary O'Neill: in the Danger Zone

Cary O'Neill is an 85-year-old man with heart failure (CHF), chronic obstructive pulmonary disease (COPD), and Parkinson's disease. He is quite frail and has difficulty with activities of daily living. He requires the help of a personal care assistant from the Everford private care company to shower and dress. He takes 15 medications, some of which make him dizzy and he has fallen several times. Cary lives with his 80-year-old wife, Caroline, who is his primary caregiver.

His two daughters help the couple out, but live several hours away and are not available on a daily basis. Cary is part of the Everford Medicare Shared Savings program. Cary, in his younger days, was much like Martina and chose to stay disconnected from the healthcare system. Unfortunately, he did not adopt effective self-care and continued to smoke, live a sedentary lifestyle, ignore his hyperlipidemia, and eat a high-fat diet. The result was several heart attacks and the eventual onset of CHF and COPD.

Cary is very resentful of the need to "constantly be seeing doctors and going the hospital." He insists on managing his own medications, which he often mixes up. He sometimes refuses to use his walker which typically results in a fall. Luckily, none of these falls has resulted in serious injury. Caroline, who has some chronic illnesses herself, finds it exhausting to deal with his resistance and is showing signs of severe stress.

Cary is well known to all the entities in the Everford continuum, including the hospital, the skilled nursing facility (SNF), the home healthcare agency, and the private care company. After his last hospital admission, Cary tried to leave the SNF against medical advice, refusing help and home care. A call to state protective services helped facilitate a risk contract, which the home care agency required before admitting him to service.

The staff in the Everford continuum find Cary to be a serious challenge and are concerned about the potential risks for Caroline. Cary is also considered a very high risk and expensive patient for the health system. Cary has developed a slight rapport with his primary care physician, Dr. Vasan, who is working hard to reduce the number of medications and to simplify his medical regimen so the burden of treatment for Cary will be less. After the SNF incident, the home care team decides to call a cross-organizational interdisciplinary case conference and to invite Cary and Caroline to join it. At the conference, it becomes clear that Cary's primary goal is to be more independent, to "be left alone more," and to be more functional.

Caroline finds the courage to express her frustration and desperation and makes it clear that one of her goals is to spend less time fighting with her husband about adhering to his medical treatment plan.

The team, with reluctant input from Cary and positive input from Caroline, comes up with a collaborative plan for Cary to enroll in a *frailty reversal program*, which incorporates regular strength training, diet, and some cognitive behavioral therapy. He agrees to create a simple personal action plan and to work with Dr. Vasan and Evette, the practice health coach, to develop a balanced care plan that he can live with. Caroline is connected with the practice social worker who provides her with emotional support and who teaches her some assertiveness and stress management techniques and helps her enroll in a caregiver support group.

Three months later, the team reconvenes with Cary and Caroline. With the help of Dr. Vasan and Evette, who help him take a hard look at his medical history, lab tests, and prognosis, Cary has come to realize that he must change his behavior if he hopes to improve his independence and reduce the cycle of readmissions. He has been attending the frailty reversal classes and is much stronger. He has had no falls or hospitalizations and is less resentful and depressed. Caroline has finally learned to assert her own needs and has enlisted the help of her daughters. With the help of the team, the couple are able to maintain their independence and their quality of life for at least the immediate future.

▶ Helping Patients in the "Danger Zone"

Patients in the danger zone quadrant of Table 7-5, who because of poor experiences with the health-care system, cultural beliefs, mental illness, substance abuse, dementia, or a variety of other reasons, strongly resist partnerships with professionals but are involuntarily tied to the health system because of very serious health problems and symptoms.

These are the patients who take up a significant amount of health professional time, energy, and patience and contribute to anger, anxiety, frustration, and often patient safety concerns, especially in postacute care settings. In settings such as skilled nursing facilities and home health care, this resistance to care is often fueled by a strong fear that a "too close" association with health care will result in a one-way trip to the long-term unit of a nursing home and a permanent loss of independence.

An example is the elderly patient with heart failure who falls frequently and calls 911 to be picked up off the floor by the emergency medical technicians, but who refuses to get help at home. While the health professional's natural instinct in these circumstances is to "wrestle" the patient into compliance, a patient-centered approach, identification of goals and fears, coupled with motivational interviewing and if necessary contracting and risk agreements, usually yields far better results.

▶ The Origins of Professional Patient Self-Management Support Techniques

We have now explored some of the complex issues that surround a patient's self-care choices. In the rest of this chapter we will focus on the tools and techniques that health professionals can use to help patients self-manage serious health conditions.

A 2004 Institute of Medicine *Crossing the Quality Chasm Symposium* provided a now-classic definition of patient self-management support: "Self-management support is defined as the systematic provision of education and supportive interventions by health care staff to increase patients' skills and confidence in managing their health problems, including regular assessment of progress and problems, goal setting, and problem-solving support. Self-management is defined as the tasks that individuals must undertake to live well with one or more chronic conditions. These tasks include having the confidence to deal with medical management, role management, and emotional management of their conditions" (p. 57).

An AHRQ (2014) review of self-management support programs identifies the many tasks that patients with chronic illnesses must perform to self-manage, including:

- Monitoring symptoms
- Responding with appropriate action when symptoms change
- Making healthier lifestyle changes such as diet or exercise
- Adhering to medication regimens and managing side effects and interactions
- Coordinating care with visits to doctors and getting lab tests (modified from AHRQ, 2014)

Not listed, but also important to self-management, is the need to coordinate insurance coverage, pay medical bills, and cope with the emotional aspects of a chronic illness. Patients may also be asked to coordinate their own care, conveying information about their care and treatment to each of their healthcare providers when these professionals fail to communicate.

The tools and techniques of patient self-management support have been well researched. Most programs draw on psychological models of behavior change related to persuasion, skills training, provision of information, stages of change, behavior modeling, goal setting, and problem solving around barriers and difficulties (AHRQ, 2014).

Wagner (1998) originated the concept of the "chronic care model," which provides a structural framework for many self-management programs. This theory assumes that interactions between informed and engaged patients and a prepared and proactive practice team that uses evidence-based best practices and works within a patient-centered environment will produce better outcomes. The

original elements of the chronic care model included the community, the health system, self-management support, delivery system design, decision support, and clinical information systems. In 2003, five additional elements were added to the model: patient safety, cultural competency, care coordination, community policies, and case management (Improving Chronic Illness Care, 2017). Many of the tools currently used in patient self-management support and health coaching have their origins in motivational interviewing (MI), a counseling technique originally developed to help substance abusers find their own internal motivation to change.

Other self-management support techniques come from the pioneering work of Dr. Kate Lorig of Stanford University who developed the Chronic Disease Self-Management Program (CDSMP). This program is based on self-efficacy theory, which proposes that confidence in achieving a desired outcome will predict actual behavior. Lorig (2014) describes how the theory was incorporated into the CDSMP: "SE (self efficacy theory) can be enhanced through skills mastery, modeling, reinterpretation, and social persuasion (1). All of these are used throughout the program. For example, participants in the CDSMP program made action plans (skills mastery) and shared with other participants their confidence in achieving their plan each week. If a participant's confidence was low, then the leaders and other participants helped them problem-solve (2). Insight: theories are useful—but only if theories are translated into programmatic elements" (p. 1).

Participants meet weekly and are guided by a certified instructor (who is often a layperson) to set personal goals, to assess their own level of confidence and motivation, to learn symptom control techniques, and to create action plans. Participants support each other in achieving these action plan goals. A randomized trial of the program demonstrated an improvement in the adoption of healthy behaviors, symptom reduction, and reduction in hospitalizations (Lorig, 2014).

🔍 CASE STUDY

A Personal Experience with CDSMP

The author, who was at one time a certified CDSMP instructor, facilitated a class of 10 participants. One participant, Mary, had heart failure and chronic obstructive pulmonary disease (COPD). She was barely able to walk into the class from the parking lot without becoming seriously short of breath. Her personal health goal was to endure a 5-hour car ride from Connecticut to Maine to visit her son and to be able to climb the steps into his house.

During the course of the program she learned how to set small strength and endurance goals, completed a supervised exercise program with a physical therapist, and controlled her shortness of breath with stress reduction and breathing techniques. Her classmates supported her, challenged her, and gave her practical, and some impractical, suggestions. By the time the 6-week class had ended, Mary was able to achieve her goal. There was not a dry eye at the table a few weeks later when the group had a luncheon and Mary described her hard-won personal triumph—with the help of her own inner motivation, her classmate/cheerleaders, and effective patient self-management support techniques from the CDSMP program.

The *Chronic Disease Self-Management Program* (Better Choices, Better Health™ Workshop) offers a book and stress management CD, which can be purchased online and a training program curriculum and leader's guide, which is available to certified facilitators. The *Chronic Disease Self-Management Program* is available to healthcare organizations under a licensing arrangement. See the Stanford website for further details, at http://patienteducation.stanford.edu/programs/cdsmp.html. Many Area Agencies on Aging throughout the United States also offer the CDSMP, using community volunteer instructors, free of charge to participants (Lorig et al., 2012).

Motivational Interviewing— The Backbone of Clinician Self-Management Support

"Motivational Interviewing (MI) is a collaborative conversation style for strengthening a person's own motivation and commitment to change" (Miller and Rollnick, 2013, p. 12). MI has been mentioned many times in the course of this book and is part of the theoretical framework of connected care. This technique was developed by psychologists William Miller and Stephen Rollnick, and has been adapted to health care. There is a strong evidence base for the effectiveness of MI which has been verified in multiple studies (Rubak, Sandbæk, Lauritzen, & Christensen, 2005).

Both the attitudes and techniques of MI can be applied throughout the clinician/patient relationship to achieve the best patient-centered outcomes. There are two aspects of MI: the spirit and the technique. "Without this underlying spirit, MI becomes a cynical trick, a way of manipulating people into doing what they don't want to do" (Miller & Rollnick, 2013, p. 14).

The Spirit of Motivational Interviewing

The spirit of MI, which is strikingly similar to the spirit of patient-centered care, incorporates four themes:

- **Partnership.** Help the person you are working with find their own motivation to change by doing things "with," not "to" them. In an MI relationship, the clinician is not solely the expert; rather he or she uses the tools of MI to help the patient identify what is really important to him and to work through ambivalence about change.

- **Acceptance.** Recognize the inherent worth of the patient, practicing empathy, honoring autonomy, and affirming strengths.
- **Evocation.** The MI model works not from a position of assessing deficits, but from assuming that patients already have within them what is needed and the clinician will help them find it.
- **Compassion.** In the MI sense, this connotes actively promoting the patient's welfare and putting his or her needs first. This attribute is included within the spirit of MI because someone could theoretically use the MI method in a manipulative way to make people change for their own ends, not for the patient's ultimate welfare.

The Four Phases of Motivational Interviewing

The four phases of MI which are illustrated in **FIGURE 7-4**:

- **Engaging.** This is the process of establishing a personal connection and a working relationship between patient and clinician. It can happen in the first few seconds of a single appointment or over a period of months or years for more complex care coordination or treatment relationships.
- **Focusing.** This is the process of uncovering what is important to the patient and of helping the patient frame a personal goal.
- **Evoking.** This phase focuses on the change that the patient wants or needs to make, managing ambivalence toward change, and helping the patient to use his own ideas, emotions, and experiences to make the change.
- **Planning.** Once the patient has conquered ambivalence and becomes ready for change, the focus shifts to how the change will happen. This is the action planning step of MI.

Rowing Toward Change with OARS

The core techniques of MI are called "OARS" and "Change talk." OARS is a four-part technique very similar to active listening.

The key elements of OARS are:

- **Open-ended questions** can't be answered with a "yes" or "no."
- **Affirmations** are direct statements of support.
- **Reflection** is listening carefully, then paraphrasing what was heard.
- **Summarizing** is listing the key points that the patient has made.

BOX 7-1 provides an example of the use of OARS in a clinical visit.

Ambivalence and Change in MI

Ambivalence is considered to be normal and natural in MI. Take the case of Mrs. Diaz. It might seem obvious to health professionals that Mrs. Diaz will end up having a heart attack if she doesn't lose weight, stop eating high-fat

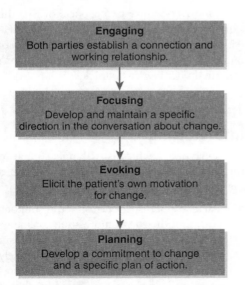

FIGURE 7-4 Four Phases of Motivational Interviewing

Modified from Miller, W., & Rollnick, S. (2013). *Motivational interviewing: Helping people change* (3rd ed.). New York, NY: Guilford Press.

BOX 7-1 Using OARS in a Clinical Encounter

Open-ended question: The home care nurse asks the patient, "What would you like to accomplish as a result of our work together?"

Reflection: The nurse listens carefully and reflects: "You want to be able to have more endurance and walk to the mailbox every day. You also want to feel less depressed and have a better outlook on life."

Affirmation: The nurse affirms positive statements: "You are trying to walk a few more steps every day, the way the PT showed you. You are also trying to fight dark thoughts when they come into your mind and tell yourself 'I can do this.' Given what you are dealing with, that shows a lot of courage and effort."

Summary: The nurse lists the key points that the patient has made: "Your goal is to be able to have more endurance, and at least to be able to walk to the mailbox before you are discharged from home care. You want to feel mentally better and not so down and sad on a day-to-day basis. You are doing some work on your own to achieve these things, but you would like some help from me, the physical therapist and the social worker."

foods, and smoking. However, these things are normal and natural to Mrs. Diaz. She enjoys her current diet and smoking relaxes her. Since she has had no real symptoms, the idea of a heart attack is theoretical and does not motivate her to change. This concept is illustrated in **FIGURE 7-5**.

If you hear "yes, but" assume that the patient is ambivalent about behavior change:

- *I should exercise; BUT it makes me tired.*
- *I want to stop eating candy, BUT when I am stressed it just calls me.*
- *I know I need to cut down on salt, BUT my family won't eat low-salt food.*
- *I know it is important to take my Lasix, BUT it keeps me in the bathroom.*

Encouraging Change Talk

Change talk is a statement that the patient makes to indicate an interest in making a behavior change. Affirming change talk is a more complex MI skill that involves listening for and reinforcing verbal clues that show that the patient is moving toward a commitment to change. Clinicians support change talk by listening for clues, even tiny ones that indicate interest in change. The clinician then uses affirmations to support

Understanding patient ambivalence – "Yes, But"

- People usually **know why they should change.**
- They also **know that they like the status quo.**

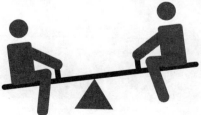

The pro/con arguments cancel each other out and the person gets **stuck in the middle.**

FIGURE 7-5 Understanding Ambivalence in Motivational Interviewing

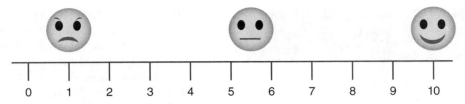

FIGURE 7-6 Change Ruler Example

this budding willingness to change. Some types of change talk are:

- Desire: *I wish I could lose some weight.*
- Ability: *I might be able to. . . .*
- Reasons: I *would probably have more energy if I exercised.*
- Need: *I have to. . . .*

Another technique is "Pros and Cons," in which the patient is asked to list the pros and cons of either continuing an unhealthy behavior or adopting a healthy one.

Change rulers are another tool in helping a patient assess readiness for change. The clinician might ask: "On a scale of 1 to 10, with 1 being low and 10 being high, how ready are you to start a regular exercise program?" If the patient says "5," the clinician reinforces the partial motivation for change by asking, "Why did you pick a 5 and not a 1?" This approach forces the patient to make a positive statement about reasons why he might change. Some clinicians use an actual change ruler diagram as part of this technique. **FIGURE 7-6** illustrates a change ruler diagram.

Motivational Interviewing Styles

Many practitioners think that MI is only concerned with the patient's motivations, goals, and change issues and that it precludes giving advice. This is not the case. MI theory describes three communication styles that are applied in different circumstances. **FIGURE 7-7** lists the components of each style:

- **The directive style** is a teaching, telling style that would be most appropriate in risky health situations or those in which the patient has little capacity to act. A cardiologist giving a patient who has just had a heart attack instruction on medications is an example.
- **The guiding style** is a coaching, evoking, exploring style that works best when the patient is in the midst of defining goals, dealing with ambivalence, and creating small action plans.

    This style would be appropriate when the patient who has had a heart attack sees a nurse health coach a month after the episode. In this encounter the coach helps the patient set goals for exercise and diet

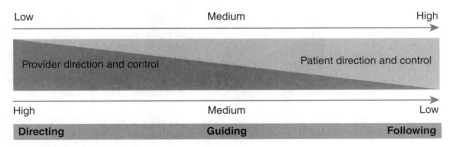

FIGURE 7-7 Three Motivational Interviewing Styles

Data from Miller, W., & Rollnick, S. (2013). *Motivational interviewing: Helping people change* (3rd ed.). New York, NY: Guilford Press.

change and uses change talk strategies to help him overcome ambivalence.

In some situations, giving advice may be appropriate within the guiding style, but only after asking the patient's permission: "Would you like some suggestions on how to get more fresh vegetables into your diet?"

- **The following style** is a more passive affirming and encouraging style that is best used when the patient is in the mastery phase of self-care and needs affirmation and encouragement to stay the course that he or she has embarked upon. This style would work best 6 months after the patient has had a heart attack, when he has adopted a healthier lifestyle and needs only occasional support to change behavior.

Some MI Tips

MI practitioners are fond of using certain phrases and tips to remind themselves of the key principles as they wade into the complexities of patient ambivalence and wavering commitment. Three of these are:

- *Roll with resistance:* Don't confront or direct. Express empathy and help the patient see how behaviors conflict with goals.
- *Resist the righting reflex:* This means becoming aware of and resisting your own need to direct, correct, or offer alternatives unless the patient asks you to.
- *You'll know if MI is working if it feels like dancing and not like fighting.*

One Obstacle to Clinician Use of Motivational Interviewing

MI, while widely used in health care, is not always an easy technique for health professionals to master. This system of communication assumes that practitioners have a patient-centered, nonjudgmental attitude and a basic competency in communication techniques such as active listening and clinical interviewing. The author's own experience in teaching MI is that many clinicians, especially those who are task oriented and provider centered, do not possess these basic competencies and often struggle to acquire basic MI skills. In these cases, some remedial work on attitude and basic communication skills may be in order prior to implementing a MI framework into the connected care process.

The MINT Network—A Key Resource for MI Information and Training

MI courses and online training are offered by the Motivational Interviewing Network of Trainers. Their website (www.motvationalinterviewing.org) provides a calendar of training events, videos, articles, and other highly useful resources.

▶ Patient Self-Management Support Tools and Techniques

We have already explored MI and shared decision making for patient self-management support. There are a variety of other tools and techniques that are frequently used in clinical practice to support patients in self-management.

These techniques cluster into several categories:

- Patient goal and agenda setting
- Assessments of readiness to change (described under discussion of MI)
- Action planning
- Health literacy and patient education
- Health coaching
- Tools for symptom management and self-tracking and reporting
- Technology to support self-management

FIGURE 7-8 illustrates these self-management tools and techniques.

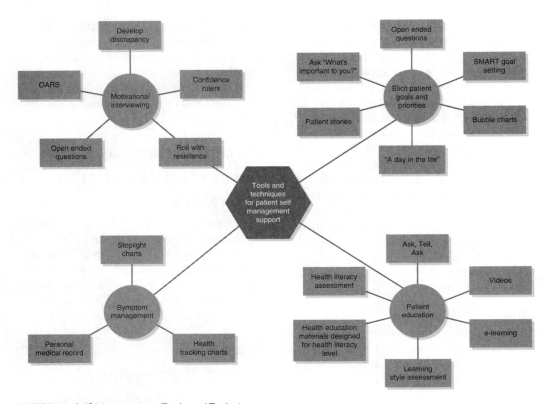

FIGURE 7-8 Self-Management Tools and Techniques

Putting Self-Management Support in Context

The use of self-management support tools and techniques is best done within the framework of a patient-centered clinical encounter in which the clinician adopts the attitudes and uses the techniques of MI. The clinician uses support techniques from the self-management toolkit with the patient's permission and in partnership with the patient. The clinician must also monitor and affirm the patient's own care strategies, many of which are part of the patient's "hidden" personal healthcare system. One way to do this is to periodically ask permission and ask the patient for input during the course of a visit or encounter: "Is it okay if we talk about or do . . .?" or "Tell me about how you do or plan to do. . . ." or "What else are you doing about this that we haven't discussed?"

▶ Helping Patients Articulate Their Wants, Needs, and Goals

What Matters to You?

A simple way to open a discussion about patient goals is to ask, "What matters to you?" as well as "What is the matter with you?" (Barry & Edgman-Levitan, 2012). Healthcare providers in Scotland have adopted "What Matters to You" as the topic of an extensive campaign to improve patient-centered care. The movement has sponsored "What Matters to You Days" in which provider teams offer ideas, pictures, posters, T-shirts, and stories that have helped to make their organization more open to the patient voice and more patient centered. The "What Matters to You" website at http://www.whatmatterstoyou.scot/activities/ offers a number of stories and photos that show how different healthcare teams have implemented the concept.

One compelling story tells about the visit of an executive officer from Healthcare Improvement Scotland to a ward at the Royal Alexandria Hospital. The visitor's first impression was of a poster about "partners in care" and open visiting hours which set the tone for the whole visit. Staff enthusiastically explained the "what matters to you boards" that are displayed above the patient's bed. These boards contain anything that the patient considers to be important such as how he takes his tea, what sports he likes, and information about his family. The boards help staff get to know the real patient and not just the patient's clinical conditions. Patients often use the boards to strike up conversations and make connections with each other. One staff person described the board of a gentleman with dementia who had "Elvis Presley" written on it. The

nurse would sing Elvis songs to him each time she saw him. Although the patient was nonverbal, he eventually started singing with her when she came to the room. To read this story in full go to the "Ward 5 Story" at http://www.whatmatterstoyou.scot/blog/.

An important technique described in the Scottish website is *deep listening*, in which the practitioner moves beyond listening from habit to listening with an open mind, an open heart, and ultimately from the source. The levels of deep listening are illustrated in **FIGURE 7-9**.

Patient Goal Setting

Patient goal setting is a next step in the process that starts with "what's important to you." In a medical setting, clinicians use this technique at the start of a visit, in a self-management class, or during an episode of care to determine the outcome that the patient hopes to achieve as a result of the care received. Mauksch and Safford (2013) suggest in their article, "Collaborative Care Plans," a scripted approach:

- "Help the patient focus on a specific goal."
- Tip: Make it the patient's goal more than yours.

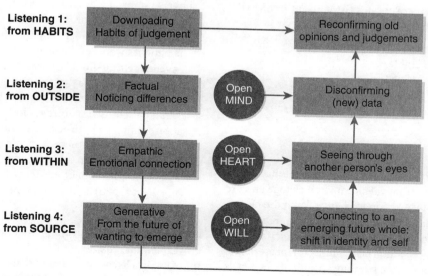

FIGURE 7-9 Deep Listening

- Script: "Can you think of a goal to improve your health? We want to help you."
- Example: "Weight control." (p. 37)

Some other examples of goal-setting questions might be:

- *Are there particular things that you would like to accomplish during the time we will be working together?*
- *Are there things that you can't do now that you would like to be able to do?*
- *What would you like your life to be like 6 months from now?*

Goal setting in a self-management class or health coaching situation is more directed and focused on what the patient herself intends to achieve, either alone or with the help of a coach or support group. Goals in this context involve specific, long-term outcomes, such as "being able to walk 20 steps without a walker," "losing weight by eating a healthier diet," or "building exercise into my daily routine."

Action Planning

Long-term patient goals are achieved through structured action planning. This type of action planning incorporates the concept of SMART goals, which are:

- Specific
- Measurable
- Achievable
- Realistic
- Timely

Steps in Action Planning

Action planning assumes that patients have overcome their ambivalence toward change and are ready to take action to change. With the help of a clinician or coach, the patient then breaks her goals into much smaller, achievable action steps and writes an action plan. During this phase of goal setting and action planning, health professionals should be following the "guiding" or "following" MI styles described earlier in this chapter. Writing

the goal and action steps is important, because it makes the plan more formal and serves as a reminder when commitment wavers.

The Chronic Disease Self-Management Program book, *Living a Healthy Life with Chronic Conditions* (Lorig et al., 2012), helps participants develop an action plan by asking themselves a series of specific questions:

- **This week I will do (specific action):** *Get exercise on the elliptical.*
- **How much are you going to do?** *10 minutes per day*
- **When will you do it?** *At 6 pm when I get home from work*
- **How often will you do it?** *Monday, Wednesday, Friday, and Sunday* (modified from Lorig et al., 2012, p. 20)

Agenda Setting

Agenda setting uses simple, open-ended questions to start a conversation about what is important to the patient in the current interaction or over the course of the episode of care. This question is most commonly phrased as, "What would you like us to talk about today?" or "What issues are important for us to work on?" The clinician then uses the tools and techniques of active listening to truly understand the dimension of the patient's wants and needs.

Agenda setting should be used at the beginning of a clinical visit so that the visit addresses issues or topics of concern to the patient. It ensures that patient issues don't get lost in a conversation dominated by the clinician questioning the patient about symptoms or medical history and giving information and instructions. The handbook, *Smith's Patient-Centered Interviewing* (Fortin et al., 2012), describes the sequence of visit agenda setting:

- **Indicate the time available:** *We have about 20 minutes today.*
- **Obtain a list of all the issues that the patient wants to discuss:** *It would help me to get a list of all the things you want to discuss today.*

- **Ask:** *Is there anything else?* (until the patient has described all his questions and concerns)
- **Summarize and finalize the agenda:** *You mentioned three things today. I think we can cover all of them in this session.* (Modified from Fortin et al., 2012)

Bubble Charts for Agenda Setting

Another agenda setting tool that helps patients with chronic conditions to pick priorities for self-management is called a *bubble chart*. This type of chart is a diagram that shows bubbles with listings of specific topics relevant to the patient's self-care goals. Patients look at the chart and choose the agenda item that they want to address first. There is usually a blank bubble which allows the patient to write in his or her own agenda item. **FIGURE 7-10** shows an example of a bubble chart.

Health Literacy

Patient-centered connected care meets patients where they are, and tailors clinical care to their particular strengths, capabilities, and needs. Understanding the patient's level of health literacy is key to selecting the most effective approaches to patient communication and education. Lower health literacy has been associated with less positive chronic illness outcomes and can be a real handicap in self-management. Health literacy is often, but not always, a problem for people with less education. Since health care is specialized, complex, and constantly changing, even, many well-educated people may harbor pockets of misunderstanding about health issues.

Any self-management support program should use an evidence-based assessment of health literacy. A simple and commonly used technique is to ask:

How confident are you about filling out medical forms?

A. Extremely B. Quite a bit C. Somewhat D. A little bit

A "somewhat" or "little bit" response indicates a lower level of health literacy (Chew, Bradley, & Boyko, 2004).

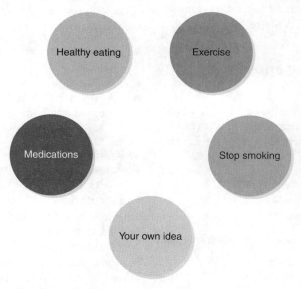

FIGURE 7-10 Bubble Chart for Choosing a Self-Management Agenda

Data from Bodenheimer, T., MacGregor, K. and Sharifi, C. (2005). *Helping patients manage their chronic conditions.* Oakland, CA: California HealthCare Foundation.

Health Literacy and Patient Education Materials

The AHRQ publication, *Health Literacy Universal Precautions Toolkit* (Brega et al., 2015), suggests that health professionals act as if every patient has a low health literacy so anything that is taught or explained is understandable by all patients. Health education materials should be clear, visual, and written at the sixth-grade level. Materials should be written in the active voice, and should contain short sentences and words. Limit the message to two to three key points (chunking information). Substitute plain language for medical jargon (yellow instead of jaundice). Give examples of medical terms. For example, instead of saying "Your test came back negative," say "Your test shows no sign of cancer." Use illustrations and diagrams when possible. Make the materials visual and readable with a serif typeface such as Times New Roman and a font size of 13 or 14 points. Large amounts of white space also keep the materials more readable. Finally, have patients review the piece and tell you how understandable it is. Use their suggestions for improvement (Mayer & Villaire, 2009).

Patient Teaching and Health Literacy

In her article, "Health Literacy: Hidden Barriers and Practical Strategies," Davis (2015) provides health teaching suggestions from patients:

- Tell me what's wrong (briefly)
- What do I need to **do** and why
- Emphasize **benefits** (for me)

If you are teaching about medications, **break it down for me**:

1. What is it for?
2. How do I take it (very specifically)?
3. Why do I take it (benefit)?
4. What should I expect?

Some other techniques for better health education are similar to those for creating materials for low health literacy learners:

- Stick with "need to know" information.
- Limit your explanation to the two or three most important points.
- Use simple words and short sentences.
- Avoid medical jargon. If you have to use a medical word, explain it simply.
- Draw or show pictures or diagrams. Repeat and summarize.
- Provide supporting written or picture information.

Teach-Back and Return Demonstration

Another key concept in health education for patient self-management support is teach-back in which the clinician asks the patient to repeat back what was explained to ensure understanding. Ask, Tell, Ask is a commonly used teach-back method. The American Medical Association provides a tip sheet that explains the technique this way:

- Ask what they know and what they want to know.
- Tell them what they want to know.
- Ask them if they understand and what else they want to know.

The first **ASK** includes asking permission to teach, asking the patient to describe what she knows, and asking what she wants to know. "Mrs. Jones, would it be okay to talk with you about your HbA1c test?" "Can you tell me what you know already?" "What more would you like to know?"

TELL: Provide the patient with the information that she wants and needs using simple language and short sentences.

ASK again: Confirm understanding by asking the patient to repeat back what she has heard. Ask if she has any additional questions.

Return demonstration is a form of teach-back in which a patient sees a demonstration of a medical procedure such as drawing up insulin. In return demonstration, the patient performs the action that was taught while the health professional watches and coaches (American Medical Association, 2016).

ASK YOURSELF

How well do clinicians in your organization typically:

- Assess health literacy?
- Develop or purchase education materials that meet health literacy standards?
- Provide health information in a way that patients can understand?
- Conduct patient teaching using teach-back and return demonstration?

Providing Health Coaching Advice

As noted, there is a role for giving advice in self-management support if the patient needs it and gives the clinician permission to provide it. This can be done by asking, "Would you like some suggestions or do you want to work this out yourself?" One source of self-management advice is the book, *Living a Healthy Life with Chronic Conditions* (Lorig et al., 2012), which provides extensive explanations of tools for patient symptom control and self-management advice. Another good source of advice for patients is a research study on treatment burden and the strategies that patients themselves use for coping and self-management (Ridgeway et al., 2014). Through a series of interviews and focus groups with over 70 patients at the Mayo Clinic and at a clinic for low-income, vulnerable patients, researchers identified five coping strategy themes:

Problem-focused strategies such as routinizing self-care with calendars, utilizing schedules and tools like pill boxes, enlisting help from others, using technology such as online portals for communicating with providers and online organizing tools, and planning for the future such as financial planning and developing advance directives.

Emotion-focused coping strategies to cope with negative emotions about illness such as maintaining a positive attitude, focusing on life priorities, and establishing spirituality and faith.

Social support includes three types:

- Informational support in which the patient got ideas for self-care from friends or other patients
- Instrumental support which includes help with tasks like making healthy meals or organizing medications
- Emotional and companionship support in which family and friends who understand the patient's health burdens provide encouragement and support

Questioning the whole issue of treatment burden by making self-care a "normal part of life" and not something that is perceived as intrusive.

Positive aspects of care like beneficial relationships with providers, getting care from a well-coordinated health system with convenient services.

Resources for Learning the Tools and Techniques of Patient Self-Management Support

Patient self-management support encompasses a complex set of skills for clinicians including teaching and coaching that enables patients to gain the skills, knowledge, and confidence to care for their own health. A number of programs are available to help master the skills of self-management. Many of these resources can be used for self-learning:

- **YouTube** offers a number of videos that demonstrate specific self-management tools (e.g., a variety of these videos demonstrate the Ask, Tell, Ask method of health teaching).

- **The Institute for Healthcare Improvement** offers a free online toolkit called "Partnering on Self-Management Support" for clinicians. The toolkit provides a handbook of techniques for clinicians and tools such as visit preparation worksheets, bubble diagrams for goal setting, a body outline diagram, among other practical tools. Registration at the IHI website is required before accessing the toolkit at http://www.ihi.org/resources /Pages/Tools/SelfManagementToolkitfor Clinicians.aspx.
- **The Health Sciences Institute** (https://health sciences.org/) provides online certifications in health coaching and motivational interviewing.
- **The Sutter Center for Integrated Care** provides a comprehensive program in patient self-management support, chronic disease evidence-based best practices, and MI. The program offers "train the trainer"

options for organizations and online training for individuals. Program descriptions and pricing are available at www.suttercenter-forintegratedcare.org/.

The Flow of Self-Management Support Interactions

When patient needs are relatively minor, practitioners can use self-management tools such as Ask, Tell, Ask as needed. Extensive chronic illness self-management support coaching requires ongoing engagement, over a period of months, with a provider or health coach.

For this reason, self-management support is usually embedded into a structured framework such as a telephonic population health program, a 60-day home healthcare episode, or a series of appointments with a nurse health coach in a medical practice.

🔍 CASE STUDY

Patient Self-Management Support in Clinical Practice

Orleanne is an embedded nurse health coach for one of the Everford internal medicine practices. The practice participates in the Medicare Shared Savings Plan and is responsible for achieving improved outcomes and lowering the cost of care for patients who are attributed to the Shared Savings program. About 100 patients have been identified as high risk through the practice's care management software tool and these are the patients assigned to Orleanne for self-management coaching. Orleanne was trained and certified as a health coach prior to taking her current position. Practice physicians and mid-level practitioners first interest patients in the idea of self-management, and then provide a warm handoff in the form of a personal introduction to Orleanne. Orleanne is responsible for assessing these high-risk patients for self-management needs, strengths, deficits, and willingness to change. She must then try to engage them in long-term health behavior change using motivational interviewing, health coaching, and self-management support tools and techniques. She has achieved considerable success by routinely and consistently using a set of patient self-management tools and best practices, employing the systematic workflow shown in **TABLE 7-6**.

TABLE 7-6 The Flow of Patient Self-Management Support

Previsit data review	■ Review the medical record. ■ Review records of recent hospitalizations. ■ Speak with the primary care provider and other clinicians.
Assessment	■ In an initial patient interview, use the "day in the life" technique by asking the patient to describe a typical day from waking up to going to bed. ■ Begin to identify what is important to the patient. ■ Use clinical interviewing to identify self-care strengths and deficits. ■ Interview family caregivers. Ask for their view of the patient's situation and assess their caregiving strengths and deficits and their own needs. ■ Assess the burden of treatment and identify what needs to be simplified.
Apply health literacy tools and techniques	■ Use a simple, evidence-based, health literacy assessment question. ■ Choose words and teaching materials based on patient health literacy level.
Patient goal setting	■ Ask the patient, "What's important to you?" ■ From there, help the patient decide what he or she wants to accomplish in the health interaction. "Can we work on setting some goals together so you can achieve what is important to you?"
Address ambivalence	■ Assess level of willingness and readiness to change using change rulers. ■ Use OARS and other tools of motivational interviewing to help the patient explore and overcome ambivalence.
Help the patient create an action plan	■ Help the patient set SMART goals. "This action plan form might be helpful to you. Let's go through it step by step." ■ Help the patient write down the action plan. That includes what you plan to do, when you will do it, and how often.
Continue reviewing results, using MI, and coaching to overcome obstacles as needed	■ Review action plans at the beginning of each visit. ■ Affirm success. ■ Use coaching techniques and a guiding style to help overcome obstacles. Coaching primarily consists of guiding questions such as, "How have you dealt with problems like this is the past?" and "How have you seen other people successfully deal with things like this?"

(continues)

TABLE 7-6 The Flow of Patient Self-Management Support *(continued)*

Provide self-care advice if the patient gets stuck or asks for help	■ If the patient gets stuck, ask permission to give advice: "There are some techniques that people use to get better control of chronic illness. Would you like me to tell you what some of them are?" ■ Provide advice in simple, concrete chunks of information. ■ Ask the patient his or her thoughts about the advice you have provided.
Summarize, affirm, and end the coaching relationship	"We have worked together for 2 months and you have been able to get your weight down, cut down on cigarettes, and start exercising. You have done an amazing job! Thank you for letting me work with you on these things. I will be very happy to report your success to Dr. Smith. I think you are well prepared to continue on your own, but call me if I can help you further."

ASK YOURSELF—HOW IS MY ORGANIZATION DOING?

How is your organization doing on patient self-management support? Using the Organizational Assessment Tool in **BOX 7-2**, check off all the techniques that your organization is using and identify gaps and potential opportunities for improvement.

BOX 7-2 Patient-Centered Care and Self-Management Support—How Does Your Organization Rate?

How well does your organization assess and provide patient-centered care and self-management support? Check off all the techniques that your organization uses.

☐ We have a method to assess patient requirements for the type of care that we provide.
☐ We have a system for measuring how well we are meeting patient-specific requirements.
☐ Improving the patient experience is a key part of organizational goals and organizational culture.
☐ Clinicians demonstrate competency in, and the regular use of, patient-centered clinical interviewing and motivational interviewing.
☐ Patient-centered care competencies are embedded in the performance appraisal document.
☐ Clinician patient-centered attitudes and actions are reinforced, rewarded, and celebrated.
☐ In case conferences and patient huddles, patient goals vs. provider goals are always the focus.
☐ We consistently use and teach patients techniques for identifying and managing symptom changes.
☐ We use the tools and techniques of shared decision making and reducing the burden of care for patients.
☐ Our systems and processes have been designed to meet patient requirements, not just staff requirements.
☐ Patients and families have a formal voice in our organization through structures such as patient/ family advisory councils.

❑ The tools and techniques of patient self-management support are embedded into our best practices and are consistently used by clinicians. (Star the following tools your organization uses.)
- Health literacy assessment
- Health education material that is appropriate to patient health literacy levels
- Patient goal setting and agenda setting
- The use of Ask, Tell, Ask and return demonstration in patient teaching
- Use of change rulers
- Use of patient action plans
- Help patients develop personal medical records
- Stoplight charts for symptom management

❑ We have methods for orienting new clinicians to the tools and techniques of patient-centered care and patient self-management support.

❑ We have structured processes and methods for including family caregivers in care planning and provide support for family caregivers.

❑ We have methods for managing situations in which patient goals and behaviors are in conflict with health professional goals and regulatory requirements.

▶ Chapter Summary

To achieve connected care, health professionals must understand patient requirements and develop clinical processes and clinician behaviors that meet those requirements. Research reveals that patient requirement themes include:

- Care that is accessible and reasonably priced
- Professionals who give me time, attention, and listen to me
- Care that is focused on patient-specific wants and needs
- Coordinated care in which nothing falls through the cracks
- Shared decision making and tools and information for self-management

Qualitative research on the "voice of the patient"—particularly the use of patient stories—provides richer insight into the patient point of view. Research also reveals that the U.S. healthcare system, while not terrible, does not consistently meet patient requirements, especially for cost-effective care and patient-centered care systems. Health disparities are a huge issue in the United States and are closely related to patient satisfaction with cost and access to care. The patient experience is measured in multiple settings

through the Consumer Assessment of Healthcare Providers and Systems (CAHPS) survey family (there are multiple variants, depending on setting) mandated by CMS for use in hospitals, home health care, and many other settings. The use of these measures in value-based payment has captured the attention of providers who are starting to put more effort into improving the patient experience.

Studies of care integration find that many patients, even those with serious chronic illness, experience a lack of coordinated care, with fragmented follow-up and a lack of teamwork among their healthcare providers who often practice in silos and do not work together to share information or collaborate on treatment plans.

Patient-centered care systems and patient self-management support meet many patients' key requirements for care personalized to their needs, for shared decision making, and for getting information necessary for self-care. Developing patient-centered systems is often complicated by the persistence of a health professional "compliance culture" and differing patient and provider wants and needs. Patients have various levels of tolerance for engagement with health professionals and often manage their own health outside the boundaries of the healthcare system which may, if not well managed, create serious conflict with health professionals.

Patient-centered care systems include interpersonal, clinical, and structural dimensions that all hinge on understanding patient wants, needs, and goals. Patient self-management support, a subset of patient-centered care, offers a robust array of tools and techniques for partnering with patients. A core technique is motivational interviewing, a communication style that helps patients deal with ambivalence and find their own motivation to change. Shared decision making helps patients understand the pros and cons of treatment choices and options, often through the use of decision support aids. An offshoot of shared decision making, minimally disruptive medicine, addresses the issue of burden of treatment and simplifying treatment regimens. Another self-management support approach is "What Matters to You?", a program that elicits patient's core health values and desires using techniques such as "deep listening." Other techniques include patient goal setting, agenda setting for medical encounters, and action planning using SMART goals.

Health literacy assessment and the use of teaching methods and materials that match the patient's level of health literacy are essential to self-management support. Patient teaching in self-management support uses teach-back techniques such as Ask, Tell, Ask and return demonstration to ensure patient mastery. Health coaching techniques use questions and advice (with permission) to help patients find strategies for health behavior change. Many organizations provide training and resources for health professionals who wish to master the art and science of patient self-management support.

References

Agency for Healthcare Research and Quality. (2014). *Self-management support programs: An evaluation.* Rockville, MD: AHRQ. http://www.ahrq.gov/research /findings/final-reports/ptmgmt/index.html

Agency for Healthcare Research and Quality. (2017). 2016 National healthcare quality and disparities report. Publication No. 17-0001. Rockville, MD: AHRQ.

American Medical Association. (2016). Ask, tell, ask sample dialogue. *AMA Steps Forward.* Retrieved from https:// www.stepsforward.org

Barry, M. J., & Edgman-Levitan, S. (2012). Shared decision making—The pinnacle of patient centered care. *New England Journal of Medicine, 366*(9), 780–781. doi:10.1056 /NEJMp1109283

Berry, L. L., Danaher, T. S., Beckham, D., Awdish, R. L., & Mate, K. S. (2017). When patients and their families feel like hostages to health care. *Mayo Clinic Proceedings,92*(9), 1373–1381. doi:10.1016/j.mayocp.2017.05.015

Brega, A. G., Barnard, J., Mabachi, N. M., Weiss, B. D., DeWalt, D. A., Brach, C., . . . West, D. R. (2015). AHRQ health literacy universal precautions toolkit (2nd ed.). (Prepared by Colorado Health Outcomes Program, University of Colorado Anschutz Medical Campus under Contract No. HHSA290200710008, TO#10.) AHRQ Publication No. 15-0023-EF. Rockville, MD: AHRQ.

Chesanow, N. (2014, January 16). Why are so many patients noncompliant? Retrieved from www.Medscape.com

Chew, L. D., Bradley, K. A., & Boyko, E. J. (2004). Brief questions to identify patients with inadequate health literacy. *Family Medicine, 36*(8), 588–594.

Davis, T. (2015). Health literacy: Hidden barriers and practical strategies (slide presentation). Agency for Health Care Policy Research. Retrieved from https://www.ahrq.gov /professionals/quality-patient-safety/quality-resources /tools/literacy-toolkit/tool3a/index.html

Deloitte. (2016). Findings from Deloitte's 2016 Consumer Priorities in Health Care Survey. Retrieved from www2 .deloitte.com/us/en/pages/life-sciences-and-health-care /articles/healthcare-consumer-experience-survey.html

DiNardo, A. (2015, February 17). Pushing beyond patient-centered design. *Healthcare Design.* Retrieved from https://www.healthcaredesignmagazine.com/trends /perspectives/pushing-beyond-patient-centered-design /Healthcare design

Fegraus, L., Taylor, H., Colamonico, J., Morrison, I., & Pearl, R. (2016). Better together: Patient expectations and the accountability gap. Washington, DC: The Center for Total Health, Council of Accountable Physician's Practices. Press Conference Presentation, June 15.

Fortin, A., Dwamena, F., Frankel, R., & Smith, R. (2012). *Smith's patient-centered interviewing: an evidence-based method* (3rd ed.). New York, NY: Lange Medical Books, McGraw Hill Publishing.

Frampton, S., Guastello, S., Hoy, L., Naylor, M., Sheridan, S., & Johnston-Fleece, M. (2017). *Harnessing evidence and experience to change culture: A guiding framework for patient and family engaged care.* Washington, DC: National Academy of Medicine.

George, T. (2013). How nurses can encourage shared decision making. *Nursing 2013, 43*(8), 65–66. doi:10.1097/01 .NURSE.0000431767.44118.c3

Gerteis, M., Edgman-Levitan, S., Daley, J., Delbanco, T. L., & Picker, Commonwealth Program for Patient-Centered Care. (1993). *Through the patient's eyes: Understanding and promoting patient-centered care.* San Francisco, CA: Jossey Bass.

Greene, S., Tuzzio, L., & Cherkin, D. (2012). A framework for making patient-centered care front and center. *The Permanente Journal, 16*(3).

Harvard T. H. Chan School of Public Health. (n.d.). Patient perceptions of integrated care (PPIC). Study Design. Retrieved from https://www.hsph.harvard.edu/ppic /about-our-research/study-design/

Improving Chronic Illness Care. (2017). Chronic care model elements. Retrieved from http://www.improving chroniccare.org/

Institute of Medicine. (2004). *1st annual crossing the quality chasm summit: A focus on communities.* Washington, DC: The National Academies Press. https://doi.org /10.17226/1108

Koven, S. (2013, April 29). In practice: Why patients don't always follow orders. *The Boston Globe.* Retrieved from https://www.boston.com/culture/health/2013/04/29 /in-practice-why-patients-dont-always-follow-orders

Lee, J. I., Cutugno, C., Pickering, S. P., Press, M. J., Richardson, J. E., Unterbrink, M., . . . Evans, A. T. (2013). The patient care circle: A descriptive framework for understanding care transitions. *Journal of Hospital Medicine, 8*: 619–626. doi:10.1002/jhm.2084

Leppin, A., Montori, V., & Fionfriddo, M. (2015). Minimally disruptive medicine: A pragmatically comprehensive model for delivering care to patients with multiple chronic conditions. *Healthcare, 3*(1), 50–63; doi:10.3390 /healthcare3010050

Lorig, K. (2014). Chronic disease self-management program: Insights from the eye of the storm. *Frontiers in Public Health, 2,* 253. http://doi.org/10.3389/fpubh.2014.00253

Lorig, K., Holman, H., Sobel, D., Laurent, D., Gonzalez, V., & Minor, M. (2012). *Living a healthy life with chronic conditions* (4th ed.). Boulder, CO: Bull Publishing.

Mauksch, L., & Safford, B. (2013, May/June). Collaborative care plans. *Family Practice Management.* www.aafp.org/fpm

Mayer, G., & Villaire, M. (2009). Enhancing written communications to address health literacy. *The Online Journal of Issues in Nursing, 14*(3).

Mayo Clinic, Center for Innovation. (2015). Uncovering the burden of treatment. Blog post. https://blog.centerforinnovation. mayo.edu/2015/07/20/burden-of-treatment/

McCormack, B., Dewing, J., & McCance, T. (2011). Developing person-centred care: Addressing contextual challenges through practice development. *Online Journal of Nursing, 16*(2).

Miller, W., & Rollnick, S. (2013). *Motivational interviewing: Helping people change* (3rd ed.). New York, NY: Guilford Press.

National Public Radio, Robert Wood Johnson Foundation, Harvard T. H. Chan School of Public Health. (2016). Patients' perspectives on health care in the United States, a look at seven states and the nation. Retrieved from www .npr.org/assets/img/2016/02/26/PatientPerspectives.pdf

National Quality Forum. (2013). Patient reported outcomes (PROs) in performance measurement. Retrieved from www.qualityforum.org/Publications/2012 /12/Patient- reported_Outcomes_in_Performance_ Measurement.aspx

NEJM Catalyst. (2017a). Measuring what matters and capturing the patient voice. Roundtable report. www .Catalyst.nejm.org

NEJM Catalyst. (2017b). What is patient-centered care? Blog post. www.Catalyst.nejm.org

Patient's View Institute. (2017). gopvi.org

Proceedings of Patient Reported Outcome Measures (PROMs) Conference, Oxford 2017: Advances in Patient Reported Outcomes Research. (2017). *Health and Quality of Life Outcomes, 15*(1):S18. doi:10.1186/s12955-017-0757-y

Rickert, J. (2012). Patient centered care, what it means and how to get there. Health Affairs blog. Retrieved from http://healthaffairs.org/blog/2012/01/24/patient -centered-care-what-it-means-and-how-to-get-there./

Ridgeway, J. L., Egginton, J. S., Tiedje, K., Linzer, M., Boehm, D., Poplau, S., . . . Eton, D. T. (2014). Factors that lessen the burden of treatment in complex patients with chronic conditions: A qualitative study. *Patient Preference and Adherence, 8,* 339–351.

Rubak, S., Sandbæk, A., Lauritzen, T., & Christensen, B. (2005). Motivational interviewing: A systematic review and meta-analysis. *The British Journal of General Practice, 55*(513), 305–312.

Schleifer, D., Silliman, R., Rinehart, C., & Diep, A. (2017). Qualities that matter, public perceptions of quality in diabetes care, joint replacement and maternity care. Public Agenda. Retrieved from https://www.publicagenda.org /media/qualities-that-matter

Singer, S. J., Friedberg, M. W., Kiang, M. V., Dunn, T., & Kuhn, D. M. (2012). Development and preliminary validation of the patient perceptions of integrated care survey. *Medical Care Research and Review, 70*(2), 143–164. doi:10.1177/1077558712465654

Stacey, D., Légaré, F., Lewis, K., Barry, M. J., Bennett, C. L., Eden, K. B., . . . Lee, J. I. (2017). Decision aids to help people who are facing health treatment or screening decisions. Cochrane Collaboration. Retrieved from http:// www.cochrane.org/CD001431/COMMUN_decision -aids-help-people-who-are-facing-health-treatment -or-screening-decisions

Wagner, E. H. (1998). Chronic disease management: What will it take to improve care for chronic illness? *Effective Clinical Practice, 1,* 2–4.

Walker, K. O., Labat, A., Choi, J., Schmittdiel, J., Stewart, A. L., & Grumbach, K. (2013). Patient perceptions of integrated care: Confused by the term, clear on the concept. *International Journal of Integrated Care, 13,* e004.

Wexler, R. (2012). *Six steps of shared decision making.* Boston, MA: Informed Medical Decisions Foundation.

Wolf, J. (2017). The state of patient experience 2017: A return to purpose. Beryl Institute. Retrieved from http:// c.ymcdn.com/sites/www.theberylinstitute.org/resource /resmgr/benchmarking_study/2017_Benchmarking _Report.pdf

CHAPTER 8

Pulling Together for the Patient—Teamwork in Health Care

CHAPTER OBJECTIVES

After completing this chapter readers will be able to:

- Define "teamwork" in health care and explain why it is vital to good patient outcomes
- Identify types of healthcare teams and when they should be used
- Describe team effectiveness measures
- List key elements of successful healthcare teams
- Describe evidence-based best practices for healthcare teams
- Assess the reader's own team effectiveness and implement improvement strategies
- Identify common obstacles and barriers to teamwork

▶ Introduction

Health care, when practiced optimally, is a team effort. In the current complex healthcare world, only rarely can one individual health professional or even a single profession achieve excellent patient outcomes. Teamwork is at the very core of connecting the dots and reducing fragmentation for patients. It is also an essential element in ensuring patient safety. Teamwork among health professionals, or the lack of it, is a key theme in *Crossing the Quality Chasm*. In its rules for redesign of healthcare processes, the Institute of Medicine (IOM) states: "Clinicians and institutions should actively collaborate and communicate to ensure an appropriate exchange of information and coordination of care" (IOM, 2001, p. 9). A key principle of connected care is "We're all in this together" for the good of the patient.

An older, classic definition of teamwork from one of the pioneers of healthcare teamwork research states that "a team consists of two or more individuals, who have specific roles, perform interdependent tasks, are adaptable, and share a common goal" (Salas, Dickinson, & Converse, 1992, p. 3). Two nurse authors define teamwork in health care in another way: "A dynamic process involving two or more health professionals with complementary backgrounds and skills, sharing common health goals and exercising concerted physical and mental effort in assessing, planning, or evaluating patient care. This is accomplished through interdependent collaboration, open communication and shared decision-making. This in turn generates value-added patient, organizational and staff outcomes" (Xyrichis & Ream, 2008, p. 232).

Work groups often call themselves teams, but many are simply a collection of health professionals working side by side without a common purpose, a structure, or a commitment to each other. Hackman (2004), an authority in the field of teamwork, describes "real" teams as having "clear boundaries, interdependence among members, and at least moderate stability of membership over time."

A functional healthcare team is an intentional creation that involves management support, leadership, clear roles and responsibilities, structures, and processes to support teamwork. Much of the research also indicates that intentional, structured teamwork is somewhat rare in American healthcare organizations, although it is becoming more common as integrated care delivery evolves. This chapter will explore some of the key elements of teamwork, measures of teamwork effectiveness, structures and methods that enhance team function, and training methods that help develop positive team behaviors. Readers will learn the basics of team leadership and how to assess and improve the effectiveness of their own teams with evidence-based tools and techniques.

TEAMWORK PART 1— TEAM RESEARCH

▶ Why Teamwork Is Essential in Health Care

Prior to the late 20th century, teamwork in health care certainly happened but was not considered particularly important except, perhaps, for care delivered on the battlefield. Today teamwork is an essential factor in delivering safe, effective, patient-centered care for a variety of reasons.

▶ The Proliferation of Knowledge in Health Care

Providing patients with the full benefits of modern health care requires a wider range of knowledge and skills than any one professional can provide. An IOM publication on teamwork describes the problem this way: "A driving force behind health care practitioners' transition from being soloists to members of an orchestra is the complexity of modern health care, which is evolving at a breakneck pace. The U.S. National Guideline Clearinghouse now lists over 2,700 clinical practice guidelines, and, each year, the results of more than 25,000 new clinical trials are published. No single person can absorb and use all this information" (Mitchell et al., 2012, p. 2).

▶ Teamwork Is a Key Factor in Patient Safety and Medical Error Avoidance

Study after study has shown that many medical errors have their roots in communication problems and a lack of concerted teamwork by the clinical staff caring for a patient. A 2009 article summarizes research on teamwork from 277 studies that were conducted between 1970 and 2007.

The authors found that teamwork played an important role in preventing adverse events. Staff perceptions of teamwork and team-related safety behaviors contributed to the quality and safety of patient care (Schmutz & Manser, 2013).

A retrospective study of 54 medical error and malpractice incidents in emergency departments found an average of 8.8 teamwork failures per case. In 20% of cases, lack of teamwork was judged to be the primary contributor to the medical error (Risser et al., 1999).

In its *2017 Adverse Event Alert*, the Joint Commission (TJC) makes a recommendation for the use of teams in creating a safety culture: "Embed safety culture team training into quality improvement projects and organizational processes to strengthen safety systems. Team training derived from evidence-based frameworks can be used to enhance the performance of teams in high-stress, high-risk areas of the organization—such as operating rooms, ICUs and emergency rooms" (TJC, 2017, p. 5).

▶ Effective Teams Produce Improved Patient Outcomes

Many studies indicate that care delivered by effective teams produces better clinical results for patients than professional care that is not delivered by teams. Two Canadian researchers reviewed 33 studies of team effectiveness. The authors note: "There is some evidence that team care can lead to better clinical outcomes and patient satisfaction across health care settings than can poorly or uncoordinated sequential care" (Lemieux-Charles & McGuire, 2006, p. 270). Several studies of geriatric care that were reviewed by the researchers found that team care achieved results such as better functional status, lower mortality rates, and better mental health status. A 2013 review of 28 studies of teamwork found

that "team process behaviors do influence clinical performance and that training results in increased performance" (Schmutz & Manser, 2013, p. 529).

One study that analyzed the impact of employee engagement activities, communication skills training, and coaching on an inpatient nursing team found that after the training was completed patient falls on the team hospital unit decreased, patient satisfaction increased, staff ratings of the level of teamwork increased, and staff turnover on the unit was lower after the training (Kalisch, Curley, & Stefanov, 2007). An extensive Agency for Healthcare Research and Quality (AHRQ) study of patient safety and pressure ulcer prevention in skilled nursing facilities (SNFs) describes a variety of studies on preventing pressure ulcers through the use of specialized teams (Sullivan, 2013).

▶ Teamwork Can Produce a Better Experience for Patients and for Professionals

A study of patients cared for by teams in 125 Veterans Health Administration hospitals found "a significant and positive relation between teamwork culture and patient satisfaction for inpatient care" (Meterko, Mohr, & Young, 2004, p. 492). A study of 400 teams in the U.K. National Health Service found that nurses and other professionals who worked in higher functioning teams experienced less stress and were less likely to leave their jobs over the 1-year period of the study (Aston Centre for Health Service, 2011).

▶ The History of Healthcare Teamwork Research

While teamwork has long been studied in the social sciences and in business, most serious healthcare team research began at the turn of the 21st century, shortly after the publication of the IOM report *To Err Is Human* (Kohn, Corrigan, & Donaldson, 2000).

This publication shocked the healthcare community by revealing the widespread incidence of medical errors and their sometimes deadly consequences, many of which resulted from lack of teamwork.

A key contribution to healthcare teamwork research was found in the aviation industry, which had pioneered the concept of crew resource management (CRM). This intensive teamwork training approach was adopted to achieve a high level of safety in commercial aviation. The objective of CRM training is to "reduce the risks that crews will make fatal errors or permit a fatal chain of errors to unfold because they failed to foster teamwork, solve problems, communicate, and manage workload" (Risser et al., 1999, pp. 373–374). Applying this concept to health care proved to be more complex than it first appeared, but it is the basis for the premier evidence-based healthcare team-building program TeamSTEPPS (AHRQ, 2018). The CRM teamwork model has now been successfully replicated in high-acuity healthcare environments such as emergency rooms and operating rooms to reduce medical errors.

A 2017 publication from AHRQ looks back on lessons learned from 10 years of disseminating TeamSTEPPS. Some key findings are relevant to organizations hoping to improve teamwork:

- **A variety of studies have proved that care coordination and teamwork are indeed linked to better outcomes** and have overcome initial widespread skepticism.
- **Organizational culture change continues to be a key barrier.** Behaviors taught in programs like TeamSTEPPS are not yet the norm in healthcare organizations. This requires organizations to change the culture to embed the behaviors taught. Organizations continue to struggle with the time and resources needed to implement the program.

- **Physicians** have emerged as leaders and advocates of team training. While many initially resisted this training as an affront to physician authority the program has come to be widely used and accepted in the medical world.
- **Interprofessional education, especially in medical and nursing schools, is gaining ground** as cross-functional teamwork moves into the mainstream of health care. (Modified from Baker, Battles, & King, 2017)

Much of the research on healthcare teams has focused on high-acuity settings such as hospitals, intensive care units, and operating rooms. TeamSTEPPS has been by far the program most used and most studied. Miller and colleagues conducted the first exhaustive study of team-building methods used in nonacute settings. A review of 14 different programs and methods of team building revealed that most, aside from TeamSTEPPS, which has a strong evidence base, were validated by a single study and much of the research was not particularly rigorous. While these findings were somewhat discouraging, the paper does provide a good conceptual framework called the Team Effectiveness Pyramid (**FIGURE 8-1**), for teams outside the acute care setting (Miller, Kim, Silverman, & Bauer, 2018).

Because TeamSTEPPS is the only strong evidence-based healthcare team-building program, it will be heavily referenced in this discussion.

ASK YOURSELF

- How extensive is teamwork in your organization?
- How has teamwork had an impact on patient outcomes, patient satisfaction, staff satisfaction, and efficiency in your organization?
- Are there teams in your organization that could perform better?
- Does your organization devote resources to team development?

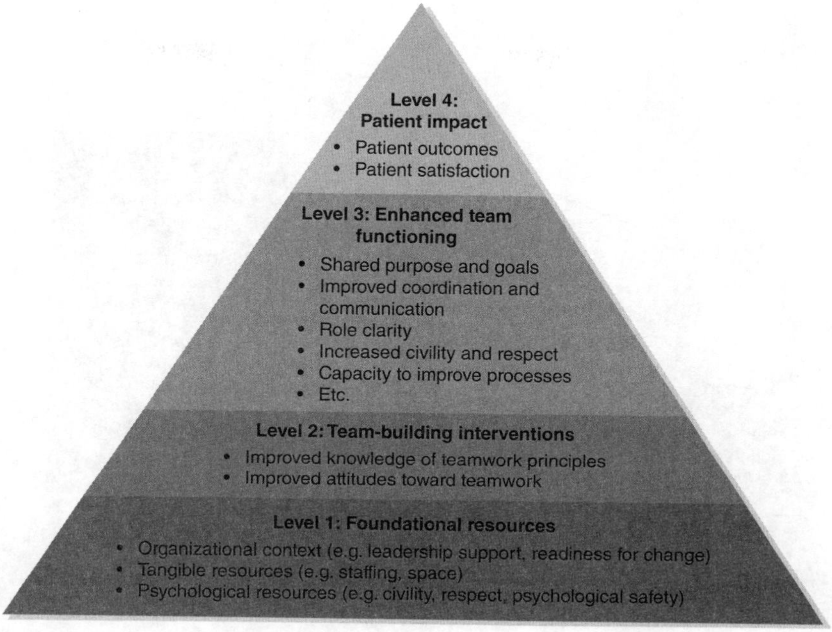

FIGURE 8-1 The Team Effectiveness Pyramid

Miller, C. J., Kim, B., Silverman, A., & Bauer, M. S. (2018). A systematic review of team-building interventions in non-acute healthcare settings. *BMC Health Services Research, 18*(1). doi:10.1186/s12913-018-2961-9

▸ What Is the Right Level of Teamwork for the Situation?

While teamwork is vital in health care, it is important to determine whether a team is actually necessary and, if it is, what level of team development and cooperative intensity is required. Organizational development expert Donald Brown suggests that there are three types of work situations: simple, complex, and problem

situations. In Brown's model the level of teamwork should be matched to the type of situation. **FIGURE 8-2** illustrates different situations and the amount of teamwork needed (Harvey & Brown, 2003).

Types of Healthcare Teams

Healthcare teams are highly variable in size, task orientation, and structure. Some teams consist of a single type of health professional such as a team of nurses on a single inpatient unit. Others are cross functional (e.g., a team of doctors, receptionists, nurses, and medical assistants in a primary care medical home).

In contrast to teams in many other settings, healthcare teams are often dynamic with changing membership (Weaver, Dy, & Rosen, 2014). One observational study of 25 healthcare teams identified four types of teams, based on the stability or variability of roles and personnel types. These teams ranged from very stable

ASK YOURSELF

- In which types of situations does your organization use teams?
- Are there other situations in which teamwork might be helpful?

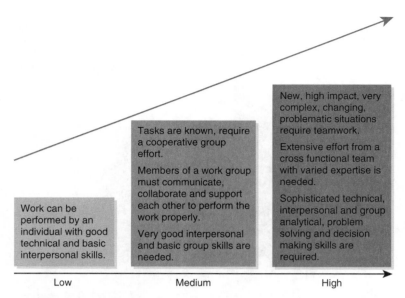

New, high impact, very complex, changing, problematic situations require teamwork.

Extensive effort from a cross functional team with varied expertise is needed.

Sophisticated technical, interpersonal and group analytical, problem solving and decision making skills are required.

Tasks are known, require a cooperative group effort.

Members of a work group must communicate, collaborate and support each other to perform the work properly.

Very good interpersonal and basic group skills are needed.

Work can be performed by an individual with good technical and basic interpersonal skills.

Low   Medium   High

FIGURE 8-2 How Much Teamwork Is Needed?

Data from Harvey, D., & Brown, D. (2003). *An experiential approach to organizational development* (6th ed.). Upper Saddle River, NJ: Prentice Hall, p. 282, Figure 10.1, Situation determines teamwork.

🔍 CASE STUDY

Do We Need More Teamwork?

The Everford Senior Management Team, in its quest to better integrate the parts of the system continuum and to achieve the quadruple aim, found that the issues of teamwork kept coming up in meetings. The group identified several "near miss" patient safety issues that had occurred in the acute care hospital because of poor teamwork, and also found that employee surveys had identified a lack of teamwork as a source of dissatisfaction. After some discussion, senior managers decided that while certain parts of the continuum did pretty well on teamwork, others did not.

There was a clear structure and a set of trained facilitators for quality assurance/process improvement projects, but not for other types of teamwork in clinical departments and no consistent organizational teamwork model or processes.

The senior management team decided to charter a team committee composed of clinical and business managers, as well as representatives of human resources and clinical education, to study the issue of teamwork and to make recommendations for an organizational team effectiveness framework. As a first step, the group looked at the research on team-building effectiveness and on types of healthcare teams and team structures to determine what might work best in the Everford System. The next section of this chapter details the research that the Everford Team Committee reviewed.

with consistent roles for personnel in a pediatric medical practice to the highly variable roles and changing personnel on the crew of an emergency transport flight team in which staff had to perform multiple functions and

substitute for each other as circumstances dictated (Andreatta, 2010).

The author makes the point that one size does not fit all and that each type of team may require different processes and training to achieve its specific goals. The most common types of healthcare teams are:

- **Intact work groups.** A group of health professionals, and sometimes support personnel, who work together consistently over time and perform the same types of tasks on a regular basis. These teams have consistent membership and group norms and are usually considered real teams.
- **Quality improvement or project teams.** Temporary teams formed for the purpose of achieving an improvement goal that have a mostly stable membership and meet over time using structured group and quality or planning tools and techniques.
- **Management teams.** Formal groups of managers who are accountable for organizing and coordinating specific organizational units and personnel and for achieving organizational goals.
- **Ad hoc or variable teams.** Teams formed based on circumstances and patient care needs. These teams may have shifting membership and may perform a variety of tasks depending on patient care or project needs. These types of teams are extremely common in health care.

Amy Edmondson of the Harvard Business School, who has written extensively about healthcare teams, details the negative impact of healthcare silos and describes ad hoc teams eloquently: "The solution to these problems is to shift focus from the *structure* to the *activities* of teamwork—what I call 'teaming.' Teaming involves fluid, collaborative, interdependent work across shifting projects and with a shifting mix of partners, often across organizational boundaries. Think of it as teamwork on the fly" (Edmondson, 2015, p. 1).

An example of a team formed "on the fly" in response to patient care needs is a code team that gathers quickly to respond to a cardiac arrest.

These teams can perform well despite their shifting membership if the organization creates "templates" that specify ad hoc team roles, task responsibilities, communication methods, and team leadership. Clinical staff are "pretrained" in the use of these templates and they simply spring into action using a standardized approach when an ad hoc team is formed. This approach eliminates the missed handoffs and miscommunication that would occur with strangers working together without guidelines.

"Knotwork"

Another type of common, and often problematic, structure that is common in health care but not in other settings is what Mosser and Begun (2014) describe as a "knotwork." This is a group of professionals who jointly care for a single patient. These professionals may consider themselves a team or they may take accountability only for their part of the care process. An example is a group of clinicians who are caring for a cancer patient. These doctors, nurses, social workers, pharmacists, and technicians may have little contact with each other outside of reading orders or clinical notes. Without some sort of organizing principles knotworks can be the source of "dropped balls," "disconnected care," and medical errors.

One method for improving communication in knotworks is service agreements. These documents are executed by clinical organizations that work together frequently and they detail the type of clinical communication and collaboration that should occur. For example, a primary care group might execute a service agreement with a preferred surgical group that clarifies expectations of each party and details standardized communications (Mosser & Begun, 2014).

Self-Managed Work Teams

Self-managed work teams are a rare and interesting structure that is seldom seen in health care. These teams are the ultimate form of employee involvement and engagement. The team is an autonomous unit. It does not have a formal leader and all task and many management functions are handled by team members themselves.

🔍 *CASE STUDY*

Self-Managed Work Teams

A published case study describes self-managed work teams at the Ararat Care Center, a skilled nursing facility. This facility uses self-directed resident care teams. These teams care for a specific group of residents. The team includes a CNA (certified nursing assistant) team leader, CNAs, laundry team leader, environmental services team leader, and food and nutrition team leader, and some shifts have social services and therapeutic activities representatives. The team members are empowered to make their own decisions, to handle issues such as staffing, and to problem solve patient care issues. This facility also has a five-tiered career ladder, with tiered raises for CNAs. At the time the reference case study was written, Ararat was a Medicare Five-Star facility (Mayfield, 2010).

▶ Teamwork Structures

Healthcare organizations have evolved a variety of tools and techniques for fostering clinical teamwork. All of these structures involve some type of patient-centered, interdisciplinary communication. Some examples of these structures are:

- **Team huddles.** These are short (15 minutes or less) meetings that occur at the beginning of the workday to review potential at-risk patients or to deal with currently pressing team operational issues (Institute for Healthcare Improvement [IHI], 2017). Sentara Health, a large chain of hospitals and postacute care providers, uses huddles to improve patient safety in both its hospitals and SNFs.

  Nursing staff members attend these meetings at the start of the day and at the end of the shift and after an adverse event. Nurses describe patients whose condition might be deteriorating and label them as

watchers. Senior clinicians coach nurses on how to integrate their perceptions into an informal severity of illness assessment. Nurses are asked to use the information to develop a plan for at-risk patients. Potential patient safety concerns are also discussed at the huddle (Yates & Federico, 2013).

In primary care, huddles are used to plan the team day. Team members review the patient list to identify special patient situations, anticipate care needs, and learn of staffing issues, policy updates, or other practice changes (Yates & Federico, 2013). The Healthy Huddles webpage from the Center for Primary Care Excellence at University of California San Francisco (UCSF) contains a variety of tools for using huddles (Center for Excellence in Primary Care, 2013).

- **Cross-functional complex case conferences.** As hospital and SNF stays get shorter, healthcare teams must quickly plan care and devise solutions to complex patient situations. These situations usually require the expertise of a full multidisciplinary team. The complex case conference is a meeting requested by the patient's primary clinician. This meeting brings all members of the patient's care team as well as quality assurance and clinical management staff together to discuss the patient's medical, psychosocial, caregiver support, and emotional situation. Team members evaluate patient risk for decompensation or repeat hospitalization and devise a plan that leverages the strengths of each discipline. These case conferences should be driven first by patient goals and secondarily by health professional goals. A home care agency encourages nurse or therapy case managers to call a complex case conference when they are caring for challenging patients and need more professional support.

- **Patient care planning meetings.** SNFs are required by Medicare and other insurance companies to do detailed patient care and discharge planning. The Office of the Inspector General (OIG) has detailed a number of deficiencies in SNF care planning and has focused on the need for cross-functional care plan and discharge plan development. Some best practices for team-based care planning in the SNF setting include a sequence of team meetings to plan patient care and discharge.

These team meetings start on the day of admission and progress through periodic interdisciplinary meetings and several discharge planning meetings. At these meetings, SNF clinical staff are directed to develop care plans, assess the patient's progress, and discuss medications, patient pain, and ability to perform activities of daily living. A final meeting just prior to discharge is to be used for medication reconciliation, to provide vital phone numbers, and to ensure that equipment has been ordered (OIG, 2013).

- **Clinical rounds.** This is a time-honored method for reviewing and communicating about patient care plans. The IHI (2015) defines rounds as: "A model of care in which multiple members of the care team representing different disciplines come together to discuss the care of a patient in real time" (p. 04). Rounds include a structured routine in which a leader facilitates a discussion about patients being cared for by the team. Patients may be included in the discussion. Topics for rounds may include care coordination, ensuring that patient goals are understood and honored, patient status updates, opportunities to update the care plan, and identification of safety or readmission risks.

Rounds originated on inpatient units but are now commonly used in SNFs, home care agencies, and ambulatory care settings. AHRQ provides a tool for assessing the effectiveness of communication in patient care rounds called "Observing Patient Care Rounds" (AHRQ, 2012; IHI, 2015).

- **Rapid case reviews.** One novel method for conducting short, complex case conferences was pioneered by Christiana Home Care. In this highly patient-centered model, home healthcare nurses meet weekly to revise the care plans of high-risk patients. Using the SBAR (Situation, Background, Assessment, Recommendation) reporting method nurses have 5 minutes to describe the patient's goals and discuss what the team has done to meet or fail to meet those goals. Suggestion ideas are generated from the team and implemented by the case manager (Huertas, Glasheen-Wray, & Price, 2016).

- **Cross-organizational reporting and problem solving.** Many accountable care organizations (ACOs) conduct regular "rounds" on high-risk patients. For example, one nurse care coordination department conducts regular telephone "virtual rounds" in which the status and care plans of high-risk patients are discussed with care coordinators in its partner SNFs and home care agencies. Participants on the call review the care being delivered and generate strategies to improve patient outcomes and reduce readmissions.

🔍 CASE STUDY

Everford Team Committee

After reviewing the research on team types and team structures, the Everford Team Committee decides to adopt the structures described in **TABLE 8-1**.

ASK YOURSELF

- What types of teamwork structures does your organization employ?
- How well do these structures function to "connect the dots" for patients?
- Which other teamwork structures might help your organization provide more connected care?

TABLE 8-1 Revised Teamwork Structures Adopted by the Everford Health System

Type of Structure	Clinicians	Clerical Support	Clinical Leaders	Patient and Family
Daily Huddles – Each entity will do a quick daily review of the status of the unit, practice or caseload and will triage high-risk situations, manage work assignments, and address potential problems, issues, or special events.	X	X	X	
Interdisciplinary Conferencing All professionals, including primary care physicians and specialists, who are involved in the patient's care must communicate and collaborate on the care plan and must communicate to each other when the patient's condition or care plan changes. This communication can be electronic, by phone, in writing, or in person, but each communication about patient care must include an acknowledgment and response.	X		X	
Rounding Traditional rounds that include representatives of each profession on the team will continue in inpatient settings. Patients and families must be given the opportunity to participate and ask questions during rounds. The home care agency will use the "rapid case review" method for rounds.	X		X	X
Complex Case Conferences This meeting can be called by any clinician if he or she feels overwhelmed by or unsure of what to do with the care of a complex patient. The meeting is attended by the whole patient care team, all of whom provide feedback and suggestions. If there are other clinicians, such as the primary care clinician, who are involved with the patient's care, they should be offered the opportunity to join the conference by phone or by videoconference. In most cases, the patient and family members should be invited to join the conference to discuss their goals and care issues.	X		X	X

Type of Structure	Clinicians	Clerical Support	Clinical Leaders	Patient and Family
Quality Improvement Teams Various quality improvement teams are chartered to deal with process problems or clinical outcome deficiencies. These teams are always cross functional and are usually cross departmental. Examples are a team to improve intake department capability, nurse scheduling effectiveness, and order cycle time improvement.	X	X	X	
The Clinical Steering Committee This team which is composed of senior clinical leadership, reviews agency clinical outcome data, monitors the work of other quality-related teams, and develops structural or process changes. The team may recommend that an improvement team be chartered.			X	

▶ Teamwork Processes

Besides the specific clinical or administrative tasks that make up the concrete work activities of the team, team members must perform process activities to foster mutual support and achievement of team goals. Common types of team process activities include:

- **Information gathering.** Team members must find out about the current status of their patient population or the details of the work they are performing. Team report meetings where the status of the patients' condition is exchanged is an example of information gathering.
- **Planning.** Teams must develop an orderly process for achieving their goals, sequencing their tasks, and following up on activities. Teams without planning are teams living in chaos. Planning group activities in advance will ensure that meeting time is well spent.

For example, teams that conduct formal meetings should always plan an agenda and end with an action plan.

- **Communication.** Team members exchange information using "closed loop communication" to ensure that the message was sent, received, and properly interpreted. Teams also need strategic communication that provides each member of the team with understandable information about team logistics, follow-up activities, reference materials, and team minutes. Communication to those affected by the work of the team is also an important part of the team's work.
- **Problem solving.** Teams will spend much of their time together solving problems. Depending on the level of group process sophistication and group cohesion, this can be a very painful or a very fruitful process.

  Teams that master problem-solving tools will achieve their goals faster and more easily. Some of the more commonly used tools are brainstorming, nominal group process, ask why five times, and forcefield analysis.

■ **Analyzing data.** To take teamwork beyond the realm of opinion and instinct, team members should have measurable goals and should review data about their own progress toward their goals. For example, a clinical team may have the reduction of 30-day hospital readmissions as its goal. The team would regularly review its progress toward this goal by looking at clinical data in graphic form. In the course of the team's work, it should be reviewing clinical, operational, or financial data about key elements of the readmission problem to diagnose causes of the problem. The team should also test solutions and collect data to measure results.

■ **Making decisions.** Team members must decide how to manage tasks, how to solve concrete problems, and how to improve team processes.

These decisions require good communication and in many cases the use of structured decision-making techniques to ensure that all views of the issue have been aired and each group member is given a fair opportunity to be part of the decision. We will discuss various methods of decision making later in this chapter.

■ **Providing mutual support.** The essence of "team" is mutual aid and support. This support might come in the form of helping with tasks, providing encouragement, filling in information gaps, or coaching a fellow team member.

■ **Giving feedback to other team members.** As teams mature and relationships between team members become more trusting, individuals start to give each other feedback. In situations in which patient safety is at issue, feedback is absolutely essential.

In other cases it helps team members develop and sometimes to hear messages that can only be delivered by a peer.

■ **Resolving conflicts.** Whenever humans work in groups some degree of conflict is almost inevitable. In fact, in teamwork, surfacing and resolving conflict is an essential step in moving beyond politeness to authentic interactions between team members. Team conflict must be constructively handled by the leader or facilitator or it can permanently damage the team's cohesiveness.

▶ Research on Team Success Factors

Practical experience and research indicates that certain conditions must be met for teams to develop and work effectively:

■ Tasks should be more suitable to teamwork than to individual health professional work.
■ The team must include the right people to perform the task.
■ Team members must pool their resources and work cooperatively to complete the task.
■ The organization must provide support for the work of the team (Dow, 2013).

A classic work on team building, *The Team Handbook*, lists additional conditions that teams need to succeed:

■ Clearly defined purpose and goals
■ Clearly defined boundaries
■ Access to people in the know
■ Access to resources (Scholtes, Joiner, & Streibel, 2003)

Hackman, the Harvard Business School authority on teams, suggests asking five questions to determine whether the factors for team success are present.

The first question, described previously, is whether the group meets the criteria for a real team (boundaries, interdependence, stability of membership). Other key questions are:

■ "Does the team have a compelling direction, a purpose that is clear, challenging,

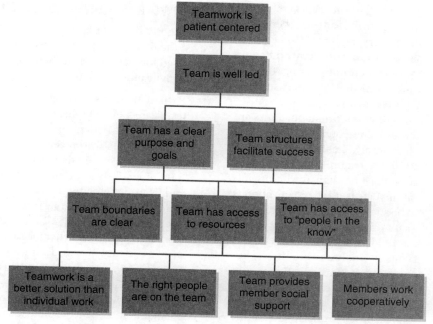

FIGURE 8-3 Building Blocks of Team Success

Data from Dow (2013); Scholtes, Joiner, and Streibel (2003); and Hackman (2004).

and consequential—and that focuses on the ends to be achieved rather than the means the team must use in pursuing them?

- Does the team's structure—its task, composition, and core norms of conduct—enable rather than impede teamwork?
- Does the team's social system context provide the resources and support that members need to carry out their collective work?" (Hackman, 2004)

FIGURE 8-3 describes the essential components of team success.

▶ Measures of Health Team Effectiveness

There are no uniformly accepted standard measures of team effectiveness in health care, but there are four areas of focus in team effectiveness measurement:

1. **Clinical results.** Ultimately clinical teams are responsible for achieving good clinical outcome measures and improved satisfaction for patients

ASK YOURSELF: WAS YOUR LAST TEAM DESIGNED TO SUCCEED?

- Thinking of a team that you have most recently led or been a part of, think about how many key success factors listed in the previous section were present.
- How many success factors were missing?
- How did these factors impact the success of the team?

served by the team. Patient safety and the incidence of adverse events also form a very important (some would say the most important) outcome measure for teamwork since the root cause of medical errors is so often poor teamwork.

Other important outcomes are those that are publicly reported by Medicare or accrediting agencies such as 30-day readmission rates. Team goals must be aligned with organizational goals if the organization is to be successful overall.

2. **Team process or task quality measures.** These types of measures typically include timeliness, accuracy, cost, and effectiveness in meeting customer requirements. A team process measure in an intact clinical work group might be the percentage of cases in which team members completed documentation of interdisciplinary communication in the timeframe required by regulation.

3. **Organizational measures.** These measures include costs of care, utilization, creation of service capacity, patient access to care, reduction in duplication of effort, and process cycle time. All are important elements of team success and part of the quadruple aim goal of reducing the per capita cost of care.

4. **Team member ratings of team effectiveness.** These team self-assessments usually focus on process issues such as team communication, effectiveness of decision-making practices, and team members' own satisfaction with the work of the team and their place on the team. The TeamSTEPPS survey instrument in **FIGURE 8-4** is one such team effectiveness rating tool.

Teamwork Benefits Research

In a slightly different approach, Mickan surveyed the literature on team effectiveness and described four categories of "benefits" that result from healthcare teamwork:

- **Patient benefits.** Patients who received team care had better health outcomes and an improved patient experience. In one study, patients who received care from a coordinated team in a designated stroke unit were more likely to be alive, independent, and living at home 1 year after their stroke (Stroke Unit Trialists' Collaboration, 2001).
- **Team member benefits.** Employees who worked in teams had better job satisfaction, more role clarity, increased self-esteem, more work sharing, better understanding of other professions, and less isolation.
- **Team benefits.** Teamwork produced better communication, better coordination and less duplication of care, efficient use of health services, and more positive interactions among team members.
- **Organizational benefits.** Teams achieved reduced costs of care, reduced readmissions, fewer unanticipated admissions, and better patient accessibility. The author notes: "Four team processes (shared objectives, participation, quality emphasis, and support for innovation) were the best predictors of team effectiveness, accounting for 23% of the variance, with shared objectives having the biggest single effect" (Mickan, 2005, p. 212).

▶ "The Big Five" Hallmarks of Effective Team Behavior

Eduardo Salas, an authority on the work of healthcare teams, has taken the vast conceptual and theoretical literature on teamwork and compressed it into a concise and useful model that

TeamSTEPPS®**2.0**

Team Assessment Questionnaire

INSTRUCTIONS:
This assessment is a statistical measurement of your impressions of team behavior as it relates to patient care in your current work setting. Please answer all 55 questions so an overall score may be calculated.

Facility _____ Unit _____ Date _____

	Strongly Disagree	Disagree	Undecided	Agree	Strongly Agree
Team Foundation					
1. The team has a clear vision of what it is supposed to do.					
2. The team's activities are guided by a clear Mission Statement/Charter.					
3. The team's goals are closely aligned with the goals of the organization.					
4. The team has adequate skills and member resources to achieve its goals.					
5. Everyone on the team has a clear and vital role.					
6. The team has adequate meeting time, space, and resources to achieve all objectives.					
7. Team meetings are well attended by all team members.					
8. The team can measure its performance effectively.					
9. The team understands its customer requirements (internal and/or external).					
10. This team is promptly informed of changes in policy or new developments.					
11. The department or unit has clear expectations of this team.					
12. The team receives adequate training to function effectively.					
Team Functioning					
13. Team meetings are run efficiently.					
14. Everyone on the team participates at an acceptable level.					
15. This team works well together.					
16. This team works well with other teams/departments in the organization.					
17. The goals and objectives of this team will have a positive impact on the organization.					
18. The team is on a continuous improvement curve.					

Please continue on next page

FIGURE 8-4 TeamSTEPPS Team Assessment Questionnaire

(continues)

TeamSTEPPS® 2.0

	Strongly Agree	Agree	Undecided	Disagree	Strongly Disagree
Team Performance					
19. The team uses an effective short and long-term strategic planning process.					
20. The team meets its (internal and/or external) customer requirements.					
21. The team is productive.					
22. Team functioning doesn't interfere with getting my own job done.					
Team Skills					
23. The team members communicate well with one another.					
24. Constructive feedback is given by the team.					
25. Team members are familiar with each other's job responsibilities.					
26. The team uses effective decision making processes and problem solving skills.					
27. The team monitors and progresses the plan of care.					
28. The team can change or improve the way it goes about working on its tasks.					
Team Leadership					
29. My boss/supervisor promotes participation by the team in key decisions.					
30. My boss/supervisor shares responsibilities with team members.					
31. My boss/supervisor is an effective leader.					
32. I share my ideas/suggestions whether or not my boss/supervisor agrees with my input.					
33. My boss/supervisor focuses on building team's technical and interpersonal skills.					
34. My boss/supervisor coaches and supports individual team members.					
35. My boss/supervisor promotes individual problem solving and intelligent risk taking.					
36. My boss/supervisor leads by example.					
Team Climate and Atmosphere					
37. Team members trust each other.					
38. Morale on this team is high.					
39. Team members support each other.					
40. There are no feelings among team members which might pull this team apart.					
41. The team resolves conflicts soon after they occur.					
42. I feel free to express my opinions.					
43. I have an influence on team decisions.					
44. Team members can openly discuss their own problems and issues.					
45. Team members show consideration for needs and feelings of other team members.					
46. Team members receive recognition for individual performance.					

Please continue on next page

Team Assessment Questionnaire   TeamSTEPPS 2.0

FIGURE 8-4 *Continued*

TeamSTEPPS 2.0

	Strongly Agree	Agree	Undecided	Disagree	Strongly Disagree
Team Identity					
47. I know why I am on a team.					
48. I am pleased to be on a team.					
49. The team subscribes to a clear set of values.					
50. This team is fun to work with.					
51. No individual, group or gender dominates team activities.					
52. The team has a positive self image.					
53. The team recognizes the patient as a critical team member.					
54. The team is a safety net for patients.					
55. I am a member of a team in which the leader promotes teamwork.					

THANK YOU FOR FILLING OUT THIS FORM

Quality Values Research and Consulting Services
http://www.qvresearch.com

TeamSTEPPS 2.0

Team Assessment Questionnaire

FIGURE 8-4 *Continued*

Reproduced from Agency for Healthcare Research and Quality. (2012). Team Assessment Questionnaire. Retrieved from https://www.ahrq.gov/sites/default/files/wysiwyg/professionals/education/curriculum-tools/teamstepps/instructor/reference/tmassess.pdf

🔍 CASE STUDY

A large internal medical practice within the Everford System is divided into interdisciplinary teams consisting of physicians, nurse practitioners, medical assistants, receptionists, a nurse care coordinator, and a behavioral health specialist. Each team has a physician or advanced practice registered nurse (APRN) team leader. Teams have had training in team development, use a structured meeting format, and frequently use quality improvement tools to improve their work processes. Every year, the team completes the TeamSTEPPS assessment tool to monitor function. Teams are measured on patient outcomes such as lead time for patient appointments, measures of HbA1c for diabetic patients, 30-day readmission rate by team, level of accuracy in medical visit coding, and costs of care. Teams benchmark their results and those with good results share best practices with other teams.

The Everford Team Committee decides to adopt the approach used by the medical practice team as an internal best practice. Each entity or unit within the system will have an interdisciplinary team structure with a clinical or business team leader. Each team will have its own outcome measures (based on corporate metrics) and will do an annual assessment of team effectiveness using the TeamSTEPPS assessment tool.

Team leaders will receive training in team building and meeting management. Trained facilitators from the quality assurance department will be available to help with consultation about team leadership, team dynamics, and meeting management.

ASK YOURSELF

- How is the work of teams in your organization measured?
- How is measurement data used to improve the performance of team tasks and team processes?

identifies the characteristics of effective team behavior. Salas, Sims, and Burke (2005) call this model "The Big Five" of teamwork. There are two components to this model: five essential dimensions of teamwork and coordinating mechanisms. The five essential dimensions are:

Team Leadership

The leader helps teams create a shared understanding of the team's goals and the ways that the goals should be accomplished. The leader monitors the environment and shares information with the team to avoid surprises. He or she also shares organizational information with the team.

The leader sets behavioral and performance expectations and intervenes to improve performance when team members don't meet these expectations. For example, if an SNF is planning on shifting staff to other floors to cover staff shortages, the nurse manager must make contingency plans for her floor and inform the staff about what is being done and why. She should also ask for suggestions on how to make the impending changes more workable.

Mutual Performance Monitoring

Within a cohesive and trusting environment, team members instinctively monitor each other's work and identify lapses, mistakes, and gaps that might compromise the team's ability to meet goals and expectations. For example, if members of an SNF clinical team are planning a patient discharge and some team members have not discussed the plan with the patient and his or her family, other team members might notice that there is a gap in the plan and tactfully point it out to their teammates.

Backup Behavior

This is the helping behavior that occurs when another team member is having a problem with performance (identified through mutual performance monitoring). Team members might provide feedback and coaching, help a team member complete a task or step, and actually finish the task if a teammate is overloaded and at the limit of his or her capacity to keep working. One member of a home care intake team, for example, might be overwhelmed with electronic referrals from a single hospital that are coming in so fast she cannot respond to them. Another member of the team might put aside what she is doing to sign on to the computer to keep the referral flow going.

Adaptability

The ability of team members to change their behavior in relation to the behavior of other team members or to respond to factors in the team's work environment is called adaptability. For example, if a key team member is out sick, the rest of the team must decide how to reallocate that person's work.

Team Orientation

Orientation means that members of the team take other's behavior into account during group interactions and believe in the importance of team goals over individual goals (modified from Salas et al., 2005).

▶ Coordinating Mechanisms of the Big Five

Shared Mental Models

In shared mental models team members have a shared vision of two things: the specific work tasks that the team must perform and the way that the team works together. Simply put, shared mental models is about team leaders and all team members "being on the same page" about the work of team. These shared mental models allow team members to anticipate and predict each other's needs and to identify changes in the team's work and adjust their behavior accordingly. For example, nurses in an outpatient dermatologic surgery clinic have a shared understanding that their work is to admit patients to care, keep patients and family members informed, assist the physicians, perform clinical procedures and patient assessments, and do patient-centered teaching. All team members are clear that the way they do their work ultimately helps the team achieve better clinical outcomes and provide a good patient experience.

Team members know that if one team member is delayed with a frail or complex patient, other nurses must jump in to cover remaining patients, keep the clinical flow going, and maintain service levels.

Closed Loop Communication

This method of communication is much like the teach-back or return demonstration model of patient teaching. A member of the team communicates to another team member. The receiving team member verifies that he or she has received the communication. The original sender or communicator of the message "closes the loop" by ensuring the message that was received was the one he or she intended. For example, a home healthcare nurse might refer a patient to physical therapy for interventions to prevent falls. The therapist would acknowledge the referral by phone or email. The nurse would then have a conversation with the therapist about her fall risk assessment and verify that the therapist intends to do her own risk assessment using standardized fall risk testing and that she will implement an exercise program to reduce the patient's risk. Closed loop communication is an essential patient safety technique because it ensures that vital information about patient care has been sent, received, and interpreted in the correct way.

Mutual Trust

Salas and coworkers (2005) describe the need for mutual trust succinctly: "Without sufficient trust, team members will expend time and energy protecting, checking, and inspecting each other as opposed to collaborating to provide value-added ideas" (modified from Salas et al., 2005, p. 568).

This type of protecting and checking is a far cry from the mutual performance monitoring that characterizes effective team behavior. Trust enables team members to interpret each other's behavior accurately to share information and work cooperatively.

Bullying and acting out by high-status health professionals in certain environments are extreme examples of the lack of trust in teams and its negative consequences.

▶ Validating the Big Five Model

Kalisch also validated the use of The Big Five model in an inpatient setting. Kalisch, Weaver, and Salas (2009) studied teamwork on five inpatient nursing units and interviewed registered nurses (RNs), licensed practical nurses (LPNs), nursing assistants, and unit secretaries about teamwork using a focus group model. The themes identified in these groups validated the use of a Big Five framework to improve teamwork. In this study, researchers collected concrete examples of presence or absence of Big Five teamwork elements.

INTERVIEW WITH ANNE ELLWELL, RN, MPH, FORMER PRINCIPAL AND VICE PRESIDENT OF COMMUNITY RELATIONS AT QUALIDIGM

Anne Ellwell has worked for Qualidigm, a Medicare Quality Improvement Organization and consulting firm that serves the Northeast. Anne was the co-leader of the team that established Connecticut Communities of Care, a statewide collaborative initiative involving 12 hospitals and a variety of community partners to improve transitions between healthcare settings and decrease preventable hospital readmissions for patients with heart failure. This coalition has been highly successful in reducing readmission rates across the state.

Anne talks about the need to develop trust and teamwork across the continuum of care. She says that when one part of the care community sends a patient to the next step in care there must be trust that the patient will be well cared for. She also believes that healthcare providers must focus on the social determinants of health if they are to achieve better outcomes.

Anne has done extensive work with patient-centered medical homes (PCMHs) across New England. She finds that nurses have a vital role to play in achieving better outcomes through teamwork at the primary care practice level.

She uses the example of a diabetic who needs help with lifestyle change. The most effective team model in these PCMHs includes nurse care coordinators, medical assistants, and practice secretaries. This model is built on the idea of the right staff providing the right level of care at the right time. For example, the practice secretary would call all diabetic patients who have not had a HbA1c test and asks them to have one done. This is enough to get many patients back into the program. When the patient comes in, the medical assistant may ask questions according to practice guidelines, do some assessment of the patient's knowledge/adherence, and provide education according to practice guidelines.

The nurse gets involved with high-risk or nonadherent patients who need more help with diet, other lifestyle changes, and medications. "Using a soft touch," the nurse may also start goals of care conversations with patients who have serious illness and frequent readmissions. In this model, the nurse is "working to the top of her license" and the physician can say "I trust her to care for these patients so I can move on."

An example of positive charge nurse leadership behavior was: "The charge nurse watches over all of the staff, determining when they need assistance." An absence of leadership was defined as: "We don't get our assignment for the shift until 9 and even later. We never catch up" (modified from Kalisch et al., 2009, p. 301).

▶ Stages of Team Development

Like human beings teams pass through stages of growth and development (Scholtes et al., 2003). As they pass through the developmental stages, successful teams slowly develop Big Five team dimensions and the "coordinating mechanisms" described by Salas et al. (2005). Bruce Tuckman (1965), a group dynamics expert, devised the classic list of team development stages:

Forming

This is the startup, getting-to-know-you stage of the team. Members are trying to understand how to change from individuals to team members. The team is defining its goals and tasks.

The team leader is developing team structures and logistics for meetings. The team is beginning to define acceptable behaviors and norms.

This is typically a period of uncertainty with group members being tentative and polite with each other. Some members may be excited about the team and happy to be part of it, while others may feel some suspicion and hang back to see what develops as the team's work progresses. At this stage, team members may be impatient with group process work, such as setting ground rules, and will want to jump right into describing problems or proposing solutions to problems.

Storming

This is the second and most difficult stage of team development. As the team begins to explore its work more fully, as different team member personalities manifest themselves, and as the enormity of the team's tasks and the list of obstacles surfaces, panic may ensue. Team members may become irritable with each other, conflict may flare, and some team members may become hyperfocused on the task while they try to ignore the emotions being expressed. Individuals may become competitive with each other during this stage. Arguing, defensiveness, withdrawal, and confrontational questioning are all hallmarks of the storming stage. Team leaders need patience and skill, which we will explore later in this chapter, to navigate the team through this stage.

Norming

In the norming stage, team members settle down and get to work on achieving their goals. Competitiveness subsides and cooperation surges. Team members have fallen into the routine of team meetings and have grown comfortable with ground rules, meeting structures, and group processes. Members of the team are beginning to think of themselves as a cohesive unit with an identity and are adopting behaviors consistent with team culture. At this stage, team members are more open with each other, there is more casual conversation and joking, and team members are starting to confide in each other and to raise differences constructively.

Performing

Members have now developed a level of respect for and confidence in each other. Team members are demonstrating Big Five team behaviors (leadership, mutual performance monitoring, supportive backup behaviors, adaptability, and team orientation) and the coordinating mechanisms. Tasks are being performed well and the team is achieving its goals.

Adjourning

When a team, such as a quality improvement team, has a more time-limited mission, there is a fifth stage of teamwork. In this stage, members sum up their work, present it to management, and make arrangements for gains to be maintained. Group members may simultaneously feel a sense of sadness and satisfaction as the team's work ends. At this stage, organizational recognition of the team's work is essential to maintaining the positive spirit of the team and ongoing team member relationships in other settings.

Modified from Tuckman, Bruce W. (1965) and Scholtes (2003)

🔍 CASE STUDY

Adopting a Framework for Effective Teamwork

The Everford Team Committee, in consultation with the team facilitators from the quality assurance department, decide to adopt a Big Five framework as goals for all their teams. They also decide to study the methods and tools that help teams constructively move through the stages of team development. Eventually, the facilitators incorporate this material into a longer team leader development course and into "just-in-time" training for team members.

TEAMWORK PART 2— BUILDING AN EFFECTIVE HEALTHCARE TEAM STEP BY STEP

In the rest of this chapter we will discuss the practical application of teamwork theory. If you are developing a new team or tuning up an existing team, you can tip the scales for success by following an organized set of team-building steps:

1. Develop and apply team leadership skills.
2. Structure for success.
3. Create a team focus.
4. Manage meetings and organize team tasks.
5. Pay attention to process.
6. Develop team member capability.
7. Build group cohesiveness.
8. Troubleshoot team problems.

▶ 1. Develop and Apply Team Leadership Skills

Teams need good leadership to achieve their goals. This leadership is not military style command and control (which is mostly suited to emergency situations) but is more like the coaching role used in developing sports teams in which each player develops his or her unique skills while working cooperatively with team members for a successful outcome. At the most basic level, team leaders need to accomplish two things:

- **Task work.** Organize the team's work with goal setting, managing meetings, organizational advocacy, and obtaining resources so the team can complete its tasks and achieve its goals in the most efficient and effective way.
- **Teamwork.** Facilitate the development of the team group process, identity, skills, and norms so that individual team members and the team as a whole has more capacity and capability to perform tasks, solve problems, and achieve goals. Teamwork should help team members to work together more productively outside team meetings.

Qualities of Effective Healthcare Team Leaders

Accomplishing the two team leadership goals is no easy task and doing so requires a specific mindset and skillset. One well-designed study used transcripts from focus groups that were conducted with members and leaders of teams in five different organizations to paint a clear picture of team leader success factors (Bachiochi, O'Connor, Rogelberg, & Elder, 2000):

- **Background and expertise.** Job knowledge and knowledge of organizational issues and success factors help build respect from team members and make them feel that their team has the kind of leadership that it needs.
- **Task-oriented skills.** Planning, organizing, delegating/sharing power, problem solving, and motivating help to get the team's job done.
- **Interpersonal skills.** Conflict management, persuading and influencing, understanding/supporting, and coaching/mentoring help to knit team members together and to defuse conflicts.
- **Communication skills.** Listening, communicating information, providing feedback, and communicating a vision form a solid skillset. Communicating information was the most widely mentioned skill in the research focus groups.
- **Liaison skills.** Acting as a liaison and advocate for the team with senior management and taking ultimate accountability for team's work are important.
- **Personal characteristics/traits.** Self-confidence, emotional stability, consistency/trust, and flexibility in a team leader foster team effectiveness.

In another view of effective team leadership skills, Mosser and Begun (2014) describe three key roles for healthcare team leaders:

- **Enable the work of the team.** This competency includes maintaining a clear and common understanding of team goals, developing shared accountability for achieving the goals, assuring that the team has enough authority, defining team membership, establishing interdependency among members, keeping the team unified, controlling "rogue" operations, and relating effectively to team sponsors/senior management.
- **Developing the team.** Team leaders must recruit and orient team members, establish group values and norms, foster team identity, create a safe climate for discussion

and debate, and develop a common understanding of how the team does its work.

- **Coaching/guiding.** The leader gathers impressions of and data about team and individual performance, identifies performance deficiencies, and gives feedback, suggestions, and support to close performance gaps.

Two other key team leadership success factors are mentioned in a number of research studies and are often mentioned by employees who serve on teams. One is transparency and good communication about the work of the team and about organizational issues that affect the team. The other leadership success factor is creating a safe environment so team members can speak their minds, freely suggest ideas, and give feedback about organizational issues without fear of reprisals. This is a particularly important factor in teamwork for patient safety.

Learning Team Leadership Skills

Leading a team is a complex task that requires a specific attitude and skillset. There are team leadership courses available and much team leadership material is available online. Most team leaders will need to use self-learning strategies in addition to formal training to develop their skills. Following are some ideas for a team leader self-learning action plan:

- **Observe team leaders in action.** One of the best ways to start mastering team leadership is to consider the behavior of team leaders you have worked with. Think of the teams that were most functional. What method did the leaders of these teams use? What about the least effective teams you have seen? What did the leaders of those teams do or not do that created obstacles to team success?
- **Take a course on team leadership.** Intensive courses in healthcare team leadership are available from universities and organizations such as the Institute for Healthcare Improvement (2015). Other team leadership courses that require less time and are less costly, but are not specific to health care, are provided

by many national seminar companies such as Dale Carnegie (www.dalecarnegie.com) and Skillpath (www.skillpath.com).

■ **Read books and articles on team leadership.** See the References section for ideas. While books on healthcare team leadership will be most helpful, there is a much wider literature about teamwork in business and learning and development publications. The American Society for Talent Development is one rich source of such information (www.td.org).

■ **Use social media to identify resources for developing your leadership skills.** Facebook and LinkedIn can be good sources of information about team-building leadership skills. LinkedIn's *Slide Share* feature offers minicourses on various aspects of team leadership and meeting management. Often, consulting firms that specialize in team building will post free content on social media sites or on their own websites.

■ **Practice in a setting outside work.** Practicing team leadership skills in a community or other professional group setting such as running a sports team booster club, or a garden club meeting, or becoming a committee chairperson for one of your professional organizations can help you develop team leadership and meeting management skills in an environment that may be less intimidating than your own workplace.

■ **Use publicly available resources to help you develop your skills.** YouTube has a variety of short videos on team leadership and managing team meetings. An example is "The Five Stage Team Building Model" (https://www.youtube.com/watch?v=nRYRZg8YSso). Two other major resources for comprehensive team building are the U.S. Army Handbook (2015) and the TeamSTEPPS program from AHRQ (2018).

■ **Learn from a mentor or coach.** If you know of a health professional with good team leadership skills within your own organization or from within your professional networks, ask for guidance and advice about your own team-building efforts. Many good team leaders and group facilitators are willing to share what they have learned and will help you adapt their "tricks and tools" to your own team challenges. Co-leading some meetings with a more experienced leader can be a good way to get some guided practice.

■ **Practice team leadership.** The only way to actually master team leadership is to practice. Start with concrete goals, the right team members, and a good meeting structure. Let planning and structure carry you along in the beginning of your team leadership efforts. Teams in the forming stage will focus mostly on tasks; and as the group begins to coalesce and your skills mature, both you and team members will focus more on effective team processes. In the early days of your team leadership experience it can be helpful to have a colleague with team leadership experience sit in and give you feedback. If you are comfortable doing so, you can ask team members for feedback about how they feel you are doing at running meetings and keeping things moving forward. As you and the team progress in your work, you should try to adjust your leadership style to the stage of team development.

▶ 2. Structure for Success

Teams work best if they have clear structures and they understand their place in the context of the organization and its work. Structure within the organization is more important for teams that have a specific purpose and a short time horizon, such as quality improvement teams, than for intact work group teams. We will call these project teams.

Successful project teams need two levels of structure: The first is the structure that supports the team within the context of the organization (sponsorship, goals, resources, reporting, etc.). The second level of structure is at the team level and is usually managed by the team leader. Team structure consists of team meetings, team tools, action plans, team meeting documents, and team communications.

Organizational Level Structure That Supports Teamwork

Although there are many articles in the literature about teamwork, actual high-level commitment to teamwork and alignment of organizational activities to support it are relatively rare. This is no surprise given that although teamwork has been proved effective as a way to achieve quadruple aim goals, it is also time consuming and an expense to the organization. When the external climate is tumultuous and senior management is dealing with competing priorities, teamwork often drops to the bottom of the list. Smart organizations that are building capacity and capability don't let this happen. Key elements of organizational structure for project teams include:

- **A senior management sponsor.** This manager must have a willingness to foster the work of teams in his or her area of responsibility. This senior manager must wield the levers of power, help the team obtain resources, and advocate on behalf of the team and its work.
- **A clear definition of the type of team and its requirements and limits.** Improvement teams will need a much more highly organized structure than intact work groups. Work groups will need regular meetings and follow-up activities, while ad hoc teams need standardized roles and rules about dividing functions and communication methods but they will not meet in an ongoing way outside of specific patient care situations.
- **A clear statement of team goals.** While the team may further refine its goals and decide on tactics to achieve them, senior management should set a clear direction that is aligned with the organization's strategic goals.

- **An understanding of the team's relationship to other teams and organizational departments.** Organizations with long histories or those with senior managers who compete with each other for power and status often have rigidly segmented departments and teams that seldom communicate or interact. In these situations, miscommunication and frustration are likely to occur—often to the detriment of patient care. Clarifying boundaries and responsibilities (sometimes with senior management) can help resolve these issues.
- **A definition of team boundaries and authority.** This is a definition of which work processes the team can address, where their work begins and ends, and the level of decisions the team is allowed to make before seeking approval.
- **Roles and responsibilities.** When team roles are clearly defined, teams function much better. Lack of role clarity can precipitate team conflict. Types of team roles include:
  - Task roles, the specific work tasks that members of a team perform such as administering medications or performing medical procedures
  - Formal group roles such as facilitator or recorder
  - Informal group roles that arise out of the personalities of group members or circumstances such as helping, information seeking, and questioning. There are also negative group roles that must be managed or suppressed

TABLE 8-2 details formal roles and responsibilities in teams.

Criteria for Team Membership

Team members should be invited to join formal improvement teams for either their task expertise or their group process expertise. Team sponsors should define criteria for team membership, assess potential team member strengths and

TABLE 8-2 Team Roles and Responsibilities	
Team leader	Leads the team in accomplishing goals, completing tasks, managing group processes, and developing as a cohesive group.
Team sponsor	A role that is most commonly used in improvement teams. The sponsor is a senior manager who maintains overall authority and accountability for team's efforts. Team sponsor provides team direction, resources, advocacy, feedback coaching, and course corrections if the team is not achieving its goals.
Participating team member	Individual members are an active and engaged part of the team. The member attends meetings, listens, offers opinions, analyzes data, supports fellow team members, and performs follow-up assignments. The member acts as a content expert for his or her area of expertise.
Facilitator	Manages the group process with the team leader, using structured group tools, and group listening, coaching, summarizing, and participant management skills.
Recorder or scribe	Records minutes from team meeting. May act as the recorder for group activities like brainstorming or end of meeting evaluations.
Resource or consultant	A content expert who may be brought into the team to analyze or advise about specific clinical or business problems when team members do not have sufficient expertise to address the issue.
Process consultant	Observes group processes, surfaces issues, or reinforces positive group behavior.

🔍 CASE STUDY

Structuring Teamwork in a Complex Environment

One of the home care agencies in the Everford Health System's network set a goal of achieving a Medicare Home Health Compare five-star rating. As a step toward that goal, clinical teams have as a goal to reduce their 30-day readmission rates to below the national benchmark of 12%. To do this, two types of team structures were developed.

First, a management quality improvement team was chartered to design a more advanced case model that utilizes population health tactics, better care transitions, improved care coordination, patient self-management support, and the use of data to achieve goals. This team had a senior management sponsor (the chief operating officer), a team charter, defined boundaries, a team leader, a facilitator, and team members who were clinical experts.

Second, clinical teams consisting of nurses, therapists, social workers, and home health aides who worked with a defined population of patients in a geographic area, met monthly to address team issues, to review team data, to consider trends in readmissions, and to generate ideas for improvement.

weaknesses, and ultimately develop a roster of team leaders and members. Often, the lowest ranking employees are excluded from teams. This is usually a mistake as these front line workers may perform narrow but vital tasks. They may also have very practical improvement ideas and are often the closest people to the patient and his or her concerns.

Resources to Do the Team's Work

These resources will include time away from work for team meetings; coverage while team members are absent; access to meeting space, equipment, and supplies; access to data; and a method for obtaining help from support departments such as information systems or human resources.

Check-in and Reporting Mechanisms

Structured reporting mechanisms ensure that the team's work continues to be tied to organizational goals and priorities and that it has not veered off course. Check-in meetings are also an opportunity to obtain resources and get help with team issues or concerns. Check-in/reporting can

be as simple as a regular meeting between the team leader and the senior management sponsor or as formal as a structured report to a quality steering committee with documents and data.

▶ 3. Create a Team Focus

Setting Goals and Direction for Teams

Clear goals must be a driving force for healthcare teams. An Institute of Medicine publication on teamwork states this concept clearly: "Shared Goals: The team—including the patient and, where appropriate, family members or other support persons—works to establish shared goals that reflect patient and family priorities, and that can be clearly articulated, understood, and supported by all team members" (Mitchell et al., 2012, p. 6). Team goals should be clearly aligned with organizational goals.

See **FIGURE 8-5** for an example of how this is done.

One clear set of goals for the healthcare organization should focus on reducing fragmentation in care and ensuring positive care transitions and coordinated care for patients.

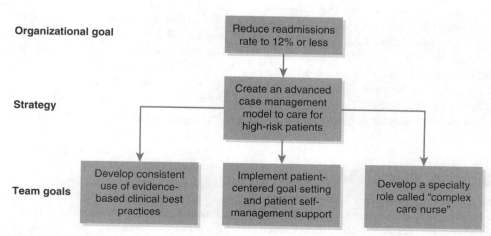

FIGURE 8-5 Aligning Organizational and Team Goals

Data from Scholtes, P., Joiner, B., & Streibel, B. (2003). *The team handbook* (3rd ed.). Madison, WI: Oriel Incorporated, pp. 3–39.

Some of these goals and measures for connected care might include:

- Reducing 30-day hospital readmissions
- Eliminating medical errors due to communication problems and lack of teamwork
- Improving the effectiveness of care transitions
- Engaging patients in making decisions about their care
- Ensuring that all follow-up tasks from an inpatient admission, outpatient surgery, home care visit, or medical office visit are completed
- Coordinating patient teaching and engaging patients in effective self-care activities to improve outcomes

Careful thought and analysis should go into how to translate these goals into actionable items for a team. Goals must be concrete enough that team members will clearly recognize when the goal is being met and when it is not. Goals must also be clear and realistic if team members are to be willing to adopt them. If team members can be involved in goal development they are more likely to accept the goals and work to achieve them.

When a team is framing a goal it can be very helpful to ask the question, "What would a good job look like?" to eliminate vagueness and create more concrete and actionable goals. It is also helpful to ask, "What is the difference between what we want and what we have?" Goals must also be translated into individual competencies and expectations that team members can articulate. One way to do this is to show team members the measurement goal for their team and then ask them to flesh out the actions that the team will need to take to achieve the goal.

Example of a Simple Team Goal

Every patient record will contain documentation that the clinician has elicited the patient's key personal goals. Care plan charting will demonstrate that the clinician has taken action to help the patient achieve his or her goal at every encounter.

Currently, 60% of team records meet this requirement. The goal is to achieve 85% adherence to this goal.

Staying Focused

As the team's work proceeds a wide variety of issues, problems, opinions, and solutions will arise. When this happens, it is very easy to get seduced by interesting ideas or problems peripheral to the team's work. Team leaders, facilitators, and team members must all take responsibility for staying focused on team goals and ensuring that precious team meeting time is not spent in digressing and discussing issues that are ultimately irrelevant to achieving team goals. One way to do this is to post the team's goal statement at the beginning of the meeting and to have a team ground rule that any team member can alert the team to digressions and ask, "Should we be getting back to working toward our goal?"

▶ 4. Manage Meetings and Organize Team Tasks

In team building, organization is half the battle. Teams that do not maintain the discipline of planned meetings with agendas, follow-up action plans, and minutes typically do not achieve their goals. Maintaining this structure is the job of the team leader and facilitator, sometimes with help from clerical support staff.

- **Team meeting logistics and planning.** Team meetings work best if they are held at a consistent day and time. This creates predictability in team members' schedules, and attending meetings becomes a habit. Before selecting team meeting times, the leader should consider the flow of the workday, times that are most convenient for team members, and the availability of staff coverage if needed. Coverage is important because if team members feel they will be punished with a backlog of work after attending the meeting their motivation to be part of the team will ebb.

- **A location for meetings.** Team meetings work best if there is a comfortable room, stocked with needed equipment and supplies (such as a flipchart with paper and markers). There should be enough room for all team members to sit at a table without crowding. Refreshments are a draw for attendance.
- **Team launch communications.** New teams and those that are refocusing will benefit from a clear explanation about the context of the team's work in the organization, the purpose of the team, team boundaries and authority, why members were selected, and some idea of how work will be accomplished. This type of communication is best done with a short explanation followed up by a discussion. For example, senior managers at an SNF met with nursing and aide staff to describe the new market environment and new expectations of staff and to discuss preliminary ideas and the vision for an improvement team that would simplify and redefine work.
- **Team communication channels.** Teams that meet regularly need to share meeting records, data, and documents. This might be done with a team book, or better, in a shared team folder on the corporate server.

Teams may also use email to communicate minutes, team tasks, information, and data. In highly structured teams, such as those planning a new product, members may use project management software to document and update activities and milestones. Someone on the team must be accountable for communicating to team members and to those affected by the team's work.

Team Meeting Essentials

Meetings with at least a minimal structure will run better and will make team members feel

more confident and competent. Team meetings, especially if they are trying to achieve challenging goals, must be planned in advance.

Each activity should be mapped and timed so that the meeting runs smoothly and achieves the desired objectives in the time available. The recipe for team meeting success includes (Pigeon & Khan, 2017):

- **Ground rules.** These are rules for meeting behavior that are adopted and agreed upon by all team members. "No side conversations" is a common ground rule. One way to set ground rules is to ask, "What positive and negative meeting behaviors have you observed in your past experience?" The ground rules should be posted in the room where meetings are held. Any team member should feel free to evoke the ground rules if someone on the team behaves in a way that is not consistent with accepted team behaviors: "Don't we have a ground rule about not interrupting?"
- **An agenda or meeting objectives.** An agenda is a list of things that the team wants to talk about. Objectives are descriptions of what the team needs to achieve. The latter are more difficult to formulate, but when used can make a meeting far more productive and effective. Here is an example of the difference:
  - Agenda: Discuss elements of patient-centered care

- Objective: Develop a list of specific staff patient-centered care competencies
- **Review of minutes and activities since the last meeting.** This review maintains the continuity between meetings and ensures that "nothing falls through the cracks." Team members are also asked what ideas or issues have come up since the last meeting.
- **Discussion and decision making.** The bulk of the meeting should be team discussion and problem-solving activities. This might consist of a facilitated discussion about data, issues facing the team, or possible solutions. It might also include individual reporting or the use of group tools such as flowcharting, forcefield analysis, or multivoting.

  Team leaders must use specific communication skills to achieve productive discussions. We will cover these skills in the section on paying attention to process.
- **Develop an action plan.** No meeting should end without some follow-up action. A simple action plan contains five elements:
  - What action will we take?
  - How will we know if it was successful?
  - Who will do it?
  - Who needs to be informed?
  - When will it be done? (Timeline with due dates)
- **Meeting debrief.** This is a process technique that takes the temperature of the team and quickly evaluates the meeting's level of success. Simply draw two columns on a flipchart. Label one side "Benefits," label the other side "Concerns." Start by asking meeting members: "What were the benefits of today's meeting?" and writing the answers exactly as stated. When all benefit ideas have been exhausted move on to ask, "What were your concerns about this meeting?" Again list the concerns as stated. Finish by summarizing key issues that were expressed.

▶ # 5. Pay Attention to Process

For newer team leaders, managing group process is one of the most daunting aspects of team building. For team leaders with more dominant personalities it is always tempting to simply take over, drive the discussion, and tell the team what to do. More reticent team leaders may be tempted to hang back and let the discussion take its course, probably steered by the most dominant members.

A better way to handle group process is *facilitative team leadership* in which the team leader manages the content/task part of the discussion and develops group process using group active listening skills. This approach takes some practice because it requires the leader to be thinking with both the right and left sides of the brain. The logical side of the brain is listening to and clarifying content and task discussions while the instinctive side of the brain is observing group interactions, body language, and voice tone. In the beginning, it can be helpful to have a second person who has group facilitation skills sit in and identify group process issues for the leader.

Group Facilitation Tips
Adopt a Neutral Attitude and Behavior

The team leader or facilitator must take an emotional step back from the issues at hand to develop team member capability and empowerment. Team members feel safer when the leader/facilitator presents a calm, businesslike, and nonemotional demeanor. This is easier for someone who is acting purely as a facilitator and who has no stake in the issue being discussed. It is harder for a team leader who is part of the team's actual task work and may have a big stake in team results, but it can be done with focused, conscious intent.

Leaders and facilitators can maintain a neutral stance by:

- Being aware of their own emotional reactions, but suppressing any expression of emotion
- Using neutral body language and comments (say "okay" instead of "good")
- Not favoring or calling upon any one team member too often
- Taking all comments and suggestions seriously

Use Group Active Listening Techniques

Group facilitation uses active listening—the same techniques you would use in a discussion with one person, except using these techniques with multiple team members in a team meeting. This is not as hard as it seems because you are simply using the techniques with different team members in sequence. The core techniques of active listening are (Bens, 2018):

- **Ask open-ended questions.** Open-ended questions are at the heart of effective group facilitation. Questioning can be thought of as a funnel. The questioning process starts with very open-ended questions (ones that **cannot** be answered with a "yes" or "no") such as, "What are the various aspects of this issue?" At the end of the discussion period use closed-ended questions (ones that **can** be answered with a "yes" or "no") to clarify what has been said: "So is the group saying that employees not believing in the efficacy of best practices are a major root cause of this problem?" Some good all-purpose questions to fuel discussions are "Help me understand. . .." and "Can you say more about that?"
- **Listening.** Active listening is the counterpoint to asking questions. In active listening the team leader gives full attention to the person who is speaking using gestures and words of encouragement ("okay"

or "go on"). The leader uses open body language by leaning slightly forward and making intermittent eye contact to signal that he or she is paying attention. This also means that the leader must control other team members who may interrupt or talk over the first speaker: "Could you hold up a minute and let Jane speak? Then we can hear what you have to say." Active listening is usually interspersed with asking clarifying questions and paraphrasing what was said.

- **Paraphrasing.** This technique means restating what you have heard from the team member either verbatim or in your own words. By doing this the leader validates the person who has spoken and ensures that he or she has heard the message correctly. This is an element of the "closed loop communication" aspect of Big Five teamwork.
- **Summarizing.** Summarizing is recapping key points of the discussion for the group. This can either be done by the team leader/facilitator or by a member of the team after prompting by the team leader: "Can someone summarize what we have decided?" Team members can then elaborate or correct the summary statement. It is easier to summarize if key points have been captured on a flipchart or if the leader has been taking notes during the discussion.

Using Structured Group Process Tools

Team leaders have access to a large toolbox of group prioritization, analysis, and decision-making tools. These structured tools, if used correctly, can both move the team forward more quickly and effectively and engage and empower team members and foster team development. There are literally hundreds of these tools and instructions for using them are readily available and mostly free on the internet. **TABLE 8-3** provides

TABLE 8-3 A Sample Listing of Team Tools and Techniques

Meeting Management Tools	Description
Ground rules	A list of behaviors that are acceptable in team meetings.
Meeting objectives or agendas	A description of what the team intends to accomplish in a meeting. Objectives use action words to describe agenda items.
Check-in	A brief discussion at the beginning of a meeting to determine what has happened between meetings and how people feel about it.
Brainstorming	Team members generate a list of ideas on a specific topic. Each idea is written verbatim on a flipchart. While the brainstorming is underway no one questions or analyzes ideas.
Action plans	A list of team action steps describing what will be done, who is accountable, when the task is due, and how success will be measured.
Benefits and concerns statement	A list of the "benefits" of the meeting and "concerns" about the meeting. This is a brainstorming technique with answers listed in two columns.
Values clarification	A set of incomplete sentences that members silently complete. For example "When I think about using data to make decisions, it makes me feel. . . ." This technique is used to explore group feelings and concerns.
Decision-Making Tools	**Description**
Nominal group process	Group members brainstorm and narrow a set of choices. They then vote for their first, second, and third choices.
Multivoting	A form of voting in which each member gets a certain number of votes to allocate among several choices.
Affinity diagram	Used when a large topic needs to be sorted and narrowed. A silent brainstorming with groups of post-it notes. Members generate ideas on a specific topic and then silently move the notes around until categories emerge.

Decision-Making Tools	Description
Forcefield analysis	A brainstorming technique that generates a list of factors that will support a goal and those that will oppose it. The team selects factors to modify as part of an action plan.
Selection matrix	A tool for evaluating choices on multiple factors using a grid. Members give a numeric score to factors such as cost and ease of implementation and then each grid is tallied for total score.

a list of the tools that are most commonly used in healthcare team meetings.

Some sources for structured team tools and techniques include:

- MIND TOOLS (www.mindtools.com)
- The Team Handbook (Scholtes et al., 2003)
- Facilitating with Ease (Bens, 2018)

Barriers to Using Structured Team Tools

New team leaders and facilitators are sometimes reluctant to move beyond simple discussion to using structured tools because they are concerned about getting the sequence right or are fearful of making a mistake. Preparation can go a long way to overcoming these fears. Most of the reference materials on team tools give detailed instructions and, in many cases, timing tips. YouTube provides many examples of the tools being used in actual teams. Seeing an experienced facilitator use the tools can be helpful. You can also prepare by creating a mental picture of each step of the group activity and then practicing it prior to the meeting by yourself or with one or two trial participants. Just remember, it is very likely that team members are far less familiar with the tools than you are. You may know that you have made a mistake, but they probably will not realize it.

Making Team Decisions

Decisions are the heart of every team's work. Good decision-making processes foster team cohesion and ensure that decisions are of good quality—meaning that they take all important factors into account including data, team opinions, management input, and information from authoritative sources.

The end result should be a decision that is in the ultimate best interest of patients, the organization, and team members. Decisions should lead the team step by step toward the goal. The *Team Handbook* (Scholtes et al., 2003) suggests three key guidelines for good decisions:

- **Understand the context of the decision.** What exactly are team members being asked to decide? Check for decision deadlines. Consider the impact of the decision on achieving the ultimate team goals, and on the function of other work units.

- **Gather relevant data.** This should include information about related past, current, and pending decisions. If previous decisions ended in a lack of improvement, find out why.
- **Decide who should be involved.** People who have the authority, those who are accountable for the decision, those who are critically affected by the results, and those who have vital information should be included at least through interviewing or being asked to act as resources, if they are not on the team.

Team Decision-Making Methods

Several common types of decision-making processes are used in healthcare teams. Each is suitable to different types of team structures and situations.

- **Leader-directed decisions.** This common type of decision making is suited to emergency situations or those in which one person's knowledge is clearly superior. It is not recommended as an ongoing method of decision making for a team because it does not elicit all viewpoints and does not develop or empower team members. Eventually (and sometimes quickly) this method can develop considerable resentment among team members.
- **Discussion ending in compromise.** This is the default decision-making choice for many teams who simply talk through meetings, generating many ideas and never really critically evaluating them or using any criteria to select a final choice. By the end of the meeting, some people may suggest moving ahead with one of the alternatives proposed. Other members of the group may not agree but because of time constraints or an unwillingness to engage in deeper discussion or generate controversy they go along. This method is not conducive to good results and often ends in the "silent disagreers" who sabotage or ignore the decision that was made.

- **Voting.** This method is quick, but it creates winners and losers and can create a disgruntled minority. Effective teams do not typically use a "one person, one vote" method, but rather use more nuanced methods such as multivoting. In multivoting, team members each get a certain number of points to apply to decisions (usually 3 points for their top choice option, 2 points for the second choice, and 1 point for the third choice). Members write their vote score next to the various choices on the list. The leader tallies up the votes and the one with the highest score is the team choice. When using this method it can be helpful to have a "devil's advocate" or "pros and cons" discussion of the top choices to ensure that issues and concerns are aired in depth.
- **Consensus.** In this method, the group comes to a decision as a whole, but the decision does not have to be unanimous. Individuals who do not fully agree with the decision can decide to "stand aside" and let the group proceed to implement the decision. If those who disagree are not willing to stand aside the decision cannot be adopted.

  Consensus is the result of extensive group discussion, active listening, paraphrasing, and testing alternatives for flaws. It is not a speedy method of decision making but it is one of the best in terms of effectiveness and likely positive outcomes. Consensus is often confused with compromise, but it is not the same thing. In a consensus decision everyone thoroughly understands the decision and sees the reason for it being accepted. Those who stand aside often do so because of personal views that they feel should not interfere with the team moving ahead. Team member maturity is a necessary prerequisite to successful consensus.

Methods for Improving Decision Making

- **Using evidence.** Obtain data that might shed light on the decision from other teams, the literature, or contacts with other healthcare organizations. Ask for reports or other data from the electronic medical record or billing system if it will help the team.

■ **Devil's advocate.** Encourage members to critique each option to tease out possible limitations, negative impact, or logic flaws.

■ **Elicit minority viewpoints.** Teams tend to focus on information that is known and shared. With the minority viewpoint approach, team members with special knowledge, differing viewpoints, or from other professions weigh in to enrich the discussion of alternatives.

■ **Negative brainstorming.** Once the decision is made, the team should brainstorm all the reasons it might not work and any drawbacks that members see. This ensures that the decision making is truly comprehensive and not the product of "groupthink" (members agreeing to a decision in the interest of harmony or team cohesiveness or because they have all developed a similar viewpoint).

■ **Involving a neutral outside source.** Sometimes, when attitudes harden and the team finds it hard to move forward, bringing in a neutral person from outside the team to weigh in can break a stalemate (Mosser & Begun, 2014).

▶ 6. Develop Team Member Capability

As teams evolve, team members typically fall into certain roles that are natural to their personalities, inclinations, or jobs. Dr. Meredith Belbin has formulated a commonly used list of positive informal roles in teams. Belbin defines team roles as a tendency to behave, contribute, and interrelate with others in a particular way. The Belbin types are somewhat self-explanatory and include the resource investigator, teamworker, implementer, coordinator, evaluator, the plant (creative problem solver), completer/finisher, shaper, and specialist. A balance of these types

within the team membership is necessary to produce the best results (Belbin.com, 2017).

Team leaders can help team members develop positive and functional roles both within team meetings and outside meeting time. Within team meetings, leaders can encourage positive contributions by using reflection and paraphrasing. Team members can be given more challenging assignments to help them grow. Having team members circulate through formal team roles such as recorder and asking them to summarize discussions can help develop communication and analysis skills. Encourage team members to explain their work roles and the contributions they make to the team effort. This will help to develop team respect and will encourage members to call on each other for help. Give formal recognition and rewards for work well done. You can help team members finish challenging assignments by doing some coaching outside meetings.

Use questioning and active listening to guide the team member in thinking through the project. Ask provocative questions such as "What are the pros and cons of using the technique that you are suggesting?"

The leader can use direct constructive feedback techniques to reduce the incidence of negative behavior by team members: "I see that you are texting. Do you need to leave the meeting to take care of something?"

Team Training

Every authority recommends team training as a key element in team building. One survey found that team training has increased in recent years and that this training can improve both teamwork itself and the patient outcomes that result from good teamwork (Weaver et al., 2014). The primary evidence-based program for training in health care is the now familiar Team-STEPPS program. This seven-session program (with five supplemental sessions) is available online from the TeamSTEPPS website (www.ahrq.gov/teamstepps/) for free. The website includes a curriculum, training materials, videos, and participant materials. Topics included in the TeamSTEPPS model are those that are seen in most team-building education including:

- Teamwork principles
- Team structure
- Communication
- Leading teams
- Situation monitoring (monitoring patient status, the environment, and fellow team member ability to function)
- Mutual support

Team training programs typically use classroom techniques, online learning, and videos or a blended approach that uses two or more of these methods.

Participants typically receive "quick guides" or participant manuals. Most other team training programs have been developed for critical inpatient teams such as operating rooms and obstetric teams.

These training programs often use simulations in which the team uses actual medical equipment in an artificial medical environment to practice on theoretical cases.

In health care and especially in smaller organizations, the time, the money, and the will to do extensive training are not always present. If this is the case in your organization, consider just-in-time training in which small chunks of content and some exercises are presented as part of regular team meetings. The TeamSTEPPS material is well suited for this type of training as it is divided into modules and can be broken into learning "chunks."

▶ 7. Build Group Cohesiveness

Shared mental models develop and are reinforced when there is a clear team identity. In some cases, this identity develops naturally over time and in some instances team leaders and members use intentional activities to reinforce identity. Clear team identities are most common in intact work group teams and in improvement teams that have worked together over a long period of time. In intact work groups, identity develops as team members work together, accomplish tasks, and recall shared experiences.

While all of the team-building activities previously mentioned foster group identity, a shared culture, symbols, and language help foster the development of group cohesion and identity. Team identity can involve activities as varied as team names, rituals, workplace decoration, storytelling, celebrations of success, posting pictures, use of social media, and visible team participation in company activities. For example, one SNF team intentionally developed a very clear identity by decorating their physical space with amusing stuffed animals and bringing in home-cooked snacks for every conceivable occasion.

Team identity activities like these should arise spontaneously from the team and not be imposed. Artificially contrived team identity activities may create cynicism about activities that do not seem relevant or sincere to team members. Another way to develop team cohesiveness is to deliberately foster team effectiveness characteristics such as backup behavior. As team leaders encourage members to mentor, coach, support, and jump in to help each other, cohesiveness will develop.

Shared success in problem solving is another component of team cohesiveness development. Nothing builds mutual respect like a job well done. As an example, a team of medical secretaries in a medical practice joined an improvement team designed to reduce the cycle time for returning signed orders. Prior to the start of the team there had been considerable conflict between members of the group and frequent instances of individuals saying "that's not my job." After a grueling 6 months of data analysis and testing solutions, the team was able to reduce the order cycle time by half and save the company thousands of dollars. The team received extensive public recognition for its efforts. Over the course of the group's work, members coalesced as a team, helping each other with training, collecting data, and pitching in when another team member was overloaded. A team identity and cohesiveness developed and persisted long after the team finished its work.

▶ 8. Troubleshoot Team Problems

Any time that health professionals with different training, different personalities, and different life experiences work together in groups, issues and conflicts will arise. Indeed, as we have seen, "storming" is one of the normal stages of team development. Some of the more common team problems and obstacles include:

- **Fuzzy goals and team frustration.** Teams that do not have clear goals will spend meeting after meeting "just talking" and not accomplishing anything. If this happens, the team leader must return to the goal statement or the work team's purpose and expected outcome measures and refocus the team or enlist a senior manager to help.
- **Lack of role clarity.** This issue creates confusion and sometimes conflicts with other team members. The leader must be alert to confusion and must better define roles or work assignments. Roles can also interfere with communication if there is a status difference between group members. The leader must use effective group process to overcome these difference, creating a space for support staff or lower ranking professionals to offer ideas.
- **Team meeting dysfunction.** The most common dysfunction is "free for all" meetings in which there is endless talk without any structure or any issue resolution. The consistent use of team meeting structures will prevent this problem. In other cases, the team may wander off the topic and get embroiled in irrelevant issues. An inability to come to closure on decisions is another

meeting dysfunction that frequently occurs. Some solutions include looking at data, having more focused discussion, using a "pros and cons" or forcefield analysis chart to help the team sort out its options, and bringing in a neutral outsider to weigh in on the decision.

- **Negative or destructive team member behaviors.** This is the most dangerous type of team problem and one that must be managed decisively by team leaders. The team leader must give immediate feedback to members who make frequent negative comments, who attack other team members, who do other work in team meetings, who are on their phones during the meeting, or who refuse to participate in team activities or action plans.

  It is the job of the team leader to ensure that members feel safe within the boundaries of the team and that all team members are treated fairly. Of particular importance is safeguarding the feedback process. In situations in which team member feedback is essential to patient safety, the leader must ensure that all team members have an opportunity to be heard and that no one is ridiculed or ignored during team discussions.

- **Lack of organizational support.** Teams that do not get needed time, resources, encouragement, and feedback from higher level managers will not be able to achieve their goals and will most likely leave the team feeling resentful or even bitter and distrustful of the organization. Team leaders must sell the benefits of their teams' work and advocate for adequate team resources.

▶ Take the Team Tune-Up Assessment

Now that you understand the basic principles of team building, take the Team Tune-Up Assessment in **TABLE 8-4** to see how well your team rates on key elements of effective teamwork.

TABLE 8-4 Team Tune-Up Assessment

Team Success Factors	Rate how well your team is doing by answering "yes," "partially," or "no" to each question.	Improvement Ideas
The team leader and facilitator support effective teamwork.	Yes Partially No	
The team has had training in teamwork competencies.	Yes Partially No	
Management has provided support and resources.	Yes Partially No	
The team has clear and measurable goals.	Yes Partially No	
Data indicate that goals are being met.	Yes Partially No	
The team has functional structures and regular, productive meetings.	Yes Partially No	
Team member satisfaction is high (using TeamSTEPPS or other assessment tool).	Yes Partially No	
Patients are involved in clinical teams or are the focus of the team.	Yes Partially No	
The team demonstrates effective group process.	Yes Partially No	
Team member contributions are maximized and supported.	Yes Partially No	
Team member challenging behaviors are minimized and managed.	Yes Partially No	
Team issues, concerns, and dissatisfaction are well managed.	Yes Partially No	
The team is doing well on Big Five teamwork.	Yes Partially No	
The team relates and coordinates well with other teams and departments.	Yes Partially No	

🔍 CASE STUDY

Tuning Up the Teams

The Everford Team Committee adopted a series of team structures and decided to loosely adopt the TeamSTEPPS program framework for its team-building efforts. After learning more about the elements of effective teamwork, committee members attended various project and work group teams to observe teamwork in action.

They found an uneven level of team meeting and team function effectiveness. One issue of particular concern was the shallowness of the decision-making process being used in most teams. With the help of the quality assurance department facilitators, the committee decided to embark on more extensive group dynamics and decision-making training for team leaders.

In the case of some dysfunctional groups, the trained facilitators were deployed to assess the reasons for team dysfunction and suggest remedies. In several instances, the issues were lack of clarity about goals, poorly managed meetings, and underlying issues of interpersonal conflict. In each of these situations, the facilitators, acting as process consultants, role modeled and coached the team leaders for more effective behaviors. In one instance, a serious issue of conflicts between professional groups of two different cultures came to light. This issue required intervention from both human resources and senior management.

The Team Committee presented its final report to senior management after a year of team-building work. The problems of teamwork had by no means been fully solved, but audits were showing fewer communication and teamwork-related patient safety issues, scores on corporate metrics were improving, and employee satisfaction survey scores rated teamwork more positively.

▶ Chapter Summary

Teamwork has proved to be an essential element in achieving connected care and ensuring patient safety. Teamwork in health care has evolved since the turn of the 21st century, particularly with the development of evidence-based team training techniques based on those developed in the aviation industry. Healthcare teams vary in size and composition from simple interdisciplinary communication between two clinicians to multitiered improvement teams. A particular challenge for health care is ad hoc teams that consist of individuals who happen to be caring for the same patients at the same time and in the same place but without team identity. Solutions such as standardized processes and roles help to achieve effective teamwork in these circumstances.

Team effectiveness in health care is measured by clinical outcomes and patient and clinician satisfaction. Special instruments that measure team cohesion and effectiveness are also used. Team success factors include effective team leadership, team training, clear goals, roles and boundaries, and structures such as team huddles or complex case conferences that support clinical teamwork. Effective healthcare team building requires good meeting structure, management of team process and task work, and good facilitation skills. There are a variety of structured team tools and techniques that can be employed to improve team decision making and action planning. Team development in health care faces a number of obstacles such as lack of time for training or team meetings and lack of support within the organizational culture. Organizations that plan to succeed at achieving the quadruple aim embed teamwork into their culture and allocate the resources necessary to achieve it successfully.

References

Agency for Healthcare Research and Quality. (2012). *Observing patient care rounds*. Rockville, MD: AHRQ. Retrieved from http://www.ahrq.gov/professionals/education /curriculum-tools/cusptoolkit/toolkit/obsrounds.htm

Agency for Healthcare Research and Quality. (2018). TeamSTEPPS® 2.0. Rockville, MD: AHRQ. Retrieved from http://www.ahrq.gov/teamstepps/instructor/index .html

Andreatta, P. B. (2010). A typology for health care teams. *Health Care Management Review, 35*(3). 345–354. Retrieved from http://journals.lww.com/hcmrjournal/Fulltext/2010 /10000/A_typology_for_health_care_teams.7.aspx

Aston Centre for Health Service. (2011). Organisation research team working and team effectiveness in health care. *Findings from the Health Care Team Effectiveness Project*. Retrieved from http://homepages.inf.ed.ac.uk /jeanc/DOH-glossy-brochure.pdf

Bachiochi, P., O'Connor, M., Rogelberg, S., & Elder, A. (2000). The qualities of an effective team leader. *Organization Development Journal, 18*(1).

Baker, D., Battles, J., & King, H. (2017). New insights about team training from a decade of TeamSTEPPS. PS (Patient Safety) Net. Retrieved from psnet.ahrq.gov/perspectives/perspective /218/new-insights-about-team-training-from-a-decade -of-teamstepps

Belbin.com. (2017). About team roles. Retrieved from http:// www.belbin.com/about/belbin-team-roles/

Bens, I. (2018). *Facilitating with ease!* Hoboken, NJ: John Wiley & Sons.

Center for Excellence in Primary Care. (2013). Healthy Huddles. University of California San Francisco. Retrieved from https://cepc.ucsf.edu/healthy-huddles

Dow, A. (2013). Applying organizational science to healthcare, a framework for collaborative practice. *Academy of Medicine, 88*(7), 952–957. doi:10.1097/ACM.0b013e31829523d1

Edmondson, A. (2015, December 15). The kinds of teams health care needs. *Harvard Business Review*.

Hackman, R. (2004). What makes for a great team? American Psychological Association, Psychological Science Agenda. Retrieved from http://www.apa.org/science/about/psa /2004/06/hackman.Hackmanaspx

Harvey, D., & Brown, D. (2003). *An experiental approach to organizational development* (6th ed.). Upper Saddle River, NJ: Prentice Hall.

Huertas, A., Glasheen-Wray, M. B., & Price, N. (2016). It takes a village to stay at home. Christiana Care VNA, Poster Session, Visiting Nurse Association of America Leadership Conference.

Institute for Healthcare Improvement. (2015). How-to guide: Multidisciplinary rounds. Retrieved from IHI.org

Institute for Healthcare Improvement. (2017). Use regular huddles and staff meetings to plan production and to optimize team communication. Retrieved from http://www .ihi.org/resources/Pages/Changes/UseRegularHuddlesand StaffMeetingstoPlanProductionandtoOptimizeTeam Communication.aspx

Institute of Medicine. (2001). *Crossing the quality chasm: a new health system for the 21st century*. Washington, DC: National Academy Press.

The Joint Commission. (2017, March 1). The essential role of leadership in developing a safety culture. *Sentinel Event Alert, 57*. Retrieved from www.jointcommission .org/assets/1/18/SEA_57_Safety_Culture_Leadership _0317.pdf

Kalisch, B., Curley, M., & Stefanov, X. S. (2007). An intervention to enhance nursing staff teamwork and engagement. *The Journal of Nursing Administration, 37*(2), 77–84.

Kalisch, B. Weaver, S., & Salas, E. (2009). What does nursing teamwork look like? A qualitative study.. *Journal of Nursing Care Quality, 24*(4), 298–307. doi: 10.1097 /NCQ.0b013e3181a001c0

Kohn, L. T., Corrigan, J. M., & Donaldson, M. S. (2000). *To err is human: Building a safer health system*. Washington, DC: National Academy Press, Institute of Medicine.

Lemieux-Charles, L., & McGuire, W. (2006). What do we know about healthcare team effectiveness? A review of the literature. *University of Toronto Medical Care Research and Review, 63*(3), 263–300. doi:10.1177/1077558706287003

Mayfield, M. (2010). Case study: The business of caregiving, Ararat Nursing Facility. PHI, Quality Care Through Quality Jobs. Retrieved from http://iwer.mit.edu/wp -content/uploads/2016/11/Arat.pdf

Meterko, M., Mohr, D., & Young, G. (2004). Teamwork culture and patient satisfaction in hospitals. *Medical Care, 42*(5), 492–498.

Mickan, S.M. (2005). Evaluating the effectiveness of health care teams. *Australian Health Review, 29*(2), 211–217.

Miller, C. J., Kim, B., Silverman, A., & Bauer, M. S. (2018). A systematic review of team-building interventions in non-acute healthcare settings. *BMC Health Services Research, 18*(1). doi:10.1186/s12913-018-2961-9

Mitchell, P., Wynia, M., Golden, R., McNellis, B., Okun, S., Webb, C. E., . . . Von Kohorn, I. (2012, October 2). Core principles & values of effective team-based health care. Discussion Paper. Washington, DC: Institute of Medicine.

Mosser, G., & Begun, J. (2014). Understanding teamwork in healthcare. New York: McGraw Hill Medical.

Office of the Inspector General. (2013). SNF Discharge Planning PowerPoint. Retrieved from https://oig.hhs. gov/oei/reports

Pigeon, Y., & Khan, O. (2017). Leadership lesson: Tools for effective team meetings—how I learned to stop worrying and love my team. American Association of Medical Colleges. Retrieved from https://www.aamc .org/members/gfa/faculty_vitae/148582/team_meetings .htm

Risser, D., Rice, M., Salisbury, M. L., Simon, R., Jay, G. D., & Berns, S. D. (1999). The potential for improved teamwork to reduce medical errors in the emergency department. *Annals of Emergency Medicine, 34*(3), 373–383.

Salas, E., Dickinson, T. L., & Converse, S. A. (1992). Toward an understanding of team performance and training. In: R. W. Swezey and E. Salas (Eds.), *Teams: Their training and performance* (pp. 3–29). Norwood, NJ: Ablex Publishing Corporation.

Salas, E., Sims, D. E., & Burke, C. S. (2005). Is there a "Big Five" in Teamwork? *Small Group Research, 36*(5), 555–599. http://dx.doi.org/10.1177/1046496405277134

Schmutz, J., & Manser, T. (2013). Do team processes really have an effect on clinical performance? A systematic literature review. *British Journal of Anaesthesia, 110*(4), 529–544. doi:10.1093/bja/aes513. Epub 2013 Mar 1

Scholtes, P., Joiner, B., & Streibel, B. (2003). *The team handbook* (3rd ed.). Madison, WI: Oriel Incorporated.

Stroke Unit Trialists' Collaboration. (2001). Organised inpatient (stroke unit) care for stroke (Cochrane Review). *The Cochrane Library, 3.* Oxford: Update Software.

Sullivan, N. (2013). Preventing in-facility pressure ulcers. In: *Making health care safer II: An updated critical analysis of the evidence for patient safety practices.* Rockville, MD: Agency for Healthcare Research and Quality. (Evidence Reports/Technology Assessments, No. 211.) Chapter 21. Retrieved from https://www.ncbi.nlm.nih.gov/books/NBK133388

Tuckman, B. W. (1965). 'Developmental sequence in small groups.' *Psychological Bulletin, 63,* 384–399. The article was reprinted in *Group Facilitation: A Research and Applications Journal, 3*(Spring 2001).

U.S. Army. (2015). *Handbook 15-02, Leader's guide to teambuilding, building adaptive, high performance teams.* Fort Leavenworth, KS: Center for Army Lessons Learned.

Weaver, S., Dy, S., & Rosen, M. (2014). Team-training in healthcare: A narrative synthesis of the literature. *British Medical Journal, BMJ Quality and Safety, 23*(5), 359–372. doi:10.1136/bmjqs-2013-001848. Epub 2014 Feb.

Xyrichis, A., & Ream, E. (2008). Teamwork: A concept analysis. *Journal of Advanced Nursing, 61*(2), 232–241. doi:10.1111/j.1365-2648.2007.04496.x

Yates, G., & Federico, F. (2013). Huddles, developing situational awareness. Slide presentation. Institute for Healthcare Improvement.

CHAPTER 9

Digital Connections, Communication, and Collaboration

CHAPTER OBJECTIVES

After completing this chapter readers will be able to:

- List key elements of the "digital revolution" in health care
- Describe how specific technologies can either fragment or connect care for patients
- Describe connected care digital technology best practices
- Explain key obstacles and pitfalls in the use of technology to achieve connected care
- Assess the effectiveness of their organization's digital technology tools in creating connected care

▶ Introduction

The healthcare industry worldwide is experiencing a massive digital revolution. This revolution ranges from small digital solutions, such as a single medical office electronic medical record, to huge advances such as "big data," predictive analytics, artificial intelligence, and machine learning in which technology actually teaches itself to become more intelligent. In developed countries, the healthcare digital revolution promises to cure a wide variety of health system ills, ranging from patient safety problems and patient disengagement to the inconvenience of traveling in person to see a health professional. Based on the volume of emailed articles and advertising received by the average health professional, it would appear, on the surface, that most recent advances in medical care and service delivery are almost all digital. Hardly a minute goes by without an email touting "wearables," "telemedicine," "data analytics saves the day," "new tracking system guarantees value based purchasing success." The constant barrage of digital product advertising is characteristic of the first two decades of the 21st century, which have been a kind of "wild west" environment in which digital health tools are being developed, capitalized, deployed, and discarded at a dizzying rate.

In the healthcare literature, the term "connected care" is often synonymous with technology, especially in the area of patient engagement. However, newer technologies, while impressive and useful, are often optimized to achieve strategic and financial goals for the healthcare organizations that purchase them, and may be less useful in actually providing a seamless and integrated patient experience.

Since the creators and distributors of each technology seek to promote their own proprietary product, there are currently minimal incentives to link and coordinate them except at the national or integrated health system level.

In this chapter we will explore a few aspects of the vast array of technologies that are transforming the healthcare landscape. We will conduct a basic assessment of the technology's potential for connected care or worsening fragmentation. We will also examine the interface between technology and human beings—a nexus point where failure can occur, particularly when technology is simply dropped into a clinical workplace without effective optimization and support. We will consider how healthcare technologies, when properly implemented, foster achievement of the quadruple aim, especially in the areas of patient and health professional satisfaction, or when poorly managed, produce the opposite effects of patient dissatisfaction and provider burnout.

We will look at new roles for health professionals in supporting technically literate, engaged, and aware patients and in helping to overcome the digital divide for those other patients without the resources and expertise to easily access and navigate the digital world. We will also address the needs of health professionals for technology education and support. We will pay particular attention to both the role of nurses in using technology to improve patient care and the impact of technology on the work of the nursing profession.

We will consider the many pitfalls of technology implementation such as privacy and cybersecurity issues and will explore best practices in the design, selection, implementation, and utilization of digital technologies by patients and in healthcare organizations.

▶ The Landscape of Healthcare Technology

In the new world of health care, technology is now a member of the healthcare team, albeit a digital or mechanical one. Implementing new technology and constantly upgrading older technologies is now a strategic imperative for healthcare organizations that are trying to navigate the rough waters of regulatory uncertainty and the fits and starts of the volume-to-value shift.

The consulting firm Deloitte, in its *2018 Global Health Care Outlook*, unequivocally states that healthcare organizations must invest in technology to achieve quality outcomes and value. The article describes the conundrum at the heart of healthcare fragmentation: ". . .smart health care is not going to come easy. Clinicians usually have difficulty coordinating appointments and procedures, sharing test results, and involving patients in their treatment plan. In other words, care providers may be working hard but are they working 'smart'?" (p. 5). The article suggests that massive investment in electronic medical records, mobile technology, interoperability (connecting digital information systems), and big data will be necessary to achieve value-based care; however, the authors also suggest, "Organizations should consider strategic investments in people, processes, and premises enabled by digital technologies" (Deloitte, 2018, p. 21).

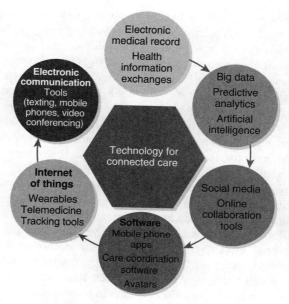

FIGURE 9-1 Technology for Connected Care

This will be a key point to remember as we further discuss the interaction between humans, machines, software, and work processes in health care. **FIGURE 9-1** describes the range of technologies that have an impact on the patient-connected care experience.

For professionals who are on the front lines of health care, technology adoption is moving at a somewhat slower pace than what might be supposed from conferences, journals, and sales pitches to senior healthcare executives. For many health professionals, older technologies such as pagers and fax machines still play a large role in communication, although smartphones are quickly becoming an essential clinical practice tool. Electronic medical records are ubiquitous, but many if not most, are not interoperable with other organizations' records and few are fully optimized for health professional use or patient access. In fact, some recent literature indicates that electronic records play a significant role in health professional burnout (Ommaya et al., 2018). Software for care coordination, patient tracking, and patient engagement management is common, but cutting-edge technologies such

as decision support fueled by artificial intelligence have not yet entered the mainstream of health professional practice.

Organizations are aggregating and analyzing their own population health data, but insights from big data gathered from thousands of patient records, diagnostic testing databases, or healthcare claims are not fully perfected. Data scientists who do this highly specialized and complex analysis are also in short supply and their services are currently too expensive for the average healthcare organization to afford.

The advance of technology in health care has also been limited by strategic and financial considerations. All but the most richly endowed or profitable healthcare organizations are struggling to stay abreast of technological advances while maintaining a viable margin in the face of declining fee-for-service revenues and the relatively slow growth of value-based payment opportunities. Making decisions about which technologies will achieve the quadruple aim and improve profit margins is a key topic in C-suites and board rooms.

Far too many healthcare organizations must use their technology budget simply to meet basic organizational and regulatory requirements rather than to advance innovative care techniques or to improve outcomes—a factor that inhibits the use of technology for connecting care.

For patients, the use of technology very much depends on the person's health problem, access to digital resources, digital literacy, and the technologies being used by the patient's healthcare organization. Researching health issues on the internet is widespread. Wearable monitoring technology (e.g., fitness trackers) is a very popular purchase, but many people abandon them when they fail to integrate the device into their daily routine. Technology can be a great help in chronic disease self-management. A diabetic who is proficient with technology may do extensive internet research, join an online support group, and fine-tune her medication after sending personal data to her health provider. Some older patients may not use digital devices at all or may use computers only for healthcare research and possibly email; but many, especially in the baby boomer generation, are digitally literate and great users of social media. Some older patients also learn to do home telemonitoring (monitoring of vital signs in the home) if they become home healthcare patients.

Families of patients with memory problems may provide personal emergency response systems and automated pill dispensers. Again, however, the patient's comfort level and willingness to use the technology determine how useful it becomes in actually providing connected care. **TABLE 9-1** describes levels of technology adoption in health care.

TABLE 9-1 Levels of Practical Technology Adoption in Health Care

Very Low	Moderately Low	Moderately High	Very High
■ Paper records ■ Phone ■ Fax ■ Pagers ■ No online organizational presence ■ A staff member doubles as information technology (IT) manager	■ Basic electronic medical record (EMR) ■ Phone ■ Fax ■ Email ■ Website and social media for promotional purposes ■ IT department ■ Clinical informatics staff person	■ EMR with patient portal ■ Email ■ Receives referrals through electronic portals ■ Smartphones for staff ■ Secure texting ■ Internal phone system with chat and video ■ Teleconferencing ■ Virtual fax and digital document indexing and storage ■ Enhanced website and intensive social media presence	■ Interoperable EMR ■ Participation in a health information exchange ■ Two-way electronic communication with referral sources during care transitions ■ Patient portal with email and patient entry of medical records data ■ Patient ability to download EMR data ■ Decision support elements embedded in EMR ■ Use of patient remote monitoring ■ Interactive website

Very Low	Moderately Low	Moderately High	Very High
		■ Use of a system that tracks patients between healthcare facilities ■ Ability to abstract and analyze population level data from EMR ■ More extensive IT support ■ Clinical informatics department ■ Data analyst available	■ Provides extensive online content, sponsors online support groups ■ Offers diagnosis and treatment via telemedicine ■ Extensive data and statistical analysis staff ■ Obtains and uses external big data for population health

ASK YOURSELF

- What are the top technologies used by your healthcare organization?
- How many of these technologies are focused on improving patient-centered connected care and how many are designed to meet regulatory requirements, extract quality data, or improve the accuracy of coding and billing?
- How far down the technology road has your organization come? Are you still mainly using older technologies and paper, or have you moved forward into the digital age?

▶ Technology Priorities for Health Care

The Health System's View of Technology Priorities

A survey of 35 of the nation's largest health systems, conducted by the Center for Connected Medicine and the Health Management Academy (2017), revealed that executives' top 2018 information technology (IT) priorities were focused on cybersecurity, but were beginning to tilt more toward patient needs. Specifically, 100% of respondents were planning, in 2018, to promote health and wellness apps to consumers; 17% expect mobile apps to be sources of valuable patient-generated data; over half of respondents (54%) intended to incorporate patient-generated

data into their electronic medical record. Home monitoring equipment, mobile apps, and wearables (self-monitoring devices worn as jewelry or clothing) were predicted to become additional sources of patient-generated data.

At some point, executives predict that patients will begin sharing lifestyle and social data. While there is interest in capturing patient-generated data from wearables there remain a host of issues around security, the lack of uniform data structures, and lack of consumer interest in certain markets.

Respondents do not seem deterred by information from other sources that indicate patients have security and privacy concerns that might seriously inhibit data sharing. Remote telemonitoring and virtual visits were areas of focus for healthcare executives, who almost unanimously believed these tools would become a major priority as health systems take more financial risk.

Reimbursement remains a barrier to more widespread use of virtual monitoring and care. Telemonitoring, which is used by many home health agencies, is not reimbursed by insurance. Telehealth, which provides virtual medical visits, is often covered by insurance. At the heart of decisions about the use of these technologies is cost and profitability, with patient-centered concerns taking a back seat.

The Patient View of Technology Priorities

In a 2016 Deloitte survey of health consumer priorities, "digitally connected to manage health care" ranked as a fourth-level priority below personal care from providers; economics of coverage; and care choice, convenience, and access. This prioritization puts the health care digital revolution into perspective, as it indicates that digital tools, while of interest to patients, lag well behind interpersonal relationships with doctors, the finances of care, and access issues on the patient priority scale. This is in sharp contrast to the sheer volume of healthcare articles and advertising that tout digital patient engagement solutions.

That said, patient interest in and skill with digital technologies is clearly on the rise. Seven in 10 consumers in the survey expressed some interest in the use of digital health care. Telemedicine is the most popular technology, particularly for postsurgical care and chronic disease monitoring. Caregivers who care for others and monitor another person remotely are an important group with an interest in healthcare technology. While there is interest in remote monitoring, only 24% of consumers in the survey used technology to monitor functions such as blood pressure, blood sugar, and breathing.

A key best practice identified by the survey is earning consumer trust by keeping health information safe. Other important actions are including patient caregivers in technology applications, having consistent providers conduct telemedicine visits, and taking consumer

preferences for learning style and type of communication into account. Another point, which is very relevant to connected care, is creating a seamless end-user experience. For example, if the system offers an automated medication list and interaction alert function but no prescription refill option, patients are unlikely to use it (Deloitte Center for Health Solutions, 2016).

▶ Specific Healthcare Technologies and Connected Care

Electronic Medical Records Overview

Electronic medical records (EMRs) are the most common and most comprehensive of the digital healthcare tools currently in use. A well-designed and well-implemented EMR can improve communication, care transitions, care coordination, and teamwork through information sharing among professionals and with patients. Electronic records can be collaborative tools if they span and connect multiple types of healthcare provider organizations.

In a 2016 review of EMR benefits and disadvantages, Alpert (2016) describes the purpose of EMRs: "Access detailed patient information, document patient progress, assist in chronic disease management, facilitate disease coding for billing and disease demographics, improve communication between health care providers with information that is easily accessible and legible, provide health care staff with decision support tools, create educational patient handouts, and help track health maintenance and preventive medical interventions" (p. 48).

An exhaustive review of the literature on the benefits and drawbacks of the EMR (Menachemi & Collum, 2011) found extensive evidence that the electronic record improves outcomes and enhances patient safety. In one example, reminders embedded in the EMR increased the use of pneumonia and flu immunizations from almost zero to 35% to 50%.

Computerized alerts that are part of a computerized order entry system prompted a 19% increase in the use of anticoagulant therapy for patients at high risk of deep vein thrombosis. An Agency for Healthcare Research and Quality (AHRQ) review of medical errors and EMRs found that in a group of Pennsylvania hospitals, those using an advanced EMR had a 27% drop in adverse events, which was fueled by a 30% drop in events caused by medication errors (AHRQ, 2016). Electronic records allow healthcare providers to share medical history as well as diagnostic and treatment information among themselves, and in some cases with patients; this approach can greatly improve the level of connected care and reduce the incidence of medical errors.

Types of Electronic Medical Records

There are two important types of digital health records. One, the EMR, is a digital version of the paper chart used in a facility or clinician office. The EMR contains the medical history, diagnostic test results, and notes from clinical visits. The EMR is usually for shared use only by physicians and other clinicians within that practice. EMRs are typically not designed to share clinical information outside the boundaries of the organization that owns them. Second, some define electronic health records (EHRs) as a different and more comprehensive type of EMR. The EHR contains information from the EMR and also from other health providers who care for a patient such as laboratories, diagnostic facilities, and hospitals (HealthIT.gov, 2011).

As of 2015, the Centers for Disease Control and Prevention (CDC) reported that 86.9% of physicians were using EMRs. Some of these physicians were still using a basic system, which is defined as a system that has all of the following functionalities: patient history and demographics, patient problem lists, physician clinical notes, comprehensive list of patients' medications and

allergies, computerized orders for prescriptions, and ability to electronically view laboratory and imaging results (CDC, 2017).

Benefits of Electronic Records

The U.S. government is a highly enthusiastic proponent of EMRs and it has gone to great lengths to encourage the widespread and appropriate use of these electronic tools. The HealthIT.gov (2018a) website touts the many benefits of EMR use:

- Improved patient care
- Improved care coordination
- Increased patient participation
- Practice efficiencies and cost savings

One of the primary benefits of the EMR, when it is used correctly, is a reduction in medical errors. The EMR accomplishes this goal through improved legibility, automated warnings about drug interactions, rapid access to lab test results, and providing complete and sequential patient information that is available to all providers who use the EMR (HealthIT. gov, 2018a).

EMR Regulations and Incentives

As part of its unreserved enthusiasm for the adoption of the EMR, the U.S. government has promulgated a number of rules, regulations, and incentives to push the healthcare industry toward universal adoption of both EMRs and interoperable EHRs. The Health Information Technology for Economic and Clinical Health (HITECH) Act of 2009, which incentivized health care (primarily doctors and hospitals) for "meaningful use" of EMRs, was the earliest and most far reaching of those regulations. New regulations for physician value-based payment, called "promoting interoperability," have replaced "meaningful use" for physicians, but the goals of the program remain the same:

- Improve quality, safety, efficiency; and reduce health disparities
- Engage patients and family

- Improve care coordination, population health, and public health
- Maintain privacy and security of patient health information

There is a variety of meaningful use criteria but some of those most relevant to connected care are security risk analysis, e-prescribing, patient access through a patient portal, and send/receive summary of care documents. To obtain program incentives, providers must use an EMR that is certified by the Office of the National Coordinator for Health IT (ONC). The certification standards ensure that the EMR has the necessary technological capability, functionality, and security to meet meaningful use criteria (HealthIT.gov, 2018b).

Patient Perceptions of Electronic Medical Records

A study by Rose, Richter, and Kapustin (2014) addressed the effect of the EMR on patient perceptions of communication in medical visits during and after a clinic transition from paper to electronic records. Focus group interviews with patients in a diabetes clinic in a major urban medical center revealed mostly positive perceptions of the EMR with some caveats. Communication was enhanced when the provider alternately looked at and talked to the patient and then consulted the electronic record and typed in information. It was important to patients that the provider made eye contact and did not turn away from the patient while typing. Some providers positioned the computer so patients could see what was in the record. Patients stated a positive preference for the EMR because it reduced the incidence of providers repeating questions that others had already asked. Patients liked the fact that the EMR provided quicker access to lab test results and they also appreciated the ability to see their data graphed to show changes over time. Patients in the study felt that information in the EMR was more likely to be accurate and would not get lost as easily as information in

paper records. Patients were somewhat disconcerted by the slowness of documentation, and sometimes confusion, that arose when providers were learning the new EMR. Once the provider became comfortable and adept with the new equipment this issue lessened.

A study of patient perceptions of EMR use by residents and attending physicians at the University of Chicago Primary Care Clinic revealed that patients liked certain aspects of EMR use. Overall 85% of patient comments were coded as positive. Patients thought that the EMR promoted efficiency by allowing doctors to read each other's notes and promoted teamwork. Patients also liked physicians engaging them in the information contained in the EMR by discussing what was written and by showing the patient charts and graphs of their lab tests or progress. Quick access to test results and readily available information about upcoming appointments was also a positive for study patients. Patients in the study perceived some major negatives in the physician use of the EMR, one being lack of eye contact, physician focus on the screen, and long silences while the physician typed. As one patient noted, "I just want my doctor's undivided attention. . .the computer takes them away from focusing on you" (p. 1317.) The other negative was a lack of transparency about what the physician was writing in the EMR. Patients perceived a decreased quality of care when this occurred. Another issue for patients was the widespread sharing of information in the EMR and perceived lack of privacy. Others worried about accuracy in what was entered into the computer (Lee et al., 2016).

Clinician Perceptions of Electronic Medical Records

The electronic record has gone from a curiosity to an almost universal tool for clinicians. For many it has become part of contemporary medical life. Those clinicians who have weathered the transition from paper to electronic systems, however, have perceived pros and cons. The cost of EMRs is high, and the level of effort to scan in old records to make the transition away from paper has been disruptive in many settings. Most clinicians feel positive about the reduction in medical errors that has resulted from the use of computerized order entry, ready access to calculators and online reference tools, and decision support systems. Clinicians also feel that easy access to lab, radiology, and medication data and notes from other clinicians is a good way to coordinate care for patients. Others find that the EMR helps them work more productively, particularly if they do point-of-service charting while they are with the patient.

For those clinicians with less well developed technical (and typing) skills and those without the patience to thoroughly learn the EMR, the electronic record is perceived as a stressor and a barrier to productivity. Technical failures, forced use of predesigned templates, and lack of support in solving technical problems are other barriers to effective EMR use.

EMR Issues and Concerns

A recent paper from the National Academy of Medicine (Ommaya et al., 2018) addresses the role of EMRs in clinician burnout. The most glaring problem identified is the huge amount of time and effort needed to enter data and to find relevant information within the EMR. Some estimate that doctors and nurses spend half their time in documentation when in the clinical setting and, as a result, perform other clinical and administrative tasks after hours.

Another issue is that templates, cut-and-paste functions, check boxes, and pulldown menus often create a hodgepodge of clinical information, some of which is repetitious and irrelevant. This leads to the process of "foraging" for relevant information—a frustrating activity that requires considerable clinician time and effort. These issues are often driven by a record that is more designed to support coding and billing than to support clinical care needs.

Apparently, EMRs have not yet solved the problem identified by Florence Nightingale in 1863: "I have applied everywhere for information, but in scarcely an instance have I been able to find hospital records fit for any purpose of comparison" (p. 173). In these situations, the electronic record is a fragmenting and not a connecting factor in patient care.

An international study of nurses' satisfaction with EMRs describes their concerns about these tools: "Two-thirds of more educated and more experienced study participants (n=283), mostly from Europe and Americas, provided alarming comments explaining low satisfaction rankings. More than one-half of the comments identified issues at the system level (poor system usability; lack of integrated systems and poor interoperability; lack of standards & standardization; limited functionality/missing components), followed by user–task issues (systems fail to meet nursing clinical needs; systems are not nursing specific) and environment issues (low prevalence of computerized systems; lack of user's training)" (Topaz, Ronquillo, Lee, & Peltonen, 2017, p. 1).

Solutions recommended by the Academy of Medicine (Ommaya et al., 2018) include making clinicians responsible only for documentation that supports patient care; designing EMRs with better capability for easy, relevant data retrieval; allowing assistants to document billing-related data after confirming their accuracy with patients; and having CMS deemphasize documentation as a requirement for payment.

Clinicians as well as patients are concerned about possible security breaches and misuse of clinical and patient data. Widespread and widely publicized data breaches have eroded patients' comfort level with EMR safety and security, creating an issue that may become an obstacle to achieving the full potential of EMRs in patient-centered connected care. An international cyberattack, using software stolen from the U.S. National Security Agency, crippled parts of the U.K. National Health System in May 2017 and certainly fanned these fears (FoxNews Health, 2017).

Telling the Patient's Story with the EMR

In an online blog post, Dr. Christopher Johnson, a pediatric critical care specialist, describes how the EMR, while vastly useful, can obscure or eliminate the patient story if clinicians rely on templates and "drag and paste" notes. He recommends a way to use electronic tools while telling the story: "For myself, even though I, of course, use the EMR, I refuse to use all those handy smart text templates. It takes me longer, but I type out my progress notes, organized as I did when I used a pen and chart paper. It takes me a little longer, but it makes me think things through. No billing coder has ever complained. More than a few colleagues have told me, that when we share patients, that they search through the EMR to find one of my notes to understand what is happening with the patient. My advice to other doctors is this: don't let the templates get in your way. Tell the story" (Johnson, 2012).

Digital Disconnects—The Interoperability Problem

The EMR is on its way to becoming almost universally used, but *interoperability,* in which records can be shared between different facilities and providers, is a work in progress and the source of much care fragmentation and frustration to both clinicians and patients. The Healthcare Information and Management Systems Society (HIMSS; 2013) defines interoperability as "the ability of different information technology systems and software applications to communicate, exchange data, and use the information that has been exchanged. Data exchange schema and standards should permit data to be shared across clinician, lab, hospital, pharmacy, and patient regardless of the application or application vendor" (p. 1).

Dr. Christine Laine, editor-in-chief of the *Annals of Internal Medicine,* described the interoperability problem in an interview with *Medical Economics*: "While EHRs offer lots of potential benefits to patient care, the biggest limitation is the lack of interoperability between different EHRs. The fact that there's a proliferation of EHRs that don't talk to each other is a barrier to realizing the true benefits you can get from HIT" (McBride, 2012, p. 1).

The 2017 update of *Vital Directions*, a roadmap for positive change in the U.S. healthcare system from the National Academy of Medicine, cites interoperability as a core project that requires sweeping solutions. The document states: "Agreeing to standards for interoperability, ensuring their systemwide application, working out use and privacy protocols, ensuring interface and personal access capacities for individuals, and embedding analytic tools for continuous learning are all feasible and their accomplishment would establish the infrastructure for transformative multisystem, multisector initiatives enabling life course–oriented strategies for health improvement" (Dzau, McClellan, McGinnis, & Finkelman, 2017, p. 60).

🔎 CASE STUDY

We All Have a Different EMR

Consider a recent gathering sponsored by a state medical society in a state that does not have any type of electronic data exchange. About 40 participants attended a seminar designed to promote participation in a new medical society–sponsored health information interchange. The speaker asked participants to describe their medical record systems. About 75% of participants had EMR systems and about 25% were still using paper records. Of those who had EMRs, nine different EMR brands were represented. Only those medical groups that were part of an accountable care organization (ACO) or which had signed on to the EPIC electronic health record used by the two large state hospital systems had any ability to communicate with the hospital medical record or with other providers. All other EMRs were completely "stand alone" and could not communicate with each other.

Health Information Exchanges

Because it is highly unlikely that every provider in the United States will ever adopt the same EMR system, health information exchanges (HIEs) provide the best interoperability solution. HIEs are electronic systems that capture, aggregate, organize, and share patient data from and between multiple clinical sources. HIE provides the capability to electronically move clinical information among disparate healthcare information systems (HIMSS, 2014). The website HealthIT.gov (2017a) explains it this way: "Health information exchange allows doctors, nurses, pharmacists and other health care providers to securely share a patient's vital medical information electronically—reducing the need for the patient to transport their medical history, lab results, images or prescriptions between health professionals." Many HIEs are sponsored and run by states. Others are private and proprietary and some are hybrid models in which an ACO and a vendor collaborate to create an exchange. The primary function of the HIE is to consolidate health information. This information usually includes the following:

- Provider clinical data (laboratory results, emergency room notes, medication lists, discharge summaries, progress notes, radiology results, and surgical notes)
- Patient encounter data by site of service
- Payer and provider cost and claims data
- Pharmaceutical data
- Quality data
- Public health data such as immunization registries and disease surveillance

The collected data can be used for the purposes of care coordination, reducing preventable readmissions, providing patient access to clinical information, informing policy decisions, determining patient outcomes, and identifying trends and patterns in data for research and clinical services design purpose (HIMSS, 2014).

HIEs, particularly those that allow both providers and patients to access the entirety of patients' personal health data, are clearly powerful tools for connected care. Exchanges can also play a key role in care transitions by tracking patient encounters through the delivery system. **FIGURE 9-2** illustrates different levels of EMR integration from the health professional's viewpoint.

Patient Access to EMRs

A personal health record (PHR) is an electronic system that allows patients to access and manage their health information in a secure environment. Personal electronic health records foster connected care by making care more patient centered, providing patients with comprehensive and current information about their care, and improving patient/clinician communication. The most common type of PHR is "tethered" to a medical office electronic record.

The tethered PHR allows patients to access their own medical information in a physician's EMR through a type of electronic window called a "portal." The tethered system or portal is currently by far the most common form of PHR (Vydra, Cuaresma, Kretovics, & Bose-Brill, 2015). Another type of PHR is "untethered." This type of record is not connected to a physician or hospital record. The untethered PHR is often an internet-based service that allows patients to obtain or enter and maintain their own personal medical information in an online system.

Recently, Apple caused a stir in the market with its announcement of an enhancement to the existing iPhone health app, that allows users to access their own medical data from participating providers. The app allows

ASK YOURSELF

Is your organization's EMR a tool for connected care or is it part of the care fragmentation problem? **BOX 9-1** allows you to see how many of the criteria are met by your EMR.

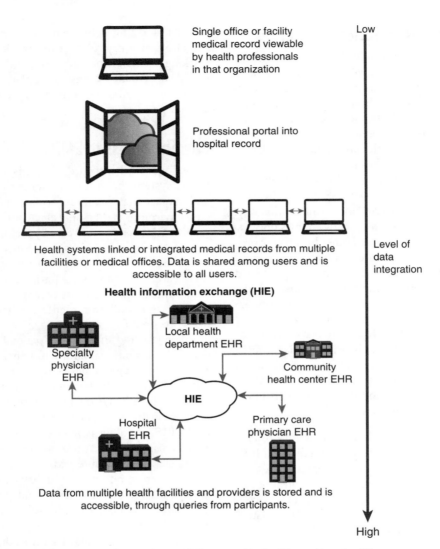

Single office or facility medical record viewable by health professionals in that organization

Professional portal into hospital record

Health systems linked or integrated medical records from multiple facilities or medical offices. Data is shared among users and is accessible to all users.

Health information exchange (HIE)

Specialty physician EHR

Local health department EHR

Community health center EHR

HIE

Hospital EHR

Primary care physician EHR

Data from multiple health facilities and providers is stored and is accessible, through queries from participants.

Low

Level of data integration

High

FIGURE 9-2 The Professional View of Electronic Medical Record Levels of Data Integration

BOX 9-1   Checklist of Factors That Make the EMR a Connected Care Tool

- ❑ Institute the most robust security and privacy controls.
- ❑ Involve clinicians in EMR configuration and optimization efforts.
- ❑ Choose and implement a system that supports clinical care needs as much as coding/billing needs.
- ❑ Optimize medical record screen design and workflows to reduce clinician level of effort.
- ❑ Utilize EMR functionality to provide charts and graphs of patient progress over time (such as vital sign or lab test result line graphs).

- ❏ Provide thorough training and mentoring for clinicians, especially those who are less technically proficient.
- ❏ Provide client-centered help desk and clinical informatics support during all hours of operation.
- ❏ Create internal knowledge bases and training programs for clinicians with cheat sheets, user-friendly reference guides, and "tips and tricks" guides.
- ❏ Set expectations for point-of-service charting and provide teaching and mentoring to help clinicians incorporate the process in a patient-centered way.
- ❏ Participate in EMR vendor-sponsored listservs, online forums, and webinars to learn about the full potential of the system and to find solutions for common problems.
- ❏ Perform recommended upgrades on a regular basis and minimize any resultant disruption to clinician workflows.
- ❏ Integrate the organization EMR with other provider EMRs or participate in a health information exchange.

patients to enter and track their own health information and can integrate information from multiple sources, giving patients a more complete portfolio of personal health data (Apple Newsroom, 2018).

Patient Portals

The tethered personal health record or patient portal is a secure online website that gives patients convenient 24-hour access to personal health information from anywhere there is an internet connection. Using a secure username and password, patients can view health information such as recent doctor visits, discharge summaries, medications, and appointment information (HealthIT.gov, 2017b).

The Advisory Board (2014) lists these "must have" features of patient portals:

- Secure messaging with providers
- View test results
- View immunizations
- View medications and allergies
- Account review and bill pay
- Explanations of medical information (e.g., Group Health of Puget Sound added an online database of plain language information about lab tests, procedures, medications, and diagnoses)
- Family access (i.e., patients also want their family members to be able to access their

medical information via their provider's patient portal)

CDW Healthcare's *2017 Patient Engagement Perspectives Study* states that 74% of patients have joined an online patient portal (up from 45% in 2016). Of patients in the study, 81% were offered an opportunity to sign up for a portal. In 2016 only 34% of patients over age 50 say they used patient portals. In the 2017 survey the percentage had risen to 53%. Of these patients, 70% said they had become more engaged with their health care in the past 2 years (up from 57%) and the main reason was greater online access to personal healthcare records and access to online patient portals.

A 2016 report from the American Hospital Association found that 92% of hospitals allowed patients to view their medical records; 84% allowed patients to download their medical records information, and 70% allowed a referral summary to be sent to a third party.

Hospital patient portals were found to help patients complete routine medical tasks online, including to refill prescriptions, schedule appointments, and pay bills.

Some (63%) of these hospital portals also allowed patients to send and receive messages from their health providers. A smaller number (37%) of hospitals allowed patients to submit data for inclusion in the EMR (American Hospital Association, 2016).

The Open Notes Movement

The Open Notes Movement is an international movement that is designed to make patient care more open and transparent by having health professionals share their notes with patients through patient portals. Open Notes is not a technology. It is an approach to sharing medical records data with patients. The Open Notes approach is a far more patient-centered type of clinical record sharing than simply having a patient sign on to a portal and then checking off one more meaningful use requirement. The Open Notes website explains the benefits of this approach to patients: "Information is power. Access to your medical information can help you ask better questions and make more confident decisions about your health. Whether you're reviewing your treatment plan or thinking through different care options, the ability to read, review, and refer back to your notes makes it easier for you and care professionals to make informed, thoughtful decisions. Having access to what your doctor writes deepens the trust between you and your health care team. It's a win-win" (Open Notes, 2017).

A study of the use of Open Notes by 100 primary care physicians published in the *Annals of Internal Medicine* found that 80% of patients read at least one note and 99% wanted the use of Open Notes to continue.

The majority of patients felt more in control of their health, better understood their medical issues, remembered their plans of care, and felt better prepared for office visits. Another significant finding was that patients who accessed Open Notes were more likely to take their medications as prescribed. Physicians in the study found that the use of Open Notes did not increase their work load or stress level. One comment from the study summarized a physician's experiences: "My fears: Longer notes, more questions, and messages from patients. In reality, it was not a big deal" (Delbanco et al., 2012, p. 467).

The Open Notes website suggests several best practices for clinicians:

- **Talk with the patient about information that is documented in the record**. This builds trust and creates clarity for both patient and clinician.
- **Avoid jargon and abbreviations that might be misunderstood.** For example, instead of writing SOB, write "shortness of breath."
- **Offer a balanced perspective.** Document the patient's strengths as well as challenges, especially when writing about mental health issues. This helps the patient and other clinicians see the illness in a broader context and may open up new methods of support.

ASK YOURSELF

- Do clinicians in your organization share notes with patients either by reviewing them at the point of service as they create notes, or through sharing notes with patients through a patient portal?
- How does your organization and your clinicians perceive the pros and cons of sharing clinical notes with patients?
- Looking at a clinical note that either you or a colleague has recently written, how might you want to rewrite it if you knew a patient was going to read it?

Patient Portal Benefits and Issues

Patient portals are clearly digital systems that can improve patient-connected care, but with some reservations. Portals provide patients with convenient access to health data at any time or on any day. Portals are also an easy way to perform healthcare tasks such as paying bills and getting prescription refills.

They can improve outcomes and reduce missed appointment and wasted provider time through automated reminders. For providers, portals are a way to reduce labor and paper by automating tasks that were formerly performed by a secretary or receptionist. On the other hand, a significant number of people do not sign up for or use portals regularly. Some are not comfortable with technology or lack access to computers or digital devices. Others are worried about the security of their data and of their privacy. Many worry about family members, employers, and government agencies getting access to their personal health information (Bandoim, 2017; Monegain, 2017). Other factors that help or hinder patients in the effective use of portals are how well the provider "sells" the use of the portal, ease of use, training, and technical support.

Too Many Patient Portals

Now that the use of portals is becoming more commonplace, most providers choose a customized portal that meets the needs of his or her office or institution. This means that patients who go to multiple physicians or healthcare organizations have access to their information, but in a fragmented form through multiple portals that each require a different password.

Fragmentation for patients rarely seems to cross the minds of providers who have been struggling to meet meaningful use criteria and promote the use of their own portals. A quote from a presentation on too many portals at the HIMSS16 conference illustrates this problem clearly: "I met a patient recently who has advanced cancer. She accesses care from multiple providers in multiple organizations. The various EHRs remain isolated and unsynchronized. She can access some of her records online, but she must log into six separate portals. After each encounter, she sends messages to five other physicians requesting they update the data in their EHR" (Mohan, 2016, p. 8).

Having access to personal medical information and test results in this fragmented fashion is a disincentive to use the portals, much less integrate information gained into personal health decision making.

The Digital Divide and Patient Portals

The use of patient portals varies widely among different segments of the population. A study of seniors in a large health plan found that adults over age 70 were much less likely to use patient portals than those between ages 65 and 69. Those groups that were less likely to use patient portals were also less likely to own computers or smartphones and did not regularly use the internet (Gordon & Hornbrook, 2016).

A study of 100 community-dwelling older adults found varying levels of interest in using patient portals and a series of themes ranging from the least to most positive views of patient portals: "(1) limited or poor relationship with technology, (2) fears and frustrations with technology and portal, (3) prefers phone over secure messaging for communication (outside of clinical visit), (4) willing to adopt the portal with support, (5) good relationship with technology, (6) Internet as source of health information, and (7) portal is helpful" (Irizarry, DeVito Dabbs, & Curran, 2015, p. 10).

Fear of and frustration with technology was an issue in all focus groups. Patients in the low literacy, no portal use typically had no experience with computers or access to them. Patients in the higher health literacy group were frustrated by trying to master the portal without technical support.

Many patients in the group felt that training, rather than just being provided with a link and password, would help them use the portal more effectively. Those who did not use computers wanted family members to be given access to the patient portal on their behalf.

ASK YOURSELF

If your organization has a patient portal, how well has it:

- Incorporated functionality that meets patient requirements?
- Promoted the use of the portal to patients?
- Provided alternative methods (say family member access) for those patients who cannot or will not use the portal?
- Provided training and user technical support to make the portal easier to use?
- Developed systems for making health information in the portal understandable to users?
- Created and explained systems for security and patient privacy?

EMR Connected Care Best Practices

The EMR is now a key element of clinical care in the United States and is certainly here to stay. Medical records that are easy for clinicians to use, that tell the patient's story, and that utilize the full power of electronic order entry and clinical decision support are a huge factor in creating connected care for patients, at least at the single institution that uses the EMR. Lack of interoperability is a key barrier to EMRs achieving their full potential in connecting care.

Lessons learned from the literature indicate that EMRs can be a powerful force in producing better outcomes and connecting care for patients if providers adopt certain patient-centered behaviors when using the EMR.

Clinicians can use the EMR to support connected care by:

- Positioning the EMR so the clinician can look back and forth from the screen to the patient.
- Not interrupting the visit to type and allowing long silences while typing.
- Engaging the patient by explaining what the clinician is writing in the record.
- Showing the patient information in the EMR, especially charts and graphs that relate to patient lab test results or outcomes.
- Explaining how the healthcare organization protects patient privacy and security.
- Using computerized order entry and decision support tools to reduce medical errors and to help coordinate follow-up.
- Reading and referencing notes from other providers so the clinician is not "asking the same questions over and over again."
- "Telling the patient's story" through short narrative notes.
- Avoiding overuse of checklists, templates, and "cut and paste" notes.

As use of the EMR becomes universal and additional best practices are developed and if security and documentation overload for clinicians can be resolved, it is likely that the EMR will be a key tool in achieving connected care.

▶ Electronic Communication Tools and Techniques

Electronic Communications Between Health Professionals

Some degree of electronic communication (think email and pagers) has been part of the healthcare workplace for many years. However, in the last decade, newer technologies such as smartphones and tablets have become members of the healthcare team.

These devices are found resting in the pockets of almost every health professional, buzzing and beeping on tables at meetings, and held squarely in the faces of doctors and nurses racing down the corridors of health facilities while simultaneously reading the screens of their devices and dodging other pedestrians.

Mobile devices have become indispensable quick medical resource guides, tools for instant communication through texting and multimedia messaging, cameras for recording visual clinical information, and a convenient way to keep in touch with personal social networks while at work. Electronic communication for health professionals is not limited to email and texting.

Many EMR systems provide functions such as tasking, which allows health professionals to send referrals, orders, and specific tasks to other members of their healthcare team and then track and report on the completion of these tasks.

More advanced phone systems meld all types of communication, allowing internal instant messaging, showing voicemail messages on email, and making conference calling convenient and easy. Meetings for members of the healthcare team who are in remote locations and consultations with specialists at major medical centers are easily possible with secure videoconferencing.

Texting Between Health Professionals

Texting is a quick and convenient way for health professionals to communicate with each other, and in some cases with patients. However, it is not without its problems. In late 2017, the healthcare community was thrown into confusion when the Centers for Medicare and Medicaid Services (CMS) seemingly banned the use of texting for clinical communication.

Later, CMS clarified its advice to state that while texting medical orders is forbidden (the preferred method is computerized order entry into the EMR), members of the healthcare team can share patient information using a secure texting platform (CMS, 2017).

Since texting is still a somewhat new innovation in health care, many health professionals mistakenly believe that patient information that is texted to other professionals is secure and compliant with the Health Insurance Portability and Accountability Act (HIPAA). It is not, unless the texting is done using a secure texting application. Use of patient initials in texting is another widespread but questionable practice.

A recent study of hospital clinicians' use of electronic communication found that 53% of clinicians reported receiving text messages about patient care at least once per day; 21.5% stated that the texts contained identifiable patient information. About a quarter of respondents indicated that their organization had implemented a secure text messaging application, but only 7% said that they were using that application for texting (O'Leary et al., 2017). Real-life experience verifies these findings. In a recent seminar, the author asked participants whether their organization had secure texting capabilities. The answer: "we have it, but how many people use it instead of just using the texting function on their phones?"

Bring Your Own Device (BYOD) Issues

As the use of smartphones and tablets as tools for health professionals has proliferated, the problem of using unsecured personal devices for clinical information exchange has arisen. In cases in which the organization does not provide a company smartphone with secure texting and email, providers often use their own devices, not realizing that their texts and emails are not secure or HIPAA compliant. A solution to this problem is encryption of personal mobile devices. This encryption must still allow healthcare organization IT professionals to access personal device data for purposes of security and support. While many organizations have policies governing BYOD use, these policies are not always uniformly clear or followed, which puts patient personal information at risk for breaches and hacking.

Secure Email

Healthcare organizations can solve the problem of secure communication between organizations by using a secure email program. These programs allow providers to enter a term in the subject line such as "securemail," which then securely sends an email and attachments. An example is monthly reporting for bundled payment in which a home care agency sends information about patient transfers to inpatient facilities about length of stay, and other data to a group of preferred provider skilled nursing facilities (SNFs) via secure email. Providers on the receiving end of the secure email unlock the email with a previously set password.

As simple as this system is, it requires different passwords for different secure email systems, which is a barrier to many busy clinicians who do not want to be troubled with matching passwords to the correct secure email system. The use of HIE eliminates the need for secure email as information is communicated securely within the exchange system. **FIGURE 9-3** illustrates the types of electronic communication

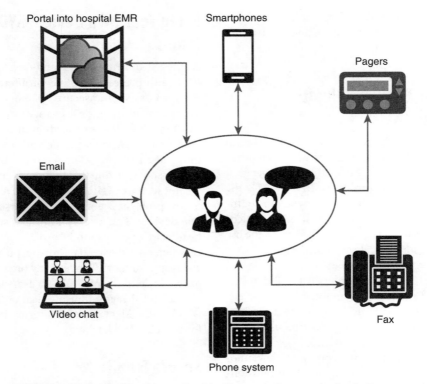

Portal into hospital EMR

Smartphones

Pagers

Email

Video chat

Phone system

Fax

FIGURE 9-3 Methods of Provider-to-Provider Electronic Communication in One Medical Community

tools that are used between healthcare providers in one medical community.

Benefits of Provider-to-Provider Electronic Communication

Despite naysayers, the fact that the majority of practicing health professionals have eagerly incorporated electronic tools into their daily workflows seems to indicate that they have some degree of value and utility in communication and patient care. Electronic communication sends messages almost instantly. The communication can be sent and then opened when the receiver is available. This speed factor can improve productivity, efficiency, and patient safety.

For a nurse caring for a rapidly declining patient, getting an immediate response from a

physician on stabilization measures can literally be a lifesaver. Electronic communication also allows clinicians to get answers to clinical questions and clarify potential misunderstandings about patient care. Electronic communication is also easier than trying to find another clinician who is available at the same time you are for a conversation.

The flip side of this ease of communication is overabundant communication, which can divert attention from the clinical tasks at hand. As one nurse put it: "I only check email three times a day, otherwise it rules me; I don't rule it."

Another benefit, or in some cases a downside, is the electronic trail left by electronic communication. Organizations can put themselves at risk if they don't develop and implement formal policies around email/text record retention. Say a patient has a bad outcome. In a lawsuit, they could reasonably demand access to any emails related to the case. Just like other parts of the medical record, there has to be a retention policy, and active removal of content which is beyond that retention policy. Electronic conversations can be recovered, tracked, referenced, and sequenced. This allows clinicians to view sequential parts of a conversation (a thread) to refresh memory. It can also provide evidence of issues, concerns, and performance problems. Electronic provider-to-provider communication can be used at inappropriate times (e.g., when managing a complex case, when a more in-depth face-to-face interaction would be more effective). Overusing electronic communication may reduce the opportunity for building personal collaborative relationships and for the kind of creative thinking and "ah-ha" moments that are sometimes sparked by live conversation with professional colleagues.

▸ Digital Communication with Patients

Digital tools have opened up a whole new world of possibilities for communication between patients, professionals, and caregivers. Most communication through patient portals is passive.

The patient can read medical record information that has been documented by the health professional. Other communication methods such as calls to physician mobile phones, email, texting, and video chat are more interactive and two way, although they are seldom instantaneous.

Each of these methods, while greatly increasing the potential for care connections, are also prone to problems and issues such as security lapses.

Many patients prefer communicating with health professionals via email or texting rather than waiting for a return phone call from the provider's office. Email is one way that providers can communicate with patients, provided certain safeguards are put in place.

A study reported in *Medical Economics* online found that many patients would prefer to get routine office communications, such as reminders for appointments or bills, via email. A case study reported in the article describes a primary care practice that depends heavily on email communication with patients to improve productivity and to respond more quickly to patients. Patients pay for the privilege of using email with the office through an annual subscription, which ranges from $395 for patients under age 55 to $595 for those over 65. The practice has found that this subscription brings in extra income and reduces time and effort spent on patient communication (Brown, 2013).

Texting is much less secure than email and is less used for patient communication, although it is not prohibited under HIPAA (Department of Health and Human Services [HHS], 2018). A policy statement on texting, published in the *Online Journal of Nursing Informatics* (Storck, 2017), provides guidelines for health professional/patient texting:

- Obtain written informed consent from patients who want to receive information by text.
- Password protect the phone that is used to send text messages.
- Ensure that the patient phone number for receiving texts is correct.
- Do not include any personal health information in the text.
- Delete texts after the communication is complete.
- Do not store patient first and last names in phone contacts; use only first name and last initial.
- Set clear expectations with patients and communicate clearly and succinctly without using abbreviations.
- Do not try to convey complex information via text. The best use is for reminders and short health promotion messages.
- Text messages, if they contain substantial clinical information relevant to the patient's care, presumably supplied by the patient, should be transcribed into the patient's medical record.

▶ Connected Care Digital Communication Best Practices

Digital communication should be subject to the same communication best practices as interpersonal communication with a few additional guidelines specific to electronic media. Connected care best practices described in earlier chapters apply to digital communication:

- **Choose a type of communication appropriate to the situation.** Simple communications, reminders, questions, and other tasks are easily managed through email or text. Complex consultations, discussions with an emotional element, or discussion of problems with many ramifications are not appropriate for electronic communication and should be conducted in person or at least by phone.
- **Drive out fear.** Contact between professionals, especially between those at different levels of the healthcare hierarchy, should not be hobbled by blame or the worry that a legitimate clinical electronic communication will be seen as an interruption or a bother. Implementing this best practice requires clinical leaders, especially in medicine and nursing, to reinforce the requirements for effective, "no-blame" communication.
- **Remember the ripple effect.** Ask yourself "who needs to know" before you communicate electronically. Few health professionals work in a vacuum, so electronic communications about patient care should always be sent or copied to all professionals and support staff who are on the patient care team. If the issue is a complaint or a problem, a clinical manager should be part of the communication chain.
- **The next step is the customer.** When there is a care handoff from one department or organization to another, communication about patient care is essential. This communication should contain information needed by the next step in care and the information must be transmitted using an electronic format that is common to both parties. For example, if a medical practice still uses paper records and does not commonly use email for interprofessional communication, phone or fax would be more appropriate.
- **Close the loop.** This means acknowledging receipt of electronic communication such as email and text and giving feedback about the message received. The most common mistakes in closed loop communication are not reading or only partially reading the written message before responding or not responding at all.
- **Express the message clearly and succinctly, using neutral words and phrases.** Tone comes through in email as well as in person. A "snarky email" can do as much to damage professional relationships as an in-person argument. Misunderstandings can arise if the words in the message are not clear or if there is no context for the message.
- **Provide and support a common set of secure digital tools** for use by all professionals in specific healthcare organizations or health systems. This use of common tools in a standard way allows for the best kind of connected care and reduces the incidence of messages "falling through the cracks" and not being received. For example, when everyone in an organization knows and uses secure email according to policy, breaches are far less likely.

▶ Patient Digital Experiences

E-Patients

The term "e-patient" was coined by the late Dr. Tom Ferguson, an early advocate for patient empowerment and self-management. Dr. Ferguson defined the e-patient as equipped, enabled, empowered, and engaged in their health and healthcare decisions (Society for Participatory Medicine, 2018). More recently, the term has come to define patients who use the internet to research a medical condition and use electronic communication tools to cope with medical conditions (Stanford Medicine X, 2014).

In an article on nursing informatics, Nelson (2016) describes the new role of e-patients and the changing role of the nurse in response to these highly empowered patients: "Healthcare is moving from a world where the educated, informed nurse offers services to patients who cannot meet their own healthcare needs to a world where the equipped, enabled, empowered, and engaged patient is becoming a peer, working together with nurses and other healthcare providers in identifying their healthcare needs" (p. 1).

The quintessential e-patient is "e-patient Dave," David deBronkart, a cancer survivor who accessed his own medical records and worked with his doctors to achieve a cure.

He is now an internationally known speaker and a passionate advocate for full transparency in medical information sharing. Dave is one type of e-patient, a nationally known speaker and consultant and something of a gadfly who tweaks the medical establishment about issues relevant to patient empowerment and information access (deBronkart, 2018).

An article by James Lytle (2017), in *Health Literacy Research and Practice,* describes another type of e-patient experience. Lytle, who is an educator, has Parkinson's disease and receives care from a major university medical center that provides patients with fairly extensive access to their EMRs. Despite his high level of health literacy and seemingly ideal access to his own medical information, he describes an experience of frustrating information fragmentation. In the course of his experience with the medical system he has found that some parts of his record are available and others not: university departments that refuse to be part of the health system electronic record and keep their own records; providers, such as his physical therapist, who are not part of the health system and can neither contribute to nor read his records; problem lists that omit his primary diagnosis; and a total lack of medical information coordination by any of his many clinicians. He asks what responsibility his many clinicians have to coordinate his medical information and questions: "Why is this whole thing so fragmented, and does anyone even care?"

After calmly summarizing the fragmentation and failings of his electronic medical information access systems, Lytle (2017) concludes: "Over time I've found that my support group, the social worker who attends the meetings, and the publications and websites of the Parkinson's Foundation (http://www.parkinson.org) and the Michael J. Fox Foundation (https://www.michaeljfox.org) are my best learning resources. I now recognize how little of what the group members share is learned from their neurologists and primary care doctors, and how much they depend on the Internet and social media discussion groups for information. I also continue to wonder how patients who have less access to health data and information than I do manage their health" (p. e1300).

This story illustrates how electronic connections do not produce real engagement and patient-connected care without a patient-centered focus. Without someone who can identify gaps in the "white space" between clinicians and various computer systems, and without a clinician to coordinate the accuracy and completeness of a patient's medical information, the patient experience, however intensely digital, remains fragmented and unsatisfactory.

The Blue Button—Patient Online Access to Personal Health Data

One example of a system designed to increase patient access to personal health data is the Blue

Button initiative. This government-sponsored effort gives patients easy online access to their health information. Patients can click a digital button⊕and download information into text and pdf formats. The blue button approach has been supported by the Office of the National Coordinator for Health Information Technology (ONC) and has been provided to many government health insurance beneficiaries.

Patients of the Veterans Administration health system can download information from their EMR and can also enter information into their medical record (e.g., information on insurance or medications, allergies, or laboratory results) (Aziz & Moshen, 2015).

Medicare's Blue Button program allows Medicare beneficiaries to sign on to their personal medicare.gov account to access their own Medicare Part A and Part B claims (CMS, 2018).

Healthcare Mobile Apps

An application (app) is a piece of software designed to perform a specific function. Most apps are accessed through mobile devices such as smartphones and tablets. The number of healthcare apps has exploded in the last decade as smartphones have become more widely used. In 2017 over 75% of Americans owned a smartphone. The percentage of both those over age 50 and lower income U.S. smartphone users has increased significantly (Smith, 2017). There are now 325,000 healthcare apps with the Android phone system offering the largest number (Pohl, 2017). The most popular apps are those related to wellness such as weight loss and exercise.

Results from Gittlen's (2017) NEJM Catalyst Survey, "What Patient Engagement Technology Is Good For," indicate that 67% of health professionals surveyed felt that "helping patients stay healthy" was one of the top three benefits of technology for patient engagement. Survey respondents rated apps as 75% effective in "engaging patients in their own care." The vast

array of medical apps includes symptom checkers, special diet choice apps, care coordination apps that help with scheduling medical appointments and reminders, and specialized apps that help patients manage diabetes, hypertension, and other chronic illnesses. Research on the quality of mobile health apps is in its infancy, so many health professionals are reluctant to recommend them to patients.

Of the respondents in the NEJM Catalyst study, 67% indicated that a top barrier to effective use of technology for patient engagement was "providers don't know what to recommend" (Gittlen, 2017).

Boudreaux and colleagues (2014) at the University of Massachusetts Medical School have developed guidance for professionals who want to help their patients select and use medical apps that are safe and effective. They recommend that professionals:

- Review the scientific literature for research about specific apps.
- Review app descriptions, user ratings, and reviews online.
- Conduct a social media query with relevant professional and patient networks.
- Pilot test the app yourself.
- Solicit feedback on the app from patients.

Apps certainly empower patients by giving them access to a huge amount of practical information and by providing useful care coordination functions. They can connect patients to new resources and knowledge. How well the app fosters connected care depends on what it does and how well it works for the user. A white paper from *Patient View* describes the results of a study of 250 patients and consumer groups (primarily in the United Kingdom) who described their requirements for a good health app. Key requirements follow:

1. Give people more control over their condition, or keep them healthy
2. Easy to use
3. Able to be used regularly

4. Allow networking with other people like them, or with people who understand them
5. Trustworthy

Some comments from the study provide more extensive information about users' specific requirements:

■ Apps with a more clinical or therapeutic nature that are evidence based

■ Apps that are culturally relevant, especially for indigenous people
■ Apps that are updated following new innovations, guidance, etc.
■ Apps that help you remember to use them

The study notes that most use of health apps did not involve recommendations or approval from health professionals, but states that such recommendations would be helpful, especially for an app that has a very clinical focus (Patient View, 2013).

🔍 CASE STUDY

A Practical App for Irritable Bowel Syndrome

I (the author) recently had dinner with a friend who has irritable bowel syndrome. We chose a restaurant where my friend said: "I can get bland broiled fish." During dinner she showed me a smartphone application that her doctor had recommended called the FODMap Diet (**FIGURE 9-4**). In one section of the app she was able to click on pictures of common foods which then lit up as red, yellow, or green for don't eat, eat with caution, or eat without restriction, respectively.

She says that since she has been using this app she has had fewer symptoms, feels more in control of her health, and is less reluctant to eat out. This simple tool has helped her to achieve the top goal of the NEJM digital patient engagement survey: "To support patients in efforts to be healthy" (Gittlen, 2017).

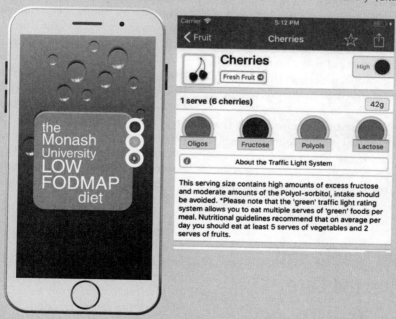

FIGURE 9-4 FodMap Diet App for Irritable Bowel Syndrome Diet Resources

Healthcare Apps and Connected Care

Healthcare mobile apps are by their nature designed to be patient centered. Only if the app design meets the needs of the population using it, is it truly patient centered. For example, a chronic disease app with a simple, color-coded screen design and a simple user interface would be considered patient centered. One that is highly complex to use and visually confusing probably better satisfies the software engineer's needs than those of the patient/user.

Apps are continually rated and reviewed by users, so developers are responsive to consumer feedback. As the Patient View study shows, patients often feel empowered and have more control over their health when using a helpful app. Information about useful apps may be shared on social media, thus improving collaboration with other people with health issues similar to those of the user. Apps for care coordination may help patients better manage healthcare transitions and keep their care more organized. If a patient discusses the use of an app, or seeks advice on its use from a health professional, there may be some element of improved patient-provider communication. Apps may help patients become more health literate and more knowledgeable about their condition, which can then improve communication with their health professionals, thus better achieving connected care.

One caveat about healthcare apps is that there may be limited quality control in terms of the health information provided, so app users must either carefully vet the source of app medical information or adopt a "buyer beware" attitude.

▶ Social Media and Connected Care

Patients and Social Media

Of all the digital technologies, social media is the fastest growing and the one with the widest reach. The website Health-Union.com, which publishes health content and hosts online communities for patients with chronic disease, conducted a 2016 survey about social media use of 2,200 people with serious medical conditions (Herbert, Makopoulos, & Lawhon, 2016).

The survey found that 70% of patients surveyed used condition-specific websites, while 59% used Facebook for health information. Hearing about other patients' experiences and getting support online were two reasons users found these sites to be valuable. Facebook, email, online support groups, and mobile apps were the most popular types of social media for participants. Patients described going online for specific reasons: 67% were experiencing new symptoms, 67% were starting a new medication, 61% were making a medication decision or change; 98% of those responding (all of whom are regular internet users) had read health-related articles or watched health-related videos in the previous year. Topics of interest were coping with symptoms, medication information, medication side effects, and lifestyle change ideas. Those surveyed actively used social media by "liking" posts, following discussions online, posting comments, and sharing health-related content (not from their own personal information). Of those who posted questions online, 87% wanted information from fellow patients; only 46% were looking for answers from doctors. Of survey respondents, 97% said they shared information from their online experience with health professionals and 65% felt that this information had at least some impact on their health decision making.

Many younger users are highly trusting of the health information that they find on social media, although the recent furor over Facebook's sharing of user personal information may change that somewhat. Trust levels vary by the source. Searchers trusted posts by physicians and nurses far more than those by pharmaceutical companies. Surprisingly, much of the research on health care and social media is older and is frequently recycled on different websites. One more recent article, from the site ReferralMD (2017), provides a list of statistics about the use of social media for health care:

- 42% of individuals viewing health information on social media look at health-related consumer reviews.
- 32% of U.S. users post about their friends' and family's health experiences on social media.
- 29% of patients viewing health information through social media are viewing other patients' experiences with their disease.

Patients also use social media such as Facebook to promote healthcare causes such as fundraising for someone with a serious illness, to find healthcare information, and to share personal health experiences and get answers to personal health questions from other likeminded social media users (ReferralMD, 2017). One example of this use of social media is the Facebook group named Rheumatoid Arthritis Forum, which describes itself as "a place for RA'ers supported by RA'ers." User posts on the site include pictures of swollen joints, rashes, and other visuals of symptoms with questions for the user community. One user posted a picture of swollen finger joints with the question, "Anyone have any suggestions for swelling and pain? I have tried ice and ibu/tylenol. Currently awaiting approval from insurance to start a new med." Over 20 suggestions from users were posted in response, including compression gloves, prednisone, biofreeze, cannabis, alternate heat and ice, and Voltaren gel. Of note: No health professional responded to this post with suggestions or any comments about the proven effectiveness of any of these symptom control methods.

Medical ethicist Art Caplan, from the Division of Medical Ethics at the School of Medicine at New York University, commented on this issue in Boachie's (2017) article on social media in health care: "The Internet is full of nonsense, hype, clickbait and ridiculous information about all kinds of health and medical elixirs and remedies that have no basis in fact." And Caplan rightly poses the question: "If you think about it, how often do you actually see a doctor, an established scientist out there, trying to correct or engage the public with scientific, verified, evidence-based information?" (Boachie, 2017).

Many people use social media to find health professionals and rate healthcare experiences. The report *Social Media Likes Healthcare* from PWC research gives an example: "When I was in the ER last night, I tweeted about the interminable wait. It seemed as though people who weren't that sick got whisked in ahead of me! Guess what? Someone from the hospital heard me! They spotted my tweet and responded. And even sent someone down to talk to me in person" (PWC Health Research Institute, 2012, p. 3).

Consumer Concerns About Social Media Data Privacy

Social media users, while often freely sharing information on the internet, do worry about the use of their own health information and social media (**FIGURE 9-5**). These concerns include

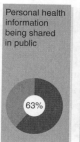
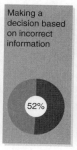
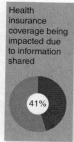
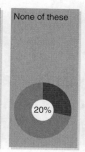
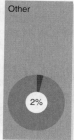

Personal health information being shared in public — 63%

Information being hacked or leaked — 57%

Making a decision based on incorrect information — 52%

Health insurance coverage being impacted due to information shared — 41%

None of these — 20%

Other — 2%

n = 1,060

FIGURE 9-5 Consumer Concerns About Sharing Health Information on Social Media

Data from PwC HRI Social Media Consumer Survey, 2012.

sharing personal information on the internet, information being hacked or leaked, making decisions based on wrong information, and having insurance status affected by shared information.

This concern is not unwarranted, as Naylor (2016) explains in an article from National Public Radio. Information shared on social media sites is collected and stored by "data brokers" who package it and sell it to other companies so they can create a digital profile of the internet user and target ads specifically to the person's profile. The article quotes former Federal Trade Commissioner Julie Brill: "Say, for instance, you do an online search for heart disease or diabetes. Depending upon the website, that information can go to ad networks and analytics companies."

If the contents of that heart disease or diabetes search end up with a data broker, that information could then be added to your digital biography, which "becomes a part of your profile and others see that and can market to you based on that information" says Brill (Naylor, 2016).

This is certainly a form of connection, but not exactly one that fosters improved care and outcomes, as it is hidden from users of social media and employed only for commercial purposes to sell products and services that are not necessarily in the best interests of the user.

ASK YOURSELF

If a patient's digital profile was available to not only the patient but also the health professionals who care for the patient, would it have a positive or negative impact on connected care?

Health Facility and Professional Engagement on Social Media

Health professional engagement with social media is increasing as clinicians and healthcare facilities realize the potential for patient engagement, patient education, and marketing their services.

The CDC (2011), in its Health Communicator's *Social Media Toolkit*, states: "Social media and other emerging communication technologies can connect millions of voices to:

- Increase the timely dissemination and potential impact of health and safety information.
- Leverage audience networks to facilitate information sharing.
- Expand reach to include broader, more diverse audiences.
- Personalize and reinforce health messages that can be more easily tailored or targeted to particular audiences.
- Facilitate interactive communication, connection and public engagement.
- Empower people to make safer and healthier decisions."

The *Social Media Toolkit* also shares a series of social media best practices and lessons learned. Among them are to use data to be strategic about the audiences you want to reach and to identify the type of social media with the largest volume of users in your target population. Start small with less-intense, low-risk tools such as videos that can easily be shared. Create portable content that can be used by your partners and make sure content is optimized for use on mobile devices such as tablets and smartphones. Make it easy for your users to share content and leverage their networks. For example, individuals often have large groups of Facebook followers.

Provide multiple social media formats and encourage participation. Finally, use information from your social media network and posts to understand your audience and how well you have met your objectives (CDC, 2011). The webpage for social media on the CDC website also contains a handbook for writing for social media and guides to using Facebook, Twitter, social media policies, and security issues. Access the webpage at https://www.cdc.gov/socialmedia/tools/guidelines/socialmediatoolkit.html

Examples of Health Facility and Health Professional Social Media Use

One example of an organization that has fully embraced social media is New York Dynamic Neuromuscular Rehabilitation and Physical Therapy.

This physical therapy practice shares information about physical therapy and rehabilitation with its thousands of followers. Recent Facebook and Twitter posts (1,500 followers) include pictures of healthy young runners and attractive older adults, and various articles. Sample articles include:

- "Why ACL Injuries Are Common in Females"
- "Ideas to Give Your Spine Special Treatment"
- "An Option for Managing Plantar Fasciitis"

The practice also utilizes YouTube for promotional videos and for instruction in the use of its virtual reality home rehabilitation program called CAREN. The owner also actively engages with Yelp, encouraging patients to share their ratings of his practice and quickly responding to any review that is even slightly negative (Boachie, 2017).

Another highly engaged medical social media user is "Dr. Mike," or Dr. Mikhail Varshavski, who describes himself as the most followed doctor on social media (3 million Instagram followers). His online biography describes him as "a practicing physician, social media personality and philanthropist" (https://www.facebook.com/realdoctormike/).

Dr. Mike is a family physician whose social media presence includes engaging photos of him in fashionable clothes and model poses, on Instagram, as well as pictures of him with his practice patients in a more traditional lab coat. His website also features a link to a YouTube recording of Dr. Mike doing a TED talk on how to question experts. Dr. Mike targets millennials for health information sharing on his Twitter, YouTube, and Facebook accounts. In an article on American Family Physician.org

news blog, "Patients Trust Social Media, So Be Their Trusted Source," Dr. Mike shares his philosophy on connecting care for patients via social media (American Academy of Family Physicians, 2017).

He acknowledges that health professionals have concerns about HIPAA, overexposure, and erosion of credibility. However, Dr. Mike feels that social media can create new lines of communication with patients and can influence "the health decisions of millions." He notes that 90% of young people trust information from their social network feeds so he suggests that it is important that they receive information from a trustworthy source.

Social Media and Connected Care Implications

The essence of social media is connection. For most people this connection means with family and friends and sometimes with health professionals. Other forms of connection such as with data brokers who capture and sell personal information from social media are far less welcome, but seldom considered by the majority of social media users. Online social networks can provide intense collaboration and much needed social support for people coping with serious conditions, but if not moderated, can lead to misinformation and misunderstanding. Many health professionals and healthcare organizations have remained reluctant to become active on social media because of concerns about crossing professional boundaries (Ventola, 2014).

Some of the risks of medical professional use of social media are accidental sharing of protected information and the potential liability of something being considered medical advice. However, if social media is used carefully, it can provide an opportunity to share valid medical information. Those who make the choice to avoid it, miss an opportunity to connect with patients and to provide scientifically correct medical information.

▶ Big Data, Predictive Analytics, and Artificial Intelligence

The newest and potentially most disruptive advance in digital health care is the broad field of big data, predictive analytics, and artificial intelligence. "Big data" is a term that appears with increasing frequency in healthcare publications and is becoming an area of strategic importance for healthcare organizations.

One definition of big data comes from John Akred, founder and chief technical officer of Silicon Valley Data Science: "Big Data refers to a combination of an approach to informing decision making with analytical insight derived from data, and a set of enabling technologies that enable that insight to be economically derived from at times very large, diverse sources of data" (Dutcher, 2014). In health care, big data consist of the billions of bits and terabytes of data contained in EMRs, radiology image files, pharmacy records, medical claims, and myriad other healthcare sources.

This huge volume of raw data can be harnessed, mined, and organized using very specialized tools to create insights into the behavior of patient populations, patient wants and needs, the effectiveness of drugs, the comparative effectiveness of different treatment methods, and the costs and benefits of different products, services, and workflows. This sorting, analyzing, and harnessing massive quantities of data is predictive analytics.

A blog post from the data analytics company Health Catalyst provides several concrete examples: Data from smart devices which are connected to the internet (the Internet of Things) such as smart pill dispensers or electronic calendars can identify missed appointments or missed doses of medication and send that data to a health provider.

Big data might analyze zip code and socioeconomic data and determine that patients in a certain zip code are unlikely to have cars and so may have difficulty with follow-up medical appointments after discharge. Big data might also use patient demographic and medical data to predict a "patient trajectory" and to identify points at which problems might occur and might cause hospital readmissions (Adamson, 2018).

The other use of big data is for marketing and "patient engagement" purposes. Large healthcare institutions work with analytics firms to identify psychographic profiles of patients (characteristics of patient psychology and likelihood of making certain choices) and incorporate these profiles into marketing campaigns and targeted online advertising.

Big data offer huge promise in the area of connected care. If, by using data, treatments and clinical activities are truly customized and targeted to individual patient needs, many unnecessary medical tests, phone calls, appointments, faxes, and paper will be eliminated, making life easier for both patient and health provider. Big data also have the potential to weed out ineffective drugs, procedures, technologies, and methods that drive care fragmentation.

While big data have huge promise, the economic impact of providing information about ineffective drugs and treatments would be huge. It is hard to imagine that manufacturers and distributors of less effective healthcare products will not try to counter, or even hide, some of the negative effects of big data and predictive analytics. Two other significant issues with big data and predictive analytics are lack of high-level expertise to extract and analyze data and problems with security and privacy. Since big data require highly specialized analytical skills, there is a concern that more amateur efforts might produce distorted or misleading predictive analytics.

Privacy and security are huge concerns, as there are few good methods for obtaining patient permission to use personal data when it is part of a huge data set. The 2018 controversy about the use of Facebook user data for political purposes without the user's permission is an example of the kinds of very troubling problems that can occur in a world where controls on the use and misuse of electronic data are still in a state of flux.

Artificial Intelligence

Artificial intelligence (AI) is another exciting (some would say the most exciting) advance in health care. One definition (among many) of AI is: "A branch of computer science dealing with the simulation of intelligent behavior in computers and the capability of a machine to imitate intelligent human behavior" (Merriam Webster, 2018).

AI is fueled by big data, machine learning (in which computer systems teach themselves new things without being programmed), and natural language processing (the ability of a computer to understand human language). For some, the definition of AI conjures up frightening visions of diagnosis and treatment by machine, white-coated robots instead of doctors and nurses, and a healthcare system devoid of human hands and human understanding. Despite these doomsday scenarios, AI has the potential to transform and connect health care in unprecedented ways. AI can be used to develop algorithms that can read digital radiographic images more accurately than humans and can aid clinicians in making more accurate diagnoses. So far, human intelligence has still been needed to take data obtained from AI and apply it in particular circumstances to specific patients.

AI also powers digital human surrogates such as Siri and Alexa (mobile phone apps) which are programmed to answer human questions. Virtual health professional avatars or software programs that are designed to mimic human interactions and to provide structured health information are also products of AI.

AI, as with any technology, has its own issues. One such issue is that research shows that when machines learn to think like humans they absorb human prejudices and biases and do not have the ability to counteract these biases. An article in a U.K. paper, *The Guardian* (2017), describes this issue:

The latest paper shows that some more troubling implicit biases seen in human psychology experiments are also readily acquired by algorithms. The words "female" and "woman" were more closely associated with arts and humanities occupations and with the home, while "male" and "man" were closer to math and engineering professions. And the AI system was more likely to associate European American names with pleasant words such as "gift" or "happy", while African American names were more commonly associated with unpleasant words.

The findings suggest that algorithms have acquired the same biases that lead people (in the United Kingdom and United States, at least) to match pleasant words and white faces in implicit association tests (*The Guardian*, 2017). Problems like the bias issue are troubling and need to be identified and addressed as the field of AI advances.

This research highlights the need for health professionals who use AI programs not to go on "autopilot" and simply accept the dictates of a piece of software that was, after all, formed by human thinking and biases.

Does AI advance the cause of connected care for patients? The answer is "maybe," if AI is used to improve the accuracy and personalization of medical care. If it is simply used as a method of decreasing labor costs by substituting machines for human health professionals, improving profits, and applying routinized protocols to care decisions that don't take individual patient needs and wants into account, then AI is a fragmenting factor in care. As with other technologies, it depends on the goals of AI use and how it is embedded into processes of care.

The Internet of Things

The use of "smart objects" that are connected to the internet, which is called the Internet of Things (IOT), has exploded in recent years. IOT is fueled by AI. Tracking devices in the form of miniature or wearable units, telemonitoring, and tracking systems within inpatient facilities are among the most popular types of IOT devices. Smart pills that can deliver medication doses precisely over time or that monitor patient adherence are a recently unveiled innovation.

Robots are smart objects that perform a variety of tasks in health care, including such repetitive tasks as phlebotomy, delivering supplies, or disinfecting a portion of the hospital. Robots perform surgery with a human operator and companion robots, such as a robot cat or baby seal, provide companionship for people with dementia.

🔍 CASE STUDY

Using IOT to Track Surgical Patients

Florida Hospital Celebration Health uses an IOT tracking device to keep families informed of patients' movement through surgery from preop preparation to the recovery room. Patients are tagged with "real-time location system badges" to track their status. Families can follow their family member's progress on a big screen TV display in the waiting room.

Patient data are kept confidential through the use of individualized ID numbers that are provided only to family members (Sutner, 2016).

Wearable Tracking Devices

Wearable fitness tracking devices such as the Fitbit or the Apple watch have become hugely popular among consumers, especially those with a bent toward physical fitness and wellness. According to the International Data Corporation (IDC): "The overall wearables market is expected to grow from 113.2 million shipments in 2017 to 222.3 million in 2021 with a compound annual growth rate (CAGR) of 18.4%.

Meanwhile, watches (both smart and basic) are on track to take the lead and are expected to grow from 61.5 million in 2017 to 149.5 million in 2021 as more vendors—particularly fashion brands—and cellular connectivity built into smartwatches help to drive growth in this category" (IDC, 2017).

Despite their widespread popularity, consumer wearables have yet to become part of the medical landscape; and data from wearables are very seldom incorporated into the EMR or used to coach patients with chronic illness, which would make it more of a tool for connected care. A survey by the online journal *Physicians Practice* (Pratt, 2017) found that only 5% of its physician readers use data from patient wearables in health counseling. One physician who is quoted in the article promotes the use of wearable data: "At the very least, the tracker serves as an educational tool, showing the patient just how little (or how much) they move" (p. 1). This same physician notes that many patients are very optimistic in self-reports of exercise levels, while wearables provide more objective and realistic information about what the patient is really doing.

Most physicians do not record or upload data into the EMR, although some give patients the option to upload their own data through a patient portal. Concerns about the accuracy of the information and the difficulty of getting it into a concise and usable format that can interface with the EMR, and concerns about liability if the data go unmanaged, are barriers to the integration of consumer wearable data into the EMR.

Some physicians recommend that patients do some degree of self-monitoring with devices such as digital blood pressure machines. Patients typically record their own results on paper and bring these to medical visits to discuss with providers.

One type of wearable has become well integrated into patient care. The medical grade wearable device, such as a remote heart monitor, is typically dispensed by a medical facility. The heart rhythm monitor collects and transmits highly accurate data in a secure manner,

⌕ *CASE STUDY*

A Digital Device Manages Patient Check-In

In a recent personal experience, the author observed the use of an IOT device for patient check-in. A provider of diagnostic testing services installed an electronic check-in system and eliminated receptionists in its waiting room. Patients were expected to come into the waiting room, see the device, read the instructions on the wall, and use it properly. No employees from the lab were in visible sight.

Some patients easily used the check-in device. Others asked for help from people in the waiting room. A third group didn't even attempt to use the device, or didn't see it, and simply knocked on the lab door until a staff member appeared. This is an example of technology employed in the service of the organization and not the patient, although it is possible that frequent users of the lab eventually mastered the device and found their waiting time decreased. A conversation with a lab employee indicated that this had indeed happened.

ASK YOURSELF

- What do you think the goal was of this technology implementation?
- How patient centered was this technology application?
- How could the technology have been used differently to improve the patient experience?

which are then incorporated into the EMR. It is very likely that wearable devices will become more accurate and more capable of transmitting data securely and in a manner that can be incorporated into the medical record in an effective way. However, medical practices will need to design workflows that allow them to manage the data effectively.

One major barrier to the widespread use of wearable devices is cost. The very patients who could most benefit from the use of wearables often do not have access (most are purchased online) or money to buy them and insurance companies do not cover these devices. If the physician does not get paid for "monitoring" wearable devices, she is much less likely to incorporate this feature into her practice. Once these issues of cost, access, accuracy, security, and acceptance by medical professionals are overcome, wearables may become a powerful connected care tool, empowering patients to monitor their own health and giving clinicians data for health coaching and chronic disease management.

INTERVIEW WITH JAKE STAR, CHIEF INFORMATION OFFICER VNA COMMUNITY HEALTHCARE

The interview began with Jake answering the question, "How does technology affect fragmentation in the healthcare system?" His answer: "The healthcare system is disconnected at every single level from patient and caregiver to providers, payer and government. For example, a patient portal isn't really a connection with a doctor. You typically can't ask a question or share data. If your blood pressure is up,

(continues)

INTERVIEW WITH JAKE STAR, CHIEF INFORMATION OFFICER VNA COMMUNITY HEALTHCARE *(continued)*

there is no meaningful electronic way to have a dialogue about it. If the blood pressure monitor was connected to the doctor's EMR, it might be more helpful, but it would also raise liability issues for the physician if he or she doesn't act on the information." It could also create the problem of "alert fatigue," which now occurs in hospitals where staff are so overwhelmed by too many alerts that they simply ignore them.

Jake talks about three promising technologies for connecting care and reducing fragmentation in health care: health information exchanges, IOT sensor devices, and predictive analytics.

Jake feels that HIEs help with the issue of fragmentation. Data from an HIE, such as about a population of diabetic patients, could really help healthcare organizations better manage a patient population. Instead of population data, we now we have data on a "project basis," which means that we are doing a project and ask for specific data such as analyzing the effect of telemonitoring on CHF patients. Registries, such as immunization registries, use continuous data entry and are a better way to analyze data from larger populations.

HIEs typically start with a admit/discharge/transfer (ADT) data element because it is so readily available and so basic. It is something that everyone can understand. Patient vital signs are another simple data element that would be desirable to store in an HIE.

Many organizations already do this, but they might have one ADT link to something like PatientPing, and another link to a different hospital, and another link to a specific ACO. The benefit of HIE is that everyone has one interface instead of many different interfaces. In an HIE that uses queries, a physician could press a button in the EMR labeled "Get vital signs from HIE."

Another useful piece of HIE information might be a longitudinal log of radiology procedures and radiation exposure for a patient over a long span of time. The HIE could be programmed to alert the provider who orders a new CT scan that the patient has already had several of these procedures recently. E-prescribing is an interesting process that provides some challenges for HIEs. For example, the HIE logs all prescriptions, but there is no "e-cancel" to show that a prescription has been discontinued, which can create a misleading and outdated patient medication list.

One of the drawbacks of HIEs concerns the question, "Who pays?" Now CMS pays 90% of the cost and the state pays 10% for design and implementation. It is less clear who will pay once the system is functional and in use. One advantage of the HIE would be having only one patient portal and not many proprietary portals with multiple log-ins and lack of data sharing. While this single portal is beneficial to the patient, it will probably create resistance among companies that sell proprietary portal software.

Another issue is interface costs, in which software companies don't share information without a fee. An example is a software company that builds interfaces with other software products and charges customers to use each interface. These fees and the limited number of interfaces available produce a disincentive to connect in the absence of an HIE alternative. Jake notes, "EMR vendors hold you hostage."

Another issue is "data blocking" in which one health system wants to "own" the patient and all information about that patient. The system would prefer that patients receive all services from system providers or contracted preferred providers. "The health system might ask why they should share the whole patient record, making it easier for another health system to 'steal the patient.' This issue really comes from that natural conflict between sharing for the good of the patient and having a competitive business strategy."

Jake talks about the advantages of IOT sensor devices. He feels that it is important to balance privacy with tracking for seniors who are not capable of being fully independent without help. He tells of a 15-year-old boy who invented GPS tracking socks to help his grandmother (https://www.nbcnews

.com/feature/making-a-difference/teen-invents-sensor-help-alzheimers-patients-n20323). IOT has the potential to provide "[t]ons of things that could be beneficial" such as smart stoves, smart thermostats, and smart houses with doors that lock and unlock electronically.

These types of devices can help people stay at home longer; and in facilities, they can help provide care with fewer staff. One problem with these devices is that because they are connected to the internet they are theoretically hackable. Lower cost devices have limited security. IOT solutions are becoming more common and the cost is coming down. As older people become comfortable with smartphones, their use of this type of technology will probably increase.

Jake is interested in the potential of predictive analytics to improve care. He uses the example of data that could predict the risk of developing a health problem 6 months in the future so that there could be earlier intervention. Analytics can show who is at risk for diabetes and allow preventive measures to be implemented. With the rise of precision medicine, genetic profiles might become part of predictive analytics if people are willing to share their data.

They may not be willing, however, because of worries that insurance companies might charge a person more because of a genetic profile.

He describes how predictive analytics can analyze data from a questionnaire about risk factors for urologic cancer. With a large enough dataset, the system can develop a model for predicting who will actually get cancer. We actually see this on a very basic level now: When you go to the MD, she might type in a bunch of factors to give you a risk score (http://www.cvriskcalculator.com/).

With a larger dataset, and one that is constantly evolving, the predictions become more reliable. This is one of those networks that has been running for more than 15 years: http://godot.urol.uic.edu/urocomp/psa_predict.html

- Predictive analytics can also help in creating more effective clinical pathways by evaluating large volumes of outcome data. "Is this making health care a factory?" Jake wonders. Another type of data analytics uses psychographic data to predict patient/consumer behavior and to target specific products and services to a certain type of patient. More data make a better and more predictive model, but because there are so many variables the predictions are never foolproof. Certain people and situations will never fit the profile, so the question is how to predict the outliers.
- Privacy is a huge issue with data sharing and data analytics. In the United States, privacy protections are relatively weak. In the European Union (EU) countries there is a "right to be forgotten" (https://www.eugdpr.org/key-changes.html), which allows users of companies such as Google to direct that their data be deleted. This is not possible for U.S. consumers, many of whom sign service agreements without knowing what they are agreeing to share.

  Jake discusses the issue of big data and its ability to use richer data sources such as natural language processing (extracting data from spoken language) and recurrent use of certain words in free text charting such as "tiredness" repeated over the course of a care encounter. Social media can actually be a rich source of health data if combined with data from the EMR, but this raises serious privacy issues.
- While predictive analytics can predict the likelihood that something will happen, such as a health problem appearing, it doesn't show how to incentivize people to behave differently. Predictive analytics can show which tests and treatments are more or less effective. While this is theoretically desirable for patients and for the healthcare system, it creates speculation about whether those companies with poorer results will attempt to suppress the data.
- Jake feels that there is great opportunity offered by technology, but the healthcare environment is too skewed in favor of big players such as insurance companies, large universities, big healthcare systems, and for-profit companies such as big pharma to allow rapid adoption.

Telehealth

The term "telehealth" encompasses a wide variety of health interactions that are conducted electronically. Telehealth is touted as an efficient method for improving healthcare access for underserved or rural populations, providing better access to high-quality specialty care, monitoring high-risk patients at home, increasing convenience for more urban populations, and lowering healthcare costs without compromising quality.

The Center for Connected Health Policy (CCHP) defines telehealth as, "A collection of means or methods for enhancing health care close up space before comma, public health and health education delivery and support using telecommunications" (CCHP, 2018).

Others make the distinction between telehealth, which is the broader term for health interactions delivered through telecommunications, and telemedicine, which is described as virtual clinical care, typically delivered through a video link between patient and provider. Telemedicine, which was originally developed to provide health care to people in remote areas, has become a way of delivering care more conveniently and without the need to travel to a health practitioner's location. The telemedicine market has exploded in recent years, but it is not without its challenges.

A survey of 5,000 healthcare consumers by the Advisory Board, reported in the online journal *Modern Healthcare* (Kacik, 2017), revealed that while over 75% of respondents would be willing to use virtual medical visits, only 20% have already done so. About 21% of respondents worried about quality of care in virtual visits and wondered if they would eventually have to seek care in person if the virtual visit was not successful. Study participants felt that telemedicine would be useful for prescription questions and refills, pre- and postsurgery care, health coaching, ongoing chronic care, and psychologist vists.

The telehealth industry is in the midst of massive change as reimbursement issues are being addressed and state-by-state regulations

created. One major impetus for the advancement of telehealth is the recent passage of the CHRONIC Care Act in February 2018.

This act "expands telehealth coverage for Accountable Care Organizations, expands flexibility for Medicare Advantage Plan use of telemedicine and provides reimbursement for telestroke care and home dialysis treatment," says a press release from the American Telemedicine Association (ATA; 2018). **FIGURE 9-6** illustrates the various types of telehealth technologies.

Types of Telehealth

The two main types of telehealth are live videoconferencing and "store and forward" technology. Live videoconferencing allows patients and providers to interact through computers, video cameras, and microphones. Since the interaction is in the digital world, patients can be connected with health professionals in a physical location remote from theirs. Store and forward technology is used when face-to-face interactions between providers and patients are not necessary.

Digital images, prerecorded video, and results of diagnostic tests can be obtained in one location, stored digitally, and then forwarded to a final digital destination for the receiving provider to access and use. This approach is most commonly used when a specialist needs to evaluate a patient who cannot travel to his or her physical location. Remote home monitoring, more commonly known as telemonitoring, allows patients to connect themselves to monitoring devices such as a blood pressure cuff, scale, and pulse oximeter; then take readings and send the readings via a secure internet connection to a remote monitoring site. This type of monitoring is most commonly done by home healthcare agencies.

Telemedicine Virtual Visits

Telemedicine is being used for visits in urgent care and in multiple medical specialties, with urgent care being the most common. Maryland Physician's Care Group, for example, recently

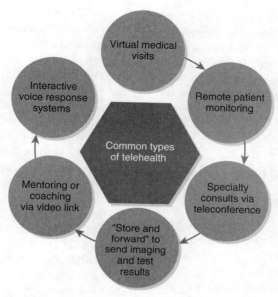

FIGURE 9-6 Types of Telehealth Technology

released a telemedicine app for its Medicaid patients (Espaillat, 2017). The app, called MyVirtualMPC, allows patients to instant message or video chat with an ER physician. A news clip shows a mother instant messaging a physician about her 3-year-old daughter's symptoms. The mother described her experience with the app: "He asked lots of detailed questions about her symptoms and her situation. He asked me to do the equivalent of FaceTime on the app, so he could see her, and she could point to the different areas of her stomach that were hurting." The physician who provided the service explained that he could give advice, triage the patient to the correct setting for treatment, or sometimes make a diagnosis remotely and call in a prescription.

▶ Telemedicine Cost and Quality

Since telehealth has only recently become a part of mainstream health care, research on the cost

and quality of these technologies is in its infancy. One review of virtual visit quality in *Managed Care Magazine* (Kirkner, 2017) finds spotty adherence to evidence-based protocols, with virtual visit vendors doing a good job in some areas but rating poorly in others. One area of concern is poor performance in visits where testing or follow-up is required. Commercial telemedicine vendors who are not connected with the patient's primary care provider adhered to clinical guidelines only 54.3% of the time. Of particular concern was that urine cultures were obtained only 34% of the time in cases of suspected urinary tract infection.

Another virtual care quality problem has been the overuse of broad-spectrum antibiotics, which fuels the growth of drug-resistant organisms. Other studies have shown little difference between virtual visits and in-person care, although the caveat is that some of these studies have been industry funded.

Virtual visits are definitely cheaper than in-person visits. According to *Managed Care Magazine* (Kirkner, 2017), the cost of a virtual visit is about $49 versus $109 for a medical office visit and $1,400 for an emergency room visit. A Rand Corporation study that was also reported in the Kirkner article, has challenged the assumption that virtual care lowers cost by finding that utilization of care increases because of the ease and convenience of telemedicine (Kirkner, 2017).

Telemedicine and Patient-Centered Care

An article about nurse practitioners and virtual visits addresses what the authors call "telehealth etiquette" best practices (Rutledge et al., 2017). This concept describes ways to use voice and visuals to establish empathy with the patient when touch is not possible.

Some techniques include reducing ambient noise, not wearing loud or distracting clothing, leaning forward, making contact with the camera and not the visual image of the patient on the screen, and using a voice tone that conveys empathy. Security and privacy in telehealth visits are key concerns for both patients and providers. Any telemedicine visit must follow HIPAA standards and data must be fully encrypted for transmittal. Providers must also ensure that the space where the encounter takes place is secure. HIPAA business associate agreements must be in place for all technical personnel involved in the telemedicine visit process (Rutledge et al., 2017).

Telemedicine and Connected Care

While telehealth technology certainly addresses patient requirements for access and convenience, there have also been concerns that it increases the digital divide by denying access to those who don't have computers or mobile devices and those without the technical skills to use such devices. Telemedicine, when delivered in a direct-to-consumer model, can be fragmenting if data from virtual visits are not shared with the patient's primary care provider and entered into the patient's primary medical record. In these instances, as in retail health care, it may be up to the patient to relay information about the virtual visit to her primary care provider, if she even chooses to do so.

Virtual care, when delivered as part of a primary care practice or a health system, can foster access and connected care and can become part of the primary medical record. When virtual care is part of the patient's regular healthcare ecosystem, it can encourage patients to engage in more health coaching, preventive care, and more frequent monitoring of chronic conditions.

Telemonitoring is used primarily in home health care to help with patient self-management support. Taking daily vital signs and weight readings can act as a kind of biofeedback mechanism, which helps patients with illnesses such as heart failure to see the connection between their behavior (eating two hot dogs) and the consequences (increased edema and dyspnea).

When the quality of care delivered via virtual visits is substandard, it can create serious fragmentation and patient dissatisfaction as patients experience continued symptoms and need to access an emergency room or physician office to correct problems that resulted from inadequate care during the virtual visit.

Virtual visits can also contribute to the depersonalization of clinical care, stripping out the elements of touch and the ability to read and respond to verbal cues and body language that occur with in-person visits and possibly making care more transactional and reducing the bond between clinician and patient. On the other hand, patients can also develop a bond with clinicians who provide virtual visits. See the upcoming interview with Tresa Marlow on telemonitoring, for an example.

▶ Nurses and the Technology Revolution

For nurses, doctors, and other clinicians, the digital revolution has opened both a whole new world of possibilities and a whole range of new frustrations. The work of hospital nurses in particular has been transformed from paper charting, one-on-one patient monitoring, and hand-poured medications to the use of electronic monitoring and medication systems and quick access to online patient care reference materials. Technology is also beginning to automate certain routine nursing tasks, raising the specter of robot nurses replacing more expensive and less predictable and controllable human RNs.

A Canadian article on AI and the future of nursing makes the point that in the near future, many tasks such as giving basic information will be transformed by technology (Glauser, 2017). Nursing professor Richard Booth of the Arthur Labatt Family School of Nursing in London, Ontario, says, "We have to plan our own obsolescence to some extent because some predictable nursing work and activities that aren't extremely complex will be automated. . . . if we don't mediate this technology, someone will do it for us."

Nursing Informatics

The digital revolution has given rise to a vital new nursing specialty—nursing informatics. The American Nurses Association (ANA) has defined the scope of practice for nursing informatics: "Nursing informatics (NI) is the specialty that integrates nursing science with multiple information management and analytical sciences to identify, define, manage, and communicate data, information, knowledge, and wisdom in nursing practice" (ANA, 2014). In practice, informatics nurses become experts in the EMR and other technology used in their organization. The nursing specialists train nurses on documentation procedures and help with practical "tips and tricks."

Informatics nurses are also involved in modifying computerized workflows when processes change, testing new tools and workflows for flaws, helping clinicians find the best electronic tools to solve a clinical problem, and developing queries to extract data needed for managerial or clinical work. For example, an informatics nurse might become part of a clinical team that is implementing a new set of fall risk best practices.

Informatics nurses may work with the IT team to embed cues into the record, to develop templates or checklists that remind nurses or therapists to follow all fall risk reduction steps, to provide instructions for the use of evidence-based fall risk assessment tools in an organizational database, and to help create reports for assessing the level of compliance with best practice use. Once the planning phase of the project is completed, informatics nurses would conduct clinician training and help the quality assurance department and nursing managers run reports on the success of the initiative. They would also continue to train and coach clinicians who are having difficulty mastering the new process.

Nursing and the EMR

As mentioned, the EMR has had a profound influence on the practice of nursing. On the one hand, this tool provides instant access to patient information, diagnostic test results, hospitalization data, and other vital information necessary to developing and implementing an effective nursing care plan—all activities that support connected care. On the other hand, nurses often find themselves wading through a thicket of random information to find data that are relevant to the current patient care situation. When the EMR is optimized for clinician use and patient-centered care, it is a powerful tool for telling the patient's story over time, providing insight into care delivered by all the patient's clinicians and offering data vital to the nurse's critical-thinking processes.

EMRs that provide longitudinal information on clinical measures such as vital signs through the use of charts and graphs can enhance connected care by helping the nurse visualize the patients' clinical progress over time. However, if the EMR is simply a coding/billing and data extraction tool, clinicians may be tempted to use standard phrasing and cut-and-paste narratives which do not tell patients' stories and do not enhance patient-centered care.

When documenting in the EMR is a highly labor-intensive effort and does not provide information relevant to daily patient care or if there is insufficient EMR support and training for clinicians, it can become a major factor in clinician burnout for nurses as well as physicians and other clinicians (Ommaya et al., 2018).

As value-based payment becomes more common, data extracted from the EMR will become very relevant in providing aggregate data about nursing practices and their impact on outcomes and in evaluating individual nurse performance. For example, in home care, many agencies track individual nurse outcomes on publicly reported data such as readmissions, timeliness of care starts, and improvement in activities of daily living.

Providing this data to individual nurses, especially when individual data are benchmarked against peer results, can be a powerful factor in performance improvement. This individual performance data must be combined with an analysis of caseload characteristics and some degree of case mix adjustment to avoid false assumptions that the nurse's performance is the only factor that influences outcomes.

▶ Electronic Monitoring and Nursing

In previous eras all patient monitoring was done by hand at the patient's bedside or home. In the modern era, much patient monitoring is electronic and the nursing role often includes setting up the monitoring system, educating patients on its use, doing the actual monitoring, and responding to the results.

Telemetry monitoring in hospitals is the best known monitoring system. In skilled nursing facilities, bed alarms alert nurses to patients who are trying to get out of bed without assistance. In home health care, the nurse case manager implements and responds to telemonitoring, in which patients self-monitor vital signs and weights and send them to a centralized monitoring station.

INTERVIEW WITH TRESA MARLOW, AMERICAN TELEHEALTH

Tresa Marlow, RNC, is director of hospice/telehealth for Advanced Telehealth Solutions (ATHS), which provides a telemonitoring call center service for home health agencies and other organizations that provide remote patient monitoring.

ATHS started in 2002. The company is a URAC-accredited medical call center. The program began with its own home health agency telemonitoring program. They eventually expanded to provide call center services to other organizations across the United States. The company sought URAC accreditation in August 2014 because they wanted to offer a standardized and quality program. They were recently reaccredited and received a 100% score. ATHS works with agencies across the United States.

The ATHS call center employs both clinical and nonclinical staff. It is an around-the-clock operation, open every day of the year. The clinical staff are all nurses and the nonclinical support staff are trained as EMTs, CNAs, or roles in other medical settings.

The program is designed so that agencies that contract with ATHS for call center services can choose their own telemonitoring equipment vendor and install this equipment in patient homes. The home care agency also uses its own electronic medical record (EMR) and gives ATHS staff access to the individual patient record and to the schedules of staff who see telemonitoring patients. The telemonitoring equipment usually consists of a unit that measures weight, blood pressure, heart rate, blood glucose, and blood oxygen.

Patients take their own measurements at specified times and then send their data over a secure internet connection to ATHS.

Each telemonitoring patient is assigned to an ATHS team that consists of clinical and nonclinical staff. There is also a weekend and evening team. Patients have consistent contact with their assigned nurse.

A hallmark of the ATHS program is the use of standardized workflow protocols. These workflows are implemented at the start of the contract between the agency and ATHS. Workflows are designed to address commonly encountered issues such as patients not transmitting data, an inability to locate the patient, and responses to abnormal data.

ATHS has protocols for responding to alerts and abnormal data. If they cannot reach a patient, they have protocols for how many times to contact before calling EMS. ATHS has honed workflows through years of experience and they continue to evolve. When ATHS and the home healthcare agency mutually agree on the use of these workflows and agency staff are educated about using them, the communication process is seamless.

ATHS has different levels of contractual responsibility for responding to abnormal data. The lowest level contract might involve the call center clinician simply contacting the nurse case manager at the home care agency. The highest level contract would empower the ATHS nurse to act as the case manager who contacts the physician in the case of an abnormal reading after completing education and extensive triage.

The telehealth team regularly monitors patient transmitted data. If the data are abnormal, the ATHS nurse will contact the home care clinician using the standardized workflow process and remotely enter the information into the EMR.

Call center staff also documents conversations between ATHS clinicians, patients, and agency clinical staff. Tresa says that it is important for ATHS staff to know who the case manager is and the scheduled visit frequency.

Call center clinicians can see home health agency clinician's schedules. "If we know a visit is coming up and we see a trend, or if the patient has communicated something important, we reach out to the clinician proactively. If, for example, a visit is scheduled and the patient's heart rate and blood pressure are up and blood oxygen saturation is down, it may affect the patient's ability to exercise. If call center clinicians see a problem, they might suggest that, based on the planned schedule, the case manager visit sooner. Sometimes clinicians reach out to Advanced Telehealth staff to get patient trend data to send to the physician when a patient has a visit scheduled or to adjust their schedule."

In most cases, ATHS clinicians communicate and collaborate very well with home care clinicians. ATHS has escalation protocols that can be employed if the telemonitoring nurse feels that the agency is not able to mount an appropriate response to abnormal readings. An example might be a home health agency on-call nurse not making an after-hours call or a visit to a patient with abnormal vital signs.

Tresa discusses how telemonitoring affects patient outcomes: "Patients on the telemonitoring program have 7 days a week nurse oversight. There are always eyes on them. Telemonitoring provides 24/7 immediate access to a clinician."

ATHS encourages patients to call them first with all medical needs: "In some cases, patients go to the ER because they are scared or lonely. Having a nurse to talk with can avoid that type of situation."

Telehealth also prevents readmissions by helping patients gain increased knowledge of their disease process. If things are abnormal, the ATHS staff do education right then and there. Constant education improves independence. It causes patients to be more secure. These interactions with call center clinical staff help to build confidence in patients. Tresa states, "If you spend a little time on the phone, you can probably can talk patients through many problems. Sometimes patients call at 1 a.m. just to talk. They don't need to go to the hospital, they are just lonely."

(continues)

INTERVIEW WITH TRESA MARLOW, AMERICAN TELEHEALTH *(continued)*

ATHS does patient experience surveys. They are required by URAC to do a semiannual survey of patient service and the telemonitoring program as a whole. Tresa notes that "patients enjoy telemonitoring. They don't like it when it ends. It is like knowing that someone is watching." Patients say, "I know that if something is wrong, I will get a call so I don't worry." When asked about obstacles, Tresa replies that the biggest obstacle is an agency that has someone involved in setting up the program who is not on board. That is an immediate road block. Field nurses may be fearful that telemonitoring will take their job. Tresa finds that these problems are becoming less and less as time goes on.

Another barrier is home health agency staff lack of knowledge of outcomes and how telemonitoring helps. Tresa's own agency, when testing the technology, developed champion nurses. The champions had success and told their peers. The champion might say, "Mrs. Jones hasn't been in the hospital for 3 months. You can schedule better and work less because someone else is watching. You can call and ask, 'What is going on with my patient?'"

Another obstacle is the patient fear of using the equipment. This is happening less as patients use technology more. "People aged 100 can use it," Tresa says. "If age is a barrier, it is because we allow it to be. If the patient refuses, you need to look at your presentation. Present it as the standard of care. If there are many refusals then the nurse is not excited about getting this kind of help. If you are enthused the patient will be enthused."

Tresa ends by describing the rewards of being a telemonitoring nurse: "One reward is one-on-one time with the patient. We get to call and talk to them. If I spend 2 minutes or 10 minutes, I get one-on-one time. We have a team of patients and keep them until discharge. We have the same group of patients all week long. We get to see patient progress. We see if they are getting better. Typically patients interact with one to two nurses and an assistant. We also have a weekend team. Patients get to know us. We have found that we develop relationships. I call Mrs. Adams to ask why she didn't check her vital signs." Patients say, "Tresa knows my habits and I know she will call me." If someone else calls, they ask, "Where is Tresa?" Tresa ends by saying, "I love talking to the patients. Sometimes we are the only call these patients get."

On the surface, it would seem that electronic monitoring is a strong factor in providing more connected care for patients by giving clinicians a more constant picture of the patient's condition and allowing for real-time response. However, monitoring in certain settings has created some problems of its own.

Monitoring has reduced physical labor involved in checking on patients and has helped provide early warning systems for patient condition changes. "Alarm fatigue," in which clinicians become desensitized to constant ringing and beeping alarms and false alarms (some estimates of hospital telemetry false alarms are as high as 85%), has become a serious patient safety problem (Ensslin, 2014). Clinicians are constantly required to check on the status of the alarm and may falsely assume that the device is not working properly and disconnect it. This has resulted in patient deaths as an arrhythmia occurs when the alarm is not operational.

The use of electronic monitoring, if not fully integrated into a patient-centered care approach, can result in clinicians treating the monitoring equipment and not the patient, who may feel more like a part of a science experiment than a human being. It is particularly important for nurses to explain how the monitoring devices work and what the alarms mean.

The nurse must allay patient fears about alarms by explaining what is going on when an alarm sounds, especially for those patients who are already anxious.

Nurse Avatars

Nurse avatars are a disruptive new development in technology that may come to have a huge effect on the nursing profession. Avatars, which are also known as "relational agents," are AI programs that are used to provide virtual care for patients. Avatars are typically animated figures on a screen that look like nurses and are programmed to use the language that a real nurse would use. Avatars can be programmed in different forms to meet the needs of different populations. For example, some programs come in two forms: a white nurse and a black nurse avatar. Avatars could conceivably be constructed to mimic the physical characteristics and language of any ethnic group.

The avatars are programmed to perform some nursing activities, including giving patients information such as discharge instructions, assessing patient health status through questioning, providing health coaching advice, and exhibiting simulated compassion through the use of facial expressions such as smiling, body language such as nodding, voice tone, and the use of the patient's name (Abbot & Shaw, 2016).

Studies of patient satisfaction have produced mixed results, but most demonstrate at least a moderately high level of satisfaction. In some cases, patients seemed to feel that the avatar was real and some actually preferred the avatar to a human nurse as illustrated by quotes from some patients who participated in a study with avatars that provided hospital discharge instructions. One patient commented, "It's more helpful than talking to a person; it's just like a nurse, but she explained everything to the T."

Another said, "It was just like a nurse, only better, because sometimes a nurse just gives you a paper and says 'here you go.'" Another concluded, "She cared about me, you know?" (Bickmore, Pfeifer, & Jack, 2009, pp. 6–7).

A virtual nursing platform created at the Université de Montréal is designed to coach patients in behavior change for chronic conditions. Patients answer a series of online questions which then prompts the system to use algorithms to select from a series of coaching videos the patient then watches. The developer of the technology says it does not replace nurses and it works best when it is embedded into interactions with real nurses who encourage patients to use the system at visits and then have the videos build on advice given in face-to-face meetings (Glauser, 2017).

ASK YOURSELF

The discussion of nursing avatars raises an interesting question about connected care. Based on some patient reactions to the technology, it does provide a more cohesive and coherent experience for some patients. It also helps connect the patient to advice, support, and in some cases perceived empathy. But is it connected care when the patient is connected with a piece of software and not a human healthcare professional?

Nurses, Social Media, and E-Patient Support

In their role as health educators, nurses could be expected to play a large role in helping patients, especially those who are less sophisticated about technology use, to find and interpret health information from the internet. Nurses can also participate in social media activities by posting useful health information or sharing articles on Facebook and LinkedIn, for example.

Many YouTube patient education videos are produced by nurses or feature nurses explaining health issues to the public or to patients.

Some internet sites actually provide the public with access to nurses who answer questions posed by site users. However, rather than a focus on the potential of social media, much of the nursing literature focuses on the dangers of overstepping professional boundaries, sharing protected information inappropriately, and not using good security protocols for technology. Social media is used extensively by nurses

BOX 9-2 Summary of Techniques for Supporting Patients in Using Technology for Connected Care

- Involve the patient in point-of-service charting, showing what is being charted and any graphic information that shows longitudinal information about test results and clinical measurements.
- Give information on sources of reliable web information.
- Evaluate new technologies from the patient vantage point.
- Do a digital use assessment at the start of care: Ask patients how they use internet research, social media, wearables, and other technologies in their own self-care.
- Help patients evaluate internet information that they have gathered themselves.
- Provide education and technical support in the use of patient communication technologies such as patient portals.
- Electronically communicate patient information to the patient's other providers. Don't expect the patient to do it.
- Direct patients to relevant online support groups.
- Ensure that any remote treatment is communicated to the patient's primary care provider and is entered in the primary medical record.
- Use social media to post information and advice relevant to your patient population.
- Monitor social media and patient support group sites for the patient view of treatments, gaps, and patient information needs.

for professional reasons such as joining online support groups for nurses, posting useful tips and tricks on nursing blogs, and finding employment opportunities.

Despite the potential for a significant nursing role in e-health, there is very little in the literature about the role of nursing in coaching e-patients, those who are empowered, want their own information, and may use self-monitoring devices (wearables) to track their own health.

Theoretically this should be a very rewarding, if demanding, practice for nurses in health coaching roles. With the right training and experience, nurses could help patients on both sides of the digital divide achieve more connected care.

For less digitally literate patients, the nurse might help the patient find local, free technical instruction, say at a senior center, and might explain how to use a few reliable internet sites for health research.

These patients may need the help of a nurse to access and use a patient portal and to interpret the information they find there. Nurses who themselves are very digitally proficient could help more sophisticated e-patients track

and interpret data from wearables, could recommend reliable healthcare apps, and could help e-patients use evidence-based criteria to evaluate online information and new technology.

BOX 9-2 summarizes actions that professionals can take to support patients in using electronic tools for connected care.

Using data from research and from experiences in the field we can summarize a series of best practices.

Using Technology to Improve Connected Care—An Organizational Checklist

❏ Does the organization have a comprehensive technology strategy that includes improved patient outcomes and patient experience?

❏ Is patient input incorporated into the design and deployment of new organizational technologies?

❏ Is clinician input incorporated into the design and deployment of new technologies?

- Does the organization assess how current technology impacts the patient experience?
- Are there robust security and privacy controls in place to safeguard patient data?
- Are all technology-based workflows optimized for the least number of steps and the best outcomes?
- Are the number of organization technology bugs, glitches, outages, and failures managed and minimized?
- Does the organization have policies and procedures for the use of communication tools and methods such as the use of personal cell phones and texting for conveying patient care information?
- Does the organization help optimize technology for clinician use through the use of training, reference materials, mentoring, clinical informatics consultation, and a customer-oriented help desk?
- Does the organization rigorously evaluate each technology that is implemented to determine its impact on quadruple aim outcomes?
- Does the organization have a user-friendly EMR?
- Does the EMR meet current regulatory criteria and does it have built-in clinical decision support tools?
- Does the organization have best practices for point-of-service charting?
- Does the organization have one patient portal that is easy to use and that gives patients access to the largest possible amount of patient health information?
- Can patients use the EMR portal to perform routine care coordination tasks such as making appointments, finding lab test results, and filling prescriptions?
- Does the organization participate in any type of interoperable EMR or health information exchange?
- Are IOT and AI technologies part of a lean and customer-oriented process that includes adequate training and support for users?
- Are there organizational processes and policies for ensuring that electronic communications are secure and HIPAA compliant?
- Do the organization website and social media postings provide true, useful content for patients and other users, or are they simply a marketing tool?
- Does the organization help clinical and medical staff participate in social media to provide accurate content?
- Does the organization use technology such as telemedicine visits to improve patient convenience?
- Does the organization assess and improve the interconnections between its various technologies?
- Does the organization have a robust data analysis function that can provide data turned into information for improved individual and patient population outcomes?

🔍 CASE STUDY

The Everford Health System Improves Digital Care Connections

Sue Chang, newly appointed chief executive officer (CEO) of the Everford Health System, sat at her desk with her mind churning. Sue, who had recently been promoted from her role of chief nursing officer when the former CEO moved on to a larger system, had been analyzing how she was spending her time. In the few months since she started her new position Sue had been keeping records on the number and types of problems she was asked to solve. Her data analysis had revealed that technology issues were taking up a disproportionate amount of her time and effort and were a constant source of agitation and conflict within the system. Sue, who had recently completed her doctorate in population health, was very aware of the technology revolution and the newest technologies being employed by health systems.

(continues)

Sue's first impression of the technology problems she was asked to address was that the health system seemed to have acquired a hodgepodge of technologies that were not optimized or well connected. These technologies were costing the system millions of dollars in hardware, software, security, support, and data analysis, but had not yielded promised results in terms of quadruple aim outcome improvements. Sue decided that one of her top priority goals would be to guide the health system to optimize its digital tools and processes. Sue knew that this was no task for the faint of heart.

Although Everford had made considerable progress on patient-centered connected care, technology had not yet been a key focus and each "owner" of a technology within the system had his or her own cherished goals and priorities. Sue's first action was to convene the senior management team and discuss chartering an analysis of Everford's digital toolkit and processes.

She particularly cultivated the support of the chief information officer, the new chief nursing officer, and the chief medical officer, all of whom had large constituencies and a large stake in the outcome.

After several weeks of discussion and debate, the senior management team commissionsed a group of internal experts with technology expertise to collect data and to assess the current state of technology use at Everford. The assessment team returned with the promised report within a month. To the surprise of no one on the senior management team, the analysis revealed considerable room for improvement. Specific findings included:

- Computer systems were optimized for regulatory, billing, and marketing purposes but not for staff use or patient care.
- There were small-scale security problems, such as the use of nonsecure texting for exchanging patient information between clinicians.
- The EMR was full of complex templates, disconnected sections, and hard-to-use features, but did not "tell the patient story." It had become a source of frustration and burnout for certain clinicians.
- Some degree of animosity existed between the clinical staff and the IT help desk staff, primarily around issues of perceived "user errors."
- There was a robust nursing clinical informatics service, but no comparable service for other disciplines.
- There was a lack of interoperable EMRs. Medical practices in the system still used paper records or had purchased EMR systems that were not compatible with the hospital system.
- Postacute care system partners (skilled nursing facilities and home health agencies), labs, and outpatient facilities were disconnected from the hospital. They had access to the hospital system through a portal, but could not share their data with the hospital.
- There was no rational system for using digital tools to engage and support patients. The hospital had a patient portal, but it did not allow patients to enter data. The system medical practices either had no portals or each practice had its own portal.
- System social media and online content were being used primarily for marketing purposes and not to support patients with useful information and guidance.
- There had been no staff or patient input into the types of technology that were chosen and the workflows that were used to embed the technology into the clinical system.
- A variety of communication tools were being used to connect healthcare providers with each other and with patients, including texting, portals, email, and phone. There was no corporate policy about closed loop communication.
- Some system medical practices were using telemedicine for remote visits and two of the systems' home health agencies were using telemonitoring. There were no coherent policies and procedures for the use of these technologies.

- There was a mix of disparate IOT solutions that had never been fully evaluated, including a patient tracking system for one surgical service, but not others; an interactive voice response system for discharged patients; and a nurse avatar software for patient education on the cardiac service, but nowhere else. For a subset of patients, a physical therapy avatar was being used for postsurgical care at home.

As soon as the report was presented, and Sue saw the variety of tools being used and the number of disconnects between parts of the system, she understood why she had been so consumed with technology issues.

After a period of analysis, discussion, considerable debate, and not a little bargaining, the senior management team decided to reapply the concept of the quadruple aim and pillars of connected care to integrate and focus its technologies. All agreed that there had been too much emphasis on business goals and revenue generation and not enough on the patient and staff experience. Higher level system IT work around hardware and software choices, security issues, and the use of data continued in parallel to the effort.

Over the next year, the Everford system implemented a variety of initiatives to move toward a more integrated and patient-centered technology system. Integrating EMRs became priority one. Everford decided that all owned and affiliated entites must participate in the enterprise EMR. Medical group contracts were rewritten to include this stipulation at contract renewal time. While some practices dropped out of the system, more agreed and interoperability became a reality.

Postacute and outpatient providers were incorporated into the system, and their notes became part of the system medical record, making it a true integrated system. All system entities also agreed to offer a uniform patient portal and to adopt the use of Open Notes. The system became a participant in the statewide health information exchange and both provided information and obtained information from other health systems and providers in the state.

The system assessed the impact of IOT implementations and only kept those that demonstrated value in improving outcomes. For example, while the physical therapy avatar for joint replacement had been helpful to patients who were more fit and more technologically capable, it had failed and resulted in readmissions for patients who were sicker and less able to master the technology. Putting guidelines in place for the use of all IOT technology selections and implementations helped resolve this type of problem.

Everford created best practices around communication, requiring providers to use the system secure texting app rather than their own device for texts. Interdisciplinary communication was standardized and closed loop communication became a requirement.

The IT department held a series of focus groups with users, did some customer service training with help desk representatives, and conducted "tips and tricks" forums for clinical staff.

Nursing informatics became clinical informatics and all professions benefited from the expertise of these clinical/IT professionals. The newly formed clinical informatics group was able to simplify the EMR and, after having researched best practices with other users of the same EMR system, was able to implement new best practices that reduced clinician documentation time and frustration.

An expert in "design thinking" was hired to get input from both staff and patients about how to improve the use of current technologies. These events produced a number of suggestions that were used to redesign workflows to make technology more user friendly for both patients and staff.

The system website and social media functions were evaluated and redesigned to provide content, online support groups, and chat functions that supported patients and family caregiver self-care and wellness rather than just marketing system products and services.

(continues)

The system reevaluated its telemonitoring and telemedicine programs and found that while they improved patient service and improved outcomes in some cases, they needed to be better integrated with clinical workflows and the EMR. These programs became the object of further study and improvement.

At the end of an intense year of review, analysis, and critical thinking, Everford had vastly improved connected care through the use of digital tools. No longer were clinical staff and patients at the mercy of a vast, complex, and fragmented technical system that no one really controlled and that had evolved without their interests in mind.

Sue and the senior management team had had their share of conflict over the integration of their technical systems, but with the support of the board, they had done it. While no one expected their work to be the ultimate answer, most felt that their foray into connecting the dots of technology would better equip Everford for a value-based future.

▸ **Chapter Summary**

Digital technologies have the potential to vastly improve connected care for patients. Various tools and mobile apps can help foster patient centeredness and build the pillars of connected care: communication, transitions, coordination, collaboration, and teamwork. Digital technologies such as the EMR, patient tracking systems, and health information exchanges allow health professionals to share and communicate information about patient care. They also reduce the incidence of medical errors and waste through the use of electronic order entry, decision support tools, and alerts and warnings.

Digital tools have allowed patients to take more control of their health. Health information on the internet, social media, mobile apps, wearable devices that can track personal health data, and patient portals provide patients with multiple methods for accessing and managing health information and making health decisions. Services such as telemedicine have improved patient access to health care and convenience.

The leading edge of digital health care such as big data, predictive analytics, IOT, and AI holds tremendous promise for personalizing patient care, validating the outcomes of treatments, and reducing labor in health care. These technological advances, however, are mostly in the developmental stages and have not yet made a major impact on the day-to-day practice of patient care.

Technology, while very useful, can also foster serious fragmentation and can actually inhibit connected care when it does not function as intended, when the patient is on the far side of the digital divide, or when it requires an extraordinary level of clinical effort to manage technical devices or complex pieces of software. Recent studies on EMR-induced health professional burnout provide a cautionary tale about this issue.

Is technology the magic answer to the fragmentation problem in health care? It is certainly framed that way in the healthcare industry, with many articles in the medical press using the term "connected care" to describe any digital product that connects individuals or organizations.

The reality is, of course, far more complex. The healthcare technology revolution has actually had a paradoxical effect on connected care (in the context used in this discussion) in the healthcare industry. When technology is chosen with the goal of meeting key patient-connected care requirements, uses patient and provider input in design and implementation, is thoughtfully integrated into existing clinical processes and information sources, and is extensively supported, it can be a powerful force for connected care.

On the other hand, technology chosen and implemented purely for strategic and competitive reasons, and not carefully integrated and linked to the patient and his or her health record in a cohesive way, can be highly fragmented and dissatisfying to both clinicians and patients.

One huge driver of technology development, sales, and implementation in the United States is competition and ultimately profit. Technology developers, driven by venture capital requirements, must aggressively sell their product as the best and only solution to a variety of healthcare ills. Healthcare facilities that are in the grip of a chaotic and competitive market, and trying desperately to drive down costs, may see a particular technology solution as a competitive edge and a magic answer to a value-based payment delivery system transformation.

Ultimately, the effectiveness of technology for connected care hinges not on the hardware, the software, the lifelike avatars, and the eye-catching screen displays, but on the hard work of considering human needs, rigorously evaluating tools for their capability to help patients, and the will, the skill, and the resources to create work processes and support systems that can extend and enhance the work of the human mind and human hands in support of good patient care.

References

Abbot, M., & Shaw, P. (2016). Virtual nursing avatars: Nurse roles and evolving concepts of care. *Online Journal of Issues in Nursing, 21*(3). http://www.nursingworld.org /MainMenuCategories/ANAMarketplace/ANAPeriodicals /OJIN/TableofContents/Vol-21-2016/No3-Sept-2016 /Articles-Previous-Topics/Virtual-Nursing-Avatars.html

Adamson, D. (2018). Big data in healthcare made simple: Where it stands today and where it's going. Retrieved from www .healthcatalyst.com/big-data-in-healthcare-made-simple

The Advisory Board. (2014). Getting patients to use your portal (poster). Retrieved from www.advisory.com /research/quality-reporting-roundtable/getting-patients -to-use-your-portal

Agency for Healthcare Research and Quality. (2016). Can electronic health records prevent harm to patients? Rockville, MD: AHRQ. http://www.ahrq.gov/news /blog/ahrqviews/020916.ht

Alpert, J. S. (2016). The electronic medical record in 2016: Advantages and disadvantages. *Digital Medicine, 2*(2), 48–51. doi:10.4103/2226-8561.189504

American Academy of Family Physicians. (2017). Patients trust social media, so be their trusted source. Retrieved from www.aafp.org/news/blogs/freshperspectives/entry /patients_trust_social_media_so.html

American Hospital Association. (2016). Individuals' ability to electronically access their medical records, perform key tasks is growing. *AHA Trendwatch.*

American Nurses Association. (2014). *Nurse informatics, scope and standards of practice* (2nd ed.). Silver Spring, MD: ANA.

American Telemedicine Association. (2018). American Telemedicine Association applauds landmark expansion of medicare telehealth coverage. Retrieved from https://thesource.americantelemed.org/blogs /jessica-washington/2018/02/09/american-telemedicine -association-applauds-landmar?CommunityKey=a19668dd -1d45-44c2-8c38-318adc561770&tab.Bick

Apple Newsroom. (2018). Apple announces effortless solution bringing health records to iPhone. Retrieved from www.apple.com/newsroom/2018/01/apple-announces -effortless-solution-bringing-health-records-to-iPhone/

Aziz, H., & Moshen, M. (2015). *The blue button project, engaging patients in healthcare by the click of a button. Perspectives in health information management.* Chicago, IL: American Health Information Management Association.

Bandoim, L. (2017). How online patient portals are transforming health care. Retrieved from http://theweek.com/articles/737128 /how-online-patient-portals-are-transforming-health-care

Bickmore, T., Pfeifer, L., & Jack, B. (2009). Taking the time to care: Empowering low health literacy hospital patients with virtual nurse agents. *Proceedings of the ACM SIGCHI Conference on Human Factors in Computing Systems (CHI).* Boston, MA. Retrieved from http://relationalagents. com/publications/CHI09.VirtualNurse.pdf

Boachie, P. (2017). Three ways social media revolutionized medical care. Retrieved from www.adweek.com/digital /pius-boachie-guest-post-3-ways-social-media -revolutionized-medical-care/

Boudreaux, E., Waring, M., Hayes, R., Sadasivam, R., Mullen, S., & Pagoto, S. (2014). Evaluating and selecting mobile health apps: Strategies for healthcare providers and healthcare organizations. *Translational Behavioral Medicine, 4*(4), 363–371. https://doi.org/10.1007/s13142 -014-0293-9

Brown, J. (2013). How to master electronic communication with patients. Retrieved from http://medicaleconomics .modernmedicine.com/medical-economics/news/tags /health-insurance-portability-and-accountability-act /how-master-electroni

CDW Healthcare. (2017). 2017 Patient engagement perspectives study. CDW Healthcare. www.cdwnews room.com/wp-content/uploads/2017/02/CDW-Patient -Engagement-2017-Fact-Sheet_3.pdf

Center for Connected Health Policy. (2018). What is telehealth? Retrieved from www.cchpca.org/what-is-telehealth

Center for Connected Medicine. (2017). *Top of mind for top US health systems, 2018*. Pittsburgh, PA: The Center for Connected Medicine and The Health Management Academy.

Centers for Disease Control and Prevention. (2011). Health communicator's social media toolkit. Retrieved from https://www.cdc.gov/socialmedia/tools/guidelines/socialmediatoolkit.html

Centers for Disease Control and Prevention. (2017). Electronic medical records/electronic health records (EMRs/EHRs). National Center for Health Statistics, Fast Facts. Retrieved from www.cdc.gov/nchs/fastats/electronic-medical-records.htm

Centers for Medicare and Medicaid Services. (2017). Memo to state surveyors regarding: Texting of patient information among healthcare providers. Retrieved from www.cms.gov/Medicare/Provider-Enrollment-and-Certification/SurveyCertificationGenInfo/Downloads/Survey-and-Cert-Letter-18-10.pdf

Centers for Medicare and Medicaid Services. (2018). Download claims with Medicare's blue button. Retrieved from www.Medicare.gov

deBronkart, D. (2018). About: E-patient Dave—A voice of patient engagement. Retrieved from http://www.epatientdave.com/about-dave/

Delbanco, T., Walker, J., Bell, S. K., Darer, J. D., Elmore, J. G., Farag, N., . . . Leveille, S. G. (2012). Inviting patients to read their doctors' notes: A quasi-experimental study and a look ahead. *Annals of Internal Medicine, 157*, 461–470. doi:10.7326/0003-4819-157-7-201210020-00002

Deloitte. (2018). 2018 global health care outlook; the evolution of smart health care. Retrieved from https://www2.deloitte.com/global/en/pages/life-sciences-and-healthcare/articles/global-health-care-sector-outlook.html

Deloitte Center for Health Solutions. (2016). *Will patients and caregivers embrace technology enabled health care? Findings from the Deloitte 2016 Survey of US Health Care Consumer*. Westlake, TX: Deloitte University Press.

Department of Health and Human Services. (2018). Does the HIPAA privacy rule permit health care providers to use e-mail to discuss health issues and treatment with their patients? Retrieved from www.hhs.gov/hipaa/for-professionals/faq/570/does-hipaa-permit-health-care-providers-to-use-email-to-discuss-health-issues-with-patients/index.html

Dutcher, J. (2014). What is big data? Retrieved from https://datascience.berkeley.edu/what-is-big-data/

Dzau, V. J., McClellan, M., McGinnis, J. M., & Finkelman, E. M. (Eds.). (2017). *Vital directions for health & health care: An initiative of the National Academy of Medicine*. Washington, DC: National Academy of Medicine.

Ensslin, P. (2014). Do you hear what I hear? Combating alarm fatigue. *American Nurse Today, 9*(11). https://www.americannursetoday.com/hear-hear-combating-alarm-fatigue/

Espaillat, R. (2017). Maryland care physicians offers app for emergency care. Retrieved from www.localdvm.com/news/maryland/maryland-care-phycisians-offers-app-for-virtual-emergency-care/764881762

FoxNews Health. (2017). Ransomware's cyberattack cripples hospitals across England. Retrieved fromhttp://www.foxnews.com/health/2017/05/12/uk-hospitals-turn-away-patients-after-ransomware-attack.html

Gittlen, S. (2017). NEJM catalyst survey snapshot: What patient engagement technology is good for. Retrieved from www.catalyst.nejm.org/patient-engagement-technology-goo

Glauser, W. (2017, May/June). Artificial intelligence, automation and the future of nursing. *Canadian Nurse*. https://www.canadian-nurse.com/articles/issues/2017/may-june-2017/artificial-intelligence-automation-and-the-future-of-nursing

Gordon, N. P., & Hornbrook, M. C. (2016). Differences in access to and preferences for using patient portals and other ehealth technologies based on race, ethnicity, and age: A database and survey study of seniors in a large health plan. *Journal of Medical Internet Research, 18*(3), e50. http://doi.org/10.2196/jmir.5105

The Guardian. (2017). AI programs exhibit racial and gender biases, research reveals. Retrieved from www.theguardian.com/technology/2017/apr/13/ai-programs-exhibit-racist-and-sexist-biases-research-reveals

Healthcare Information and Management Systems Society. (2013). What is interoperatiblity? Retrieved from www.himss.org/library/interoperability-standards/what-is-interoperability

Healthcare Information and Management Systems Society. (2014). HIE FAQ. Retrieved from https://www.himss.org/library/health-information-exchange/FAQ

HealthIT.gov. (2011). EMR vs. EHR, what is the difference? Retrieved from www.healthit.gov/buzz-blog/electronic-health-and-medical-records/emr-vs-ehr-difference/

HealthIT.gov. (2017a). Health information exchange. Retrieved from www.healthit.gov/topic/health-it-basics/health-information-exchange

HealthIT.gov. (2017b). What is a patient portal? Retrieved from www.healthit.gov/providers-professionals/faqs/what-patient-portal

HealthIT.gov. (2018a). Benefits of electronic medical records. Retrieved from www.healthit.gov/providers-professionals/benefits-electronic-health-records-ehrs

HealthIT.gov. (2018b). Meaningful use. Retrieved from www.healthit.gov/providers-professionals/meaningful-use-definition-objectives

Herbert, L. P., Makopoulos, C., & Lawhon, L. (2016). Social media and health, what socially active patients really want. Retrieved from https://health-union.com/news/online-health-experience-survey/

International Data Corporation. (2017). IDC forecasts shipments of wearable devices to nearly double by 2021 as smart watches and new product categories

gain traction. Retrieved from www.idc.com/getdoc
.jsp?containerId=prUS4340851

Irizarry, T., DeVito Dabbs, A., & Curran, C. R. (2015). Patient
portals and patient engagement: A state of the science
review. *Journal of Medical Internet Research, 17*(6), e148.
http://doi.org/10.2196/jmir.4255

Johnson, C. (2012, October 10). Thoughts on the electronic
medical record and the disappearance of patients'
stories. *Health Beat Blog by Maggie Mahar.* http://
www.healthbeatblog.com/2012/10/the-electronic
-medical-record-and-the-disappearance-of-patients
-stories/

Kacik, J. (2017). Telehealth market poised for growth, but
use remains low. Retrieved from www.modernhealthcare
.com/article/20170620/NEWS/170629995

Kirkner, R. (2017). Telehealth: Some thumbs up, some
down, on quality of care. Retrieved from www.managed
caremag.com/archives/2017/4/telehealth-some
-thumbs-some-down-quality-care

Lee, W. W., Alkureishi, M. A., Ukabiala, O., Venable, L. R.,
Ngooi, S. S., Staisiunas, D. D., . . . Arora, V. M. (2016).
Patient perceptions of electronic medical record use
by faculty and resident physicians: A mixed methods
study. *Journal of General Internal Medicine, 31*(11),
1315–1322. doi:10.1007/s11606-016-3774-3

Lytle, J. (2017). A patient's perspective on health information
management. *Health Literacy Research and Practice,
1*(1), e11–13. doi.org/10.3928/24748307-20170307-03

McBride, M. (2012). The disconnect between EHRs and
health information exchange. Retrieved from www
.medicaleconomics.modernmedicine.com/medical
-economics/news/modernmedicine/modern-medicine
-feature-articles/disconnect-between-ehrs-and-h?
pag

Menachemi, N., & Collum, T. (2011). Benefits and drawbacks
of electronic health record systems. *Risk Management
and Healthcare Policy, 4,* 47–55.

Merriam Webster. (2018). Artificial intelligence. Retrieved
from www.merriam-webster.com/dictionary/artificial%20
intelligence

Mohan, S. (2016). Too many patient portals—What can
you do about it? HIMSS16 Conference and Exhibition
Presentation, February.

Monegain, B. (2017). Health care's digital divide is getting
bigger and other bad news from Black Book. Healthcare
IT News.

Naylor, B. (2016). Firms are buying and selling your information
online, what can you do about it? Retrieved from www
.npr.org/sections/alltechconsidered/2016/07/11/485571291
/firms-are-buying-sharing-your-online-info-what
-can-you-do-about-it

Nelson, R. (2016). Informatics: Empowering epatients to
drive health care reform—Part I. *The Online Journal
of Issues in Nursing, 21*(3).

Nightingale, F. (1863). *Notes on hospitals.* London: Longman,
Green, Longman, Roberts and Green.

O'Leary, K., Liebovitz, D. M., Wu, R. C., Ksheeraja, R.,
Knoten, C., Mengxin Sun , M. P. P., . . . Reddy, M. (2017).
Hospital-based clinicians' use of technology for patient
care-related communication: A national survey. *Journal
of Hospital Medicine, 7,* 530–535.

Ommaya, A., Cipriano, P., Hoyt, D., Horvath, K., Tang, P.,
Paz, H., . . . Sinsky, C. (2018). Care-centered clinical
documentation in the digital environment: Solutions
to alleviate burnout. National Academy of Medicine.
https://nam.edu/care-centered-clinical-documentation-
digital-environment-solutions-alleviate-burnout/

Open Notes. (2017). Website front page. Retrieved from
Opennotes.org

Patient View. (2013). What do people want from health
apps? Retrieved from https://alexwyke.files.wordpress
.com/2013/10/health-app-white-paper-to-go.pdf

Pohl, M. (2017). 325,000 mobile health apps available in
2017—Android now the leading mHealth platform.
Retrieved from www.research2guidance.com

Pratt, M. (2017). Making wearables valuable to physician
practices. Retrieved from www.physicianspractice.com
/technology-survey/making-wearables-valuable-medical
-practices

PwC Health Research Institute. (2012). Social media
likes healthcare, from marketing to social business.
Retrieved from www.pwc.com/us/en/health-industries
/health-research-institute.html

ReferralMD. (2017). Facts & statistics on social media
and healthcare, 2017 update. Retrieved from https://
getreferralmd.com/2013/09/healthcare-social-media
-statistics/

Rose, D., Richter, L.T., & Kapustin, J. (2014). Patient
experiences with electronic medical records: Lessons
learned. *Journal of the American Association of Nurse
Practitioners, 26*(12), 674–680.

Rutledge, C. M., Kott, K., Schweickert, P. A., Poston, R.,
Fowler, C., & Haney, T. S. (2017). Telehealth and eHealth
in nurse practitioner training: Current perspectives.
Advanced Medical Education Practicum, 8, 399–409.
doi:10.2147/AMEP.S116071

Smith, A. (2017). Record shares of Americans now own
smartphones, have home broadband. Pew Research
Center. http://www.pewresearch.org/fact-tank/2017/01/12
/evolution-of-technology/

Society for Participatory Medicine. (2018). About us. Retrieved
from http://e-patients.net/about-e-patientsnet

Stanford Medicine X. (2014). 2014 Stanford Medicine
X ePatient scholarship program information. Retrieved
from http://medicinex.stanford.edu/2014-stanford-
medicine-x-epatient-scholarship-program-information
/#about

Storck, L. (2017). Policy statement: Texting in health
care. *Online Journal of Nursing Informatics, 21*(1). http://
www.himss.org/ojni

Sutner S. (2016). The internet of things improves
patient experience, IOT agenda. Retrieved from

http://internetofthingsagenda.techtarget.com/feature /Internet-of-Medical-Things-improves-patient-experience

Topaz, M., Ronquillo, C., Lee, Y. L., & Peltonen, L.-M. (2017). Nurse informaticians report low satisfaction and multi-level concerns with electronic health records: Results from an international survey. *AMIA 2016 Annual Symposium Proceedings, 2016,* 2016–2025

Ventola, C. L. (2014). Social media and health care professionals: Benefits, risks, and best practices. *Pharmacy and Therapeutics, 39*(7), 491–520.

Vydra, T., Cuaresma, E., Kretovics, M., & Bose-Brill, S. (2015). Diffusion and use of tethered personal health records in primary cCare. AHIMA Foundation. *Perspectives in Health Information Management.*

CHAPTER 10

High-Risk Gaps and Cracks I: Social Determinants of Health, Health Disparities, and Mental Health

CHAPTER OBJECTIVES

After completing this chapter readers will be able to:

- Identify gaps in care related to social determinants of health, health disparities, and mental illness
- Describe measures for assessing patient requirements and care effectiveness
- List evidence-based best practices for each focus area
- Describe successful models that apply connected care techniques to close care gaps
- Explain the role of nursing in providing holistic, connected care in high-risk focus areas
- Assess their organization's status on successfully integrating care to reduce high-risk gaps

▶ Introduction

Visualize a true connected care system as a giant jigsaw puzzle. All needed services, communications, and resources are pieces of the puzzle and they fit together snugly to create a coherent and holistic treatment and support system for patients and families. Now picture the reality of the U.S. healthcare system. The jigsaw puzzle is missing pieces everywhere, and in some cases, the pieces aren't even designed to fit together. **FIGURE 10-1** illustrates this concept.

For patient populations with needs that don't fit well into the fee-for-service, private

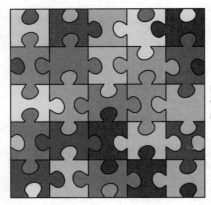

Holistic, connected care system with medical care and all related services integrated and coordinated.

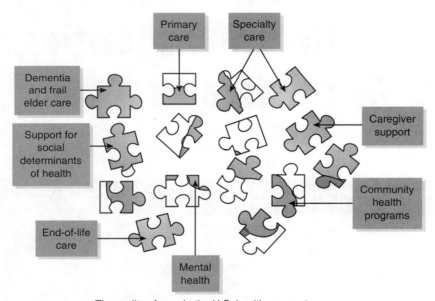

The reality of care in the U.S. healthcare system.

FIGURE 10-1 High-Risk Gaps and Cracks in Care

insurance, medical model of the U.S. health system, this puzzle has even more missing pieces. These populations include those who are socioeconomically disadvantaged and those of a different racial, ethnic, or gender identity group from the perceived majority population. Many of these patients are simply cut off from access to regular health care by lack of insurance, by immigration status, or by virtue of the patient's location in relation to health facilities.

In many cases, health professionals see only their own piece of the puzzle and not the holes or disconnected pieces. Patients and families are often the only ones who see and feel the full extent of gaps in care and support. The culture of health care in the United States with its focus on medical treatment, procedures, and cures, to the exclusion of other health and socioeconomic issues, has worsened these disconnects.

Vital Directions for Health and Health Care, a 2017 document from the National Academy of Medicine, summarizes the challenges that the United States faces in improving the health of its citizens: "Health care today is marked by structural inefficiencies, unprecedented costs, and fragmented care delivery, all of which place increasing pressure and burden on individuals and families, providers, businesses, and entire communities. The consequent health shortfalls are experienced across the whole population, but disproportionately impact our most vulnerable citizens due to their complex health and social circumstances" (Dzau, McClellan, McGinnis, & Finkelman, 2017, p. 1).

One underlying theme in the *Vital Directions* document is the issue of "persisting care fragmentation and discontinuity." In this chapter we will look at some specific focus areas where these problems are most pressing and prominent, including the social determinants of health, health disparities, and the gaps between medical and mental health care.

While it is impossible to define all of the patient populations that fall into these care gaps, many can be characterized as "high need" or "different need" patients. For each of these areas, we will consider patient requirements and the gap between what patients want and what they actually get. We will review measures relevant to each gap area and how measures and assessments can be incorporated into clinical practice to identify individual patient or family care gaps and provide more holistic care for patients.

We will consider best practices for each focus area and give examples of models that have successfully closed care gaps and provided more connected care to patients. We will provide specific examples of tools and techniques that can be used at the organizational and clinical practice levels.

We will discuss progress that has been made as the U.S. health system moves from an entirely medical, fee-for-service model to a value-based model of payment which provides many more incentives for healthcare providers to close the gaps and fill the cracks in the care system. We will review the historical and essential role that nurses play in helping patients with health and socioeconomic conditions that don't fit neatly into the mainstream of the medical/cure model that has dominated health care.

▶ Social Determinants

Of all the high-risk gaps in the healthcare system, the lack of attention to social determinants of health may have the most impact on patient outcomes and the patient experience of care. The Centers for Disease Control and Prevention (CDC) National Center for HIV/AIDS, Viral Hepatitis, STD, and TB Prevention (2014) defines the social determinants of health in this way: "Factors that contribute to a person's current state of health. These factors may be biological, socioeconomic, psychosocial, behavioral, or social in nature."

Scientists generally recognize five determinants of health of a population:

- Biology and genetics. Examples: sex, age, gender identity
- Individual behavior. Examples: alcohol use, injection drug use (needles), unprotected sex, and smoking
- Social environment. Examples: discrimination, income, and gender
- Physical environment. Examples: where a person lives and crowding conditions
- Health services. Examples: access to quality health care and having or not having health insurance (CDC.gov, 2014)

A second and closely related concept is that of health disparities. The U.S. government report, *Healthy People 2020,* describes the concept of health disparities: "A particular type of health difference that is closely linked with social, economic, and/or environmental disadvantage. Health disparities adversely affect groups of people who have systematically experienced greater obstacles to health based on their racial or ethnic group; religion; socioeconomic status; gender; age; mental health; cognitive, sensory, or physical disability; sexual orientation or gender identity; geographic location; or other characteristics historically linked to discrimination or exclusion" (Healthy People, 2018).

Research has shown that the social determinants of health have far more of an impact on health outcomes than medical care itself. **FIGURE 10-2** illustrates this concept.

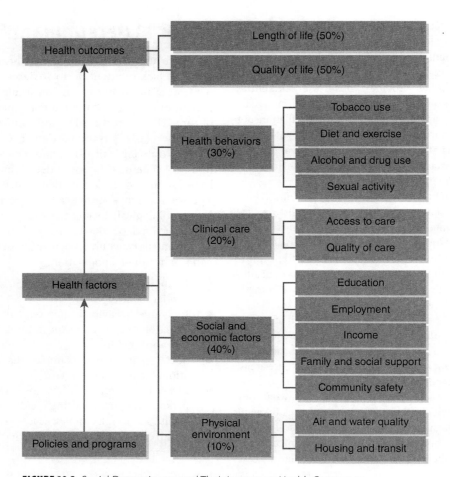

FIGURE 10-2 Social Determinants and Their Impact on Health Outcomes

Reprinted with permission from County Health Rankings & Roadmaps. Retrieved from http://www.countyhealthrankings.org/our-approach (accessed July 18, 2017).

How Social Determinants and Health Disparities Impact Care Fragmentation

Health disparities and a lack of attention to the social determinants of health are core factors in the fragmentation of health care.

Social and financial barriers to care create a fundamental disconnect—that is, a lack of access to healthcare services, without which there cannot be connected care of any kind. While a subset of health professionals has often seen the social determinants of health as part of their responsibility, most have not. Many healthcare facilities and health professionals have been more narrowly focused on procedures and processes that treat and cure. Some would say that this is as it should be. Health professionals should focus on medical care, and social services agencies should help patients with social determinants of health. One view, in fact, says that medicalizing interventions for the social determinants of health would worsen the problem by entangling social solutions with medical care systems. The paper, "Social Determinants 101," gives the example of a social worker who sees a patient in a healthcare setting but who determines that what the patient really needs is social support and a friend (Magnan, 2017).

Another fragmenting aspect of the social determinants of health is secrecy. Many patients, without significant help and prompting from health professionals, fail to reveal social or emotional issues that are closely related to health (e.g., domestic violence or drug abuse). These issues are clearly root causes of many medical and emotional ailments. Without full disclosure, health professionals are treating with pills what might be best helped by social services, support groups, and legal advice. This is the worst kind of fragmentation in health care.

Much of the research agrees that the real solution to the negative impact of the social determinants of health is at the policy level (better jobs, access to nutritious food, communities with open space and areas for walking and recreation, affordable housing, etc.). Two major barriers at this level are the lack of political will to solve these problems and a lack of funding.

One interesting view of the latter issue comes from the *Vital Directions* document, which notes an estimated 30% of healthcare costs are wasteful and unnecessary. These funds could be much more effectively redirected to more effective care delivery and to social, behavioral, and other essential services necessary for good health outcomes. Many policy makers argue that health professionals who want to help patients with social determinants of health become active in local and national policy debates and that they advocate for programs and funding that alleviate poverty and provide social supports to vulnerable populations.

In this chapter we will focus more narrowly on the types of things that health professionals themselves can do to help their own patients overcome barriers to connected care that have their roots in the social determinants of health.

Assessing Social Determinants of Health

Much of the work of measuring social determinants of health has been done with large populations at the city, state, regional, or national level. This data, while helpful for organizational planning and for developing collaborations between health and social services agencies, is less useful in modifying clinical care to effectively address the social determinants of health.

Traditional clinical practice focuses on assessment of physical, and to some extent psychological, aspects of health, but has typically not done a good job of assessing the impact of social determinants of health on individual patients. In recent years a variety of assessments, some of them evidence based, have been developed to help clinicians assess the impact of social determinants of health on both an individual patient and patient population levels.

One widely used evidence-based tool is the standardized *Protocol for Responding to and Assessing Patients' Assets, Risks, and Experiences* (PRAPARE), developed in 2013 through a collaboration between the National Association of Community Health Centers, the Association of Asian Pacific Community Health Organizations, the Oregon Primary Care Association, and the Institute for Alternative Futures.

The Oregon Community Health Information Network has also released a set of electronic health record (EHR)–based tools that use PRAPARE to identify and address patients' unmet social needs. The National Association of Community Health Centers (2016) offers a full implementation toolkit for assessment users, including information about integrating PRAPARE into the electronic medical record. The PRAPARE tool assesses issues such as housing, education, work situation, stress level, transportation, refugee status, safety at home, incarceration history, and social supports. To view the PRAPARE tool in depth, go to http://www.nachc.org/wp-content/uploads /2018/05/PRAPARE_One_Pager_Sept_2016.pdf. Billioux, Verlander, Anthony, and Alley (2017) provide an example of an extensive screening tool utilized by accountable health communities (a Medicare innovation model) to screen for social determinants of health.

Health Leads, an organization that works with healthcare organizations to manage social needs interventions, has created a screening toolkit that guides providers in how to uncover underlying social needs and assesses the impact of the answers on health issues. Health Leads lists five criteria for a great screening tool:

1. Make it short and simple.
2. Choose clinically validated questions at the right level of precision.
3. Integrate the tool into clinical workflows.
4. Ask patients to prioritize social needs that matter most to them.
5. Pilot before scaling.

Health Leads provides a sample screening tool which addresses social determinants of health such as food insecurity, potential utility shut-offs, child care, transportation, cost barriers to healthcare access, health literacy, and personal safety. The instrument also asks whether any current need requires urgent assistance. **FIGURE 10-3**

Recommended Screening Tool

This is a sample social needs screening tool – please tailor it based on your population, scope, and goals.
This work is licensed under a Creative Commons Attribution-ShareAlike 4.0 International License

Example introductory text: This form is available in other languages. If you do not speak English, call (800) 555-6666 (TTY: (800) 777-8888) to connect to an interpreter who will assist you at no cost.

Name:__________ Phone number: __________

Preferred Language:__________ Best time to call:__________

	YES / NO
In the last 12 months, did you ever **eat less than you felt you should** because there wasn't enough money for food?	Y N
In the last 12 months, has your **utility company shut off your service** for not paying your bills?	Y N
Are you worried that in the next 2 months, you **may not have stable housing?**	Y N
Do problems getting **child care make it difficult for you to work** or study? *(leave blank if you do not have children)*	Y N
In the last 12 months, have you needed to see a doctor, **but could not because of cost?**	Y N
In the last 12 months, have you ever had to go without health care because you didn't have **a way to get there?**	Y N
Do you ever need help **reading hospital materials?**	Y N
Are you **afraid you might be hurt** in your apartment building or house?	Y N
If you checked YES to any boxes above, **would you like to receive assistance** with any of these needs?	Y N
Are any of your needs urgent? For example: I don't have food tonight, I don't have a place to sleep tonight	Y N

FIGURE 10-3 Health Leads Recommended Screening Tool.

Reproduced from Health Leads. (2016). Health Leads screening toolkit. Retrieved from https://healthleadsusa.org/tools-item/health-leads-screening-toolkit/

shows the sample Health Leads Recommended Screening tool (Health Leads, 2016).

The Health Leads screening toolkit is available to any user through a Creative Commons license. You can access it at https://healthleadsusa .org/wp-content/uploads/2016/07/Health-Leads -Screening-Toolkit-July-2016.pdf.

In 2014, the Institute of Medicine's (IOM) *Committee on the Recommended Social and Behavioral Domains and Measures for Electronic Health Records* recommended that, at minimum, 10 patient-reported social and behavioral domains and one neighborhood/community level domain should be documented in EHRs. The domains included in this framework are alcohol use, race and ethnicity, address, median income, tobacco use, education, depression, dietary patterns, physical activity, financial resource strain, intimate partner violence, physical activity, stress, and social isolation. The recommendations provide benchmarks for prioritizing social issues in clinical assessments (IOM, 2014).

Using Social Determinants of Health Assessment Tools in Clinical Settings

A review of the clinical assessment tools described in this chapter reveals many similarities, but no total agreement on which domains are most important and which questions should be asked.

Healthcare organizations that choose to create their own instruments rather than using a validated tool such as PRAPARE must ask themselves which of the social determinants of health are of most importance to their particular patient population. This may require the healthcare organization to acquire population data from national data sources or from public health agencies or other nonprofits that collect local and regional health data. For example, in an impoverished inner-city community, food security, transportation, safety, and housing may be of paramount importance.

An example of a data gathering nonprofit network is the National Neighborhood Indicators Partnership (NNIP; 2018). This project works with local "data intermediaries (organizations that collect and process community data) to:

- Build and operate an information system with recurrently updated data on neighborhood conditions across topics
- Facilitate and promote the practical use of data by community and government leaders in community building and local policymaking; and
- Emphasize the use of information to build the capacities of institutions and residents in low-income neighborhoods."

BOX 10-1 provides a simple "home-grown" social determinants of health questionnaire that is used by home healthcare hospital nurse liaisons when visiting hospitalized patients who are about to be discharged. The template is used to identify socioeconomic factors that might interfere with a safe discharge and recovery at home.

Thomas-Henkel and Shulman (2017) describe the various ways that organizations participating in the Transforming Complex Care Initiative, a multisite project funded by the Robert Wood Johnson Foundation, use social determinants of health assessment tools:

- OneCare Vermont, a statewide accountable care organization (ACO), has embedded its screening tool, the *Vermont Self-Sufficiency Outcomes Matrix*, into its electronic care coordination software.
- Theda Care, a health system in Wisconsin, has created an electronic tool for paramedics who provide care to home-based patients.
- The Redwood Community Health Coalition, a collaboration between 17 California community health centers, uses customized versions of the PRAPARE tool at each center.
- Access Health in Spartanburg, South Carolina, has created its own assessment tool, which asks unique questions such as information about connections to a faith-based community.

BOX 10-1 Hospital Liaison Nurse Discharge Question Template

Liaison Visit Note

❑ Liaison visit made to patient at the hospital and instructed on home care services.
❑ VNA Community Healthcare brochure and contact information given to patient.
❑ Verified with patient the demographic, insurance information, and primary MD who is: _____.
❑ Verified patient or caregiver will schedule next MD appointment within 1 to 2 weeks post discharge.
   MD appointment is scheduled for: _____.
❑ Assessed that patient has transportation home from hospital and to MD appointments.
❑ Verified the patient's primary caregiver and pharmacy, and that patient has a plan to obtain
   medications the same day as discharge.
❑ Assessed who will be assisting patient with medication administration.
❑ Verified that patient has food in the home and who assists with meal preparation.
❑ Notified patient that there may be a copay with the insurance plan and to contact the insurance
   company with any benefits questions.

Instructed patient on homebound status and patient verbalized understanding.
Name/Title:

Courtesy of Janine Fay, CEO, VNA Community Healthcare and Hospice.

These projects have identified a series of strategies that make the use of social determinants of health screening tools more effective and help create more connected care for patients (Thomas-Henkel & Shulman, 2017):

- Collect and integrate social determinants of health information into the medical record.
- Administer the instrument at intervals, especially after a transition of care, to track progress or deterioration of the patient's situation over time.
- Create workflows to track patient needs and referrals to social service agencies.
- Identify community resources and close the referral loop to find out if the patient/client actually accessed resources and obtained needed services.
- Communicate appropriately with patients about social determinants of health, first building rapport and avoiding any inkling of condescension or judgment.
- Build an adequate local referral network.
- Break down silos and effectively collaborate with local social services agencies.

ASK YOURSELF

- How does your organization assess social determinants of health?
- How is the data from these assessments incorporated into clinical care practices?
- How is the data from these assessments aggregated and analyzed to guide organizational policy decisions and program planning?

Clinical Responses to Social Determinants of Health

The negative impact of health disparities on health outcomes has been widely researched and validated. Lower income and minority patients typically have more chronic illnesses, worse clinical outcomes, and shorter lifespans. A quote from an article in the *Harvard Gazette* (Powell, 2016) describes the problem succinctly: "Health inequality is part of American life, so deeply entangled with other social problems—disparities in income, education, housing, race, gender, and even geography—that analysts have trouble saying which factors are cause and which are effect. The confusing result, they say, is a massive chicken-and-egg puzzle, its solution reaching beyond just health care. Because of that, everyday realities often determine whether people live in health or infirmity, to a ripe old age or early death" (p. 1).

Professional Support for Managing the Social Determinants

Reducing the impact of health inequity is often seen as strictly a political, policy, or health system issue, but healthcare providers have an ability to influence social determinants of health at an organizational and individual patient level. In areas of practice such as public health, skilled nursing facilities, and home health care, working with the social determinants of health is a part of daily practice. Public health nurses, epidemiologists, and sanitarians have whole jobs that focus on environmental and social determinants of health issues such as clean water, food sanitation, mass immunizations, infestations of vermin and insects, outbreaks of infectious disease, and outreach to at-risk pregnant women, mothers, and babies. These professionals, while mostly invisible to clinicians in direct clinical practice, provide a vital service in preventing serious illnesses within local communities. It might even be said that the lack of communication between public health agencies and medical facilities is another factor in the fragmentation between health care and programs that address social determinants of health.

Since social work is a covered service under Medicare Part A, both skilled nursing facilities and home health agencies employ social workers who assist patients with transportation, insurance, benefits and entitlements, and psychosocial and family issues. In primary care and specialty medical practices, there have typically been few professionals whose work is dedicated to the social determinants of health. As medical practices hire patient advocates and embedded nurse care coordinators, this is starting to change. We will discuss another type of healthcare support (community health workers or health advocates) later in this chapter. The professionals whose job it is to address social determinants of health are still relatively rare in clinical organizations, so direct care clinicians are still on the front lines of managing both medical and psychosocial issues in patient care.

Integrating Social Determinants of Health into Medical Practice Settings

DeVoe and colleagues (2016) describe basic practices for effectively integrating the social determinants of health into primary care practice:

- Standardize the collection of social determinants of health data by adopting the social determinants of health domains recommended by the National Academy of Medicine (cited earlier).
- Integrate social determinants of health assessments into the patient medical record.
- Make the data available to clinicians in ways that can enhance care such as identifying relevant screenings, implementing more customized treatment, coordinating care, and making appropriate referrals.
- Automate the use of social determinants of health information into decision support tools such as popup reminders or prompts to take specific clinical actions based on social determinants of health data.

An opinion paper from the American College of Obstetrics and Gynecology (ACOG; 2018) offers a list of best practices for addressing social determinants of health in reproductive health:

- Inquire about the social determinants of health.
- Maximize social service referrals to help patients in managing social determinants of health.

- Provide access to interpreter services when the patient's language is different from the practitioner's language.
- Acknowledge that race, institutionalized racism, and other forms of discrimination serve as social determinants of health.
- Recognize that stereotyping patients based on the patient's cultural beliefs can have an adverse effect on the patient-clinician interactions.
- Advocate for policy changes that positively impact social determinants of health for patients.

Dr. Anne Andermann (2016), from the Canadian CLEAR Foundation, offers a series of practical best practices for clinicians to constructively support patients in overcoming negative social determinants of health:

- Once a "social diagnosis" has been made, use "social prescribing" to connect patients within and outside the health system.
- Beyond referrals, advocate for patients by writing letters or calling social service agencies.
- Help patients find local benefit programs to which the patient is entitled.
- Reduce barriers to underserved patients by doing simple things such as providing bus fare for transportation to appointments, providing interpreter services, and setting practice hours that are convenient for patients.
- Provide simple materials such as a one-page guide to local resources.
- Treat patients with dignity and respect, and create safe spaces for disclosure.
- Take extra time in visits to address complex health and social needs.
- Become personally familiar with local resources that are needed by patients. (Modified from Andermann, 2016)

The *CLEAR Toolkit* from the McGill University Clear Collaboration is a simple tool with infographics that can be used to remind clinicians of four simple steps to helping patients with social determinants of health:

1. Treat illness in a way that is compassionate and respectful.

2. Ask about social determinants of health in a respectful and friendly manner.
3. Refer your patient to local resources and support networks.
4. Advocate through community involvement, political action, and raising awareness of local social determinants of health issues.

Access the toolkit at https://www.mcgill.ca/clear/files/clear/clear_toolkit_2015_-_english_1.pdf.

Models of Care That Incorporate Social Determinants of Health Supports

While many health professionals are still stuck in the "only medical problems are my responsibility mindset," many other facilities and individual professionals have taken responsibility for integrating help for social determinants of health into the fabric of clinical practice. There are also new, more holistic models of care that have arisen from the Affordable Care Act (ACA) and the Center for Medicare and Medicaid Innovation (CMMI) and multiple regional and national collaborative social determinants of health efforts that are grant funded.

Community Health Centers

Community health centers have been at the forefront of combining primary care with a multidisciplinary team, care coordination approach to care for low-income, underserved populations. The top three nonclinical services health centers offer to their community are health education, eligibility assistance, and outreach.

Community health centers also leverage their partnerships with local communities by hiring local residents and utilizing their boards and community advisory committees. Many community health centers expand their services far beyond the boundaries of medical care to include food, diet, exercise, housing, safety, and job assistance (National Association of Community Health Centers [NACHC], 2012).

Vermont Blueprint for Health

This statewide program provides multidisciplinary care teams that support 85% of Vermont primary medical practices in managing the social determinants of health. These teams include nurse care managers, social workers, behavioral health counselors, dietitians, and health educators.

Integrated Delivery Systems

An example of a health system that is addressing social determinants of health issues head-on is the Montefiore Health System in the Bronx borough of New York City, which serves a large underserved population.

The system has hired about 600 care managers, including nurses, social workers, and health educators, who address the chronic diseases of high-cost patients and link them with community resources (Terry, 2017).

Accountable Care Organizations

On the surface, it would seem that ACOs, which are driven by a value-based payment model, would fully incorporate processes to manage the social determinants of health into their systems. According to a recent article in *Health Payer Intelligence* (Gruessner, 2017), this seems not to be the case. Most ACOs, driven by payments that focus mostly on medical outcomes and by a need to control all the factors that contribute to financial risk, have largely avoided integrating responses to social determinants of health into their operations. The ACOs that have done work on social determinants of health tend to be funded by Medicaid and have a high needs population.

Gruessner (2017) suggests that insurers add funds for social determinants of health and that providers accept global capitation to enable them to pay for a broader range of social services support.

Accountable Care Communities

Accountable health communities are a new health model currently funded as grant programs through the CMMI. These initiatives include multiple stakeholders working together to improve the health and well-being of their communities by addressing social determinants of health. Stakeholders include healthcare delivery systems, public health organizations, and community organizations (Plescia & Dulin, 2017).

According to CMMI (2016), this model will promote clinical-community collaboration through:

- Screening of community-dwelling beneficiaries to identify certain unmet health-related social needs
- Referral of community-dwelling beneficiaries to increase awareness of community services
- Provision of navigation services to assist high-risk community-dwelling beneficiaries with accessing community services
- Encouragement of alignment between clinical and community services to ensure that community services are available and responsive to the needs of community-dwelling beneficiaries

State Medicaid Innovations

Many states are experimenting with ways to reduce health disparities and impact the social determinants of health through various structural and programmatic changes. "The Massachusetts state Medicaid agency, MassHealth, through its Medicaid 1115 demonstration waiver, is investing in accountable care organizations and community partners to integrate physical health, behavioral health, and long-term services and supports. The state is also funding certain approved 'flexible services' that address health-related social needs that are not otherwise covered as MassHealth benefits" (Freda, Kozick, & Spencer, 2018, p. 2).

🔍 *COLLABORATION CASE STUDY*

Collaborating to Address the Social Determinants of Health

In a real community, health responses to social determinants of health are far more variable and complex than would appear from research papers. In the author's own New England community, which consists of two smaller cities with large low-income, minority populations and mostly white affluent suburbs and small towns, a variety of organizations and individuals work on social determinants of health issues, sometimes alone and often collaboratively. These collaborations are sometimes formal and are sometimes very informal. The informal collaborations are often based simply on colleagues in different agencies calling each other for resource suggestions.

Three community health centers provide primary care to underserved populations. The local teaching hospital provides outpatient clinics for low-income patients. The community health centers are active participants in local professional networking and collaboration efforts. Most local towns have social service councils that meet regularly to discuss benefits, entitlements, and social services for local residents. The local health departments address issues such as maternal child health outreach, sanitation, and infectious disease, but mostly function alone within the state public health system. The local Agency on Aging serves as a focal point for professionals who work with low-income or isolated seniors and family caregivers. Several eldercare networking groups convene regularly and share resources.

The author participates in two hospital readmission collaboratives, one of which focuses mostly on medical issues. However, this teaching hospital has an active "community benefit" program which provides wellness programming for the local community and actively promotes community assessment of social determinants of health issues with a research organization.

The other hospital readmission collaborative incorporates some social service agencies, nursing homes, home care, and emergency services. This collaborative spends far more time discussing the social determinants of health and sharing resources.

The author's home healthcare agency has developed a Health Neighborhood, which consists of multiple stakeholders from the medical and eldercare community who do health literacy projects and address the issues of high-risk patients and better care transitions.

While a few of the larger medical groups in the community participate in these collaboration efforts, smaller medical group representation is mostly absent as these practices continue to be consumed by the need to provide a high volume of care under a fee-for-service system.

The statewide nonprofit *211* program is another resource for the public and the health and eldercare community. This program maintains a huge database of state community resources and provides toll-free phone support and internet access for residents who are looking for help with benefits, entitlements, housing, food, child care, and other resources (211.org, 2018).

Fighting Health Disparities and Social Determinants of Health at the Personal Level

An underlying theme in the literature on health disparities and social determinants of health is the pervasiveness of institutionalized racism, gender identity bias, cultural bias, and cultural insensitivity. Research has proved again and again that patients who are not heterosexual, white, English speaking, and middle class often receive inferior treatment within the healthcare system. Hardeman, Medina, and Kozhimannil (2016) describe this issue succinctly: "Most physicians are not explicitly racist and are committed to treating all patients equally. However, they operate in an inherently racist system" (p. 1).

It would be nice to believe that this is true and that bias in health care is primarily institutional and not individual, but simple observations of clinical interactions indicate that this is not always the case. Bias is one of the most inherently fragmenting factors in health care, disconnecting patients from both the caring and supportive care that they want and the most effective treatment available. The issue of combatting institutionalized bias is clearly beyond the scope of our discussion, but there are a few best practices that can be applied by organizations and individuals to counteract the worse aspects of bias.

Hire professionals and support staff who understand and can communicate with the patient population being served. Community health workers and health advocates are a new class of health support professionals who come from local communities and who are trained in techniques of patient engagement, patient advocacy, and the use of community resources. Health advocates and community healthcare workers often spend the bulk of their time helping patients manage the social determinants of health. See the interview about the work of patient navigators in a large medical practice in Chapter 6.

Become culturally competent. Many healthcare organizations are recognizing the need for more culturally competent and nonbiased care for patients. Health professionals can educate themselves about the cultures and cultural health norms of the patients they serve. This education can help to improve patient centeredness by prompting professionals to provide care in a way that fits the specific needs and expectations of patients who are from a minority group.

Fight bias and racism in our own practice. Dr. Monique Tello (2017) in *Harvard Health Blog* gives this advice: "To fight racism and discrimination, we all need to recognize, name, and understand these attitudes and actions. We need to be open to identifying and controlling our own implicit biases. We need to be able to manage overt bigotry safely, learn from it, and educate others. These themes need to be a part of medical education, as well as institutional policy. We need to practice and model tolerance, respect, open-mindedness, and peace for each other."

While this is good advice, it is not so easily done. To achieve this level of self-awareness, health professionals may need to have uncomfortable conversations about their own views of the healthcare world and may need to engage in reading about or interacting with people from minority communities inside and outside of clinical settings.

Another strategy is to speak with other health professionals who come from the patient populations that you are serving. Ask honest questions such as "How do you think our patients experience care in this setting?" or "What types of missteps do we make when caring for our patients?" or "How can I be more responsive and sensitive to our patients' cultural requirements?" Avoiding pejorative patient labels is another active way to fight bias. An example is not labeling and objectifying patients with terms such as "train wreck" as a way of describing a complex patient. Ultimately, a truly patient-centered approach is a counter to unconscious bias. As you listen to patients talk about what is important to them, monitor your own mental reactions and work collaboratively with the patient to craft a care plan that meets his or her unique needs. In this way, you are providing the kind of respectful and supportive care that transcends race, gender, and socioeconomic circumstances.

Another avenue for fighting bias in clinical care is formal education. The healthcare system is waking up to the fact that social determinants of health are at least as important as medical interventions in achieving positive health outcomes. As a consequence, professional schools are beginning to focus more resources and more training on the topics of social determinants of health, health disparities, cultural sensitivity, and patient engagement. Healthcare organizations are also providing cultural sensitivity training to help professionals develop more open and inclusive attitudes. Professionals, themselves, can seek out such training to enhance the quality of the care they provide to their whole patient population.

Nurses and Social Determinants of Health

Nurses, along with social workers, have always been on the forefront of helping patients manage the social determinants of health. In the United States, Lillian Wald, who at the end of the 19th century became a pioneering public health nurse and passionate advocate for the poor of New York City, led the way on this issue. She was instrumental in developing social services support, along with public health nursing through the Henry Street Settlement House. **FIGURE 10-4** shows a public health nurse from that era crossing the rooftops of tenement buildings to reach her patients because of congestion and filth in the streets.

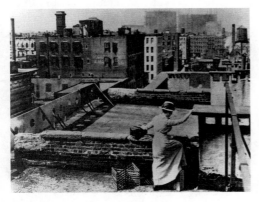

FIGURE 10-4 Public Health Nurse Crossing the Rooftops of New York City Tenements

© MPI/ Stringer/ Getty Images

Another famous example of nurses helping with both medical and social issues involves nurse midwives of the Frontier Nursing Service who rode on horseback to isolated areas of eastern Kentucky to provide care to mothers and babies.

Nurses today remain strongly committed to the principles and practice of unbiased, culturally sensitive care that underlie any effort to mitigate negative social determinants of health, although they too must continue to fight personal and institutional bias. Advanced practice registered nurses (APRNs) provide the backbone of the primary care workforce in underserved areas and community health centers. Nurses in public health, clinic, and community service organizations work on both individual patient and population health initiatives that address social determinants of health.

The American Nurses Association Code of Conduct describes the role of nursing in social determinants of health and health disparities: "The Code of Ethics for Nurses of the American Nurses Association includes principles of social justice and emphasizes the need to integrate social concerns into nursing and health policy. Nursing can lead in translating social determinants of health awareness into action by taking the following steps:

- Teach social determinants of health content in all clinical courses, with students routinely assessing for social determinants of health in clinical settings and advocating for change to improve social determinants of health.
- Develop interprofessional practice to include representatives of social work, public health, city planning, occupational health, police and fire fighters, and many others who can contribute to addressing social determinants of health.
- Prioritize nursing research on social and biomedical aspects of health to connect social determinants of health to health outcomes and develop nursing interventions that alleviate problematic social determinants of health.

- Collaborate with social and community agencies and institutions to recommend that health policy address harmful social determinants of health" (Olshansky, 2017).

Insurance Gaps and Healthcare Fragmentation

Good health insurance coverage is a strong factor in connected care. Patients with no coverage or inadequate coverage are almost certain to receive fragmented care and may possibly not receive the most effective type of diagnoses and treatment. While the ACA has somewhat alleviated parts of the problem, recent political maneuvering has weakened the program and high cost increases have threatened to partially dismantle it. Even for many patients who have insurance, very high out-of-pocket costs are barriers to care.

Insured patients with high deductibles and copays may be covered for catastrophic events and preventive care, but may avoid the use of primary and specialty care for more extensive diagnosis, treatment of chronic conditions, and elective surgery. Many patients with high deductibles find themselves seeking care from lower cost providers or avoiding care all together to keep family finances balanced. Where patients live may well determine the size of their cost-related care gaps.

Patients who live in states that did expand Medicaid as part of the ACA have seen some improvements in health outcomes and a reduction in debts, unpaid bills, and bankruptcies related to medical care. For those lower income patients who live in states that did not expand Medicaid, none of these positive outcomes have occurred (Antonisse, Garfield, Rudowitz, & Artiga, 2018).

Health professionals can help advocate for patients with health insurance gaps. A first line strategy is to help patients understand and maximize their health insurance coverage. When individuals do not have adequate coverage, professionals can help patients find alternative resources such as drug company programs to subsidize medication costs for low-income patients. Health professionals and their support staff must also understand and follow insurance company procedures to avoid unnecessary claim denials. Lastly, professionals can write appeals and conduct peer-to-peer discussions with insurers to attempt to get more coverage for their patients. Sometimes this is simply a matter of knowing how to document the "why" of patient needs rather than simply listing care and treatment procedures that were performed. Facility billing departments can help professionals understand insurer documentation and appeal procedures.

Summary of Best Practices for Integrating Social Determinants of Health into Clinical Practice

- Develop or adopt the use of evidence-based, standardized assessment tools for social determinants of health, customized to meet the needs of your patient population.
- Incorporate social determinants of health information into the medical record.
- Create decision support and reminder tools in the electronic medical record to trigger effective responses to social determinants of health issues.
- Identify insurance gaps and tailor treatment choices to patient financial circumstances.
- When feasible, offer payment plans and alternative financial arrangements for patients with financial issues.
- Develop or obtain lists of community resources, benefits, and entitlements and assign one staff member to learn and explain eligibility requirements.
- Develop collaborative relationships with local community resources.
- Make closed loop referrals to community resources; check to ensure that the patient actually contacted the resource and received service.
- Develop facility hours, locations, and services that best meet patient needs.
- Identify and address institutionalized and individual bias issues through training, facility policies and procedures, and structure redesign.

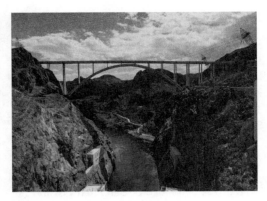

FIGURE 10-5 The Medical and Mental Health Care Gap
© Dawnie Fung/ Shutterstock

▶ Mental Health and Medical Care— The Chasm in the Healthcare System

For patients and families who are coping with mental health problems, the disconnect between mental health and medical care in the United States isn't just a gap, it is a yawning chasm (**FIGURE 10-5**). For health professionals and organizations, medical and mental health care are two parallel systems with tenuous and fragile connections that have seldom been integrated effectively or well. Research has effectively proved that chronic disease and mental health conditions are inextricably linked. However, our healthcare system is too often governed by a type of dualistic thinking in which mind and body are treated separately.

This fragmentation is fueled by the culture of medicine, organizational structures, cultural norms around mental health issues, and payment mechanisms. In a perverse way, the opioid crisis, which is tearing the social and healthcare system fabric of the country, may be bringing the huge disconnect between mental and physical health to light. The current epidemic of opioid drug abuse and subsequent emergency room admissions and drug overdose deaths is finally getting the attention of the healthcare system. The irony is that the healthcare system, at least partially, caused the crisis through deceptive pharmaceutical company marketing and overprescribing of pain medications by medical practitioners.

The correlation between mental illness and gun violence has also been the subject of a national debate and has further raised the issue of ineffective screening and engagement of people with mental illness to the forefront of the national consciousness.

PAUL'S STORY—A FIRSTHAND EXPERIENCE OF MENTAL HEALTH CRACKS AND GAPS

In 1997, I was diagnosed with bipolar condition, but the medications I was prescribed did not seem to blunt either the mania or the clinical depression I experienced. In 2002, when the grant funding my position expired, I was laid off and was placed on Consolidated Omnibus Budget Reconciliation Act (COBRA), which provides continuation healthcare coverage insurance for 18 months at considerable expense. At the close of 18 months, I was no longer eligible for COBRA insurance and my unemployment benefits had run out several months prior. Hence I was no longer able to afford medication or therapy.

I plunged into a period of deep depression and was not in a frame of mind to explore my options (e.g., Medicaid, free care under the Hill-Burton Act, or mental health services provided for the uninsured and underinsured).

Because I had been working and independent for most of my adult life I had no social/case worker or medical professional to direct me to seek treatment under my circumstances. My psychiatrist, who was in private practice, did nothing to ensure that there was no gap in service, when I could no longer afford his services.

While these circumstances are particular to me, I have heard many similar stories from peers, friends, and family in the years since. In my case, after a few months without therapy and medication and after a brief manic period, I plunged once again into a deep depression and made a dramatic suicide attempt, jumping off a 600-foot cliff in May 2004.

Miraculously, I survived intact, and a friend of mine who volunteered to serve as my conservator applied for Social Security Disability Insurance (SSDI) on my behalf.

Given the nature of my suicide attempt, along with the fact that three people in my family had committed suicide, my application for benefits was approved the first time around (as compared to many other cases, where the application is denied and benefits granted to some after one or more appeals).

Despite getting retroactive cash benefits, Medicare benefits are delayed for 2 years from the time that SSDI benefits are awarded. During this period I qualified for Medicaid only (Medicaid covers some but not all of the procedures that Medicare covers, but it also covers some dental services, which Medicare does not). Medicaid features a "spend down" for those who are deemed to earn too much from SSDI (such as myself), suspending benefits until the beneficiary has spent a designated amount of money for health care out of pocket.

In conclusion, I literally had to jump off a cliff to get the attention of clinicians and the Social Security Administration, and also of family and friends (who were concerned before the suicide attempt but coalesced as a team afterward), to qualify for health care. It shouldn't require such a dramatic step for a mentally ill person to get help, but it did. And I was one of the lucky ones. Once I had gotten everyone's attention, an effective team of advocates assembled around me. This is not always the case for others.

In my view, anyone who has been diagnosed with mental illness and is unemployed should trigger an automatic review of the circumstances prior to the expiration of COBRA benefits.

This is only one of many gaps in mental health care that needs to be filled. Here is a partial list:

1. Failure of psychiatrists and APRNs to identify effective medicine (through titration) in a timely fashion; need for intensive experimentation (sometimes inpatient) while insurance usually pays for medication administration visits once every 8 weeks.
2. Failure to educate users of mental health services that they are consumers and can exercise choice as to who provides services for them.
3. Demands placed on consumers do not always match the reality of their lives; for instance, one provider required me to attend groups during the day when I was working; they had no groups during the evenings for consumers who worked during the day!
4. Alternative medicine (e.g., acupuncture) is offered as a mental health treatment, and sometimes covered by insurance, but is not widely practiced.

ASK YOURSELF

How could both healthcare and mental healthcare professionals have been more proactive in helping Paul and his support network?

Data on Mental Health and Chronic Disease

Incidence of Mental Illness

The most recent data on the incidence of mental illness in the United States comes from the 2016 *National Survey on Drug Use and Health* from the Substance Abuse and Mental Health Services Administration (SAMHSA). The survey, which includes data obtained from over 67,500 people over the age of 12, states:

> In 2016, an estimated 44.7 million adults aged 18 or older had AMI (any mental illness) in the past year. This number represents 18.3 percent of adults in the United States. An estimated 10.4 million adults in the nation had SMI (serious mental illness) in the past year, and 34.3 million adults had AMI excluding SMI in the past year. The number of adults with SMI represents 4.2 percent of adults in 2016, and the number of adults with AMI excluding SMI represents 14.0 percent of adults. Among adults with AMI in the past year, 23.2 percent had SMI, and 76.8 percent did not have SMI. (SAMHSA, 2017a, p. 36)

Substance Abuse

Substance abuse, which has always been a problem in the United States, has spiked in recent years as a consequence of the misuse of opioids. A summary of the substance abuse section of the 2016 SAMHSA survey provides some sobering statistics:

> In 2016, 7.5 percent of Americans aged 12 or older—approximately 20.1 million people—had a substance use disorder in the past year. Of those, about 1 in 3 (36.7 percent) struggled with illicit drug use; about 3 in 4 (74.9 percent) struggled with alcohol use; and about 1 in 9 (11.7 percent) had both an alcohol use disorder and an illicit drug use disorder.
>
> Approximately 11.8 million individuals misused opioids in 2016 – or 4.4 percent of population of people over the age of 12. The vast majority, 11.5 of the 11.8 million opioid misusers, were misusing prescription pain relievers.
>
> From the period 2002 through 2016, the U.S. has witnessed a 2.35 fold

(135 percent) increase in the number of heroin users while the nation has been jolted by a 6.33 fold (533 percent) increase in the number of deaths attributable to heroin. (SAMHSA News, 2017b)

Chronic Disease and Mental Health Comorbidity

A huge amount of research indicates that mental health and chronic disease are closely intertwined. People with serious and persistent mental illness have a high rate of chronic disease and a very high mortality rate. People with chronic disease often also have some type of mental health condition, particularly depression, although it is often unclear which came first, the physical or mental health issue. A CDC (2012) Fact Sheet on Mental Health and Chronic Disease states: "Depression is found to co-occur in 17% of cardiovascular cases, 23% of cerebrovascular cases, and with 27% of diabetes patients and more than 40% of individuals with cancer" (p. 2). Serious injuries are also related to mental illness according to the CDC (2012) report, which states "injuries, both intentional such as homicide and suicide and unintentional such as motor vehicle accidents, are 2-6 times higher for persons with a history of mental illness than those without a history" (p. 2)

Jolles, Haynes-Maslow, Roberts, and Dusetzina, in a 2015 study of 3,659 primary care visits for patients with depression, found that many patients reported co-occurring chronic illnesses, with the most common being hypertension, hyperlipidemia, and arthritis. The study found patients with both chronic illness and depression were less likely to be referred for mental health services than those who presented only with depression (Jolles et al., 2015).

A report on comorbid mental health and medical conditions from the Robert Wood Johnson Foundation (Druss & Reisinger-Walker, 2011) describes data from the National Comorbidity Replication Survey (NCS-R):

- 29% of adults with medical conditions have mental disorders

- 68% of adults with mental disorders have medical conditions
- 50% of adult Medicaid enrollees with psychiatric conditions also had cardiovascular disease, pulmonary disease, or diabetes

The cost of treating combined medical and mental health conditions is high: 2.5 to 3.5 times higher than for those who do not have a mental health condition (Roeber, McClellan, & Woodward, 2016). Most of this spending is on general medical care, not behavioral health services (Klein & Hostetter, 2014).

Factors That Perpetuate the Medical and Mental Health Gap

Cultural Stigmas of Mental Health Care

The cultural stigma of mental health care discourages people from getting help and causes some providers to avoid treating patients with mental health and medical comorbidities. Pellegrini (2013) describes this issue in the *Canadian Medical Journal*: "Many patients who seek help for mental health problems report feeling 'patronized, punished or humiliated' in their dealings with health professionals," the report states. "Discrimination can include negativity about a patient's chance of recovery, misattribution of unrelated complaints to a patient's mental illness and refusal to treat psychiatric symptoms in a medical setting" (p. E17).

Health Professional Education

A 2015 American Hospital Association report on the state of the behavioral health workforce summarizes a series of issues and obstacles to integrating the treatment of both physical and mental health. The report notes that the behavioral health workforce is aging and that the primary care workforce is currently not well trained to manage mental health conditions. "Behavioral health students are siloed in education programs. For example, there is no curriculum in U.S. undergraduate or graduate psychology programs that focuses on primary care" (AHA, p. 4). More than half of patients with behavioral health issues are treated by primary care providers, yet these providers have no specialized training in treating mental health conditions (AHA, 2016). Health professional education often separates mental healthcare education into specialty courses or specialty psychiatric clinical rotations rather than incorporating mental health training into all clinical practice education. This means that medical practitioners may not feel adequately prepared to deal with basic mental health issues and often refer patients for specialty care rather than providing integrated medical/mental health care. This lack of training, coupled with a shortage of trained behavioral health workers, creates an acute workforce shortage at a time of accelerating need (SAMHSA, 2014). Postgraduate training in mental health diagnosis and treatment for medically trained physicians and nurses has been used to temporarily close the education gap until medical and other health professional schools can further integrate their curricula.

Regulatory and Payment Systems

Payment systems; licensing laws; and federal, state, and insurance company regulations have traditionally been huge barriers to closing the gaps between medical and mental health services, but some progress has been made.

According to Ross Johnson and Meyer (2017) in *Modern Healthcare*: "Mental health services became part of the Affordable Care Act's 10 essential health benefits that all health plans are required to cover. Mental health parity rules restrict insurers from placing higher limits on mental health services than ones applied to medical and surgical services." The 21st Century Cures Act, signed in 2016, provides a variety of initiatives designed to improve mental health services including new coordination at the federal level, funding of innovation initiatives, and some Medicare and Medicaid rule changes that make it easier to get funding for mental health services.

The Structure of Organizational Healthcare Systems

A study by the Behavioral Health Workforce Research Center (BHWRC) at the University of Michigan identified a series of factors that inhibit the integration of mental health and medical services: (1) insufficient number of staff; (2) disagreements about provider roles; (3) restrictions on sharing patient information, specifically for patients receiving treatment for substance use; (4) state and federal policies that hinder reimbursement for care; and (5) workflow and logistical obstacles (Buche et al., 2017).

Ambiguity About Professional Responsibility

It is clear that most mental health issues surface in primary care or emergency room settings, yet there is no agreement on who should treat these conditions once they are identified. Some believe that because of the stigma of mental health, patients will more easily accept treatment by a primary care medical practitioner.

Others argue that primary care clinicians are already overwhelmed with the volume and complexity of the patients they see and that adding responsibility for mental health would be counterproductive.

The current model, which consists of medical practitioners referring to mental health clinicians, does not seem to solve the problem, as a high proportion of patients who are referred never actually visit a mental health professional. This lack of follow-through on mental health referrals is one of the biggest gaps between mental health and medical care.

Systems for Linking Medical and Mental Health Services

According to the SAMHSA Center for Integrated Health Solutions, "Integrated care is the systematic coordination of general and behavioral healthcare. Integrating mental health, substance abuse, and primary care services produces the best outcomes and proves the most effective approach to caring for people with multiple healthcare needs" (SAMHSA, 2018a, p. 1). The agency describes six potential levels of collaboration/integration between medical and mental health practitioners and facilities ranging from minimal contact to full colocated integration and collaboration. These levels are described in **FIGURE 10-6**.

Mental Health and Medical Integration/Collaboration Programs

Throughout the United States, hundreds of pilots and research efforts are testing the best methods of integrating medical and mental health services. Some of these programs are occurring in ACOs and primary care medical homes, which participate in value-based payment initiatives and have a vested interest in successful integration (Health Affairs, 2017).

Many other programs are grant funded and organized by university or private foundation researchers. While each of these pilot projects has some core characteristics, some require adjustment to local conditions. For example, a program in Minnesota uses telehealth to connect behavioral health specialists with patients in far-flung rural areas. To date, none of these pilot projects has been fully adopted nationwide. As most are grant funded, they are not yet ready to enter the mainstream of healthcare delivery.

Nurses and the Integration of Mental Health and Medical Care

Nurses have long had a role in caring for patients with mental health issues in inpatient psychiatric facilities and in homes as psychiatric home care nurses. In recent years APRNs with specialty psychiatric training have become front

Level 1	Minimal collaboration
Level 2	Basic collaboration at a distance
Level 3	Basic collaboration onsite
Level 4	Close collaboration onsite with some systems integration
Level 5	Close collaboration approaching an integrated practice
Level 6	Full collaboration in a transformed/merged/integrated practice

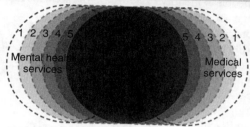

FIGURE 10-6 Six Levels of Mental Health and Medical Services Integration/Collaboration

Modified from Heath, B., Wise Romero, P., & Reynolds, K. (2013, March). A review and proposed standard framework for levels of integrated healthcare. Washington, DC: SAMHSA-HRSA Center for Integrated Health Solutions, Table 1: Six levels of collaboration/integration.

line providers of mental health services and prescribers of psychiatric medications, especially in safety net organizations. The American Psychiatric Nurses Association (APNA) provides a variety of resources on nursing and mental health on its website (www.apna.org). SAMHSA (2018b) lists five best practices that all nurses can use to encourage mental health and medical integration:

- Nurses can counteract negative attitudes and discrimination about behavioral health conditions by approaching mental health and substance use problems in the same way they deal with hypertension, diabetes, and other common medical problems.
- Nurses should routinely screen for mental illness, history of trauma, substance use, and suicide risk in all healthcare settings. Nurses in behavioral health settings should be paying special attention to tobacco use, blood pressure, and signs of diabetes.
- Nurses can advocate for increased access to specialized mental health care for both children and adults.

- Nurses should identify resources in their community to assist in crisis intervention and specialty treatment.
- Nurses can work to reduce the social determinants of health that contribute to behavioral health problems in their communities.

Peer and Family Support for Mental Health

Not all mental health support comes from professional sources. Both families and peer counselors play a vital role in bridging cracks and gaps in care by helping people with mental health issues in informal settings. The National Alliance on Mental Illness (NAMI), for example, plays a large role nationwide in educating and supporting families of people with mental illness. NAMI offers a multisession course in many community locations on understanding and supporting someone with mental illness. The NAMI toll-free helpline provides support during weekday business hours and has a crisis text service (nami.org). Many mental health self-help and support groups exist in communities around the country.

For example, the Anxiety and Depression Association of America (adaa.org) provides an online listing of support groups by state. Many local resource referral hubs can also provide information on mental health support.

Mental Health First Aid is an evidence-based, 8-hour course that teaches laypeople to identify, understand, and respond to signs of mental illnesses and substance use disorders. The training gives participants the skills to reach out and provide initial help and support to someone who may be developing a mental health or substance use problem or experiencing a crisis (www.mentalhealthfirstaid.org).

According to the American Psychiatric Association (APA), *peer support* refers to people with the same types of problems helping each other. A peer supporter is someone who has experienced recovery from psychiatric and/or substance use challenges and, as a result, can offer assistance and support to others' recovery. Peer supporters are trained to help promote recovery and improve the quality of life for individuals and their families by sharing their own recovery stories, providing encouragement, instilling a sense of hope, and teaching skills. Research has shown that peer support can reduce the stigma of getting help for some people with mental illness. Peer supporters have also been shown to foster a key element of recovery—that is, hope and a belief in the possibility of recovery. While many peer supporters are informally trained, some have formal training and certification at the state level or through a national organization such as Mental Health America (mentalhealthamerica.net, 2017). As of 2015, peer support counseling was covered by Medicaid in 38 states (APA, 2017).

Best Practices for Integrating Mental Health and Medical Care

Best practices in this area are often specific to the structure of a specific medical or integrated care setting. Many publications detail best practices for step-by-step integration.

SAMHSA's Center for Integrated Health Solutions provides an infographic flowchart that details each step of the integration assessment and implementation process, called *A Quick Start Guide to Behavioral Health Integration for Safety-Net Primary Care Providers* (SAMHSA, 2018a). An excellent resource for identifying and managing mental health conditions in general medical settings, *mhGAP Intervention Guide for Mental, Neurological and Substance Use Disorders in Non-specialized Health Settings*, is available online from the World Health Organization (WHO; 2010).

Principles of Successful Mental Health/Medical Organizational Integration

Schaps and Post (2015) list best practices for the structural integration of medical and mental health services:

- **Comprehensive scope of services** that includes physical and behavioral health
- **A patient-centered model** that is responsive to the needs, goals, and preferences of the patients served
- **Standardized care delivery through interprofessional teams** that involves professionals from different disciplines who work to understand and respect each other's roles and to use evidence-based protocols for care (Many programs have a behavioral health case manager who helps to integrate and manage care and community resource referrals.)
- **Performance measurement** of outcomes, integration, and patient perception of services provided
- **Information systems**, in which system wide integrated electronic medical records improve communication and track utilization and outcomes, ensuring that patient privacy and security concerns are accommodated

- **Organizational culture and leadership,** wherein a unified vision and leadership actions help integrate the professional cultures of medical and mental health care
- **Physician integration** that builds on informal networks and relationships and ensures adequate compensation to offset some perceived negatives of shared decision making in an integrated culture
- **Governance structure** that involves developing contractual relationships that foster coordination and collaboration
- **Financial management** that incorporates mechanisms to allow pooling of funding across services

Some commonsense best practices for supporting patients with mental health conditions in medical settings might include:

- Develop basic competence in recognizing symptoms of mental health problems through continuing education.
- Identify and address concerns and attitudes about mental health issues that might contribute to the stigma of mental health.
- Use simple screening tools such as the Patient Health Questionnaire-2 (PHQ-2) to identify patient mental health issues such as depression.
- Provide patient-centered care, assessing patient goals and learning enough of the patient's story to determine whether mental health concerns are present.
- Develop relationships with mental health providers in the community. Understand the roles and capabilities of different types of providers (psychiatrists, psychologists, APRNs, licensed clinical social workers, licensed counselors, and community outreach workers).
- Learn about and refer patients to local mental health support groups, educational programs, and peer counseling.
- Make closed loop referrals to mental health and substance abuse providers by following up with patients to check on the status of

the referral and reinforcing the reasons for getting mental health support.
- Provide basic treatment of common mental health conditions such as depression after researching current evidence-based best practices.
- Understand and respect patient privacy concerns and special considerations for sharing of mental health information.
- Carefully monitor care transitions of patients with psychiatric conditions carefully and communicate vital information to the next step in care.
- Learn to recognize and ask about symptoms of potential suicide.
- Learn to recognize signs and symptoms of substance abuse.
- Apply brief motivational interviewing strategies to engage patients in seeking treatment.

ASK YOURSELF

To what degree has your organization and individual clinicians adopted best practices for the integration of medical and mental health care?

▶ Care of Complex, High-Need Patients

A 2017 publication from the National Academy of Medicine (Long, 2017) describes certain patients as being high cost and high need: "Today, 1 percent of patients account for more than 20 percent of health care expenditures, and 5 percent account for nearly half of the nation's spending on health care" (p. 1). This population of patients has captured the attention of national funding and research organizations. In 2016, a coalition of leading healthcare foundations (Commonwealth Fund, John A. Hartford Foundation, Peterson Center on Healthcare, SCAN Foundation, and Robert Wood Johnson

Foundation) proposed three steps to meet the needs of this diverse population (Blumenthal, Chernof, Fulmer, Lumpkin, & Selberg, 2016):

- Understanding this diverse population
- Identifying evidence-based programs that offer high-quality integrated care at a lower cost
- Accelerating the adoption of these programs nationally

The foundations collaborated to maximize their individual investments and avoid duplication in efforts to scale and spread promising care models for high-need individuals across organizations participating in value-based reimbursement (Want, 2017).

In the 2 years since the collaboration was launched, there have been two major accomplishments. First, the Harvard T.H. Chan School of Public Health has conducted extensive research on the characteristics of this diverse population, many of whom have combined medical, mental health, and social determinants of health challenges. Second is the development of The Better Care Playbook, an interactive website developed by the Institute for Health Care Improvement that provides data and best practices for caring for the high-need population (bettercareplaybook.org).

What Has Been Learned About High-Cost, High-Need Patients?

This research has determined that high-cost, high-need patients fall into several distinct categories (Figueroa, 2017):

- Under 65 disabled
- Frail elders
- Patients with major complex, chronic conditions

Some important lessons that are relevant to the whole issue of connected care have been learned in the short period of time since the high-cost, high-need patient foundation collaboration was launched. One lesson is that success depends on finding the right approach for each patient and adapting the care plan to his or her needs and goals. Ineffective and inefficient care has less to do with the patients than with the system that is delivering care to them. Another lesson learned is that promising care models exist, but they are not yet universally replicable and scalable (Want, 2017).

The care models being tested range from care transitions programs to programs that integrate primary care and nonmedical care (Health Leads), to programs that provide interdisciplinary comprehensive care to frail elders (the GRACE program) and the Programs of All-Inclusive Care for the Elderly (PACE).

The nationally known Camden Coalition (camdenhealth.org, 2018), founded by Dr. Jeffrey Brenner, famously pioneered the technique of "hotspotting" (using data to geographically identify high-utilization patients) and developed a comprehensive, integrated care system for an underserved population. One cornerstone of this program is the "7-day pledge," a citywide campaign that tries to connect hospital discharged patients with a primary care provider within 7 days of discharge.

These successful, integrated, person-centered programs have some similar characteristics. These characteristics include good population segmentation data so that the specific needs of the population can be addressed by the program. Larger programs may have well-integrated medical records and data analytics capabilities. Cross-functional teamwork with a care coordinator at the center of the team's efforts is the core of these programs. Successful programs also have a strong structural coordination element, with all team members working from the same location, outreach efforts, and regular face-to-face encounters between patients and care team members. Outreach, in which care is extended to the community and into the home, is an element of these programs. Programs all have links between medical and social services. Discharge planning with prompt follow-up after hospital stays is an essential element of care for those populations with serious chronic illness (Cohn et al., 2017; Long, 2017).

While the model programs described herein have been highly successful, there are still significant obstacles to scalability and diffusion: "One obstacle to wider diffusion is the nature of the programs. They tend to be complex and novel, with many moving parts—new types of personnel, such as care managers; new information technology capabilities; new tasks, such as home visits. Some require not only changes in behavior and clinical workflow but also cultural adaptations as professionals assume new roles on the care team" (Blumenthal et al., 2016, p. 910).

▶ Chapter Summary

This chapter provides multiple examples of fragmentation in health care that is caused by lack of attention to the social determinants of health, bias, and the traditional divide between mental health and medical care. One consistent theme is the mismatch of patient populations with needs that don't match the structure of a primarily fee-for-service, medical, episodic, and acute care–focused system. Another theme is that true solutions to these problems can be achieved through integration of medical, social, and mental health services. Many of the root causes of these problems lie in our divided American culture and political system and disparate views of how much care the nation owes all its citizens, who should be able to get care, and what the responsibility of government-funded programs are in achieving positive health outcomes.

Since a resolution of these political and cultural issues any time in the near future seems unlikely, it is left to large and small health, insurance, and social service organizations to do the best they can to close the gaps. In some parts of the country, commitment, energy, and innovation are closing care gaps in a way that has been absent at the national level. Some health systems that also take insurance risk will use premium dollars to fund more integrated and comprehensive care programs. There is developing interest in integrating mental health and social determinants of health within ACOs. Some integrated delivery systems such as the Montefiore System in the Bronx, New York, have developed model programs.

Some other positive factors are an emerging consciousness in the medical community that paying attention only to medical matters is not enough to create positive patient outcomes. The work of large national funders such as the Robert Wood Johnson Foundation through its Culture of Health Initiative is another bright spot in integrating care.

Research on better cross-sector metrics of social determinants of health is also accelerating. National collaboratives such as the Network for Regional Healthcare Improvement and its affiliated online collaborative, Health Doers Network, are sharing best practices and collecting cross-sector data about social determinants of health.

The ongoing collaboration of five major health foundations on the care of high-cost, high-need patients may prove to be one of the most important efforts in developing a nationally scalable model of connected care. With the funding and the prestige of the sponsoring foundations behind them, the model projects under study may become templates for developing connected care models in the rest of the healthcare system.

Nurses who have had a historical role in integrating patient social and medical concerns through their work as public health nurses are involved in all aspects of integrated care initiatives. Nurses have continued to be on the front lines of care in safety net organizations that provide medical and often mental health services to underserved populations. Nurses also play key roles in improving the integration of care through nursing research into care integration best practices. Nursing education plays a role by training students to deliver culturally competent care and to work in interprofessional teams.

References

211.org. (2018). Help starts here. Retrieved from www.211.org

American College of Obstetricians and Gynecologists. (2018). Committee Opinion No. 729. Importance of social determinants of health and cultural awareness in the delivery of reproductive health care. *Obstetrics & Gynecology, 131*(1). doi:10.1097/aog.0000000000002459

American Hospital Association (AHA). (2016). The state of the behavioral health workforce: A literature review. Retrieved from https://www.aha.org/system/files/hpoe /Reports- HPOE/2016/aha_Behavioral_FINAL.pdf

American Psychiatric Association. (2017). Peer support: Making a difference for people with mental illness. Retrieved from www.psychiatry.org/news-room/apa-blogs/apa-blog /2017/03/peer-support-making-a-difference-for-people -with-mental-illness

Andermann, A. (2016). Taking action on the social determinants of health in clinical practice: A framework for health professionals. *Canadian Medical Association Journal, 188*(17–18). doi:10.1503/cmaj.160177

Antonisse, L., Garfield, R., Rudowitz, R., & Artiga, S. (2018). The effects of Medicaid expansion under the ACA: Updated findings from a literature review. Henry J. Kaiser Family Foundation. Retrieved from www.kff.org/medicaid/issue -brief/the-effects-of-medicaid-expansion-under-the-aca -updated-findings-from-a-literature-review-march-2018/

Billioux, A., Verlander, K., Anthony, S., & Alley, D. (2017). Standardized screening for health-related social needs in clinical settings: The accountable health communities screening tool. National Academy of Medicine. Retrieved from https://nam.edu/wpcontent/uploads/2017/05 /Standardized-Screening-for-Health-Related-Social -Needs-in-Clinical-Settings.pdf

Blumenthal, D., Chernof, B., Fulmer, T., Lumpkin, J., & Selberg, J. (2016). Caring for high-need, high-cost patients—an urgent priority. *New England Journal of Medicine, 375,* 909–911. doi:10.1056/NEJMp160851

Buche, J., Singer, P., Grazier, K., King, E., Maniere, E., & Beck, A. (2017). *Primary care and behavioral health workforce integration: Barriers and best practices.* Ann Arbor, MI: University of Michigan Behavioral Health Workforce Research Center.

Camden Coalition of Healthcare Providers. (2018). Retrieved from www.camdenhealth.org/about/about-the-coalition /history/

Centers for Disease Control and Prevention. (2012). Mental health and chronic disease fact sheet. Retrieved from www .cdc.gov/workplacehealthpromotion/tools-resources /pdfs/issue-brief-no-2-mental-health-and-chronic -disease.pdf

Centers for Disease Control and Prevention National Center for HIV/AIDS, Viral Hepatitis, STD, and TB Prevention. (2014). Social determinants of health and health disparities. Retrieved from www.cdc.gov/nchhstp /socialdeterminants/definitions.htm

Center for Medicare and Medicaid Innovation. (2016). Accountable health care communities model. Retrieved from https://innovation.cms.gov/initiatives/ahcm/

Cohn, J., Corrigan, J., Lynn, J., Meier, D., Miller, J., Shega, J., & Wang, S. (2017). Community-based models of care delivery for people with serious illness. Discussion paper. Washington, DC: National Academy of Medicine. Retrieved from https://nam.edu/wp-content/uploads/2017/04/

DeVoe, J. E., Bazemore, A. W., Cottrell, E. K., Likumahuwa-Ackman, S., Grandmont, J., Spach, N., & Gold, R. (2016). Perspectives in primary care: A conceptual framework and path for integrating social determinants of health into primary care practice. *The Annals of Family Medicine, 14*(2), 104–108.

Druss, B., & Reisinger-Walker, E. (2011). *Mental disorders and medical comorbidity.* Princeton, NJ: Robert Wood Johnson Foundation.

Dzau, V. J., McClellan, M., McGinnis, J. M., & Finkelman, E. M. (Eds.). (2017). *Vital directions for health & health care: An initiative of the National Academy of Medicine.* Washington, DC: National Academy of Medicine.

Figueroa, J. (2017). Segmenting high-need, high-cost patients: A video presentation. Retrieved from www .bettercareplaybook.org/_blog/2017/1/segmenting -high-need-high-cost-patients-video-presentation -dr-jose-figueroa

Freda, B., Kozick, D., & Spencer, A. (2018). Partnerships for health: Lessons for bridging community-based organizations and health care organizations. Center for Health Care Strategies. Retrieved from www.chcs .org/resource/partnerships-health-lessons-bridging -community-based-organizations-and-health-care -organizations

Gruessner, V. (2017). Should accountable care organizations include social services? Retrieved from www.health payerintelligence.com/news/should-accountable-care -organizations-include-social-services

Hardeman, R., Medina, E., & Kozhimannil, K. (2016, October 12). Structural racism and supporting black lives—the role of health professionals. *New England Journal of Medicine, 375,* 2113–2115. doi: 10.1056/NEJMp1609535

Health Affairs. (2017, January). Weaving whole-person health throughout an accountable care framework: The social ACO. *Health Affairs Blog.* doi:10.1377/hblog 20170125.058419

Health Leads. (2016). Social needs screening toolkit. Retrieved from https://healthleadsusa.org/tools-item /health-leads-screening-toolkit/

Healthy People 2020. (2018). Disparities. Retrieved from www.healthypeople.gov

Institute of Medicine. (2014). Capturing social and behavioral domains and measures in electronic health records: Phase 2. The National Academies Press. Retrieved from https://doi.org/10.17226/18951

Jolles, M. P., Haynes-Maslow, L., Roberts, M. C., & Dusetzina, S. B. (2015). Mental health service use for adult patients with co-occurring depression and physical chronic health care needs, 2007–2010. *Medical Care, 53*(8), 708–712. doi:10.1097/mlr.0000000000000389

Klein, S., & Hostetter, M. (2014). In focus: Integrating behavioral health and primary care. Quality Matters Archive. The Commonwealth Fund. Retrieved from http://www.commonwealthfund.org/publications/newsletters/quality-matters/2014/august-september/in-focus

Long, P. (2017). *Effective care for high-need patients: Opportunities for improving outcomes, value, and health*. Washington, DC: National Academy of Medicine.

Magnan, S. (2017). Social determinants of health 101 for health care: Five plus five. Discussion paper. Washington, DC: National Academy of Medicine. Retrieved from https://nam.edu/social-determinants-of-health-101-for-health-care-five-plus-five

Mental Health America. (2017). State of mental health in America—prevalence data. Retrieved from www.mentalhealthamerica.net/issues/2017-state-mental-health-america-prevalence-data

National Association of Community Health Centers. (2012). Powering healthier communities: Community health centers address the social determinants of health. Retrieved from www.nachc.org/wp-content/uploads/2016/07/SDH_Brief_2012.pdf

National Association of Community Health Centers. (2016). PRAPARE implementation and action toolkit. Retrieved from www.nachc.org/research-and-data/prapare/toolkit/

National Neighborhood Indicators Partnership. (2018). The NNIP concept. Retrieved from www.neighborhoodindicators.org/about-nnip/nnip-concept

Olshansky, E. (2017). Social determinants of health: The role of nursing. Viewpoint. *American Journal of Nursing, 117*(12). doi:10.1097/01.NAJ.0000527463.16094.39

Pellegrini, C. (2013). Mental illness stigma in health care settings a barrier to care. *Canadian Medical Association Journal, 186*(1). doi:10.1503/cmaj.109-4668

Plescia, M., & Dulin, M. (2017). Accountable care communities. *North Carolina Medical Journal, 78*(4), 238–241. doi:10.18043/ncm.78.4.238

Powell, A. (2016, February 22). The costs of inequality: Money = quality health care = longer life. *Harvard Gazette*. Retrieved from https://news.harvard.edu/gazette/story/2016/02/money-quality-health-care-longer-life/

Roeber, C., McClellan, C., & Woodward, A. (2016). *Adults in poor physical health reporting behavioral health conditions have higher health costs*. Rockville, MD: Substance Abuse and Mental Health Services Administration, Center for Behavioral Health Statistics and Quality.

Ross Johnson, S., & Meyer, H. (2017). Behavioral health care fixing a system in crisis. Retrieved from www.modernhealthcare.com/article/20170612/NEWS/306129999

Schaps, M., & Post, S. (2015). *Best practices in behavioral-physical health integration*. Chicago, IL: Health and Medicine Policy Research Group.

Substance Abuse and Mental Health Services Administration. (2014). Building the behavioral health workforce. *SAMHSA Newsletter, 22*(4). Retrieved from www.samhsa.gov/samhsaNewsLetter/Volume_22_Number_4/building_the_behavioral_health_workforce/

Substance Abuse and Mental Health Services Administration. (2017a). *Key substance use and mental health indicators in the United States: Results from the 2016 National Survey on Drug Use and Health* (HHS Publication No. SMA 17-5044, NSDUH Series H-52). Rockville, MD: Center for Behavioral Health Statistics and Quality, Substance Abuse and Mental Health Services Administration. Retrieved from https://www.samhsa.gov/data/

Substance Abuse and Mental Health Services Administration. (2017b, October 12). SAMHSA shares latest behavioral health data, including opioid misuse. *SAMHSA News*. Retrieved from newsletter.samhsa.gov/2017/10/12/samhsa-new-data-mental-health-substance-use-including-opioids/

Substance Abuse and Mental Health Services Administration. (2018a). A quick start guide to behavioral health. Center for Integrated Health Solutions. Retrieved from www.integration.samhsa.gov/resource/quick-start-guide-to-behavioral-health-integration

Substance Abuse and Mental Health Services Administration. (2018b). Nurses. Center for Integrated Health Solutions. Retrieved from www.integration.samhsa.gov/workforce/team-members/nurses

Tello, M. (2017). Racism and discrimination in health care: Providers and patients. Harvard Health Blog. Retrieved from https://www.health.harvard.edu/blog/racism-discrimination-health-care-providers-patients-2017011611015

Terry, K. (2017, February 25). Why physicians must step up and address the social determinants of health. *Medical Economics*. Retrieved from http://medicaleconomics.modernmedicine.com/medical-economics/news/why-physicians-must-step-address-social-determinants-health?page=0,1

Thomas-Henkel, C., & Shulman, M. (2017). *Screening for social determinants of health in populations with complex needs: Implementation considerations*. Trenton, NJ: Center for Health Care Strategies, Inc.

Want, J. (2017). Learning update: Improving care for high needs patients. Retrieved from https://petersonhealthcare.org/learning-update-improving-healthcare-high-need-patients

World Health Organization. (2010). mhGAP intervention guide for mental, neurological and substance use disorders in non-specialized health settings. Retrieved from www.who.org

CHAPTER 11

High-Risk Gaps and Cracks II: Caregivers, Dementia, and End-of-Life Care

© Manop Phimsit/EyeEm/Getty Images

CHAPTER OBJECTIVES

After completing this chapter readers will be able to:

- Identify gaps in care for frail older adults, family caregivers, patients with dementia, and those at end of life
- Describe measures for assessing patient requirements and care effectiveness for these populations
- Describe successful models that apply connected care techniques to close care gaps
- List evidence-based best practices for each focus area and assess your organization's level of adoption of these practices
- Explain the role of nursing in providing care for caregivers, frail older adults, and those at end of life

▶ Introduction

You might think that since most people get old, many get dementia, and everyone dies, the healthcare system would be prepared to deal with aging, dementia, and death in a coherent way. It would also seem that family caregivers—who play a significant role in helping patients with aging, dementia, death, and dying—would be an important target population for healthcare support. Unfortunately, this is far from true in our fragmented American healthcare system.

In our primary care system, internists, who care for the vast majority of elderly patients, have only minimal training in geriatrics, which is considered a separate subspecialty. In a culture of aggressive medical treatment, admitting that end of life is near, and that comfort care measures might best be used, is often labeled "giving up." Family caregivers and other nonrelated caregivers of elderly patients or those with chronic disease help keep patients safe and cared for; yet they receive very little recognition or support from the healthcare system (American Association of Retired Persons [AARP], 2011). Patients with dementia are seen, rightfully, as needing specialized services and support, yet they still frequently need to interact with a medical care system that is very much not designed for people who may be confused, fearful, and perhaps display behavioral outbursts.

While there are significant gaps in care for the frail elderly, those with dementia, and patients at end of life, there are at least a variety of programs and services for these populations that are somewhat more integrated with the healthcare system than services that address mental health and health disparities.

The IMPACT Act with its emphasis on care coordination and communication, creating integrated measurements, and eventually developing an integrated payment system for all postacute care patients is slowly pushing home health care, skilled nursing facilities, and rehabilitation hospitals toward more seamless connections (Centers for Medicare and Medicaid Services [CMS], Medicare Learning Network, 2017).

Nationally, there has been a surge of interest in end-of-life care. This interest has been fueled by attention from national figures such as Atul Gawande (2017), whose book, *Being Mortal*, was on the required reading list for both professionals and laypeople. However, AARP (2018) still cites a number of gaps in end-of-life care that can only be rectified by legislation and healthcare policy.

In this chapter, we will look at gaps in care for frail elders, patients with dementia, and those at end of life. We will also consider the role and struggles of the marginalized and sometimes powerless, yet vital, family caregiver. We will review measures of care effectiveness for these patient populations and will look at model programs that have successfully coordinated and integrated care for older adults and caregivers.

▶ Family Caregivers

Family caregivers are the forgotten people in the healthcare system. The lack of support for caregivers is a fault line that may, without attention, contribute to an earthquake of negative consequences in the healthcare system and the social fabric of the United States. One definition of caregiving from the Family Caregiver Alliance (2016a) is "an unpaid individual (for example, a spouse, partner, family member, friend, or neighbor) involved in assisting others with activities of daily living and/or medical tasks." It is important to note that, while the term "family caregiver" is often used, caregiving may be done by a much wider variety of people including friends, neighbors, volunteers, or members of a faith community.

Caregiving does not seem to be an issue that is top of mind for policy makers, healthcare executives, or health professionals, unless their work directly involves them in caregiver issues. Research on family caregiving and its relationship to, and impact on, health care has been sporadic and relatively sparse.

Much of the literature is older, and studies on family caregivers often seem to be an afterthought and certainly not a part of mainstream healthcare thinking and priorities. An exception to this lack of attention to caregivers is a recent landmark report by the National Academies Press (Schulz & Eden, 2016). In this report the authors describe the size and scope of the problem: "Family caregiving affects millions of Americans every day, in all walks of life. At least 17.7 million individuals in the United States are family caregivers of someone age 65 and older who needs help because of a limitation in their physical, mental, or cognitive functioning. As a society, we have always depended on family caregivers to provide the lion's share of long term services and supports (LTSS) for our elders. Yet

ASK YOURSELF

- Do you and other clinicians in your organization think of the patient and his or her caregiver as one entity (patientandcaregiver) or do you think of the patient and caregiver as connected, but having separate needs (patient + caregiver)?
- Does your patient satisfaction measurement system distinguish the caregiver experience from the patient experience in any way?

the need to recognize and support caregivers is among the most significant overlooked challenges facing the aging U.S. population, their families, and society" (p. 1).

Caregiving Statistics

The Family Caregiver Alliance (2016a) provides an exhaustive list of the characteristics of U.S. caregivers:

- Approximately 43.5 million caregivers have provided unpaid care to an adult or child in the last 12 months.
- The value of services provided by informal caregivers has steadily increased over the last decade, with an estimated economic value of $470 billion in 2013, up from $450 billion in 2009 and $375 billion in 2007.
- Upwards of 75% of all caregivers are female, and they may spend as much as 50% more time providing care than males.
- Of family caregivers who provide complex chronic care, 46% perform medical and nursing tasks. More than 96% of caregivers provide help with activities of daily living (ADLs), such as personal hygiene, dressing and undressing, and getting in and out of bed, or instrumental activities of daily living (IADLs) such as taking prescribed medications, shopping for groceries, transportation, or using technology—or both.

The reality behind these statistics is that there is a vast spectrum of diversity among caregivers. Caregiving, especially when it involves physical care, is more often performed by women. Spouse caregivers are more intensely involved in both physical and personal caregiving tasks and in advocating for their spouse. These husband, wife, or life partner caregivers put in the most time and effort and are among the most impacted by caregiving. In some cultural groups, caregivers are caught in the sandwich of caring for young grandchildren as well as older relatives.

One major shift in demographics, which has put a major strain on caregivers and the healthcare system, is the movement of many women, who were formerly available to be full-time family caregivers, into the workforce. This shift has resulted in less available caregiver time, more caregiver stress, employment issues for both caregivers and employers, and a more "patchwork" system of care support for patients with complex and serious illness.

Working caregivers, who make up a significant portion of the caregiver population, find their ability to perform their jobs and advance their careers may be seriously affected by caregiving demands: "69% of working caregivers caring for a family member or friend report having to rearrange their work schedule, decrease their hours, or take an unpaid leave in order to meet their caregiving responsibilities" (Family Caregiver Alliance, 2016b).

The Work of Family Caregivers

Family caregivers commonly provide five types of help to care recipients (**FIGURE 11-1**):

- Assistance with ADLs and personal care
- Help with medical procedures at home
- Advocacy and care coordination
- Emotional support and companionship
- Financial, legal, and household maintenance activities

Of particular interest to health professionals are the medical procedure, care coordination, and advocacy functions of caregiving. The

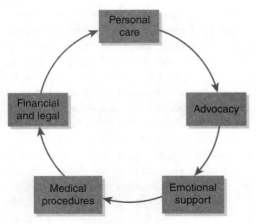

FIGURE 11-1 Family Caregiver Support Responsibilities

Modified from Schulz, R., & Eden, J. (2016). *Families caring for an aging America*. Washington, DC: The National Academies Press.

2016 caregiver study, *Families Caring for an Aging America* (Schulz & Eden, 2016), describes the frequency of medically related tasks performed by caregivers.

Care coordination type tasks such as making medical appointments, speaking with medical providers, keeping track of medications, and helping with changing health insurance or managing health insurance issues top the list of tasks performed by family caregivers. A second tier of "medical" tasks are performed less frequently, including giving injections, performing medical tasks such as tube feedings, managing medical equipment, preparing special diets, and providing wound care (Schulz & Eden, 2016).

An earlier study of a large population of caregivers (*Home Alone: Family Caregivers Providing Complex Chronic Care*) from AARP (Reinhard, Levine, & Samis, 2012) rated the difficulty of the medical tasks that family caregivers performed at home. The tasks rated as most difficult were:

■ Using incontinence equipment and supplies, administering enemas
■ Doing wound care
■ Managing medications including intravenous (IV) lines and injections

These tasks are important because some are technically complex, and if not performed correctly, can result in adverse patient outcomes and unnecessary emergency room visits and hospital readmissions. The two highest-risk medical tasks performed by caregivers are medication management and wound care.

Caregivers found managing incontinence not as technically difficult, but difficult in the sense of providing an intimate level of an uncomfortable type of personal care to someone with whom the caregiver has a long-standing personal relationship, especially when the two parties are of the opposite sex. An example would be a daughter managing incontinence and the use of adult diapers with her father.

Training in caregiver performance of medical tasks was a significant issue. Less than a third of caregivers in the study said they had received formal training in tasks such as medication management. What training there was came from outpatient providers and home healthcare nurses. Caregivers reported fairly low levels of instruction from hospital staff and very little medication instruction from pharmacists (Reinhard et al., 2012).

Caregivers and Care Transitions

Another study (Jeffs et al., 2017) showed that caregivers play a significant role in care transitions—one of the higher risk gaps in health care. In this study, caregivers provided support for relatives who were transferred from an acute care facility to a rehabilitation hospital. Some caregiver functions during transitions were:

■ **Watching.** Being a physical presence and a second pair of eyes and ears. Watching involved monitoring the health status of the caregiver's family member and checking on medication administration. The caregiver also helped the patient understand what was happening during the transition.
■ **Providing care.** Where resources were scarce, family members pitched in to provide direct care such as feeding the patient.
■ **Advocacy.** Family members advocated for the patient's preference being honored and for help with mobility, obtaining physical therapy, and ensuring that the patient was

not discharged too soon. Caregivers also acted as translators, interpreting their relative's needs to health professionals and explaining professional information and instructions to their relative.

- **Navigating the healthcare system.** Caregivers took on the responsibility for arranging follow-up care for their relative and for asking practical questions such as, "My mother can't get in the car, how is she going to get to the appointment?"

Jeffs and colleagues (2017) identified a key gap in care for caregiver and patient alike. While professionals saw family members as indispensable to the transition process, they seldom engaged them or involved them in care without the caregiver actively inserting oneself into the process. The authors describe this as "active involvement in care while struggling to gain influence" (p. 1448). The study concludes that caregivers play a vital role in preventing medical errors and in creating a more effective discharge process yet are not well supported by health professionals. This is a key theme found throughout the literature on caregiver involvement in the healthcare system on behalf of their loved ones.

HELENE'S STORY—FAMILY CAREGIVING

Helene has been a family caregiver for her son, who was born with cystic fibrosis (CF). He is now an adult and is managing his own care. Helene has also cared for both her mother and her mother-in-law. Helene is now an RN, but when her son was born she was not in the healthcare field.

Helene's son has needed both primary and specialty care since he was born. Maintaining insurance has always been central to her caregiving. At one point, she and her son were covered by a staff model health maintenance organization (HMO) and had to prove to them that their staff couldn't provide the type of specialty care he needed and that out-of-network care was necessary. Every job she has had in her career as a nurse has been selected for the quality of its insurance coverage.

She says that "specialty care is an overarching issue." Having to find a CF specialty clinic that was compatible with her insurance was sometimes a challenge. The insurance wanted her to use a clinic at a local teaching hospital, which worked well for a while. The CF clinic had consistent physicians, social workers, and nutritionists. When the head physician retired, "things fell apart," and Helene had to find another source of care for her son. She had to "fight with the insurance company" to get them to cover care at a better organized CF clinic in another part of the state.

When asked about how much support she as a caregiver had received from the healthcare system, she had to stop and think. She finally replied that the CF clinic, when it was functioning, was supportive. She also received supportive counseling from a genetic testing service at the hospital, which she consulted before the birth of her daughter.

Helene says that at age 21, she learned to be a case manager for her baby. "I learned to be resourceful, be on the phone, push the envelope." She notes that it is easier to do these things for your child than it would be to do them for yourself.

When her son was first born, Helene was on Medicaid. While Medicaid offered good insurance coverage, "there were some mean people in the system, who made judgments." For example, there often were not enough chairs for people to sit when at the Medicaid office.

She received some great help from several sources, however. One was a local independent pharmacy that delivered medical supplies such as colostomy bags for her son. She also got great support from other parents at a local cooperative daycare center where her son attended. She says, "That was my support, not the healthcare system." Many of the parents "swapped child care" and helped one another. When her son was young, her mother moved closer to help support Helene.

Helene had plenty of experience with specialty care and visits to the ER. Every time her son developed a symptom the specialists would say "go to the ER." Sometimes they would "call ahead and

(continues)

HELENE'S STORY—FAMILY CAREGIVING *(continued)*

grease the wheels" and other times they wouldn't, which then made the visit harder. During this time, she was juggling care of a chronically ill son and attending nursing school.

Helene says that her pediatricians were a bright spot for her. "They would do anything for us to make things easier." They would often consult with her about her son's symptoms on the phone rather than making her bring him to the office. They would refill specialty prescriptions and provide convenient office hours.

As her son's CF progressed, he developed more symptoms, including diabetes. This necessitated visits to even more specialists. He also became depressed and needed counseling. Helene notes that high copays were a barrier to him getting mental health help.

The need for insurance kept him from getting a full-time job and forced him to stay on Helene's insurance well into his twenties, which made him feel less of an adult.

Her son eventually got married, but at first it was not a legal wedding, because marriage would have caused his insurance to lapse. After his wife got a job with good insurance, they were able to marry legally. Helene notes, "Care never seemed to be driven by the patient's medical needs, but only by insurance requirements." Helene's son is now in his early forties and is in a pre–lung transplant program. He has done well medically and is independent and working.

Besides caring for her son, Helene cared for her mother at the end of her life. She is also currently caring for her mother-in-law, who is 99 years old and mentally alert, but who has vision and hearing problems. Helene notes that "a lack of geriatricians is huge." Her experience is that several of the internists who her mother-in-law has seen want to do unnecessary medical testing. For example, they want to do a carotid ultrasound on her mother-in-law, despite the fact that she is not willing to have any treatment if something is found.

She feels that primary care physicians sometimes show a "lack of thought about what to do and what not to do with elderly patients." She speaks of her mother, who when in the terminal phase of cancer was sent for a CT scan. "She couldn't lay on the table, the tech was not kind and my mother started crying. I just said 'we are out of here,' and took her home." She also mentions that once her mother was diagnosed with cancer, the internist "washed his hands of her" and turned her care entirely over to a specialist despite Helene asking him to remain involved because he was the doctor who her mother knew best. Helene gives an example of another health systems problem, which is that her mother-in-law's advance directives and her papers designating a healthcare agent have been lost many times. She says that she now just carries the papers with her when her mother-in-law has a medical procedure.

Helene talks about her experience with hospice care for her mother and home health care for her mother-in-law. Her mother had home hospice care for 10 days before her death. Helene was surprised at how little supportive help was available. A home health aide came in the morning for several hours and then the expectation was that the family would do all the other physical care. Helene feels that she received good supportive help from hospice staff, however.

She found home health care to be helpful to her mother-in-law, who had problems with mobility and ADLs. However, her mother-in-law did not see the value of it because the therapists failed to connect the exercises to ADLs by saying such things as, "If you do your exercises, you will be able to reach that shelf." She has gotten practical support and eldercare advice from a friend who works in a home health agency and from some of the aides. Just having someone to sit and talk is helpful.

She ends by saying that her mother-in-law does not believe in doctors and medications. However, when she was prescribed medication that stopped her incontinence, allowing her to go out more, she was amazed. However, she has asked Helene, "Why can't I take just half a pill? It would probably work just as well." Helene knows that if she wasn't around to be the caregiver, her mother-in-law actually would take just half the pill.

Caregiver Willingness to Perform Medical Tasks

An important issue for caregivers and the healthcare community is caregiver willingness and ability to perform medical care tasks.

Both the AARP report and the National Academy of Sciences caregiver report indicate that many caregivers feel that they have no choice in the performance of medical tasks for their care recipient (the patient). This lack of choice may have adverse consequences for the health and well-being of caregivers.

Of caregivers, 57% report they do not have a choice about performing clinical tasks, and many feel that this lack of choice is self-imposed; 43% feel that these tasks are their personal responsibility because no one else can do it, or because insurance will not pay for a professional caregiver (Family Caregiver Alliance, 2016a). Schulz and colleagues (2012), in a study of 1,397 caregivers, found that lack of choice is associated with stress and negative health impacts.

Observations from the field indicate that in recent years, with reduced payments and the incidence of shorter hospital and skilled nursing facility stays, caregivers are simply expected to take on complex medical tasks, with only minimal (and often no) consideration of their willingness or ability to do so. Health professionals have begun to assume that many tasks that were formerly the responsibility of health professionals can now be done by family caregivers. Unfortunately, family caregivers are generally unaware of these shifting expectations and many are amazed and shocked at health professionals' casual expectation that the caregiver can and will give injections, manage IV lines, manipulate medical equipment, and do complex wound care in the home. When the caregiver resists, professionals, who have no recourse other than to discharge quickly under Medicare and other insurance payment rules, can become frustrated with the caregiver. This situation creates a serious mismatch between family and professional expectations, considerable stress, and conflict. It also sometimes causes huge gaps in care, particularly in transitions from inpatient facilities to care at home.

A good example is a patient who needs personal care, medication management, and wound care at home. If the patient is lucky enough to be referred to home care, clinical staff will perform these functions for a short period of time until the family can be taught to do it themselves. Some caregivers, caught in the trap of low finances and too little time, or job and other family pressures, will agree to take on medical tasks and then not follow through, creating patient harm.

Caregivers and Resource Gaps

Even caregivers who want to pay for help with medical procedures find resources to be scarce or nonexistent. Private duty nurses filled this function at one time, but this type of service is now seldom available. For example, a spouse caring for a husband with dementia and recurrent urinary tract infections was not able to do IV therapy at home. Despite her willingness to pay for this service, she could not find an agency or individual nurse to do it because of the time commitment and liability issues. She was eventually forced to pay for transport to an outpatient clinic where the IV therapy could be administered. State regulations often thwart the caregiver in getting help with home medical procedures. In some states, nonmedical aides who work for home care agencies cannot perform any type of medical procedure. Caregivers are forced to hire private aides, who are not subject to any state regulations and who may have no medical training other than that provided by the family, to perform this function.

Another common gap is the now widespread use of *observation stays*, in which a patient appears to be admitted to a hospital but is actually considered an outpatient. When a patient is admitted in observation status, he or she does not meet Medicare criteria for admission to a skilled nursing facility stay, again leaving family members to provide care for a fairly acutely ill person at home. These gaps, because they are largely invisible to healthcare providers, are the source of fragmentation, communication disconnects, frustration, and often adverse patient outcomes.

An additional issue is the rise of Medicare Advantage plans, which are required to cover the same services as regular Medicare, but that sometimes limit access to these services through prior authorization to reduce costs.

Caregiver Advocacy and Decision Making Support Obstacles

Family caregivers are often intimately involved in helping family members make healthcare decisions. In some cases, they are welcomed by health professionals as valued partners in care plan development. In other cases, they are ignored or their involvement is minimized. This is a complex issue that involves the patient's willingness to involve family members, the number of family members, their own goals for patient care, and the health professional's perception of the caregiver role.

Health professionals walk a fine line in providing connected care to patients in these circumstances. While the role of the family caregiver is crucial, the patient, if he or she is mentally competent, has the right to decide how much medical information to share with the caregiver and how much to involve this person in the decision-making process. A truly patient-centered approach can sometimes create dissonance when the patient and caregiver do not agree on the level of caregiver involvement.

A common circumstance is a very ill patient who does not want to worry family members or who wants to control his or her own response to an illness in a way that is different from what family members want.

This problem becomes particularly acute when it involves not adhering to recommended medical treatment. For the patient, holding information and decision making close may be a connected care experience.

For the family it may be fragmented and agonizing; but it is truly the patient's choice. In these cases it is up to health professionals to support both patient and family in a highly emotional situation.

A statement from the American College of Physicians Center for Ethics and Professionalism provides a list of best practices for physicians who work with patients and family caregivers. One part of the statement addresses the issue of caregiver involvement in decision making about treatment choices. The essence of these recommendations is that while the family caregiver should be a valued member of the team, his or her involvement should always be authorized and controlled by the patient. Clinicians should not turn their attention to the caregiver to the exclusion of the patient and they should allow patients to choose the level of caregiver involvement in their care planning (Mitnick, Leffler, & Hood, 2010).

The Health and Well-Being of Caregivers

Family caregivers themselves are a highly vulnerable patient population. Research shows that the caregiving experience, while highly fulfilling for many caregivers, can have an adverse effect on caregiver mental and physical health. Often, the family caregiver who is caring for an identified patient becomes the patient, too. The Family Caregiver Alliance (2006) has summarized the research on health issues related to the burden of caregiving:

- Caregivers show higher levels of depression.
- Caregivers suffer from high levels of stress and frustration.
- In response to increased stress, caregivers may turn to alcohol or prescription or psychotropic drugs.
- Caregivers are in worse health and suffer from more physical ailments than noncaregivers.
- Caregivers have lower levels of self-care than noncaregivers.
- Caregivers pay the price in increased mortality. In one striking statistic it was found that spouse caregivers who are under stress experience a 63% higher mortality rate than noncaregivers of the same age.

The National Academy of Medicine report referenced earlier devotes 19 pages of text and citations to the various negative emotional and physical effects of high-stress caregiving (Schulz & Eden, 2016).

Health Professional Attention to Caregiver Distress

Because the caregiver is often so focused on the care recipient, who is the identified patient, he or she often neglects his/her own health. Health professionals may unconsciously collude in this neglect by focusing solely on the identified patient and not on the caregiver, who may be showing physical and emotional symptoms, too. Dr. Pauline Chen (2010), in a poignant article about supporting family caregivers, describes this scene of a middle-aged man who had brought his 90-year-old father for medical care: "Later outside the exam room, the son pulled me aside. I noticed the dark circles around his eyes. 'You're tired, aren't you?' I asked him. The man's dark eyes began to fill with tears. I immediately, reflexively almost, started apologizing for not being able to do more for his father. But he stopped me. 'No, no,' he said, wiping the tears away with the back of his hand. 'It's not that. It's not that at all.' He paused and looked toward his father, still lying on the table in the room and smiling at the lights. 'It's just that no doctor has ever asked me if I was tired'" (p. 2).

Supporting Family Caregivers

Caregivers want and need support from government, healthcare, and social service agencies. These supports fall into several categories, as illustrated in **FIGURE 11-2**.

Legislation

Until recently, caregivers had no official status in medical facilities and were not guaranteed the ability to advocate for their care recipient, even if the patient requested that the caregiver be involved. In many instances, this lack of

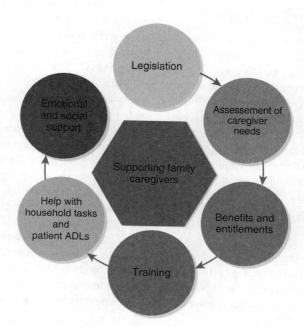

FIGURE 11-2 Categories of Support for Family Caregivers

official caregiver status has created huge gaps in care for patients. The Caregiver Advise, Record, and Enable (CARE) Act is one remedy for this problem. Through the lobbying efforts of AARP, this legislation has been passed by 75% of states. The act requires hospitals to:

- Let patients identify a family caregiver when they're admitted.
- Notify the family caregiver in advance when the patient will be discharged.
- Instruct the family caregiver about any necessary ongoing treatment. (Morris, 2017)

In 2017, the Recognize, Assist, Include, Support and Engage (RAISE) Family Caregivers Act was passed. This act directs the Department of Health and Human Services (HHS) to create an advisory council charged with making recommendations on strategies to support family caregivers.

The blueprint, which was to be developed within 18 months, would address financial and workplace issues, respite care, and other ways to support caregivers (Hackett, 2018).

Family Caregiver Assessment

As noted, caregivers are often ignored or marginalized by the healthcare system with the result that caregiver capabilities and their own health and emotional needs are not recognized or supported. Formal caregiver assessments can help identify the specific physical and emotional challenges that caregivers face. The National Academy of Medicine caregiver report suggests that caregiver assessments should include specific caregiver needs and strengths, caregiver emotional and physical health, the caregiver's ability to help meet the needs of the family member, and caregiver relationships with the healthcare team (Schulz & Eden, 2016).

Unfortunately, because caregivers' lack official status within the healthcare system, and care for them is not covered by health insurance, their needs are seldom assessed separately

from the identified patient. This may change, as value-based payment systems force healthcare organizations to take a more holistic view of the patient's care system. A simple assessment tool that can be used in medical settings is the evidence-based Caregiver Self-Assessment Questionnaire from the American Medical Association. This simple, 18-question form allows caregivers to self-assess the impact of caregiving on their life, health, and well-being (Epstein-Lubow, Gaudiano, Hinckley, Salloway, & Miller, 2010).

Benefits and Entitlements

The financial stress of caring for an ill or elderly relative is well documented and contributes to a highly fragmented and disconnected care experience for caregiver and patient.

Many people have the illusion that Medicare will pay for long-term care, but this is a fallacy. Other than limited coverage for temporary rehabilitation in a skilled nursing facility and some coverage for home health care, Medicare does not cover any type of long-term care. In 2018, CMS announced that Medicare Advantage plans will be allowed to cover nonmedical supportive services. This may be a first step in providing more substantive support for family caregivers (Moeller, 2018).

Since, prior to this new benefit, there was no system of insurance for long-term care outside private long-term care policies, many patients and families impoverished themselves when long-term support for personal care and ADLs were required. Caregivers who reduce their work hours or who quit their jobs to care for an ill relative experience a huge reduction in income as a result of their decision to become a caregiver.

There are benefits and entitlement programs that help family caregivers, but they vary greatly by state. Most of these programs require means tests and are only available to those patients who truly have low incomes. Some states actually pay family members to care for a relative under programs with titles such as "consumer directed care programs." Through Medicaid waiver programs, other states offer home- and community-based supports and coverage for personal care and help with household tasks to avoid nursing home placement and reliance on state Medicaid programs. Short-term caregiver respite grants are available in other states. The Veterans Aid and Attendance benefit provides long-term care support for veterans who qualify. BenefitsCheckUp, a service of the National Council on Aging, allows seniors to search almost 2,500 benefits online. The program provides data on federal, state, and local benefits for housing, food, tax relief, medications, employment, and more (BenefitsCheckUp, 2018).

Resource and Referral Hubs

Most communities have referral hubs for seniors and people with disabilities. Some resource hubs are online and others are available by phone or in person. Agencies on Aging, which are funded by the Older Americans Act, are one source of information for caregivers and exist in all 50 states. Senior centers and city and town social service departments are another source of program information for caregivers. The National Family Caregiver Alliance provides a 50-state Family Caregiver Navigator, which allows caregivers to search all benefit, entitlement, and support programs in their state (www.caregiver.org/state-list).

Not surprisingly, many healthcare providers who are focused on the medical aspects of care are often unaware of social services and resource hubs in their communities. Primary care medical homes and organizations that are part of an accountable care organization should have a robust system for identifying and referring to community resources. If the organization does not have nurse care coordinators or health navigators, a best practice for support of caregivers is to become aware of one resource hub or to assign a staff member to develop a small list of resources for elderly and high-need patients. Clinical staff should then practice the closed loop referral process described in the social determinants of health section of Chapter 10.

Training and Support Groups

The AARP paper on caregivers performing medical tasks highlighted the serious problem of spotty and inadequate training for caregivers.

In states that have passed the CARE Act, training and instruction for family caregivers is mandated as part of discharge planning. However, in the rushed and stressed discharge process, health professionals, caregivers, and patients are often too distracted for optimal learning.

Written instructions or access to online videos can be a helpful way for caregivers to get the information they need once the patient is settled in at home. Much of the instruction given to caregivers occurs in medical offices and health clinics. The quality of this instruction varies greatly and is dependent on the type of professionals available to do it and their skill in patient education. The quality of written and online educational materials also plays a role. Some caregiver organizations have developed courses for caregivers that provide instruction in performing medical tasks and in the tools and techniques of caregiver self-care. One example is the Building Better Caregivers program from the Veterans Administration (2018). This 6-week online course developed by Stanford University covers a variety of topics:

- Managing stress
- Problem solving/effective communication
- Taking care of yourself
- Utilizing technology

Many community organizations offer family caregiver support groups which are professionally facilitated and which provide both education and peer emotional support to stressed family caregivers.

⌕ CASE STUDY

Comprehensive Support for Family Caregivers

VNA Community Healthcare has provided a Caregiver Resource Center and Consultation Service since 2008. Developed to support both community family caregivers and caregivers of patients under care by the agency, this program consists of the following:

Caregiver consultations. A geriatric care manager, who is also trained in Medicare and other benefit and entitlement programs, provides short phone and in-person assessments, support and information, and referral for both community caregivers and family caregivers referred by agency clinicians.

Caregiver support groups. The agency runs family caregiver support groups in community locations, senior centers, and assisted living facilities.

A toll-free help line. The "VNA Help Line," which is staffed during regular business hours, answers caregiver questions and provides information and referrals to services within the organization's continuum (home health care, nonmedical home care, hospice, and adult day center) and in the community.

A volunteer network and a "buddy match" program. A strong network of volunteers provides help with caregiver educational events, mailings, and in the past, delivery of roses and notes to family caregivers during caregiver month. A buddy match program connects current and former caregivers for socialization and peer support.

The Caregiver School. This program is a series of classes and videos that teach family caregivers both medical and self-care skills. Originally funded by the South Central Connecticut Agency on Aging, this program includes topics such as body mechanics and mobility assistance, incontinence and skin care, care coordination, coping with challenging dementia behaviors, and creating a positive home environment (dementia care). The program was developed based on focus group interviews with members of the agency's caregiver support groups. The agency also offers single-session classes with such titles as "The New Balancing Act" on caregiver stress management and self-care skills.

Clinician Resource Guide. The agency researched and developed an online resource guide of pharmacies, food programs, used medical equipment sources, and other useful links. The guide is available to agency clinicians on agency smartphones and is shared with local hospitals, medical practices, and social service agencies.

Technology Help for Family Caregivers

As the U.S. population ages and the availability of both family and paid caregiving support becomes less available, technology must step into the care gap. Technology for aging and disabilities falls into several categories (Saltzman, 2017):

■ **Sensors.** These devices are installed on beds or around the home and can track the movements of an elderly person within a home or facility. This aids caregivers in knowing whether the person is sleeping, wandering during the night, or going to the kitchen to eat. Another type of sensor can automatically shut off a stove if the person leaves the kitchen and doesn't return in a specific time period.

■ **Emergency alert and fall detector systems.** Emergency buttons, watches, and pendants allow people who fall to push a button to call for help. The alert system is typically connected to a remote call center where trained dispatchers can assess the situation and alert family members or emergency services. Some alert systems can sense that the patient has had a fall and can contact emergency services without the patient needing to press a button.

- **Medication reminders and dispensers.** These systems consist of a preprogrammed alert system that uses an audible signal to tell patients that it is time to take a particular medication. Some systems also provide locked medication boxes that can be prefilled. The system uses flashing lights or an audible alert to cue the patient and unlocks the needed pills so the patient can take them at the correct time.

- **Video connections** allow families to connect seniors or disabled patients with family members or professionals for socialization and as a way to monitor the patient's status without being physically present.

Health professionals, unless they are specialists in geriatrics, are usually not familiar with the various "aging in place" technologies. There is no centralized hub for information about this topic, so internet searches are the best way for caregivers to find it. Many Agencies on Aging can provide local contacts for technology vendors. As of this writing, there is some evidence that AARP and Amazon may be discussing possible opportunities for providing aging in place technologies in a more coordinated manner.

INTERVIEW WITH MARIO D'AQUILA, ASSISTED LIVING TECHNOLOGIES, INC.

Mario D'Aquila is vice president of Assisted Living Technologies, Inc. (www.assistedlivingtechnologies .com), which was established in 2010. He is also director of business development for Assisted Living Services, Inc., a provider of nonmedical home care services that is affiliated with the technology company. The company provides primarily wireless, sensor-based, technologically advanced products that provide seniors and individuals with disabilities with an improved quality of life and the ability to age in place.

Mario explains that Assisted Living Technologies was developed as a "technology hub" for the senior market. This hub helps seniors and family members choose the technology that best meets their needs and then teaches them how to use the products they buy. This advisor function, along with a rigorous program of product evaluation and testing, have given Assisted Living Technologies a unique market niche.

Mario initially reached out to manufacturers and began a rigorous evaluation of each product—a practice the company has continued. Each product is evaluated on several criteria:

Reliability. Does the product consistently work as it is supposed to? In this market, reliability is a vital criterion, because someone's life might depend on reliability of a piece of equipment such as a fall detector or wandering sensor.

Ease of use. The senior population is hesitant to use technology, so it must be easy to use. Technology that requires many complex steps is not practical for Mario's customers. He says, "It must be a one button thing."

Visual appeal. Customers of Assisted Living Technologies want products that "don't look super medical" or that would "make them feel old" or "remind them of something you would see in a hospital." They want the product to look good and be comfortable to use.

Assisted Living Technologies sells four types of products:

- **Personal emergency response systems.** These are medical alert systems that can be activated with the touch of a button. The call goes to a centralized emergency dispatch center, which evaluates the problem and sends help. Some systems include a fall detector and some are wireless and use GPS so they can be used outside the home.

(continues)

INTERVIEW WITH MARIO D'AQUILA, ASSISTED LIVING TECHNOLOGIES, INC. *(continued)*

- **Medication management systems.** Some products simply cue the user to take medication with sound or lights. Other products dispense medications. Some products log activity so family members can view compliance levels. Many people who forget to take their medications will agree to use these systems as an alternative to moving into a facility.
- **Remote monitoring devices.** These devices do "passive activity monitoring" to track when the senior wakes and gets out of bed, uses the bathroom, goes to the kitchen, etc. This monitoring can help supplement home caregiving and sometimes the device can prove that there is a need for a caregiver. In one case the state would not pay for a client to have 24-hour care. When the sensor technology proved that the client was up most of the night, the state relented and provided more help.
- **Home and facility safety devices.** Sensor bed pads can send a signal to a mobile phone to let a family member know that an older parent is getting out of bed frequently. An automated stove shutoff system monitors the kitchen for movement when a stove is on. When the person who is cooking leaves the kitchen, it tracks the time and automatically shuts the stove off after a certain interval. This type of system allows seniors with memory impairment to still do some limited cooking. Systems that track people within a building such as a tracker for residents in a dementia facility are popular with assisted living facilities.

Mario describes how his technologies fill gaps in care for seniors and their families. He feels that these technologies do not replace human help; they supplement it. Having technology means that less care is required, and people can avoid institutionalization and can remain independent in their own homes longer.

Mario describes his most successful clients as those who "want to get out and stay healthy. They have busy lives and they don't want things like forgetting medications to hold them back." To be successful, however, they must admit that they need a "little more help."

When asked about the advising function of his business he says that most customers come in having some idea of what they need. He asks them to describe the problem they want to solve which is usually described as, "Mom is wandering," "Dad is socially isolated," or "Mom gets out of bed." One of the technology advisors then suggests a technology that can help with the specific problem and with the special needs of the client. If the company does not carry a product that a client needs, Mario says that he can usually find it for them.

He says that he has learned from his mistakes and is not quick to recommend a technology until he really understands the client's needs.

When asked about challenges, Mario says that the most common one is the level of acceptance by the client. Often, a care manager will make a referral, but unless the client and family are both involved and are willing to pay attention and use the device properly, it doesn't work. "Technology is only as good as the people who use it," Mario says. "If the daughter can't find the time to fill the medication dispenser, the system won't work for the client." Assisted Living Technologies improves its success rate by doing its own local installations and by providing instruction on how to use the equipment. They have a learning lab and will invite families to come in by appointment and try different types of technology. Assisted Living Technologies created metrics to analyze its success in preventing falls and hopes to measure the effectiveness of other technologies.

Mario ends by saying that the business has become very successful and is soon to open a branch office in another county. As for himself, Mario describes his business as "absolutely fascinating and satisfying."

Nurses and Family Caregiver Support

Nurses are on the front line of support for family caregivers. Since nursing takes a holistic view of patient care, support for family caregivers is often woven into daily nursing practice as a matter of course. A publication from the Robert Wood Johnson Foundation (2015) describes this important nursing role: "Nurses are providing more care for the sick and elderly in their homes and communities, which alleviates burdens on family caregivers. They are training caregivers to provide skilled care so their loved ones can live longer in their homes and avoid expensive long-term care facilities. And they are teaching caregivers how to stay healthy and well. Supporting family caregivers is a 'major focus for nurses across the health care system and especially in the growing fields of palliative and hospice care,' said J. Taylor Harden, PhD, RN, FAAN, executive director of the National Hartford Centers of Gerontological Nursing Excellence."

Nurses educate family caregivers to perform medical tasks. Nurses are often the voice on the end of the phone when a distraught family caregiver calls for advice about a patient's declining condition. It is the ambulatory care nurse who so often notices caregiver stress, fatigue, and potential health issues. Nurses provide telehealth and remote monitoring for patients. Woven into these interventions are listening and emotional support that nurses routinely offer to family caregivers as part of the delivery of care to patients (Reinhard & Young, 2017). Structured nursing interventions for family caregivers tend to involve education and training. A good example is a series of articles and videos on key caregiver training topics published in the *American Journal of Nursing*. The program is described in this way: "This article is part of a series *Supporting Family Caregivers: No Longer Home Alone*, published in collaboration with the AARP Public Policy Institute. Results of focus groups, conducted as part of the AARP Public Policy Institute's *No Longer Home Alone* video project, supported evidence that family caregivers aren't given the information they need to manage the complex care regimens of family members. This series of articles and accompanying videos aims to help nurses provide caregivers with the tools they need to manage their family member's health care at home" (Kirkland-Kyhn, Generao, Teleten, & Young, 2018, p. 63).

Cross-Functional Teamwork to Support Caregivers

Other professionals also provide family caregiver support. Social workers in healthcare facilities are often asked to support family caregivers through counseling and helping them find and enroll in benefit and entitlement programs. Support staff may develop a rapport with family caregivers and are often able to address their practical needs and concerns as well as or better than professionals.

Physical and occupational therapy professionals help caregivers find practical strategies for mobility and improving ADLs. Cross-functional teamwork between physicians, nurses, social workers, therapists, and support staff is the best way to fully support stressed and overwhelmed family caregivers. Pharmacists, especially those in community pharmacy settings, are a common source of medication advice for family caregivers.

Nonmedical home care agencies are another source of support for caregivers. These companies typically provide homemakers, companions, personal care assistants and live-in aides to help frail or elderly patients with ADLs and household management. Many of these programs are private pay, while others may be state funded.

Best Practices for Family Caregiver Support

While legislative, policy, and insurance factors play a big role in healthcare fragmentation or connection for caregivers, individual healthcare organizations and clinicians can play a big role in supporting caregivers in their difficult task by using a series of simple best practices. **TABLE 11-1** describes these best practices.

TABLE 11-1 Some Best Practices for Supporting Family Caregivers

- Don't categorize patients and caregivers as one entity. Identify the caregivers as members of the patient's care team with separate needs from those of patients.
- Adopt policies, procedures, and training for maximizing the family caregiver role in patient care.
- Train staff to assess and support family caregivers.
- Develop clinical processes for identifying patient requirements for their family caregivers' involvement in patient care and decision making.
- Create processes for sharing vital information about patient care with family caregivers.
- Interview family caregivers about their needs and obstacles to caregiving.
- Adopt and utilize a caregiver assessment tool.
- Use assessment results to identify at-risk family caregivers.
- Develop clinical processes for identifying dysfunctional or abusive relationships between caregivers and care recipients (the patient).
- Identify key community resources for caregivers.
- Provide instructions and training for caregivers, using health teaching best practices such as teach-back and return demonstration.
- Instruct caregivers in how to identify patient changes in condition and how to respond to or report these changes.
- Use closed loop referrals for referring caregivers to community resources.
- Encourage at-risk caregivers to obtain needed medical care.
- Provide or refer caregivers for emotional support or support groups.
- Develop and implement measures of caregiver satisfaction (separate from patient satisfaction).

Care Gaps for Frail Older Adults

Frail older adults are often part of the population of high-cost, high-need patients. These patients consume many medical resources and often strain a system that lacks integrated medical, mental health, and social supports that can address their specific needs. This population is characterized by specific characteristics (Want, 2017):

- "Over 65 years with two or more of the following frailty indicators: gait abnormality, malnutrition, failure to thrive, cachexia, debility, difficulty walking, history of falls, muscle wasting, muscle weakness, decubitus ulcer, senility, or durable medical equipment use.
- Frailty is one of the highest indicators that a patient will require high-cost care that could otherwise be avoided.
- Overall, this group spends the most on post-acute and long-term care, with Part D spending representing only a small portion of the frail elderly's total spending" (p. 8).

One promising approach to the high need senior population is the Creating Age-Friendly Health Systems from the John A. Hartford Foundation. This approach builds on characteristics of model geriatric programs, including addressing ageism, specialized training for staff, a systematic approach to coordinating care, high performance teamwork, engaging patients and families, and using patient goals to set priorities. **TABLE 11-2** describes the 4 M model of age-friendly interventions: what matters, medications, mobility, and mentation (Mate, Berman, Laderman, Kabcenell, & Fulmer, 2018).

Mental Health Care Gaps for Older Adults

In addition to many gaps in the medical care system, older adults often face mental health challenges and difficulty in accessing geriatric mental health care. In *U.S. News,* Newman (2017) quotes Dr. Dilip Jeste, director of the

TABLE 11-2 Age-Friendly Systems 4 M Model		
		Specific High-Level Interventions
What matters	1	Know what matters: health outcome goals and care preferences for current and future care, including end of life
	2	Act on what matters for current and future care, including end of life
Medications	3	Implement standard process for age-friendly medication reconciliation
	4	De-prescribe and adjust doses to be age friendly
Mobility	5	Implement an individualized mobility plan
	6	Create an environment that enables mobility
Mentation	7	Ensure adequate nutrition, hydration, sleep, and comfort
	8	Engage and orient to maximize independence and dignity
	9	Identify, treat, and manage dementia, delirium, and depression

Reproduced from Mate, K. S., Berman, A., Laderman, M., Kabcenell, A., & Fulmer, T. (2018). Creating age-friendly health systems—A vision for better care of older adults. *Healthcare, 6*(1), 4–6.

Stein Institute for Research on Aging at the University of California–San Diego School of Medicine, to illustrate the seriousness of this problem: "The way we treat and take care of people, especially older people, with mental health illnesses is certainly an embarrassment and a shame to society. This is one of the most disenfranchised segments of our society." Suicide is also a significant risk for older adults. The World Health Organization (WHO) estimates that 15% of older adults suffer from a mental health or neurological problem. The most common of these problems are depression and dementia (WHO, 2017).

Older adults with mental health issues suffer from a double stigma, ageism and the stigma of mental illness. Another issue is the lack of geriatric psychiatric professionals. Older adults may be in denial about mental health issues, and their many complex medical problems may take precedence at medical visits. Referral to the small number of geriatric psychiatric services that are available and integration and colocation of medical and mental health services are probably the most promising solutions to the older adult mental health gap (Newman, 2017).

▶ Medical Care for Patients with Dementia

Medical care in the United States is typically not designed to accommodate the special needs of patients with dementia and their caregivers. This care gap produces frustration for health professionals and support staff, and in some cases, results in medical errors and negative outcomes for patients and caregivers.

Older adults with dementia typically receive care from a primary care physician. Most primary care practices do not specialize in

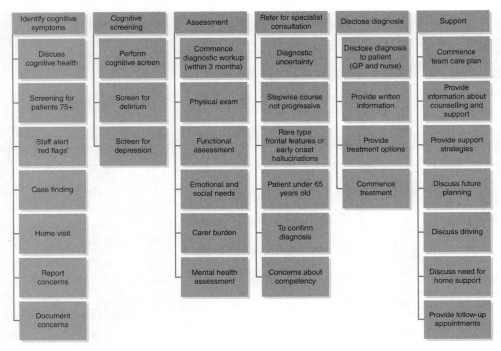

FIGURE 11-3 Dementia Screening, Assessment, and Support Pathway, Australia

Reproduced from Alzheimer's Australia. (2015). Four Steps to Building Dementia Practice in Primary Care. Retrieved from https://www.dementia.org.au/files/VIC/documents/Building -Dementia-Practice.pdf

dementia care and typically have a relatively small number of patients with dementia. Callahan and colleagues (2014) describe the basic principle of care for dementia patients as "support for a patient-caregiver dyad" (p. 1). They then describe the challenges of the current care model: "For a primary care practice to adhere to the key components of best practice care, providers would need to redesign their clinical practices to focus on team-based and population-based care and accept care for the patient's entire panoply of multimorbidity. Barriers to such redesign include financial, technical (e.g. information systems), cultural, and workforce constraints" (p. 4). Primary care practitioners may need specialized training in the care of geriatric and dementia patients to avoid common mistakes and poor outcomes. An example is the overuse of antipsychotic drugs in the treatment of dementia.

In some other countries, primary care practices take significant responsibility for managing the care of dementia patients. See **FIGURE 11-3** for a pathway for dementia care in primary care practice from Australia. In this model, the whole responsibility for care from symptoms through diagnosis, treatment, and support is done within a modified and dementia prepared primary care setting.

In the United States, many communities offer a parallel system of geriatric care that supplements primary care and long-term care and provides consultation to clinicians and caregivers.

An example is the Dorothy Adler Assessment Center at Yale New Haven Hospital, which offers geriatric assessments by board-certified geriatricians and ongoing care coordination and advice for patients and caregivers from a team of physicians, geriatricians, APRNs, and social workers (https://www.ynhh.org/services/aging.aspx).

A NURSE CARE MANAGER HELPS FAMILIES COPE WITH DEMENTIA

Interview with Kathy Heard, APRN

Kathy Heard, APRN, is a geriatric care manager at the Dorothy Adler Geriatric Assessment Center of Yale New Haven Hospital. She is dedicated to supporting patients with dementia and their family caregivers.

Kathy describes her role as "doing the Alzheimer's walk" with patients and families. Over the course of the months or years that symptoms progress, Kathy conducts a psychosocial assessment and provides education about dementia and emotional support. Additionally, another important part of her role is helping families find resources to support the care of their family member, to maintain a quality of life at home.

Working cooperatively with program physicians, Kathy helps families navigate the healthcare system and access care. In one instance, she was called by an inpatient physician dealing with one of her patients who had developed delirium. She was able to provide information and suggestions that produced better outcomes for the patient. Kathy often works with families on advance care planning and decision making about palliative or hospice care.

A key element in her success has been an intimate knowledge of community resources to which she can refer patients and families. Kathy explains that she feels fortunate to live in a state that has a number of entitlements, but identifies that barriers to success are plentiful in this work. Patients who have dementia and are under age 65 (thus not eligible for Medicare) are a huge challenge. Kathy notes that financial barriers, insurance limitations, and burdensome regulations (such as the Medicare requirement that patients must be homebound and have a "skilled need" to receive home care) are all problems that limit patient and family access to home healthcare services.

Financial barriers are a particularly serious problem: "People think twice about service if they have high deductibles," she says. Affordable alternatives to nursing home care and transportation are other big barriers to effective care. Helping families cope with the emotional stresses and strains of dementia caregiving is another key element of her role that helps "prevent families from burning out." Some are in denial and some are financially dependent on the person with dementia, which makes care choices even more difficult.

Kathy continues to experience a great deal of satisfaction in caring for this population and is constantly impressed by the many dedicated caregivers and families she has had the honor of working with over her three decades of practice.

▶ Other Types of Medical Care and Dementia

Medical care, especially when it involves invasive procedures, often meets none of the requirements for effective care of dementia patients. While comprehensive dementia-friendly medical care is not common, individual health facilities and practitioners often develop their own specialized services to close this particular care gap. For example, geriatric dentists specialize in providing dental care for older adults and those with dementia. Optometrists, podiatrists, and audiologists may also specialize in geriatric care. There is no central hub for identifying practitioners who specialize in dementia care. The Alzheimer's Association, local geriatric clinics, the internet, and professional organizations are the best way to find these types of services for patients. Some hospitals have also redesigned their facilities to accommodate geriatric patients and those with dementia by providing geriatric emergency rooms and geriatric units with senior-friendly designs and staff who are specially trained in geriatrics and dementia care.

Meeting the Needs of Patients with Dementia in General Medical Settings

While there are a wide variety of specialized medical care and care coordination programs for people with dementia, they are not widely available in every community. This means that each healthcare organization or medical practice that serves older adults must adopt some best practices for identification, care, and referral of patients with dementia. Most postacute settings such as skilled nursing facilities, assisted living facilities, and home care agencies serve populations with a relatively high incidence of dementia. These healthcare organizations have typically developed specialized staff training, care pathways, and multidisciplinary team structure to deal with patients suffering from dementia and their caregivers.

> ### ASK YOURSELF
>
> - If you asked a patient with dementia or a caregiver of someone with dementia how well your services work for them (or don't) what would they be likely to say?
> - How could you implement some simple patient/caregiver research to answer this question?
> - What methods could your organization use to implement a more dementia-friendly environment using the information obtained from patient and caregiver responses?

Modifying the Clinical Interaction for Patients with Dementia

The experience of medical care can be particularly difficult for patients with dementia and their caregivers. These patients typically need routine, a simplified and calm environment, and visual and verbal clues to function well.

Too much stimuli, loud noise, bright lights, undressing, touching by strangers, and quick movements can increase confusion and sometimes provoke fear and behavioral outbursts in dementia patients. Some thoughtful conversation with family caregivers may provide constructive suggestions for making the environment more age and dementia friendly.

Most of the literature on dementia care emphasizes the role of the family caregiver in coordinating care and advocating for the patient with dementia in medical settings. This implies that the responsibility for accommodating the dementia patient's needs falls to the caregiver.

Why Should This Be So?

In a connected care world, clinicians assess patient needs and change their practice to accommodate the patient and caregiver, rather than the opposite. There is a dearth of research on this topic, with few studies or articles considering the role of general healthcare facilities in providing dementia-friendly medical care and medical procedures.

> ### ASK YOURSELF
>
> What if healthcare organizations took the advice given to caregivers and reversed it to create processes to accommodate patients with dementia and to prevent potential problems?

An example is a document from the Mayo Clinic (2016), which gives caregivers advice about how to manage medical appointments, including scheduling, taking notes, asking questions, and asking for referrals.

Handley, Bunn, and Goodman (2017) used a "realist" perspective to study the implementation of dementia-friendly practices in inpatient units. Their findings indicate that organizations need to provide clinical staff with, "awareness, authority and resources to provide personalised care with support from staff with the relevant expertise. Educational interventions should focus on how staff can identify with the experience of being a patient living with dementia, combined with opportunities for staff to share their experiences of addressing behaviours they find challenging and accommodating person-centered practices within ward routines and priorities" (p. 11).

TABLE 11-3 provides suggestions for how a medical facility could take responsibility for modifying its actions to proactively address dementia care issues rather than putting the full responsibility on an already busy and stressed caregiver (Act on Alzheimer's, 2017).

Consider this issue in light of the "burden of treatment concept," in which the health professional's treatment recommendations often determine the level of effort required of patients and caregivers (Spencer-Bonilla, Quiñones, & Montori, 2017).

Resources for Improving Care and Outcomes for Dementia Patients

Many family caregivers have an incomplete understanding of dementia and the changes that it creates. The Alzheimer's Association is the best comprehensive resource on dementia care for patients, caregivers, and providers. The organization website and 24-hour toll-free help line (800-272-3900) provide a huge range of resources and training materials.

Another excellent resource comes from ACT on Alzheimer's: Minnesotans Working Together on the Impact of Alzheimer's. This program provides a full spectrum of materials for medical practices that wish to improve dementia care. The toolkit includes clinical practice protocols, a video on delivering the dementia diagnosis, electronic medical record decision support tools, and a variety of training programs on dementia-related topics (ACT on Alzheimer's, 2017).

The American Geriatrics Society (AGS) offers a variety of practical resources for clinicians

through its site at www.geriatriccareonline.org. One such tool is a *Clinician Guide for Assessing and Counseling Older Drivers* (AGS, 2015).

The AGS provides clinician information on topics as varied as feeding tubes, geriatric medications, and the management of geriatric patient surgery.

Some Best Practices for the Management and Support of Dementia Patients and Caregivers

- Research specialized dementia care programs in your community, including program design, eligibility, and the referral process.
- Refer patients and families to the Alzheimer's Association chapter in your community (www.alz.org). If all else fails, a referral to this organization can provide some level of advice and resources for families dealing with dementia as well as professional resources.
- Mandate that all clinical and support staff who deal with older adults, as part of their regular professional education, obtain some basic training in dementia.
- Ensure that medical staff understand current medical treatment protocols for patients with dementia.
- Assess and modify clinical practices to accommodate the needs of patients with dementia and their caregivers.
- Identify and eliminate any barriers to the care of dementia patients.
- Use complex case conferences or consultation with geriatric specialists if dealing with a patient who needs complex medical care and who has a diagnosis of dementia.

▶ End-of-Life Care

The Ideal and the Real

One would hope that end-of-life care would epitomize patient-centered, compassionate, and

TABLE 11-3 Changing Clinical Practices to Accommodate Dementia Patients and Family Caregivers

Advice to Caregivers	Clinical Practice Modifications
Be prepared. Make a list of medications, symptoms, and issues you want to discuss. List information about your relative's specific needs to share with providers.	■ Identify patients with dementia through some type of alert or template in the medical record. ■ Clinicians review the record in advance for information about the patient's clinical and psychosocial situation. ■ If the patient is having a procedure, assess the potential implications of dementia on the procedure and outcome. For example, dementia patients may have adverse reactions to anesthesia, procedures that require touching, or the patient holding still, all of which may provoke behavioral outbursts. ■ Ask the caregiver for advice on how to approach and manage the patient during care procedures.
Schedule wisely.	■ When a family caregiver contacts the practice to schedule the appointment, ask what time of day is best for the caregiver and patient. ■ Try to schedule dementia patients when the office is least crowded and noisy. ■ Note that dementia patients are often more alert and less stressed in the morning, but it may take the caregiver time to get the patient ready for the appointment.
Get specific instructions about medications and medical treatments.	■ Use agenda-setting best practices, asking both the patient and caregiver, "What is important for us to discuss today?" ■ Review the medication list with the patient and caregiver. ■ Conduct medication reconciliation. ■ Identify polypharmacy or the use of any medications on the Beers List. ■ Provide specific instructions for medications or medical procedures to be done at home using teach-back, written handouts, and other health teaching best practices. ■ Involve the patient to the level of his or her capabilities.
Take notes.	■ Provide the caregiver with a medical visit form that can be used for note taking. ■ Offer copies of the medical record notes, or help the caregiver to access the practice patient electronic medical report portal. ■ Provide simple written instructions for aftercare.
Consider the future.	■ Educate clinicians about the course of dementia and possible variations. ■ Offer information on future planning rather than waiting for the caregiver to ask.
Deal promptly with conflict.	■ Avoid conflict by training staff and adopting dementia-friendly policies and patient-centered and team-based care. ■ Ask caregivers and patients, "How did this visit or experience work for you?" ■ Be open, nondefensive, and compassionate when addressing issues of concern with caregivers and patients.

coordinated connected care. Articles in both the popular and professional press, stories from the field, and research reports indicate that, in the United States, this is not always a reality. In its publication *Dying in America: Improving Quality and Honoring Individual Preferences Near the End of Life*, the National Academy of Sciences (2015) describes ideal characteristics of end-of-life care:

- Seamless, high-quality, integrated, patient-centered, family-oriented care that is consistently accessible around the clock
- Considers the evolving physical, emotional, social, and spiritual needs of individuals approaching the end of life, as well as those of their family and/or caregivers
- Is competently delivered by professionals with appropriate expertise and training
- Includes coordinated, efficient, and interoperable information transfer across all providers and all settings
- Is consistent with individuals' values, goals, and informed preferences

A summary of 40 years of work on end-of-life care in the *New England Journal of Medicine* (Wolf, Berlinger, & Jennings, 2015) describes the current state:

> Nearly 40 years of intensive work to improve care at the end of life has shown that aligning care with patients' needs and preferences in order to ease the dying process is surprisingly difficult—although there has been some incremental progress. . . .
>
> This history has demonstrated the need to attack the problem at all levels, from individual rights, to family and caregiving relationships, to institutional and health systems reform. (p. 678)

The National Academy of Sciences (2015) publication, *Dying in America*, recounts the story of a 98-year-old man who received care that was inappropriate, terribly disconnected, and lacking in compassion. In one instance, the patient was even sent to a mental institution. The authors sum up the lessons learned from this story:

"This story illustrates care near the end of life that is neither needed nor desired, neither coordinated nor continuous. Those dimensions include a failure to implement advance directives, an excessive number of burdensome transitions, repeated miscommunications with the family, inadequate pain management and apparent overuse of sedation, insensitive communication with the patient, and an inordinate delay in referral to hospice" (p. 56).

A brief entitled *Quality of Life Through End of Life*, from Grantmakers in Aging (2006), provides a summary of the gap between patient/family needs and reality: "This long period of time marking the end of life points up the importance of having care that enhances functioning, enables control, avoids impoverishment, encourages relationships, supports family, assuages pain, respects spiritual growth, and otherwise generally supports having a good life despite the shadow of death. However, our care system does not yet do this well. Pain and fragmentation of care is commonplace, attention to function is unusual, and even recognition of the implacable fact of mortality seems elusive" (p. 2).

Gaps in End-of-Life Care

When considering gaps in end-of-life care, a view from the field may be instructive. In this case, the view from the field comes from the author's home healthcare and hospice agency and from 10 years of experience with a family caregiver education and support network described in the caregiver section of this chapter. Some commonly observed gaps are described in this section.

A Medicalized Culture with a Preference for Aggressive Medical Treatment

The metaphor of "fighting" a disease and even fighting death is ingrained in both the broader American culture and the culture of medicine. Many patients and families simply don't believe that nothing more can be done in the face of a terminal diagnosis. Some physicians, whose whole purpose is to cure, frame referrals to hospice and palliative care as "giving up." In home health care, clinicians frequently hear families say, "Don't you dare mention the H word [hospice] around my mother." The result of this penchant for endless, aggressive treatment may be a patient who spends her last days intubated and helpless in the sterile environment of an intensive care unit (ICU) while enduring multiple and agonizing, but ultimately futile, resuscitation attempts. For some, this is as they want it to be. For others, it is simply the sad end point of a system that doesn't always elicit or respect patient wishes.

A study presented at the meeting of the American Society of Clinical Oncology (ASCO) in 2016 showed that 75% of patients with advanced metastatic disease received aggressive treatment even when it was unlikely to help. This percentage remained the same in 2016 as it was when ASCO made recommendations to reduce the use of such aggressive treatments in 2012 (Chen et al., 2016).

Begley (2016), in the online journal *Stat News*, quoted one physician who noted that there is very little incentive for physicians to stop using aggressive treatment: "If they do, they will be accused of giving up." This compulsion to cure, rather than the profit motive, is why some believe aggressive treatment is overused.

Lack of Advance Planning and Advance Directives About End-of-Life Wishes

The American Bar Association describes advance directives this way: "The generic term for any document that gives instructions about your health care and/or appoints someone to make medical treatment decisions for you if you cannot make them for yourself. Living Wills and Durable Powers of Attorney for Health Care are both types of Health Care Advance Directives" (Sabatino, 2015, p. 6). Even among highly educated people, thinking about and planning for end-of-life wishes is not a popular activity. A recent analysis, published in the journal *Health*

Affairs (Yadav et al., 2017), studied the percentage of people who had created advance directives. The study, which was based on data from 150 studies and 795,000 people, indicated that about 37% had advance directives including 29% with living wills. The percentage of people with advance directives differed very little between those with chronic disease (38%) and those who were healthy (33%).

As a result, many people never create advance directives, and become incapacitated, with no direction for family members and medical personnel. This leads to "guessing" about what the patient might want, and in some cases, in the absence of other information, substituting a course of action that is comfortable only for family members. Good advance care planning requires thinking through what would be important to you in an end-of-life situation and how much aggressive medical treatment you might choose to have.

Doing good advance care planning is complicated by the fact that many laypeople simply cannot visualize what aggressive end-of-life treatment such as long-term ICU stays, tube feeding, intubation, and repeated resuscitations would look and feel like; and most don't care to. Another aspect of advance care planning is making provisions for those who are left behind. When patients don't order their affairs, spouses or other dependents may be left without financial protection. An example is an 87-year-old man who had been in a state of denial about a cancer diagnosis but was now being admitted for extensive cancer surgery. He had not created any advance directives before the surgery and had no plan for the care of his 83-year-old wife, who had dementia.

A good resource for thinking through end-of-life choices is the Five Wishes Program from Aging with Dignity (2018). This program provides a booklet and online program (agingwithdignity.org) to help people think through the details of end-of-life choices such as how you might want to be treated, who will be your healthcare agent, and whether you might want certain medical procedures such as tube feedings.

Advance Directives Not Honored

Even patients who have advance directives cannot count on them being honored by acute care hospital staff. Span (2015) in the *New York Times* tells a common story: A 79-year-old man, who had created a living will before he developed dementia, was treated for a nosebleed that wouldn't stop with aggressive surgery and a tracheostomy. His advance directives were in his chart but were not found until long after the treatment. The patient's son, who wanted to follow his father's wishes, didn't know the living will existed. The article also details circumstances where healthcare providers ignore the living will in favor of a relative's pressure to provide more aggressive treatment.

One solution to this problem is *Physician Orders for Life-Sustaining Treatment* (POLST), a method of codifying patient's wishes into actual medical orders. This method is not usually used unless the patient has a serious illness. Another approach is to ensure that patients have appointed a healthcare proxy or healthcare agent who can speak on their behalf if they are incapacitated and who can advocate for advance directives to be honored (National POLST Paradigm, 2018).

Diffuse Responsibility for "Having the Conversation"

So often patients and families experience a delay in referral to supportive end-of-life programs because no healthcare provider wants to "have the conversation" about a negative prognosis and end-of-life care goals. Health practitioners often use euphemisms and downplay the seriousness of a patient's condition to help the patient and family maintain hope and because of the health professional's own ambivalence about end-of-life interventions. Since families and patients often collude with providers in not wanting to discuss "bad news," the end result is, by default, unwanted and uncomfortable, aggressive end-of-life treatments that could have been avoided with some prior planning.

In the poignant article, "Whose Job Is It to Talk to Patients About Death?" hospitalist Dr. Richardo Nuila (2015) tells the story of a patient, named Pedro, who had a terminal illness and who was not told about the seriousness of his condition while doctors focused on procedures to treat his various symptoms. Nuila describes a panel discussion on palliative care he participated in soon after this incident: "One of the words that kept coming up in the meeting in Chicago was *ownership*. In the American medical system, with all its experts, shift work, and moving parts, it can be difficult to place ultimate responsibility for a patient's care on one individual. That is to say, responsibility is shared—which is how certain duties, like talking with a patient about how close he is to death, can fall through the cracks." Nuila ends the article by saying that another hospitalist did what he did not do—shared the terminal prognosis with the patient and family so they could prepare. He says, "Still, I couldn't help but feel a professional shame, one I used to feel as a younger doctor when nurses called to remind me of some routine task I had forgotten about, one that made me occasionally punch myself in the thigh and say, 'I *really* need to remember to do that next time.' For Pedro's sake, I really do" (Nuila, 2015).

Dr. Barry Baines (2014) of Stratus Health's TRUE Hospice Utilization project, which was designed to foster earlier hospice referrals, describes miscommunication that occurs around end-of-life conversations. While both patient and doctor want this conversation to occur, the patient thinks that the doctor will explain when the time is right. The doctor, on the other hand, waits to talk about end-of-life care until the patient or family brings it up. The end result is a gap of silence during which patient may be suffering while help was available. Statistics on hospice length of stay illustrate this problem:

- 30% of all Medicare beneficiaries who died were in hospice for 3 days or less
- 35% to 40% of patients enrolled in hospice died in 7 days or less

Baines (2014) suggests that this gap can be closed by teaching physicians best practices for having a "goals of care" conversation. These steps include:

- Creating the right setting
- Finding out what the patient already knows
- Learn what the patient and family are hoping for
- Suggest realistic goals and respond with empathy
- Help the patient and family create a plan
- Adjust the plan as the situation changes

The True Project webpage provides a series of resources that both patients and providers can use to start the conversation about end-of-life care. Access this page at http://www.stratishealth .org/providers/hospice.html.

Barriers to the Use of Palliative Care

Palliative care is another important approach to advanced illness and end-of-life care. The WHO (2018) defines *palliative care* as "an approach that improves the quality of life of patients and their families facing the problems associated with life-threatening illness, through the prevention and relief of suffering by means of early identification and impeccable assessment and treatment of pain and other problems, physical, psychosocial and spiritual."

Palliative care is a medical specialty, and palliative care physicians have special expertise in pain and symptom control, although general medical practitioners can integrate palliative care approaches into regular clinical practice. In many cases, palliative care is part of a hospital-based or hospice program. Palliative care programs may be directed at patients who have a serious advanced illness but who do not necessarily meet the Medicare hospice criteria for a prognosis of 6 months of life or less. Patients who choose palliative care can continue curative treatment, a fact that is often poorly understood in the medical community.

Despite extensive research that proves that palliative care has the potential to improve patient quality of life and lower costs, there are many obstacles to the widespread use of palliative care services. Aldridge and colleagues (2015) identify major barriers:

- Lack of adequate professional education about palliative care and a small trained workforce
- Challenge of identifying patients who could benefit from palliative care
- A clinical culture that does not support palliative care
- Fragmented healthcare systems, lack of reimbursement, and regulatory barriers

Hawley (2017), in another article on barriers to palliative care, lists reasons for reluctance to refer to palliative care: fear of upsetting patients, not wanting to abandon them, seeing referral as an admission of failure, and not understanding the benefits of referral. In hospitals, palliative care is typically delivered by a specialized team of physicians, nurses, and social workers with special training and expertise in palliative care techniques. In home health care, palliative care is usually a specialized kind of home care service that is often closely aligned with a home hospice program. In home care, palliative care may be delivered by hospice nurses or by regular nurse case managers with training in palliative techniques. Patients must meet the Medicare criteria of having a skilled need and being homebound to receive palliative care under the Medicare home healthcare benefit. Outpatient palliative care is available in some places, but is not common in most communities. This lack of access to palliative care services in outpatient settings is a huge obstacle to the more successful and widespread use of palliative comfort care techniques.

Lack of Care Coordination

Patients and families facing serious and worsening chronic illness or a catastrophic diagnosis of terminal illness are often totally overwhelmed and confused by the variety of treatment and end-of-life choices available. If the patient belongs to a primary care medical home or an accountable care organization, then he or she may have a care coordinator or case manager to help with these choices. If the patient has been in the hospital, then a physician, nurse, or care coordinator will sometimes make a referral to palliative care or hospice. However, for most people, this type of advice is not readily available.

By default, the primary care physician or specialist who is treating the advanced illness is left to refer and advise patients and families, but these physicians seldom have the time to fully coordinate care, leaving patients and families to do much of the work on their own.

Patchwork Reimbursement

One major barrier to effective, connected end-of-life care is a fee-for-service reimbursement system that supports some, but not all, of the services that patients and families need. Hospice care is the most comprehensively reimbursed service. Hospice care is a defined Medicare benefit under Medicare Part A and most commercial and managed insurance plans. If a patient's illness meets strict clinical criteria (including a prognosis of 6 months or less to live), patients give up their regular Medicare benefits and are then covered by hospice benefits, which cover medications and most clinical care, but do not cover any type of curative treatment. Palliative care is covered under a patchwork of fee-for-service medical billing codes, making reimbursement difficult in outpatient settings.

One hope is that value-based payments will provide incentives for more holistic end-of-life care that is tied to outcomes and less to fee-for-service billing codes. Another huge reimbursement issue is for nonmedical services. As the patient's condition worsens, there is typically more need for help with personal and household chores, and issues such as transportation to medical appointments. Only in environments where providers are receiving global capitation or perhaps through the new Medicare

Advantage coverage expansion will these services be covered.

Excessive Care Transitions at End of Life

Another surprising barrier to effective end-of-life care is excessive transitions. Because of the delay in referral to hospice and the persistence of aggressive hospital-based end-of-life care, many patients shuttle back and forth between hospitals and home or a postacute setting in the last 6 months of life.

One study (Wang et al., 2017) found that more than 80% of decedents had at least one transition within the last 6 months of life; and 218,731 (about 40% of the sample) had four or more transitions. The most-frequent transition pattern, 19.3% of all decedents, was home to hospital, back to home or skilled nursing facility, to hospital again, and then to settings other than hospital. These transitions may work for patients and families who choose acute care end-of-life treatment. For those who have not had the opportunity to make informed choices, these potentially traumatic transitions may exacerbate discomfort, the potential for medical errors, and emotional distress; and theoretically, they may even hasten death.

Best Practices in End-of-Life Care

To achieve the best quality of care at end of life, providers in all corners of the healthcare system must accept that every patient with serious and advanced illness is owed the opportunity to make informed end-of-life choices. These choices include deciding whether to continue aggressive medical treatment, to receive palliative care with treatment, or to transition to hospice for comfort care and symptom control. Integrating end-of-life care with care from familiar medical clinicians can also help create a more patient-centered experience. Key best practices include:

- Clinicians educate themselves about end-of-life treatment choices and criteria for referral to each type of program or service. "Clinicians should have access to at least generalist palliative care training and be trained to collaborate across shifts, during transfers, and with family caregivers during discharge planning" (Wolf et al., 2015, p. 681).

- Clinicians address their own feelings about mortality, end-of-life care, and responsibility for guiding patients and families.
- Clinicians learn evidence-based techniques and develop personal scripts for having a goals of care conversation.
- Healthcare organizations identify patients who are appropriate for end-of-life care using evidence-based clinical tools such as the Palliative Performance Scale (PPS) or simply using the criteria developed by Sutter Health (Hostetter, Klein, & McCarthy, 2018) to assess patients with serious advanced illness for palliative care at home:
  - One or more chronic diagnoses
  - Questionable benefit from further aggressive treatment
  - Decline in functional and/or nutritional status in the past 30 days
  - Hospice eligible but not ready for hospice care
  - Frequent emergency department (ED) visits or hospitalizations in the last 6 months
- Have a goals of care conversation with the patient and family. LeBlanc and Tulsky

(2018), in the online journal *UpToDate*, describe best practices in this area:

- Once goals of care are clear, help patients revise advance directives and create a personal health record for documenting questions, tests, medications, and other issues about the patient's care.
- Work with a physician to create a POLST document that outlines the patient's specific wishes.
- Help the patient decide on the type of service that best meets his or her needs (specialized medical care, palliative care, or hospice [home or in a facility]) and make a timely, closed loop referral (LeBlanc & Tulsky, 2018).

Best Practices for End-of-Life Care Management

The best practices for end-of-life care management are summarized in this section (Agency for Healthcare Research and Quality [AHRQ], 2013; Cohn et al., 2017). See **FIGURE 11-4**.

- **Patient- and family-centered care.** Ensure that all care is based on patient and family preferences (the goals of care conversation) and that clinicians frequently check in with patients to determine whether preferences have changed.
- **Shared decision making.** All decisions about care are made with, not for, the patient

---

Create advance directives while still capable

Appoint a healthcare agent or health proxy to advocate for your wishes

Discuss your wishes with family and healthcare providers

Provide your advance directives to your physician and family members

Update advance directives at least yearly

Revisit advance directives if chronic illnesses worsen

Work with a personal physician to create Physician Orders for Life Sustaining Treatments (POLST) when the patient's prognosis worsens to a year or less of remaining life

Referral for palliative care if treatment is still desired

Referral to hospice or home hospice when comfort measures only are desired

Minimize transfers to acute care settings during the last days of life

FIGURE 11-4 End-of-Life Best Care Practices Summary

and family using the tools and techniques of shared decision making described in Chapter 7.

- **Comprehensive coordinated care.** The healthcare organization provides a care management function that addresses both medical and social determinants of health as well as coordinated communication between all the patient's healthcare providers.
- **Financial sustainability.** Organizations that would like to provide some aspect of palliative care should research payment options and opportunities for medical billing coding that can facilitate delivery of palliative care services. For example, Medicare now allows doctors to bill for conversations with patients about advance directives.
- **Team-based care.** Patients with complex, advanced illness need help from a team that consists of physicians, nurses, social workers, chaplains, therapists (physical, occupational), aides, and volunteers. Areas of expertise and skills needed for successful teams include pain and symptom management, expert communication capabilities, and assessment and remediation of the social contributors to ill health and suffering (such as food insecurity).

- **Caregiver training.** End-of-life care places a very heavy burden on family caregivers. Any end-of-life program must have training and support for family caregivers.

  This training should address symptom management, the expected course of the illness, how to perform medical tasks at home, and how to manage emotions and stress. Emotional support for caregivers and screening of caregivers for signs of physical symptoms is another important component of end-of-life care.
- **Effective symptom management.** Clinicians must develop care plans based on patient and family goals of care. Symptom management and pain control will be important focal areas. Communication among providers to ensure a coordinated care plan is essential in end-of-life care. There should be a mechanism for consultation with a medical expert such as a hospice medical director or palliative care physician or nurse specialists.
- **Support for clinicians.** Clinicians will have their own emotional reaction to end-of-life care. While this is satisfying work, it may take its toll and healthcare organizations must implement systems to support professional caregivers.

A COMPREHENSIVE HOSPICE AND PALLIATIVE CARE PROGRAM

Interview with Dr. Nancy Guinn, Medical Director, Presbyterian Healthcare at Home, Director, CAPC Palliative Care Leadership Center, New Mexico

Dr. Guinn's home care agency is part of the largest nonprofit healthcare system in New Mexico and includes hospitals, medical groups, a health plan, and a home healthcare agency. The Presbyterian system cares for one in three New Mexicans. Her agency and other medical practices and programs in the Presbyterian system provide a fully integrated care experience for patients with serious, complex illnesses. Dr. Guinn describes it in this way: "Our system can wrap a nice blanket around you."

Dr. Guinn explains her commitment to integrating care in this way: "I started by experiencing illness as a patient, family member and caregiver. I saw first-hand how fragmented the health care system is. I went to medical school relatively later in life at age 38. As a physician, I have always been interested in innovative models that integrate care."

She describes the mission of the palliative care programs in her system as "creating a seamless safety net of care for people who are at a vulnerable point in their lives." The palliative care system at

(continues)

A COMPREHENSIVE HOSPICE AND PALLIATIVE CARE PROGRAM   *(continued)*

Presbyterian incorporates a number of connected and overlapping programs that utilize all of the tools and techniques of connected care. The key elements of the program include:

- Inpatient palliative care
- Home palliative care
- House calls (a "mobile" patient-centered medical home)
- Hospital at home (a program that provides MD, nurse, and aide visits; diagnostic testing and medical equipment in the home for acutely ill patients)
- Hospice at home
- Complete Care (a Medicare Advantage plan program that cares for the 5% of Medicare Advantage plan members with the most serious illness burden and which provides RN care management, a home foot care nurse, and one number for patients to call)
- Community paramedic program

Dr. Guinn describes the evolution of these various elements as "stitching together programs and then finding funding solutions." The comprehensive nature of these programs means that "we have enough shared work between teams that transition points are not even visible." For example, if Dr. Guinn writes an order for home palliative care, the care of the patient is reported at a home care interdisciplinary team meeting at which the "house calls and hospice" physicians and staff are present. Team members share patient stories and simply ask each other, "Can you pick them up?" if another type of expertise is needed for optimal patient care.

Other connected care techniques utilized by the Presbyterian palliative care and hospice programs include:

- Care coordination
- One number to call
- A shared electronic medical record with scanned advanced directives. Patients in palliative care programs are flagged and the team uses the electronic medical record to communicate with each other
- Programs borrow expertise from each other
- Strong team structures with membership from multiple programs
- A comprehensive program that provides multiple internal resources and minimizes transfers outside the system care continuum
- Monthly educational conferences with all present
- Complete care RNs cover phone calls for house call patients
- Night nurses for hospice cover hospice, palliative, house call, and complete care patients
- Colocation of services including primary care and behavioral health, and primary care and oncology

The palliative care team runs a report on all patients who are in Presbyterian hospitals as inpatients, applying the Charlton comorbidity score as a screening tool. If the patient meets criteria for palliative care, the team reaches out to the primary site and contacts the patient using phrases such as, "You are coping with a lot and we may have some other ways to help you."

Dr. Guinn and her team have plans to innovate and integrate even further in the future. One planned endeavor is the development of a high-risk geriatric center of excellence, which would provide multiple services in a single location to the 5% to 10% highest risk patients in the Presbyterian system population. Another effort is transition clinics, where patients with substance abuse problems would receive medical care with substantial amounts of behavioral health services and then would gradually be transitioned back to a primary care medical home. Finally, Dr. Guinn and her team want to do more to incorporate patient feedback into their design process. They have some new survey instruments to facilitate this, and hope to develop a patient advisory council. They hope to incorporate a self-rated "patient distress screening score" into their patient portal to identify patients who need more rapid intervention.

Collaboration and High-Risk Gaps and Cracks

High-risk gaps in care occur for a wide variety of reasons, as discussed in this chapter. An underlying theme is health professionals and organizations that are specialized in caring only for certain types of patients or those who are pushed into narrow types of care delivery by rigid regulatory requirements and fragmented payment mechanisms. This specialization creates a type of myopia in which the organization or individual practitioner focuses only on one type of patient, a single type of diagnosis, or the type of care that he or she is trained to provide. In this fragmented fee-for-service type of care model, the patient is not seen as a whole person with medical conditions, socioeconomic issues, feelings, and as part of a family.

Closing High-Risk Gaps—Best Practices

- Has your organizational leadership consciously taken responsibility for identifying gaps in care and developing mechanisms for closing them through integration, collaboration, or referral relationships?
- Does your organization have mechanisms for identifying patients who have additional or different needs from the bulk of your patient population, due to diagnosis, socioeconomic status, health disparities, or stage and type of illness?
- Has your organization committed to providing person-centered connected care to patients who have more intense or different needs from those of the rest of your patient population?
- Has your organization defined which services your staff can be trained to effectively deliver to these patients and which services must be provided through referral relationships, collaboration, or integrated services?
- Have staff received specific training in working with patients who are different

or have more intense needs than the bulk of your patients?
- Does your organization have a mechanism for providing cross-functional team care to high-need patients?
- Is the care provided to patients with high needs or different needs customized to that patient's goals?
- Are family caregivers integrated into the plan of care and given the training and support that they need to be effective care partners?
- Is one clinician accountable for coordinating care for patients with different or high levels of need?
- Has your organization identified specialty partners who can provide specialized services that are complementary to those that you deliver?
- Do staff in your organization know the capabilities of organizations and specialty professionals with whom you have a collaborative or referral relationship?
- Are there well-defined personal or electronic methods for information sharing and referral between collaborating organizations?
- Do collaborating organizations use evidence-based care transition practices to ensure a positive patient experience?
- Has your organization developed measures to monitor the quality of care and outcomes for patients who have high or different needs?

▶ Chapter Summary

We see the range of care gaps for older adults, caregivers, and those at end of life. While there is a system of care for older adults, it, like the rest of the healthcare system, is full of silos, myopic thinking, fragmented payment systems, and state and federal policies that act as barriers to patient-centered connected care. That said, there are many evidence-based models for integrated care for the elderly and considerable innovation in this area that is being fueled by attention to high-cost, high-need populations. The cost drain of caring for these high-need populations may well be the impetus for the development of better quality, integrated care models.

Pervasive ageism in a culture that values youth more than experience has fueled negative attitudes toward the elderly and may be an underlying reason for the lack of health professionals entering geriatric specialties.

As the population ages, the number of people with dementia is increasing, taxing the resources of both primary care practices and medical facilities. While specialized facilities such as dementia-specific assisted living programs are multiplying, the medical care system has not been widely modified to accommodate the needs of this special population and their caregivers.

End-of-life care has received more attention in recent years and there is more effort to engage people in creating their own advance directives and in the wider use of palliative care. Obstacles stubbornly persist in the form of limited health professional understanding of end-of-life care and an aggressive medical culture that is intent on cure to the exclusion of care and comfort.

Family caregivers who provide millions of hours of unpaid healthcare labor are still all but ignored within the healthcare system. This lack of recognition and support for these vital resources is an underappreciated gap in the care system and one which, if not rectified, may well have catastrophic consequences. One of these consequences is that caregivers themselves are at high risk of developing chronic illnesses. Nursing is one profession that has made some attempt to close this gap, but without a preventive approach, these caregivers may become the next cohort of high-cost, high-need patients.

AARP has been the major national voice for caregivers and through its policy division works to prompt more caregiver-friendly legislation. A potential resource for caregivers is the new-found ability of Medicare Advantage plans to pay for nonmedical support services for beneficiaries.

As more seniors enroll in these plans and if the benefit proves substantive, it may provide considerable relief for caregivers who are constrained by both time and financial resources. As technology that is targeted to support the elderly advances, it may well also become a major source of cost and labor savings for family caregivers.

Healthcare organization can contribute to closing high-risk gaps and cracks in care by becoming aware of the needs of their population and either enhancing and expanding services to meet those needs or creating effective referral relationships to do so.

References

ACT on Alzheimer's. (2017). Dementia-specific practice tools and resources for providers. Retrieved from www.actonalz.org/sites/default/files/documents/ACT-Provider-ToolsResources_0.pdf

Agency for Healthcare Research and Quality. (2013). System-integrated program coordinates care for people with advanced illness, leading to greater use of hospice services, lower utilization and costs, and high satisfaction. AHRQ Innovations Exchange. https://innovations.ahrq.gov

Aging with Dignity. (2018). Five wishes. Retrieved from www.agingwithdignity.org/five-wishes

Aldridge, M. D., Hasselaar, J., Garralda, E., Eerden, M. V., Stevenson, D., Mckendrick, K., & Meier, D. E. (2015). Education, implementation, and policy barriers to greater integration of palliative care: A literature review. *Palliative Medicine, 30*(3), 224–239. doi:10.1177/0269216315606645

American Association of Retired Persons. (2011). Public Policy Institute. Valuing the invaluable: 2011 update—the economic value of family caregiving in 2009. Retrieved from www.aarp.com

American Association of Retired Persons. (2018). Policy book 2017-2018, end of life care. Retrieved from http://policybook.aarp.org/the-policy-book/chapter-7/ss165-1.3570290

American Geriatrics Society. (2015). *Clinicians guide to assessing and counseling older drivers.* New York, NY: AGS.

Baines, B. (2014). Hospice through a community lens. PowerPoint presentation. Stratis Health Medicare.

Begley, S. (2016). Cancer patients keep getting aggressive end-of-life treatment, despite lack of benefit. Retrieved from www.statnews.com/2016/06/06/cancer-patients-end-of-life/

BenefitsCheckUp. (2018). National Council on Aging. Retrieved from https://www.benefitscheckup.org/

Callahan, C. M., Sachs, G. A., Lamantia, M. A., Unroe, K. T., Arling, G., & Boustani, M. A. (2014). Redesigning systems of care for older adults with Alzheimer's disease. *Health Affairs, 33*(4), 626–632. doi:10.1377/hlthaff.2013.1260

Centers for Medicare and Medicaid Services, Medicare Learning Network. (2017). Implementing the IMPACT

Act: Status update & activities. Retrieved from www
.cms.gov/Outreach-and-Education/Outreach/NPC
/Downloads/2017-02-23-IMPACT-Presentation.pdf

Chen, P. (2010, January 21). Offering care for the caregiver.
New York Times. Retrieved from https://www.nytimes
.com/2010/01/22/health/21chen.html

Chen, R., Falchook, A. D., Tian, F., Basak, R., Hanson, L.,
Selvam, N., & Dusetzina, S. (2016). Aggressive care at
the end-of-life for younger patients with cancer: Impact
of ASCO's Choosing Wisely campaign. Poster session
presented at the American Society of Clinical Oncology
Conference, June.

Cohn, J., Corrigan, J., Lynn, J., Meier, D., Miller, J., Shega,
J., & Wang, S. (2017). *Community-based models of care
delivery for people with serious illness*. Discussion paper.
Washington, DC: National Academy of Medicine. https://
nam.edu/wp-content/uploads/2017/04/

Epstein-Lubow, G., Gaudiano, B. A., Hinckley, M., Salloway,
S., & Miller, I. W. (2010). Evidence for the validity
of the American Medical Association's Caregiver
Self-Assessment Questionnaire as a screening measure
for depression. *Journal of the American Geriatrics Society*,
58(2), 387–388.

Family Caregiver Alliance. (2006). Caregiver health, a
population at risk. Retrieved from www.caregiver.org
/caregiver-health

Family Caregiver Alliance. (2016a). Caregiver statistics:
demographics. Retrieved from www.caregiver.org
/caregiver-statistics-demographics

Family Caregiver Alliance. (2016b). Caregiver Statistics:
Work and Caregiving. Retrieved from www.caregiver
.org/caregiver-statistics-work-and-caregiving

Gawande, A. (2017). *Being mortal*. Toronto, Ontario: Anchor
Canada.

Grantmakers in Aging. (2006). Quality of life through end
of life. Engagement. Retrieved from www.giaging.org
/documents/Quality-of-Life-Through-End-of-Life_Care
-Issue-Brief.pdf

Hackett, B. (2018). President signs law to support family
caregivers. Retrieved from www.aarp.org

Handley, M., Bunn, F., & Goodman, C. (2017). Dementia-
friendly interventions to improve the care of people
living with dementia admitted to hospitals: A realist
review. *BMJ Open*, *7*(7), e015257. doi.org/10.1136
/bmjopen-2016-015257

Hawley, P. (2017). Barriers to access to palliative care. *Palliative
Care*, *10*. doi.org/10.1177/1178224216688887

Hostetter, M., Klein, S., & McCarthy, D. (2018). Supporting
patients through serious illness and the end of life:
Sutter Health's AIM Model. The Commonwealth Fund.
Retrieved from www.commonwealthfund.org/publications
/case-studies/2018/jan/sutter-health-aim

Jeffs, L., Saragosa, M., Law, M., Kuluski, K., Espin, S., &
Merkley, J. (2017). The role of caregivers in interfacility
care transitions: A qualitative study. *Patient Preference
and Adherence*, *11*, 1443–1450. doi:10.2147/ppa.s136058

Kirkland-Kyhn, H., Generao, S. A., Teleten, O., & Young, H. M.
(2018). Teaching wound care to family caregivers. *American
Journal of Nursing*, *118*(3), 63–67. doi:10.1097/01.naj
.0000530941.11737

LeBlanc, T., & Tulsky, J. (2018). Discussing goals of care.
Retrieved from www.uptodate.com

Mate, K. S., Berman, A., Laderman, M., Kabcenell, A., &
Fulmer, T. (2018). Creating age-friendly health systems—A
vision for better care of older adults. *Healthcare*, *6*(1),
4–6. doi:10.1016/j.hjdsi.2017.05

Mayo Clinic. (2016). Alzheimer's: 7 tips for medical visits.
Retrieved from www.mayoclinic.org/healthy-lifestyle
/caregivers/in-depth/alzheimers/art-20047326

Mitnick, S., Leffler, C., & Hood, V. L. (2010). Family caregivers,
patients and physicians: Ethical guidance to optimize
relationships. *Journal of General Internal Medicine*, *25*(3),
255–260. doi:10.1007/s11606-009-1206-3

Moeller, P. (2018). This plan to add broad non-medical
benefits to Medicare Advantage is a big deal. Here's
why. *PBS News Hour Column*. Retrieved from: https://
www.pbs.org/newshour/economy/making-sense
/column-these-9-new-medicare-advantage-benefits
-are-a-big-deal-heres-why

Morris, S. (2017). Does your state have a care act? Caring.com.

National Academy of Sciences. (2015). *Dying in America:
Improving quality and honoring individual preferences
near the end of life*. Washington, DC: National Academies
Press.

National POLST Paradigm. (2018). POLST and advance
directives. Retrieved from www.polst.org

Newman, K. (2017). A look into older adults' state of
mind. *U.S. News*. Retrieved from www.usnews.com
/news/best-states/articles/2017-10-11/older-adults
-struggle-to-get-adequate-mental-health-care

Nuila, R. (2015). Whose job is it to talk to patients about
death? *The Atlantic*. Retrieved from www.theatlantic
.com/health/archive/2015/08/palliative-care-medicare
-end-of-life-ethics/400823/

Reinhard, S. C., & Young, H. M. (2017, May). Nurses supporting
family caregivers. *American Journal of Nursing*, *117*
(5 Suppl 1): S2. doi: 10.1097/01.NAJ.0000516385.05140.b0

Reinhard, S. C., Levine, C., & Samis, S. (2012). *Home
alone: Family caregivers providing complex chronic care*.
Washington, DC: AARP Public Policy Institute.

Robert Wood Johnson Foundation. (2015). Nurses help
adults manage family caregiving responsibilities.
Retrieved from www.rwjf.org/en/library/articles-and
-news/2015/11/nurses-help-adults-manage-caregiving
-responsibilities.html

Sabatino, C. (2015). Myths and facts about health care
advance directives. *Bifocal, Journal of the Commission
on Law and Aging*, *37*(1).

Saltzman, M. (2017, June 24). 'Aging in place' tech helps
seniors live in their home longer. *USA Today*.

Schulz, R., & Eden, J. (2016). *Families caring for an aging
America*. Washington, DC: The National Academies Press.

Schulz, R., Beach, S. R., Cook, T. B., Martire, L. M., Tomlinson, J. M., & Monin, J. K. (2012). Predictors and consequences of perceived lack of choice in becoming an informal caregiver. *Aging & Mental Health, 16*(6), 712–721.

Span, P. (2015, March 13). The trouble with advance directives. *New York Times.* Retrieved from https://www.nytimes.com/2015/03/17/health/the-trouble-with-advance-directives.html

Spencer-Bonilla, G., Quiñones, A. R., & Montori, V. M. (2017). Assessing the burden of treatment. *Journal of General Internal Medicine, 32*(10), 1141–1145. doi:10.1007/s11606-017-4117-8

Veterans Administration. (2018). VA offers programs for family caregivers. Retrieved from www.va.gov

Wang, S., Aldridge, M. D., Gross, C. P., Canavan, M., Cherlin, E., & Bradley, E. (2017). End-of-life care transition patterns of Medicare beneficiaries. *Journal of American Geriatrics Society, 65,* 1406–1413. doi:10.1111/jgs.14891

Want, J. (2017) Learning Update: Improving Care for High Needs Patients. *Peterson Center on Healthcare.* Retrieved from https://petersonhealthcare.org/learning-update-improving-healthcare-high-need-patients

Wolf, S. M., Berlinger, N., & Jennings, B. (2015). Forty years of work on end-of-life care—from patients' rights to systemic reform. *New England Journal of Medicine, 372*(7), 678–682. doi:10.1056/nejmms1410321

World Health Organization. (2017). Mental health and older adults fact sheet. Retrieved from www.who.int/mediacentre/factsheets/fs381/en/

World Health Organization. (2018). WHO definition of palliative care. Retrieved from http://www.who.int/cancer/palliative/definition/en/

Yadav, K. N., Gabler, N. B., Cooney, E., Kent, S., Kim, J., Herbst, N., & Courtright, K. R. (2017). Approximately one in three US adults completes any type of advance directive for end-of-life care. *Health Affairs, 36*(7), 1244–1251. doi:10.1377/hlthaff.2017.0175

Epilogue

Connected Care Trends and Collaboration Best Practices

When thinking of change in the healthcare system, an image that comes to mind is ocean icebergs and ice floes. As the temperature and the currents of policy and culture shift, some floes drift apart, some crack and break, and others float together and eventually fuse. Given the complex and constantly shifting political and cultural currents of our times, there seem to be more gaps than connections and a unified and coordinated system for patient-centered connected care seems, in the near term, nowhere in the offing. Without a very clear crystal ball no one knows what will come next.

There are, however, some hopeful signs from the highest levels of government regulatory and payment agencies to the front lines of daily clinical care and patient service. Many people in the healthcare system, both leaders and clinicians, have emerged from the "We don't know what we don't know" stage of thinking to "We know what we don't know," and some have even progressed to "We know some things that work." A good example is the recent national consensus on the need to find solutions for high-cost, high-need patients through innovation and connected care structures and processes. One thing that is very clear is, ultimately, nothing will be accomplished without collaboration between professionals, between disciplines, between health and social services organizations, and with patients themselves.

▶ Staying Focused on the Goal—Patient Requirements and the Pillars of Connected Care

The goal of this book has been to describe systems, processes, and behaviors that produce patient-centered connected care and achieve the four quadruple aim goals (lower cost per capita, better patient experience, improved outcomes for populations of patients, and a better clinician experience).

Patient requirements, described in Chapter 7, "Experiencing Connected Care—The Patient Role," should remain key drivers of healthcare delivery systems, no matter how strong the currents of change and disruption. Key requirements include:

- Personalized care from healthcare providers who listen to the patient and who build care based on the patient's individual needs and goals
- Insurance coverage that pays for the cost of care without overly high out-of-pocket costs and offers a reasonable choice of providers

- Coordinated care that meets patient and family needs without care gaps, miscommunication, or care tasks that "fall through the cracks"
- Convenient care that is available when, where, and in a form that meets patient needs
- Digital access to health information, health advice, and in some cases treatment via telehealth

In the chapters on senior management, middle management, and front line clinicians we have posed methods for achieving patient goals in an integrated way, called connected care. The base of connected care is patient centeredness and the pillars of connected care and the tools for achieving patient goals and the quadruple aim are:

- Teamwork
- Care Transitions
- Care Coordination
- Communication
- Collaboration

Current trends in health care are like a field of opposing forces. Some foster integrated, patient-centered, connected care; others have the potential to create larger and more disruptive care gaps for patients.

▶ The Currents of Change

At the beginning of 2018, the usual "trends for the year" reports appeared in healthcare publications. Many of these reports had remarkably similar views of what matters in health care in this current slice in time. The recurrent trends and forces impacting the healthcare system include:

- Patient population trends and patient empowerment issues
- A fractured political, payment, and regulatory environment
- The structure and culture of health care
- Shifting power, dominance, and relationships in health care
- The impact of technology and data analytics

Underlying all these trends is an almost overwhelming complexity that can stifle the most ardent healthcare innovator and the most well-intentioned healthcare organization. Coping with complexity and burnout among the front line clinicians who must deal with it on a daily basis is one of the biggest challenges to connected care and to an effective healthcare system in general.

Patient Population Issues

The diversity of the U.S. population is a factor in the effective delivery of health care. As patient-centered care is more universally adopted, healthcare organizations must use stratified data to identify their specific patient populations and must then communicate with these patients to understand their specific wants and needs.

An aging population with an increase in dementia and the need for family caregiving support is another population trend that is having a profound impact on health care. Employed family caregivers who struggle to juggle jobs with the care of an ill or aged loved one creates more care gaps and fragmentation. Complex chronic illnesses, exacerbated by social determinants of health and comorbid mental illness, put a huge strain on our fragmented, medically driven healthcare system. These complex populations are the ones that most need patient-centered connected care solutions and often are the ones that receive it least often. The opioid crisis, a problem partially created by the healthcare system itself, is taxing social services, law enforcement, and health care and is siphoning resources that might have been used to improve population health.

Patient Engagement

The need for patient engagement is a theme throughout the healthcare literature. The chapters on the patient experience and on digital connections address many of the issues relevant to this topic. Care has become too complex and healthcare facility stays too short to allow health professionals to do everything for patients.

While the healthcare paradigm has shifted to an assumption that patients and caregivers will assume much of the burden of care tasks, many patients do not feel that this is a reasonable expectation. This dissonance between provider and patient expectations sometimes creates serious conflict and patient and clinician dissatisfaction. Other patients have taken fairly extreme measures to manage their own care by becoming e-patients who utilize the internet, social networks, and electronic communication to manage care more independently.

New clinician skills and attitudes are creating better partnerships with patients and are enriching the patient experience as clinicians adopt advising, coaching, and support roles rather than relying solely on telling and directing. Advances in patient-centered care techniques that have been mentioned in previous chapters such as shared decision making, motivational interviewing, teach-back, health teaching that is adapted to patient literacy levels, interactive online education, clinical avatars, and conscious efforts to reduce the burden of treatment are closing care gaps and providing more connected care for patients.

Changes in the Structure and Culture of Health Care

Despite a tumultuous political climate, the volume-to-value shift continues in health care. This shift is driving care redesign, collaboration, and advances in clinical best practices. It has also created considerable turmoil as healthcare organizations struggle to overcome decades of fee-for-service, volume-based thinking to focus on outcomes. Leadership and culture change is the focus of much discussion and activity in health care. The movement of clinicians into leadership positions is helping to close the gap between clinical practice and the business of health care.

A lack of qualified healthcare executives and the impending retirements of baby boomers from the healthcare workforce are fueling efforts in recruitment, succession planning, and workforce training and engagement. A counterbalancing effect in the workforce shortage is the entrance of millennials into the health professions. These employees, with their requirements for purpose in work and work-life balance, may be a factor in the drive toward workplace redesign and connected care.

The clinician burnout epidemic looms large in the current healthcare environment and it is a factor that fuels fragmentation and care gaps. Involvement of clinicians in care redesign, the use of patient and clinician–centered automation tools, and the application of industrial process improvement and employee involvement techniques such as Lean and Design Thinking are being utilized to solve this huge problem (Groscurth, 2017; Hosthealthcare.com, 2017; NEJM Catalyst, 2018; Pollack, 2017; Sanborn, 2018).

Shifting Power, Dominance, and Relationships in Health Care

In early 2018, corporate giants Berkshire Hathaway, JP Morgan Chase, and Amazon announced a new collaborative healthcare effort that sent tremors through the healthcare industry. The details of this plan have not been revealed, but two things are known: Technology will play a key role and the companies plan to try new techniques with their own employees (Lashinsky, 2018).

In describing this alliance, *The New York Times* noted: "The alliance was a sign of just how frustrated American businesses are with the state of the nation's health care system and the rapidly spiraling cost of medical treatment. It also caused further turmoil in an industry reeling from attempts by new players to attack a notoriously inefficient, intractable web of doctors, hospitals, insurers and pharmaceutical companies" (Wingfield, Thomas, & Abelson, 2018).

Another set of jolts to the healthcare establishment occurred when CVS and Aetna shareholders approved CVS's plan to acquire the health insurer. Walmart and Humana also announced a possible merger (Graham, 2018; LaVito, 2018).

Some think that these mergers of giant corporations that deliver health care but are outside the existing healthcare establishment may be the death knell for the healthcare industry as we know it.

Since corporations involved in these new relationships have expressed frustration with the rigidity and fragmentation of health care, will they chart their own course and develop their own solutions to connected care that are built on market dominance and technology or will they build on the innovations, best practices, and solutions that are already being tried? At this point, it is anyone's guess whether these relationships will create a new era of connected care or simply a different form of fragmented care that is geared primarily toward corporate goals and reduction of health insurance costs.

Mergers, Partnerships, and Collaborations

Consolidation, mergers, and acquisitions continue within the traditional healthcare system. The success of these joined corporations often seems to be dictated by their level of cultural compatibility. In cases in which the merger creates uneasy alliances, scores of layoffs, changes in leadership, higher out-of-pocket costs, and shifts in service lines, it is highly fragmenting and dissatisfying to both patients and healthcare providers. If these changes prove to be temporary, and the merger creates a new and more functional culture with a broader array of convenient and patient-centered services, the end result may be better outcomes and a better patient and provider experience (Sanborn, 2018).

Partnerships and Collaborations

Partnerships to improve population health outcomes and to lower costs have been discussed at various points in this book, most notably in Chapter 10, on the social determinants of health. In different parts of the country hospitals, healthcare organizations, and social services agencies

such as Area Agencies on Aging are teaming up to tackle problems as diverse as diabetes and obesity and food security. An article in *Modern Healthcare* quotes Gurpreet Singh, a partner at PwC and the leader of its health services sector, "Providers who participate in more cross-sector partnerships get a 360-degree view of the consumer and all interactions they may have with social workers and from a community standpoint. . . . Having influence points outside of acute care can lower readmission rates and reduce costs" (Kacik, 2018). While these cross-sector partnerships may provide positive connected care experiences for patients, many are highly localized and dependent on uncertain funding and the shifting priorities of healthcare partners. In some cases, the lead healthcare organization may leave the partnership in a quest to improve profits in a declining profit margin environment, fueling yet more fragmented care for users of the partnership services (Kacik, 2018).

Technology

Of all the trends in health care, technology is the one most likely to disrupt or connect care for patients. Chapter 9 on digital connections explores this issue in depth. Texting, telemedicine, social media, and mobile apps all provide patients and providers with endless opportunities to gather information, to communicate, and to confer with each other. The electronic medical record, while a strong force for communication, patient safety, and teamwork, can also be a burdensome, labor intensive and frustrating tool when it is not optimized for patient care use.

Health information exchanges, which consolidate and organize comprehensive data from multiple providers, will almost certainly help with connecting care once they are more widely adopted and funded.

The Internet of Things (IOT) is revolutionizing healthcare processes and improving efficiency through tracking, monitoring, and alerting functions. Monitors that track patients through the surgical process provide peace of mind for caregivers, while smart houses and reminder tools help seniors stay independent at home. The popular movement toward wearable tracking devices has not yet resulted in large-scale transmission of patient-collected data to providers, but it may prove to be a connected care tool in the near future.

Artificial intelligence with its ability to extract information from spoken language, mimic the reactions and responses of a human healthcare professional, and better diagnose abnormalities in x-rays, scans, and laboratory testing data may at least partially replace scarce human health professionals. This insertion of technology into the health professional/patient interaction has interesting implications for a new type of three-way connected care (patient, provider, and software).

Data analytics potentially has a huge role to play in connecting care although many say it is not yet "ready for prime time." Analytics can help in stratifying patient populations so patient needs can be understood more precisely. Data help providers to assess the results of care redesign experiments and particular clinical interventions. Big data analytics with its ability to create coherent information from huge volumes of data holds the promise of confirming which treatments are most effective and of projecting the trajectory of an illness. In theory, then, data has the potential to greatly aid in connecting care.

In reality, the science of data management is not foolproof. Bias in data collection and analysis abounds and certain corporate players may have a vested interest in skewing data to achieve their own goals. As technology and data advance we will learn more about which aspects of analytics connect and which fragment care.

Collaboration and Care Coordination—The Universal Dot Connectors

While the currents of change roil the waters of health care, professionals who are interested in innovation and improved results continue to work together through personal relationships with colleagues and formal and informal collaborations. These collaborative efforts range from interdisciplinary communications about a single patient to multiorganizational collaborations and, in some cases, integration of services. Where formal care connections do not exist, case managers and care coordinators act as bridge builders, finding resources and communicating to the next steps in care on behalf of patients. So often, these collaborations are informal, loosely organized, and messy. These are the collaborative efforts that are never reported in journals.

🔍 CASE STUDY

Help Us Find Our Patients

An example is a recent conversation between two colleagues. One is a manager in a multisite medical practice of primary care providers that is also an accountable care organization. The other is a manager in a home healthcare agency. These two organizations have no electronic medical record connections.

Medical practice manager: *Is there a way you can get your staff to notify us when one of our patients is discharged from a skilled nursing facility? We only have two business days to make the transitional care calls and it is an important part of our providing continuity of care, reconnecting the patient to the responsible primary care provider.*

Home care manager: *Don't your preferred provider SNFs do that?*

Medical practice manager: *They are supposed to, but they are so rushed and crazed, they can't seem to do it consistently. We are in the process of getting tracking software, but we need a workaround until we get it. You could really help us in the meantime.*

Home care manager: *Okay, I have nurse liaisons who visit patients in the SNFs to do assessments and who go to utilization*

(continues)

🔍 CASE STUDY *(continued)*

management meetings. They know who is being discharged. If I can get the EMR to trigger an alert, or at worst, if I can get them a list of your practice physicians, we might be able to do it. Can you narrow down the phone calls to one or two care coordinators?

Medical practice manager: *Yes, we can do that. I really appreciate your help with this. Maybe someday we will have a health information exchange that will eliminate the need for these manual processes.*

Collaboration Best Practices

Collaborations between health professionals and organizations can be as simple and informal as the one described in the previous case study. More formal collaboration efforts range from agreement on a simple referral protocol to an extensive contracted integration of services. One example is the Middlesex Hospital T.I.M.E to Act collaborative. This is a monthly meeting of a hospital and its associated healthcare community partners that is designed to improve patient safety and reduce hospital readmissions.

Definitions of collaboration best practices differ but many have similar elements.

INTERVIEW WITH TERRI SAVINO, MSN, RN, CPHQ

Terri Savino, MSN, RN, CPHQ, is Manager, Patient Satisfaction and Service Excellence. Terri was a founder of the T.I.M.E. to Act Community Collaborative at Middlesex Hospital in Middletown, Connecticut. The collaborative is a monthly meeting of hospital staff and representatives of agencies and facilities that care for patients referred from Middlesex Hospital. The goal of the collaborative is to reduce hospital readmissions and help patients achieve better outcomes. The group meets monthly and consists of 30 to 40 participants. The agenda usually includes an educational presentation, a patient safety story, sharing of best practices, and case reviews of readmissions.

Terri tells the story of how the collaborative started. Qualidigm, which was then the Medicare Quality Improvement Organization for the State of Connecticut, sent a letter inviting Middlesex Hospital to participate in a heart failure readmission reduction initiative. Terri and her team began by looking at heart failure readmissions data. Terri met with the Chief Nursing Officer and the Vice President of Quality. She asked who the hospital should reach out to as partners, since they had never developed a collaborative of this type before. The team initially picked three skilled nursing facilities and two home care agencies. According to Terri, "It was a very interesting process." At the first meeting Terri asked, "What are the things we are not doing that you want us to do?" Several of the partners stated that the hospital medication reconciliation process was terrible and that the information they received on discharged patients was confusing. The hospital said to the skilled nursing facilities and home care agencies, "We don't get patient weights from you." Terri says that "the first 'ah ha' was when we did some research and found that we were sending patients out and not putting the weight on the referral document. We were asking for it but we were not sending it."

Terri feels that the collaborative has been successful because it always focuses its work on the patient. "It is not about the hospital." For example, after the comments about problems with medication reconciliation, the hospital hired a consultant to improve the medication reconciliation process. "Even when we discussed readmits, it was all about the patient and what could have been done differently."

Another success factor is having a standardized agenda. Having an educational component has kept people interested and engaged. After several years of successful work, Terri was asked to present T.I.M.E. to Act at a Qualidigm Leadership Academy Seminar. Afterward, people came up and asked to join. Terri continued to reach out to collaborative members and asked what people wanted to know. For a time, the group rotated facilities for their meetings. Terri feels that this was helpful in pulling down walls between organizations.

The group has met for a number of years and Terri says, "It is still exciting; it never got stale or stagnant." The group collaboratively came up with heart failure zone charts, which were then implemented in the hospital. They had a cross-organizational fall risk committee that researched best practices for hospitals, home care, skilled nursing facilities, hospice, and assisted living. The committee created core best practices and specialized ones for each setting. Members adopted these best practices and shared their fall rates with the hospital. Terri notes, "The fall committee was huge. It was really a cross-continuum collaboration. It was amazing hearing different viewpoints from different facilities and learning some of the best practices being used by members."

Terri says, "The networking was great. It was also great, knowing that we made a difference. We have never stopped wanting to do better for the patient. Staying focused on what is best for the patient, not the facilities, has been the major success factor."

When asked what the hospital thinks of the collaborative. Terri replies that when they had their magnet designation site visit they had SNF and home care partners at the sessions. "The magnet site team was impressed that we worked so well with our partners."

Another thing the collaborative did was to engage physicians in the group, which is something that is rarely done. They also looked to see who was missing. Pharmacy, EMT, hospice, and assisted living were added as the group realized that these services were an important part of the continuum. T.I.M.E. to Act has continually broadened the base of the group.

Terri's advice is, "Keep it simple. It is hard work, but it is worth it. If you build it they will come. We built a community of care and it just grew. We were never scared of sharing best practices. We looked amongst us to improve and to be in each other's shoes. We were eager to hear the other person's point of view. We learned more about regulations in other settings such as the use of antipsychotics in skilled nursing facilities."

Terri ends by saying, "When I came back from a meeting, I felt exhausted. I felt like we made a difference. We bonded together. We tried to have an aim or focus for the year. That helped us as engaged partners."

The Association of State and Territorial Health Officials identifies five key best practices for effective cross-organizational collaboration:

- **Identify shared goals.** Pick an issue that already has "traction," work with key influencers, understand partner priorities, and choose shared goals that meet the priorities of key stakeholders.

- **Engage partners early.** Become an asset to other organizations by helping them achieve their goals, help your partner agency do its job more easily, and understand roles and responsibilities in partner organizations.

- **Define a common language.** Use shared definitions, learn how decisions are made, and invest in alignment early in the project.

- **Activate the community.** Understand community stakeholder perspectives, educate patients or other stakeholders who are affected by the collaboration, and create incentives for positive action.

- **Leverage funding from complementary programs.** When you don't have enough money think of new ways to fund projects, use contributions or funding streams from each organization to support the project, but be sure that financial relationships are clearly defined. (Association of State and Territorial Health Officials, 2018)

Converge for Impact (2017) is an organization that describes itself as "a team of strategists and designers committed to social and environmental *impact* through collaboration and networks."

Converge for Impact (2017) frames the issues of complex collaboration in a blog post: "Something Tom Atlee recently wrote sums up for us what's happening on the planet right now. 'Things are getting better and better, and worse and worse, faster and faster, in bigger and bigger ways.' We live in a world of problems that are so complex—so tangled up with other problems, so non-linear, ambiguous, and volatile—that they defy solutions and cannot be effectively addressed by any one organization or even by any one sector." Some best practices suggested by the blog are:

1. **Clarify purpose.** Get a clear initial statement of the problem that you want to address. The best way to do this is to answer the question, "How do we…?"

2. **Convene the right people.** Involve people who, collectively, can tackle the problem. Ensure that you include people from all parts of the system you are trying to change.

3. **Cultivate trust.** Participants do not necessarily need to agree or even like each other but they must believe that the action they take together, "trust for action," is vital.

4. **Coordinate existing actions.** One way to build this trust is to share information about positive actions that have already been taken by individual organizations to meet the shared goal and then connect the dots of these actions across the participating organizations.

5. **Collaborate for systems impact.** Participants in the collaboration must identify "leverage points," where small actions can make a big impact. Once these leverage points are identified, members can work together to influence change in the right places.

Evaluating Collaboration

Once a collaboration is up and running, members can evaluate its effectiveness using the Wilder

🔍 CASE STUDY

The Everford Health System Is Recognized for Collaboration

In the 2 years since Sue Chang took the reins as CEO of Everford Health System, there have been many improvements in the level of connected care. Once the technical issues were resolved (described in the digital connections case study in Chapter 9), Sue moved forward on other issues that the health system had been unable to tackle alone. Through collaborations with specialty clinical facilities and community agencies, Everford was able to develop integrated care for high-cost, high-need patients; frail elderly patients; people at end of life; and community residents with socioeconomic challenges. The Everford System became part of a national care transformation collaborative that helped it steadily improve outcomes and lower costs.

The board, the medical staff, and the clinical staff had broadened their views and had become more inclusive and more realistic about what could be accomplished. As a consequence of these actions, Sue and the Everford team were honored for their collaborative efforts and positive outcomes by a national healthcare organization.

Sue and the team were somewhat surprised by this recognition as they still considered themselves learners and as travelers at the beginning of a long journey to fully realized, patient-centered, connected care. However, they were happy to accept the award on behalf of all the clinicians and support staff who had worked tirelessly to improve care and outcomes for patients, and in the process, learned to love their jobs again.

Collaboration Inventory. This research-based tool is available for free at www.wilder.org. The instrument looks at process factors such as willingness to compromise, flexibility, development of clear roles and responsibilities, and open and frequent communication (Mattessich, Murray-Close, & Monsey, 2001).

Of course, the ultimate test of a collaboration is whether it achieves its stated and shared purpose. In health care, measures of success will revolve around quadruple aim measures such as clinical outcomes, cost, and improved patient experience.

References

Association of State and Territorial Health Officials. (2018). Characteristics of successful collaboration. Retrieved from http://www.astho.org/NPS/Toolkit/Characteristics -of-Successful-Collaboration/?terms=characteristics +of+a+successful+collaboration

Converge for Impact. (2017). How to make complex collaborations work. Retrieved from https://blog.convergeforimpact .com/how-to-make-complex-collaborations-work/

Graham, J. (2018). Walmart, not Amazon, may turn out to be the real health care disruptor. Retrieved from https:// www.investors.com/news/walmart-humana-amazon -disrupt-health-care/04/02/18

Groscurth, C. (2017). Are you ready to respond to 2018's biggest healthcare trends? Gallup. Retrieved from http:// news.gallup.com/businessjournal/223406/ready-respond -2018-biggest-healthcare-trends.aspx?version=print

Hosthealthcare.com. (2017). Future trends in the nursing industry. Retrieved from www.hosthealthcare.com /future-trends-in-the-nursing-industry

Kacik, A. (2018). Cross sector collaborations improve care. Retrieved from www.modernhealthcare.com /article/20180108/NEWS/180109930

Lashinsky, A. (2018). Why Jeff Bezos might be the one to crack the health care challenge. Retrieved from www .fortune.com/2018/01/31/jeff-bezos-amazon-health-care/

LaVito, A. (2018, March 13). CVS, Aetna shareholders approve drugstore's acquisition of health insurer. Retrieved from www.cnbc.com/2018/03/13/cvs-aetna-shareholders -approve-merger.html

Mattessich, P., Murray-Close, M., & Monsey, B. (2001). *Wilder collaboration factors inventory*. St. Paul, MN: Wilder Research.

NEJM Catalyst. (2018). The critical role of clinical leaders. Retrieved from http://join.catalyst.nejm.org/download /clinical-leader-role-ebook2018/register

Pollack, R. (2017, October 11). 2018 environmental scan: Trends that are shaping health care. *Hospitals and Health Care Networks Magazine*. www.hhnmag.com/articles /8640-trends-that-are-shaping-health-care#Innovation

Sanborn, B. J. (2018, March 29). Merger and acquisition activity has record-breaking first quarter in 2018. *Health Care Finance News*. http://www.healthcarefinancenews .com/news/merger-and-acquisition-activity-has-record -breaking-first-quarter-2018

Wingfield, N., Thomas, K., & Abelson, R. (2018, January 30). Amazon, Berkshire Hathaway and JPMorgan team up to try to disrupt health care. Retrieved from www.nytimes .com/2018/01/30/technology/amazon-berkshire-hathaway -jpmorgan-health-care.html

Index

Note: Page numbers followed by *b*, *f*, and *t* indicated material in boxes, figures, and tables respectively.